Health Psychology

THIRD EDITION

Health Psychology

THEORY, RESEARCH AND PRACTICE

David F. Marks, Michael Murray,
Brian Evans and Emee Vida Estacio

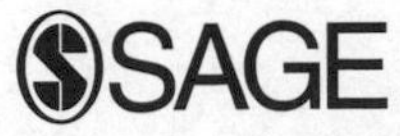

Los Angeles | London | New Delhi
Singapore | Washington DC

First edition published 2000
Reprinted 2001, 2002 and 2004
Second edition published 2005.
Reprinted Chinese edition 2006, Spanish edition 2008 and Indian edition 2008
This third edition published 2011

SAGE Publications Ltd
1 Oliver's Yard
55 City Road
London EC1Y 1SP

SAGE Publications Inc.
2455 Teller Road
Thousand Oaks, California 91320

SAGE Publications India Pvt Ltd
B 1/I 1 Mohan Cooperative Industrial Area
Mathura Road
New Delhi 110 044

SAGE Publications Asia-Pacific Pte Ltd
33 Pekin Street #02-01
Far East Square
Singapore 048763

Library of Congress Control Number: 2010936809

British Library Cataloguing in Publication data

A catalogue record for this book is available from
the British Library

ISBN 978-1-84860-621-0
ISBN 978-1-84860-622-7 (pbk)

Typeset by C&M Digitals (P) Ltd, Chennai, India
Printed and bound in Great Britain by TJ International Ltd, Padstow, Cornwall
Printed on paper from sustainable resources

Contents

Author Biographies

DAVID F. MARKS is Professor of Psychology at City University, London, UK. Previously he held positions at the University of Sheffield, UK, the University of Otago in New Zealand, and Middlesex University, London, UK. His other books include *The Psychology of the Psychic* (1980, with R. Kammann), *Theories of Image Formation* (1986), *Imagery: Current Developments* (1990, with J.T.E. Richardson and P. Hampson), *The Quit For Life Programme: An Easier Way to Stop Smoking and Not Start Again* (1993), *Improving the Health of the Nation* (1996, with C. Francome), *Dealing With Dementia: Recent European Research* (2000, with C.M. Sykes), *The Psychology of the Psychic* (revised edition) (2000), *The Health Psychology Reader* (2002), *Research Methods for Clinical and Health Psychology* (2004, with L. Yardley), and *Overcoming Your Smoking Habit* (2005). He was Chair of the Special Group in Health Psychology of the British Psychological Society, Convenor of the Task Force on Health Psychology of the European Federation of Professional Psychologists' Associations, Chair of the Standing Conference on Public Health, and a member of the Department of Health's Scientific Committee on Tobacco and Health. He is Founder and Editor of the *Journal of Health Psychology.*

MICHAEL MURRAY is Professor and Head of the School of Psychology at Keele University, Staffordshire, UK. Previously he has held positions at Memorial University, Canada, University of Ulster, Ireland, and St Thomas' Hospital Medical School, London, UK (now Kings College). He is a Visiting Professor of Psychology at City University, London, UK and has held visiting appointments at Durham University, UK and Massey University, New Zealand. His previous books include *Smoking Among Young Adults* (1988, wit L. Jarrett, A.V. Swan and R. Rumen). He has also edited *Critical Health Psychology* (2004) and *Qualitative Health Psychology: Theories and Methods* (1999, with K. Chamberlain). He is an Associate Editor of the *Journal of Health Psychology* for which he has edited several special issues on such issues as *Qualitative Research* (with K. Chamberlain), *Community Health Psychology* (with C. Campbell) and *Health Psychology and the Arts* (with R. Gray). He also sits on the editorial boards of several other journals including *Health Psychology Review*, *Psychology Health & Medicine*, and *Arts & Health*. He is a Registered Health Psychologist.

BRIAN EVANS teaches health psychology at Middlesex and City Universities, London, UK. Previously he has held positions at the University of Sussex, UK, and at Concordia University, Montreal, Canada. He is interested in the analysis of psychological research and theory in its socio-political context and his previous publications include *IQ and Mental Testing: An Unnatural Science and Its Social History* (1981, with B. Waites). He is a member of the editorial board of the *Journal of Health Psychology*.

EMEE VIDA ESTACIO is a Lecturer in Psychology at Keele University. She completed her Bachelor's degree in psychology (magna cum laude) at the University of the Philippines, Diliman and her MSc and PhD in health psychology at City University, London. She specializes in health promotion and community development and has facilitated action research with the indigenous Ayta community in the Philippines. She has also project managed community-based needs assessments and evaluation of health improvement programmes in some of the most deprived areas in London. She is a member of the editorial board of the *Journal of Health Psychology* and the International Advisory Group for the World Conference on Psychology, Counseling and Guidance. She is affiliated with the International Society for Critical Health Psychology and the Association for Heterodox Economics. As a scholar activist, she became actively involved in supporting activities for Oxfam, the Association for International Cancer Research, CRIBS Philippines and Save the Children UK. She is an honorary fellow of the Popular Education for People's Empowerment (PEPE) Philippines and the Institute for Health and Human Development (IHHD).

Publisher's Acknowledgements

The authors and publisher wish to thank the following for permission to use copyright material:

Chapter 2

- BMJ Publishing Group for Figure 2.1 World population (line) and annual increments (bars), 8000 BC to 2050 AD from Raleigh, V. S. (1999). World Population and Health in Transition. *BMJ* 319: 981–984

Chapter 4

- Elsevier for Figure 4.3 Conceptual model on cultural competence in health-care from Anderson, L.M. et al. (2003). Culturally competent healthcare systems: A systematic review. *American Journal of Preventive Medicine*, 24: 3, 68–79.

Chapter 6

- The University of Cape Town, South Africa, for Figure 6.2.
- Guildford Press for Figure 6.5 Sexual risk scores for Chinese rural-to-urban migrants for different levels of mobility, from Li, X., Fang, X., Lin, D., Mao, R., Wang, J., Cottrell, L., Harris, C. & Stanton, B. (2004). HIV/STD risk behaviors and perceptions among rural-to-urban migrants in China. *AIDS Education & Prevention*, 16, 538–56.

Chapter 7

- Wiley-Blackwell for Figure 7.1 Neighbouring areas in Liverpool with unhealthy and healthy dietary habits from Hackett, A., Boddy, L., Boothby. J., Dummer, T.J.B., Johnson, B. & Stratton, G. (2008). Mapping dietary habits may provide clues about the factors that determine food choice. *Journal of Human Nutrition & Dietetics*, 21, 428–437. Copyright © 2008, John Wiley and Sons.

- The American Psychological Association for an extract from Harris, J. L., Bargh. J. A. & Brownell, K.D. (2009). Priming effects of television food advertising on eating behavior. *Health Psychology*, 28, 404–413. Copyright © 2009, American Psychological Association.

Chapter 9

- Massachusetts Medical Society for Figure 9.2. Cumulative probability of death from any cause among smokers and non-smokers between the ages of 30 and 69 years from Jha, P. et al. for the RGI–CGHR Investigators (2008). A nationally representative case–control study of smoking and death in India. *New England Journal of Medicine*, 358, 1137–1147. Copyright © 2008 Massachusetts Medical Society. All rights reserved.

Chapter 15

- Ian Lubek for Figure 15.2 Health promotion by the local grass-roots NGO, Siem Reap Citizens for Health, Educational and Social Issues shown at Angkor Wat.

Chapter 19

- The National Academy of Sciences for Figure 19.3 Brain regions displaying different frequencies of activation between high- and low-sensitivity subgroups from Coghill, R.C., McHaffie, J.G. & Yen, Y-F. (2003). Neural correlates of interindividual differences in the subjective experience of pain. *Proceedings of the National Academy of Science*, 100, 8538–8542. Copyright 2003 National Academy of Sciences, U.S.A.
- Oxford University Press for Table 19.1. Using psychological factors in clinical practice from Eccleston, C. (2001). Role of psychology in pain management. *British Journal of Anaesthesia*, 87, 144–152. Copyright © 2001 by The Board of Management and Trustees of *The British Journal of Anaesthesia*.

Chapter 20

- Macmillan Publishers Ltd. for Figure 20.1: A schematic of cancer and the metastatic process. Steeg, P.S. (2003). Metastasis suppressors alter the signal transduction of cancer cells. *Nature Reviews Cancer*, 3, 55–63. Reprinted by permission of Macmillan Publishers Ltd: [Nature Reviews Cancer copyright 2003].

Preface

THE AIMS OF THIS BOOK

This textbook aims to provide an in-depth introduction to the field of health psychology with special relevance to health promotion, disease prevention and health care. It is suitable for advanced undergraduate and postgraduate courses in psychology, medicine, nursing and health care. The authors present an eclectic but critical view of the field, its theories, research and applications. We aim to dig below the surface to expose the underlying theoretical assumptions and to critically analyse methods, evidence and conclusions.

The importance of psychological processes in the experience of health and illness is being increasingly recognized. Evidence for the role of behaviour and emotion in current trends of morbidity and mortality is accumulating; much research has also been conducted on the effects of stress and psychological characteristics on the onset, course and management of physical illness.

In the 1970s, 80s and 90s, health psychology focused primarily on clinical issues. In the 'noughties' and, we expect, the next few decades, more effort is being directed towards creating effective interventions for disease prevention and health promotion, especially with reference to sexual health, diet, smoking, alcohol, inactivity and stress. This textbook provides a step towards that goal.

Against the view that health behaviours are an individual responsibility, governed by freely taken choices, a large amount of the burden of disease is the product of a toxic environment that pushes people towards health-aversive behaviours. Interventions must be multi-levelled, not purely behavioural or educational in kind, as the evidence suggests that such approaches alone are ineffectual and too small in scale (Marks, 1996, 2002a, 2000b).

In addition to working in clinical environments, health psychologists have a contribution to make in developing and evaluating health promotion interventions. Psychologists carry out these activities in close collaboration with communities, other health care practitioners and policymakers. Changes in policy and practice are urgently needed to increase equity and enhance the well-being of the most vulnerable members of society. This book adopts a preventive perspective with a focus on positive health enhancement through the use of multi-level strategies that take into account the whole context of health-related experience and behaviour.

Health psychology is a richly interdisciplinary field requiring an understanding of the cultural, socio-political and economic roots of behaviour and experience. The authors of this textbook apply an international, cross-cultural and interdisciplinary perspective. We suggest that social, economic and political changes have not kept pace with industrial, scientific and medical achievements. As the gaps between the 'haves' and the 'have-nots' widen, and the population is ageing, the impacts of learned helplessness, poverty and social isolation are increasingly salient features of society. The contemporary emphasis on improving health care – a significant and worthy task – at times is little more than tinkering in a way reminiscent of Nero fiddling while Rome burnt.

In preparing to deal with these issues, all those concerned with health services and disease prevention require in-depth understanding, not only of the complexities of human behaviour in its social context, but of the lived experience of health, illness and health care. By integrating quantitative, qualitative and action research approaches, this book is intended to be a step in that direction.

WHAT THE BOOK COVERS

This book places health psychology within its global, social and political context. This requires a glimpse of the 'bigger picture' using a wide-angle lens as well as giving detailed analyses of the 'nitty-gritty' of theory, research and practice. To reflect the widening interest in the field, four chapters are completely new:

Chapter 6 Theories, models and interventions applied to sexual health
Chapter 11 Information and communication
Chapter 14 Health literacy
Chapter 15 Community within health psychology

All remaining chapters have been thoroughly updated and revised. More than 20 per cent of the 1650-plus references are from 2005–10. We have selected only the best available evidence for our major review of the health psychology field. We present boxed case studies of some of the most interesting and significant international studies.

This edition is in four parts. Part 1 introduces the *broader demographic, social, economic and political context of health psychology.* The first three chapters introduce the field and place the study of health psychology within its global, social and political context. Chapter 3 discusses social inequalities and social justice as health issues. Chapter 4 gives an introductory analysis of culture and health. This cross-cultural perspective is maintained throughout the rest of the book. Chapter 5 is concerned with research methods and is designed as an introduction to methods described in more detail in a companion volume by Marks and Yardley (2004).

Part 2 covers the *principal areas of health experience and behaviour of interest to health psychologists*. The topics covered have all been researched and theorized from the perspective of *how health is influenced by the way people think, feel and behave*. These experiences and behaviours are seen as the major psychological determinants of the long-term health and quality of life of the 6.8 billion humans alive today. We examine theories and models and interventions applied to sexual health (Chapter 6), food and eating (Chapter 7), alcohol and drinking (Chapter 8), tobacco and smoking (Chapter 9), and exercise and activity (Chapter 10).

Part 3 covers *health promotion and disease prevention.* We explore many of the principal areas for the improvement of health care through psychological understanding: information and communication (Chapter 11), stress and coping (Chapter 12), immunization and screening (Chapter 13), health literacy (Chapter 14), and community within health psychology approaches (Chapter 15).

Part 4 covers *illness experience and health care*. We discuss illness beliefs and explanations (Chapter 16), illness and personality (Chapter 17), treatment concordance and patient empowerment (Chapter 18), pain (Chapter 19), and cancer and chronic diseases (Chapter 20).

MAKING THE BEST USE OF THIS BOOK

The reader can select chapters relevant to the main approaches to health psychology: clinical, community, public health or critical health psychology (see Box below). Part 1 is core reading of relevance to all students of health psychology.

Chapters can be read in any order according to your personal interests and preferences. In most cases chapters are free-standing and assume no prior reading of other chapters.

Box **Relevance of the different chapters to the four main approaches to health psychology**

Clinical health psychology	**Public health psychology**
Chapters 1–5, 16–20	Chapters 1–15
Community health psychology	**Critical health psychology**
Chapters 1–15	Entire book

Key terms are set in **blue** and emboldened and defined in the **Glossary** at the end of the book.

A useful companion to this textbook is *The Health Psychology Reader* (Marks, 2002a), which reprints and discusses 25 key articles accompanied by introductions to the main themes.

THE COMPANION WEBSITE

A companion website also has been especially developed to complement this textbook. We urge readers to use this website in combination with the text. You can keep thoroughly up to date in this rapidly changing field as we update the website with an interactive blogsite for readers' views and opinions from across the globe. The website is arranged chapter-by-chapter to enable you to deepen and extend your understanding of the topics dealt with in the textbook. The URL is: **www.sagepub.co.uk/marks3**

The website contains the following features:

- Chapter summaries
- PowerPoint slides for use by lecturers
- Video clips of the authors and key researchers discussing 'hot topics'
- Links to downloadable PDF files of relevant new articles from SAGE journals including the *Journal of Health Psychology*
- Links to websites relevant to each topic
- Interactive blog

We gratefully acknowledge the contributions of Mark J. Sparks, Toni Karic, Katie Wright-Bevans and Ashvin Sathasivam in the development of the companion website.

ACKNOWLEDGEMENTS

DFM: Thanks to my family for their continuous support. I dedicate this book to the memory of my late brother Jonathan.

MM: As always, I acknowledge the continuing support of my family.

BE: Thanks to Nick Heather.

EVE: To my parents for life, to my Andy for love, and to my mentor, DFM for guidance – thanks!

Part 1

Health Psychology in Context

The first part of the book places health psychology in its social and economic context. The first chapter introduces health psychology as a new field of inquiry. The concept of health is introduced from a historical perspective. We review theories of need-satisfaction as a foundation for health. The definition, scope and rationale of health psychology are discussed. Two epistemological approaches are described: natural science and human science. A framework for the study of health psychology is described. Finally, we critique the use of evidence-based practice as a paradigm for knowledge in health care, and suggest ideas for further research.

In the second chapter we use a wide-angle lens to explore the context for health experience internationally. We introduce the demographic, economic and societal factors that impinge upon health experience. Profound population and environmental changes add complexity to the economic and social conditions of human behaviour and health. Population growth, increasing poverty, and lack of resources, especially water, are bringing a worsening of health globally in spite of the advances in medicine. Universal gradients for health experience persist over time and space. Progress in reducing poverty and inequality has been slow and concerted, meaningful action is required from intergovernmental policymakers and planners.

There is substantial evidence linking poor social conditions with ill-health. The explanations for this include material, behavioural and psychosocial factors. Chapter 3 considers the extent of social inequalities in health within developed countries, the competing explanations and the role of health psychology in creating a healthier society. The explanation of health inequalities creates many important challenges for theory and research in health psychology.

The way people think about health, become ill and react to illness is rooted in their broader health belief systems that are in turn immersed in culture. Chapter 4 provides some examples from the work of historians and anthropologists who have investigated how health belief systems vary across time and space. We consider some of the different expert health belief systems that have existed historically in Western society and contemporary popular belief systems. We also consider several non-Western health belief systems and discuss some of the issues related with the rapid cultural changes in today's modern society and the interpenetration of cultural groups and belief systems.

Finally Chapter 5 presents a basic A–Z of research and methods within health psychology. Not all letters have a method, but those that do generally fall into one of three categories: *quantitative, qualitative* and *action research*. Quantitative research designs place emphasis on reliable and valid measurement in controlled experiments, trials and surveys. Qualitative methods use interviews, focus groups, narratives or texts to explore health and illness concepts and experience. Action research enables change processes to directly feed back into improvement, empowerment and emancipation.

1

Health Psychology: An Introduction

The desire for the prolongation of life we may take to be one of the most universal of all human motives.

Kenneth Arrow, 1963: 75

Outline

This chapter introduces health psychology as a new field of inquiry. The concept of health is introduced from a historical perspective. We review theories of need-satisfaction as a foundation for health. The definition, scope and rationale of health psychology are discussed. Two epistemological approaches are described: natural science and human science. A framework for the study of health psychology is described. Finally, we critique the use of evidence-based practice as a paradigm for knowledge in health care, and suggest ideas for further research.

WHAT DO WE MEAN BY 'HEALTH'?

It seems natural to discuss what we mean by the term 'health' in a book about health psychology. Otherwise, how do we know what the subject is really about? To understand the word 'health' we need to take a quick dip into etymology, the study of the origin of words.

Many of the words we use today have common roots in a Proto-Indo-European language. 'Health' is one of them. The word 'health' is derived from Old High German and Anglo-Saxon words meaning whole, hale and holy. The etymology of 'heal' has been traced to a Proto-Indo-European root 'kailo-' (meaning whole, uninjured, or of good omen). In Old English this became 'hælan' (to make whole, sound and well) and the Old English 'hal' (health), the root of the adjectives 'whole', 'hale', and 'holy', and the greeting 'Hail'. The word became 'heil' in German (unhurt, unharmed), 'heil' (good luck or fortune), 'heilig' (holy) and 'heilen' (to heal). In Old Norse there was 'heill' (health, prosperity, good luck). Today, 'Hello' in English, 'Hallo' in German, or 'Hi' in US English are well-known greetings.

Thus, links exist between health, wholeness, holiness, hygiene, cleanliness, sanitariness, sanity, saintliness, goodness, and godliness. An emphasis on health as wholeness and naturalness was present in ancient China and classical Greece where health was seen as a state of 'harmony', 'balance' or 'equilibrium' with nature. These beliefs are found in many healing systems to the present day. On the other side of the coin, there are strong associations between these words: disease, disorder, disintegration, illness, crankiness ('krankheit' in German), uncleanness, insanitariness, insanity, badness, and evil.

Galen (CE 129–200), the early Roman physician, followed the Hippocratic tradition in believing that *hygieia* (health) or *euexia* (soundness) occur when there is a balance between the four humours of the body: black bile, yellow bile, phlegm and blood. Galen believed that the body's 'constitution', 'temperament' or 'state' could be put out of equilibrium by excessive heat, cold, dryness or wetness. Such imbalances might be caused by fatigue, insomnia, distress, anxiety, or by food residues resulting from eating the wrong quantity or quality of food. For example, an excess of black bile would cause melancholia. The theory was closely related to the theory of the four elements: earth, fire, water and air (see Table 1.1).

In wintertime, when it is chilly and wet, we worry about catching a cold, caused by a build up of phlegm. In summer, when we are hot and sweaty, we worry about not drinking enough water because we could otherwise become 'hot and bothered' (bad tempered). Some common beliefs today are the descendents of early Greek and Roman theories of medicine.

Mass media which are pervaded by stories about health and medicine fuel a universal fascination with health and illness. There is a torrent of content about health, medicine, and illness, especially the 'dread' diseases. The Internet offers instantaneous updates on every

Table 1.1 Galen's theory of humours

Humour	Season	Element	Organ	Qualities	Personality type	Characteristics
Blood	spring	air	liver	warm & moist	sanguine	amorous courageous, hopeful,
Yellow bile	summer	fire	gall bladder	warm & dry	choleric	easily angered, bad tempered
Black bile	autumn	earth	spleen	cold & dry	melancholic	despondent, sleepless, irritable
Phlegm	winter	water	brain/ lungs	cold & moist	phlegmatic	calm, unemotional

health-related topic at the touch of a few keys. A search with two popular search engines revealed more than 12.5 billion items containing the term 'health' – *almost two items for every person on this planet.*

It is almost impossible to find a single definition in the massive literature that exists. However, in 1946 the World Health Organization (WHO) defined health as: 'the state of complete physical, social and spiritual well-being, not simply the absence of illness'. One doubts whether 'complete physical, social and spiritual well-being' can ever be reached by anyone. In reality, the state of incomplete physical, social and spiritual well-being, with the presence of illness is more familiar to many people. Apart from its idealism, the WHO definition misses key elements of human health and well-being. We would insist that *psychological, cultural* and *economic* aspects should be included in any meaningful definition of health. Psychological processes, behaviour, cognition, imagination, volition and emotion are all mediators of health experience in different ways (the main subject of this book). These processes are all embedded in our social interactions with others. For this reason, the term 'psychosocial' is used to describe the way in which human behaviour and experience help to mould wellness and illness. The role of wealth/poverty in health is evident on a wide scale. A person who knows a healthy diet should include fruit and vegetables ('5 a day') but cannot afford to buy such items. Pork is an affordable meat but against religious edicts for many. Spiritual well-being, for many people, is a primary element of what it means to be human.

With these thoughts in mind, we define health to take account of all of its key elements (see Box 1.1).

Box 1.1

Definition of health

Health is a state of well-being with physical, cultural, psychosocial, economic and spiritual aspects, not simply the absence of illness.

In this definition, health is never seen as 'complete', more like something we strive for. This definition includes the key ingredients for a recipe for health, including factors that must be considered in assessing a person's state of health. To be really useful, it needs further unpacking. In the next section we discuss what philosophers and others think it means to be 'healthy'. Then we unravel the implications for health psychology theory and practice.

HEALTH AS NEED-SATISFACTION

Different people would describe health in a multitude of ways. A fashion model in New York, a young dairy farmer in Somerset, an 80-year-old pensioner living alone, a hunter-gatherer in Southern Africa, or an abalone diver in Polynesia will quite possibly prioritize different things. Yet, people might struggle to describe the difference between health and illness, and what needs to be in place for human beings to thrive, not simply survive.

Maslow's (1943) hierarchy of needs provides initial guidance (see Figure 1.1). One is healthy if all of these needs are satisfied, starting with the most basic needs for air, food, water, sex, sleep, homeostasis and excretion. Then as our need-satisfaction moves toward the top of the pyramid, we become more and more 'satisfied', and thus physically and mentally healthy. But do human needs really fall into any such hierarchy? For example, a participant in extreme sports such as mountain climbing puts 'esteem' and 'self-actualization' well ahead of 'safety'. Also, key elements are missing from Maslow's hierarchy, for example, **agency** and **autonomy** – having the freedom to choose – and **spirituality** – the feeling that not all of experience is created by the physical world.

Philosophers have tried to improve upon Maslow's hierarchy in a variety of ways. Doyal and Gough (1991: 4) argue 'that "health" and "autonomy" are the most basic of human needs which are the same for everyone … all humans have a right to optimum need-satisfaction … For this to occur … certain societal preconditions – political, economic and ecological – must be fulfilled.' The satisfaction of three basic needs – physical health, autonomy of agency, and critical autonomy, to achieve the avoidance of serious harm – is a universal goal in all cultures. If or when a person has reached this universal goal, he/she will then be able to experience 'minimally disabled social participation' (1991: 170) and be free to participate

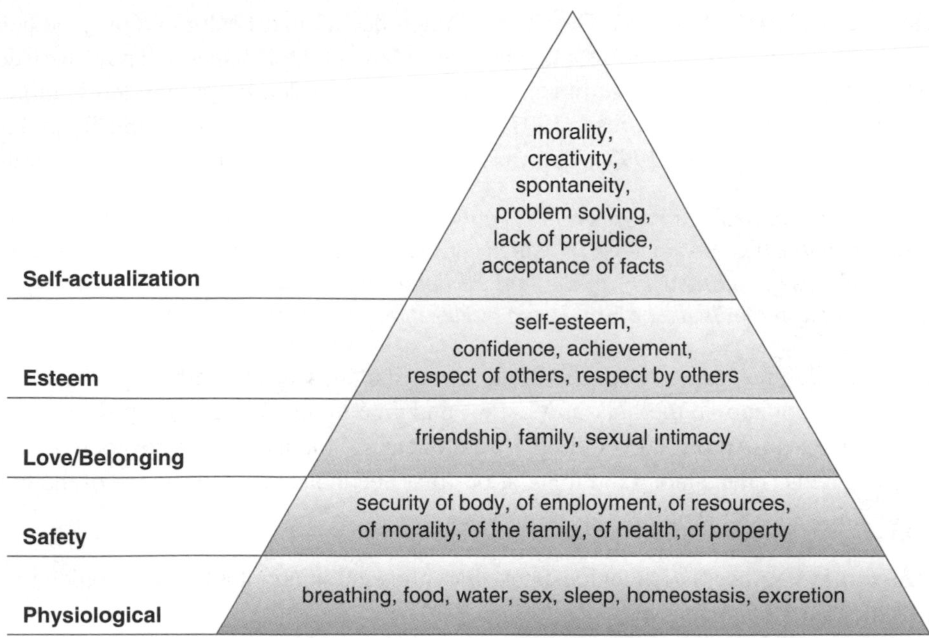

Figure 1.1 Maslow's hierarchy of human needs

in his/her chosen forms of life. The form of the latter will depend upon culture, interests and education.

There are different 'courses for horses'. If I am a Laplander I want to be free to herd reindeer and follow them on their great march through the Arctic. If I am a football fan I will want to follow my team through the various stages of the league and cup competitions. If I am a mother I will want to give my baby all the nourishment, security and comfort that I possibly can. For anybody to participate freely in their chosen 'forms of life', Doyal and Gough list 11 intermediate needs:

1 Adequate nutritional food and water
2 Adequate protective housing
3 A safe environment for working
4 A safe physical environment
5 Appropriate health care
6 Security in childhood
7 Significant primary relationships with others
8 Physical security
9 Economic security
10 Safe birth control and child-bearing
11 Appropriate basic and cross-cultural education

Rejecting the WHO definition, Doyal and Gough decide that health can only be defined negatively – as the minimization of death, disablement and disease. They also define autonomy negatively – as the minimization of mental disorder, cognitive deprivation, and restricted opportunities. Seedhouse (1997) advocates another approach – the 'Foundations theory of health promotion' (1997). This theory of health promotion is based on this premise:

> *A person's (optimum) state of health is equivalent to the state of the set of conditions which fulfil or enable a person to work to fulfil his or her realistic chosen and biological potentials. Some of these conditions are of the highest importance to all people. Others are variable dependent upon individual abilities and circumstances.* (Seedhouse, 1997: 136)

Seedhouse defines 'basic needs' as food, drink, shelter, warmth and purpose in life. All except the last appears in the lists of Maslow, and Gough and Doyal. 'Purpose in life' is a primary concept in Antonovsky's (1979) 'salutogenetic' theory. So far so good – familiar ground, one feels. Then among the foundations that Seedhouse considers 'are of the highest importance for all people' are:

1. **Information** 'Access to the widest possible information about all factors which have an influence on a person's life.'
2. **Literacy and numeracy skills** 'People need to be able to understand how the information applies to them, and to be able to make reasoned decisions about what action to take in the light of that information.'
3. **Sociality** '…an awareness of a basic duty which follows from living in a community.'

Seedhouse suggests, in addition to universal foundations, specific foundations for different individual situations depending upon living conditions and circumstances. A person with an illness, a person in a damp and dilapidated house, a prisoner, an athlete, a terminal patient, or an expectant mother will each have specific requirements and priorities. For Seedhouse, 'the devil is in the detail'. There are only four generic foundations, and a set of special foundations tailored to individual circumstances on a case-by-case basis. Any effort at health promotion therefore involves an act of discovery, to find out what any individual or group must be given to fill the gap between what they aspire to and what they currently have. Health policies must be designed to 'bolster the foundations of all' and health services need to work towards 'improving the lot of everyone' (1997: 145–6). But such idealism may be difficult to implement in real world settings.

Seedhouse compares two options that, to him, are 'fairly easy to decide'. He asks us to imagine deciding between funding a campaign to improve road safety and a life-extending treatment for Alzheimer's patients which produces no increase in the patients' quality of life. Seedhouse claims foundations theory would dictate opting for the road safety campaign which, he claims, affects every road-user, and ditching the treatment for Alzheimer's patients because they would only live longer, not gain any improvements in quality of life. The fact that road users outnumber Alzheimer's patients is a reason for opting for the road safety campaign. However, to others, this example may well be contentious. Road users who have a family member with Alzheimer's would most likely disagree that this makes a 'fairly easy' decision. Indeed they might well feel that deliberately withholding a life-extending treatment would be unethical. Who actually wants to live to a 100 anyway? Ask a 99-year-old and you may get a positive answer.

This example gives perfect illustration of the political assumptions that underlie all decision-making in health care. Contrasting points of view about resources will tend to emerge from different social groups, i.e. whether they are young or old, have aging parents with dementia, use a bus, bicycle, or walk to work. What is advocated as the *best* approach depends on *who* is making this decision, *whose* values and interests are held in mind, and *who* will be most affected by the decision.

THE NATURE OF HEALTH PSYCHOLOGY

The importance of psychosocial processes in health and illness is increasingly recognized. For example, evidence on the role of behaviour and emotion in morbidity and mortality is accumulating. Much research has been conducted to investigate the possible role of stress and psychological characteristics on the onset, course and management of physical illness. Advances in genetics, medicine oncology, and immunology are all offering exciting new challenges to health psychology. It is therefore unsurprising that health psychology is growing rapidly and health psychologists are in increasing demand in health care and medical settings. Psychologists have become essential members of multidisciplinary teams in rehabilitation, cardiology, paediatrics, oncology, anaesthesiology, family practice, dentistry, and other medical fields. In the UK and Europe, health psychology is a new profession alongside clinical and counselling psychology.

Although the primary focus for health psychology has been clinical settings, interest is now also being directed towards interventions for disease prevention, especially with reference to sexual health, nutrition, smoking, alcohol, inactivity and stress. The traditional view of Western societies is an ideology of individualism which views individuals as 'agents' who are responsible for their own health. A person who smokes 40 a day and then develops lung cancer is held responsible for causing a preventable, costly and terminal illness. Traditional health education has consisted of campaigns providing a mixture of exhortation, information and advice to persuade people to change their unhealthy habits. By telling people to 'Just say no' policymakers expect people to make the 'right' choices and change their unhealthy choices into healthy ones. Health education has succeeded to a degree. Supported by services offering treatments and techniques for behaviour change, improvements in public health have definitely been achieved. Tobacco control provides a benchmark for what may be achieved through health education and behaviour change. However, the major approach to tobacco control has been pharmacological. Millions continue to smoke because these treatments are only marginally better than no treatment at all (see Chapter 9). There is little room for thinking that we have the necessary technology to produce behaviour change on an industrial scale. However there is the potential to do so if the human side of health care is strengthened. Health care systems would become more efficient and evidence based if the benefits of scientific medicine are complemented with psychosocial and other evidence-based approaches. This could ultimately lead to a **wholistic** system offering 'health for all'.

Against the view that keeping ourselves healthy means making responsible choices, there is little convincing evidence, beyond the example of smoking control, that people who change their diet or lifestyle actually *do* live longer or have more quality of life than people who 'live and let live' and make no real attempt to live healthily. Consider a hypothetical example: an epidemiological study shows that vegetarians live longer than meat eaters. Such a study normally proves very little. This type of study usually falls well short of being a randomized controlled trial, the closest thing we have to a controlled 'experiment'. The vegetarians may differ from the meat-eaters in many ways other than their choice of diet, e.g. religious beliefs, use of alcohol, social support. A second issue is that a statistical association between two variables such as a vegetarian diet and longevity never proves causality or allows a prediction about any particular individual case. A vegetarian could still die of stomach cancer and becoming a vegetarian will not necessarily lengthen the life of any specific person. Epidemiology is purely a statistical science – it can never tell individuals what will happen if they do X, Y or Z, but only provide a statistical or probability statement.

Yet the assumption that we must 'live well to be well' is prevalent in contemporary society. The moral aspect of this assumption also leads to victim blaming. If people get ill it is often seen as 'their own fault' because they smoke, drink, eat a poor diet, fail to exercise or use screening services, do not cope with stress in a healthy way by joining a gym and so on. Health policy is run through with the blaming and shaming of individuals for their own poor health. The 'smoking evil' has been replaced by the 'obesity evil'. A person who smokes, eats fatty foods, drinks alcohol and watches TV for many hours every day is represented as a 'couch potato'. Fitzpatrick (2001) compares disease with sin, and health with virtue. Medicine is thereby portrayed as a quasi-religious quest against gluttony, laziness and lust. Diets are seen as moral choices, in which a 'balanced' and healthy diet is a moral imperative.

We may like to believe in the fiction that we are free agents with self-determination. To what degree the people who are the targets for healthy eating campaigns have the resources to choose what they eat is a matter of concern. The majority of human activity is influenced by the social and economic environment, role models among family, friends or in the mass media. The herd instinct is as strong in humans as in bees, birds or sheep. Christakis and Fowler (2007) report evidence that there is a person-to-person spread of obesity. They evaluated a database containing a social network of 12,067 people from 1971 to 2003 and found clusters of obese persons at all time points, and the clusters extended to three degrees of separation. A person's chance of becoming obese was increased by 57 per cent if he or she had a friend who became obese in a given interval. Network phenomena appear to be relevant to the biologic and behavioural trait of obesity, and obesity appears to spread through social ties. Social imitation in social networks seems to be as an important determinant of health as any individual decision to live a healthy life. A successful approach, social cognitive theory, is based on this assumption (Bandura, 1995).

The built environment, the sum total of objects placed in the natural world by human beings, is equally important to the social one. The '**toxic environment**' propels people towards unhealthy behaviours and causes large amounts of mortality and illness (Brownell, 1994). People become overweight and obese because they inhabit an **obesogenic**

environment which contains affordable but nasty, fatty, salty or sugary foods. For example, 'hot dogs' made with mechanically recovered meat can contain 0 per cent real meat. Chicken nuggets can contain 0 per cent real meat. The ready availability of such items offers consumers little real choice when income levels are low and living costs, rents and house prices are high. The poisoning begins very early in life. Garbarino (1995) discusses the 'socially toxic environment' in which: 'Children's social world has become poisonous, due to escalating violence, the potentially lethal consequences of sex, diminishing adult supervision, and growing child poverty' (Garbarino, 1995: 12). Toxicity can be extended to all of the major determinants of health and well-being.

In this book, we present evidence and arguments on different sides of the 'freedom and choice' debate. We accept that our present understanding of health behaviour is far from definitive. However we also believe that a critical position toward the discipline is warranted. Health psychology as it is currently structured as an academic discipline is based on an ideology of **individualism** based on interests and values embedded in mass culture. Educational or behavioural approaches based on internalized processes within the individual are often ineffectual and too small in scale (Marks, 1996, 2002a, 2002b). The necessary infrastructure for mass dissemination of such approaches through the health care system is lacking. The medical model remains the foundation of health care and is likely to remain so well into the future. The more wholistic approach of biopsychosocial health care is becoming more evident. Health psychologists can work within this approach at different levels of the health care system: carrying out research; systematically reviewing research; helping to design, implement and evaluate health interventions; training and teaching; consultancy; providing and improving health services; carrying out health promotion; designing policy to improve services; and, last but not least, advocating social justice so that people and communities are enabled to act on their own terms.

In the latter domain, a **communitarian** perspective to health work can lead to more effective interventions. In working towards social justice and the reduction of inequities, people's rights to health and freedom from illness are a life and death matter, a responsibility of all planners, policymakers and leaders of people wherever they may be (Marks, 2004). We return to this subject in the chapters that follow.

We suggest a definition of health psychology in Box 1.2. In discussing this definition, we can say that the objective of health psychology is to promote and maintain the well-being of individuals, communities and populations.

Box 1.2

Definition of health psychology

Health psychology is an interdisciplinary field concerned with the application of psychological knowledge and techniques to health, illness and health care.

Health psychologists generally hold a wholistic perspective on individual well-being. While the primary focus is on *physical* rather than *mental* health, in reality it is acknowledged that these are 'two sides of a coin'. When a person has a physical illness they can experience anxiety or depression. When a person has a mental illness their behaviour or treatment may well lead to a deterioration in physical health. Feeling well involves mind, body and spirit. At a practical level, the health psychologist is concerned with the behaviour and experience of the individual, the interface of the individual with the health-care system, and with society as a whole.

RATIONALE AND ROLE FOR HEALTH PSYCHOLOGY

There is a strong rationale for developing the discipline of health psychology: (1) the behavioural basis for illness and mortality requires effective methods of behaviour change; (2) the search for a wholistic system of health care requires expert knowledge of the psychosocial health needs of people. Firstly, in relation to point 1, findings from **epidemiology** suggest that *all* of the leading causes of illness and death in Western societies are *behavioural.* This means that many deaths are preventable if we can find effective ways of changing behaviour. The mortality rates for different conditions in younger and older people are shown in Table 1.2.

Table 1.2 Leading causes of mortality among adults worldwide, 2002

Rank	Cause	Deaths (000)
Mortality: adults aged 15–59		
1	HIV/AIDS	2279
2	Ischaemic heart disease	1332
3	Tuberculosis	1036
4	Road traffic injuries	814
5	Cerebrovascular disease	783
6	Self-inflicted injuries	672
7	Violence	473
8	Cirrhosis of the liver	382
9	Lower respiratory infections	352
10	Chronic obstructive pulmonary disease	343
Mortality: adults aged 60 and over		
1	Ischaemic heart disease	5825
2	Cerebrovascular disease	4689

Table 1.2 *(Continued)*

Rank	Cause	Deaths (000)
3	Chronic obstructive pulmonary disease	2399
4	Lower respiratory infections	1396
5	Trachea, bronchus, lung cancers	928
6	Diabetes mellitus	754
7	Hypertensive heart disease	735
8	Stomach cancer	605
9	Tuberculosis	495
10	Colon and rectum cancers	477

Source: http://www.who.int/whr/2003/en/Facts_and_Figures-en.pdf

KEY STUDY The Global Burden of Disease study

An important epidemiological perspective comes from measures of '**disability**' or '**disablement**'. The **Global Burden of Disease** (GBD) study projected mortality and disablement over 25 years. The trends from the GBD study suggest that disablement is determined mainly by ageing, the spread of HIV, the increase in tobacco-related mortality and disablement, psychiatric and neurological conditions and the decline in mortality from communicable, maternal, perinatal and nutritional disorders (Murray & Lopez, 1997).

The GBD uses the **disability-adjusted life year** (DALY) as a quantitative indicator of burden of disease that reflects the total amount of healthy life lost, to all causes, whether from premature mortality or from some degree of disablement during a period of time. The DALY is the sum of years of life lost from premature mortality plus years of life with disablement, adjusted for severity of disablement from all causes, both physical and mental (Murray & Lopez, 1997). The GBD study prepared figures by age, sex and region for 1990 and 2020 (see Table 1.3).

While various cancers feature highly in the causes of mortality (see Table 1.2), they do not appear in the top ten causes of disablement (Table 1.3) because people with untreatable cancer die fairly quickly with the condition. However, diseases of the cardiovascular system cause many deaths and also a large proportion of disablement. Many patients with cardiovascular disease live for a long time. The contribution of communicable maternal, perinatal and nutritional disorders to the GBD is expected to decline from 44 per cent in 1990 to 20 per cent in 2020. Meanwhile the contribution from non-communicable diseases is expected to rise from 41 per cent in 1990 to 60 per cent in 2020.

(Continued)

(Continued)

Table 1.3 Rank order of DALYs for the ten leading causes of disablement, World 1990–2020

Position	1990 Diseases or Injury	2020 Diseases or Injury
1	Lower respiratory infections	Ischaemic heart disease
2	Diarrhoeal diseases	Unipolar major depression
3	Conditions arising during the perinatal period	Road traffic accidents
4	Unipolar major depression	Cerebrovascular disease
5	Ischaemic heart disease	Chronic obstructive pulmonary disease
6	Cerebrovascular disease	Lower respiratory infections
7	Tuberculosis	Tuberculosis
8	Measles	War injuries
9	Road traffic accidents	Diarrhoeal diseases
10	Congenital anomalies	HIV/AIDS

Source: Murray and Lopez, 1997

The data in Table 1.4 indicate that nearly 30 per cent of the total global burden of disease is attributable to five risk factors. The largest risk factor (underweight) is associated with **poverty** (see Chapters 2 and 3). The remaining four risk factors are discussed in Part 2 (see Chapters 6–10).

Table 1.4 The five leading risk factors for global disease burden computed in DALYs

Risk factor	Number of DALYs (millions)	Percentage of DALYs
Childhood and maternal underweight	138	9.5
Unsafe sex	92	6.3
High blood pressure	64	4.4
Tobacco	59	4.1
Alcohol	58	4.0
Totals	411	28.3

Source: Ezzati et al., 2002

The statistics on death and disablement provide a strong rationale for health psychology. If the major risk factors are to be addressed, there is a need for effective methods of behaviour change. The mainstream ideology of **individualism** assumes that *individuals are responsible for their own health.* Health psychology is at the 'sharp end' of the quest to produce

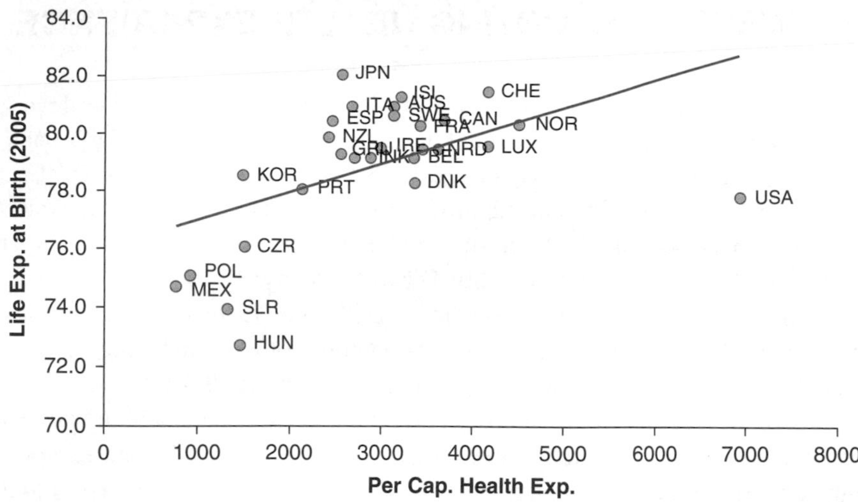

Figure 1.2 Life expectancy at birth and per capita health expenditure for different countries

health behaviour change on an industrial scale. The fact that people are highly constrained by their circumstances often militates against such changes. There are constraints on the ability of health-care systems to influence health outcomes at a population level because of the significant social and economic determinants that structure the health of individuals and communities.

A second rationale for health psychology is growing recognition that a purely medical approach to health care is failing to meet the psychosocial needs of many patients. This has led to a search for an alternative perspective which values the wholistic care of patients and attempts to improve services through higher quality psychosocial care. In spite of their very high costs (see Figure 1.2), health-care systems are often perceived to be inefficient, ineffective and unfit for purpose. This is especially the case in the US where the largest per capita expenditure is producing some unimpressive outcomes. Longevity in the US is lower than in the majority of countries in the Western world. One wonders why? The dominance of the **medical model** has been criticized since the 1970s (Illich, 1976). While medicine wants to take the credit for the decline of disease in the twentieth century, critics have suggested that health improvements are due mainly to better hygiene, education and reduced poverty (McKeown, 1979).

High costs, dissatisfaction and disenchantment, together with a growing awareness of psychosocial influences, led to concepts such as the biopsychosocial model (Engel, 1977; see Chapter 3). Since that suggestion, health psychology has developed distinctive approaches.

DIFFERENT WAYS OF STUDYING HEALTH EXPERIENCE

Epistemology is concerned with theories about how we can acquire knowledge. Traditionally, there are two major approaches to acquiring knowledge and understanding of human behaviour and experience. An approach to acquiring new knowledge is termed an 'epistemology'. The first of these is the *natural science* approach that analyses behaviour and experience in a manner similar to the way in which physicists, chemists or biologists conduct experiments to search for a single, 'true' account of reality. For example, by observing a chemical reaction in a test tube the chemist is able to use induction and extrapolate by using general laws to the whole of the natural world. Human behaviour often does not fit comfortably within the test tube model of science and another approach is found to be more illuminating. This has led to the conception of the *human science* approach that explores human behaviour and experience using a variety of methods, including qualitative ones. This approach focuses upon understanding the underlying personal meaning of events, trying to see how the world looks from the perspective of one individual, one group or one culture.

Both traditions have been influential. Table 1.5 presents contrasting features of the two approaches. From a pragmatic point of view, the two epistemologies are complementary, not mutually exclusive. The natural science approach aims to identify causal relationships between variables. It asks 'does x cause y?' and attempts to generate accurate predictive models from an objective, 'third-person' perspective. By contrast, the human science approach aims to analyse meanings and reasons. It asks 'how does y feel about x?' or 'what does y mean to x?' and produces detailed accounts of human action from a subjective, 'first-person' perspective. Both approaches deliver descriptions and explanations of what has happened in the past, and make predictions about what can be expected in future. One 'size does not fit all'. In many situations it is possible to apply both types of description. The degree of fit between each approach and a given event depends on its nature.

The natural science tradition is represented by the medical model. Health and illness are complex physical states of the body and brain. The mind is neural activity in the cerebral cortex. Engel (1977) challenged the traditional medical model by proposing a **biopsychosocial model** which assumed that health and illness have physical, psychosocial and cultural determinants.

Critics have suggested that the biopsychosocial model is essentially the medical model 'with knobs on', that it is not a proper theory which is capable of making testable or refutable predictions (Armstrong, 1987; Marks, 1996). Many textbooks have advocated the biopsychosocial model as a viable alternative to the medical model. The biopsychosocial model has been a kind of 'Trojan Horse' with which to establish health psychology as a distinctive discipline. However, the fact that the biopsychosocial model is not a coherent theory makes it an unsuitable choice for the foundation of a scientific discipline.

The second epistemology, the human science tradition, is represented by research on discourse, **narrative** and **social representations**. People's accounts of health and illness are an illuminating topic of study in its own right. Much of the research on health and illness narratives has been influenced by **social constructionism** (Stainton-Rogers, 1991). From this

Table 1.5 Contrasting the natural science and human science approaches to health psychology

Aspect	Natural science	Human science
Objective	Identifying causes: Does X cause Y?	Identifying meanings: What does X mean to Y?
Epistemology	Realism: only one true description of nature (reality)	Social constructivism: many descriptions (plurality)
Ontology	Everything has a physical structure (mind = body)	Psychological experiences (subjectivity, consciousness, etc.) are not reducible to physics (mind ≠ body)
Model	Medical model (3 Ds: disease, diagnosis, drugs)	Biopsychosocial model (3 Ps: people, prevention, psychology)
Research methods	Quantitative methods: observation, experiments, randomized controlled trials	Qualitative methods: discourse analysis, grounded theory, interpretative phenomenological analysis, narratives, diaries, art and performance
Interventions	Physical (surgery), pharmacological (drug treatments), behavioural (lifestyle change)	Social, psychological, cognitive, phenomenological

perspective, there is no single, fixed 'reality' but a multiplicity of descriptions or 'drafts', each with its own unique pattern of meanings. Mulkay (1991: 27–8) suggests the existence of 'many potential worlds of meaning that can be imaginatively entered and celebrated, in ways that are constantly changing to give richness and value to human experience'. One of the more popular ways of studying 'worlds of meaning' has been to analyse the social psychological functions of people's accounts using discourse analysis (Potter and Wetherell, 1987). Discursive psychology was influenced by Berger and Luckmann (1966), who argued that 'reality' is a social construction. Earlier intellectual forbears were Pascal, Marx and Nietzsche, who believed that conscious thinking is strongly influenced by the thinker's socio-historical context.

Social constructionists continue to engage in a lively debate regarding the extent to which social constructions are grounded in material reality (see Parker, 1998). Some are relativists, in which there is no single reality at all, while others are critical realists in which there is one reality giving rise to different descriptions or perspectives. Relativist social constructionists, inspired by Nietzsche, emphasize the flexibility of discourse and the sense in which language can be said to construct reality. Critical realist social constructionists, inspired by Marx, acknowledge that discourses construct different versions of reality, but they argue that the material world cannot accommodate all constructions equally well. Some accounts are more useful than others.

Whatever approach we choose, both are interested in developing an improved understanding of health in body and mind and the relationships between the two. We suggest that we can actually have the 'best of both worlds' by accepting the value and benefits in attempting to understand the objective and the subjective aspects of health and illness.

A CROSS-CULTURAL PERSPECTIVE

In addition to wide variations in health beliefs between cultures, there is significant within-culture diversity. Folk beliefs, knowledge and practices among individuals from different communities and social groups rub shoulders with each other and with those of health-care professionals in a Tower of Babel. These diverse beliefs meld with practices and lifestyles in accord with people's worldviews and values.

Theories in health psychology provide accounts of how psychosocial processes affect individual health experience. In reviewing such theories (see Chapter 6) it must be acknowledged that they are principally products of the USA and British Commonwealth, together with inputs from Continental Europe and Scandinavia. Many of health psychology's theories are adaptations of US/European cognitive and social psychology from the last 50 years of the twentieth century. The resurgence of research in laboratory environments used structured psychometric instruments, questionnaires and performance tests designed to reveal the mechanisms underlying human behaviour. These methods lacked **ecological validity**, or, in other words, the findings could not be generalized to the world that lies outside the laboratory. Critics have suggested that the laboratory experiment and the questionnaire are subject to more bias than their proponents are willing to admit (Harré, 1979).

Anglo-centric theory can be viewed as one large-scale **indigenous** psychology that is inapplicable to cultures outside (Heelas & Lock, 1981). This view was supported by Lillard (1998) who catalogues evidence that 'European American' folk psychology shows major differences from the folk psychologies of other cultures. One example of a cultural value that is embedded in Western societies is **individualism**, which dictates that individuals are responsible for their own health. Over-concern with personal responsibility for health can lead to guilt and stigmatization. Brownell warned that the 'tendency to overstate the impact of personal behaviour on health' could feed the victim-blaming ethos that is already strong in western societies (Brownell, 1991: 303).

Cross-cultural psychology emphasizes cultural diversity and casts a sceptical eye over the **ethnocentrism** of contemporary Western psychology. It considers national or large group samples as the unit of analysis rather than individuals. Research has focused primarily on mental health (e.g. Dasen et al., 1988) and relatively little attention has been paid to physical health. A truly cross-cultural approach to health psychology is at an early stage of development.

Case Study

INTERNATIONAL CASE STUDY 'Health psychology in African settings. A cultural-psychological analysis' (Adams & Salter, 2007)

This study reveals how the individualistic nature of mainstream health psychology is not applicable to settings in Africa. The mainstream Western approach assumes a world-view in which the causes of illness are attributed to atomistic, physiological processes within the individual. This construction of reality is associated with a view of a person as an individual with his/her own internalized assumptions that he/she is a separate individual. In African cultures, however, each person is seen as interconnected to other people, including living relatives and dead ancestors, and also to places and spiritual forces. Markus, Mullally and Kitayama (1997) refer to cultural assumptions about self hood as '**selfways**'. Selfways include what it means to be a good or bad person, and what causes us to become healthy or ill.

Adams and Salter give as an example of African selfways the idea of 'enemyship' – the belief that hatred of another can lead to bad things happening to one. The belief in the power of malevolent others is manifest through such practices as divination, infant seclusion, sorcery and witchcraft. They quote the following example: 'I don't know my enemies, but I know that I have them. One day something will happen to me, and then I will know that this person has been after me all along' (Adams & Salter, 2007: 541).

There are implications of selfways for health-care provision. In the West we assume that social support and caregiving are generally a source of comfort and coping. Indeed, social support is a major focus for health psychology research and services. We need to consider how intimate family members could also be viewed as *a source of danger, stress, worry and depression.* In highlighting enemyship, the selfways of African cultures show social embeddedness is an 'inevitable fact of social existence' (Adams & Salter, 2007: 542).

A FRAMEWORK FOR HEALTH PSYCHOLOGY

Theory in health psychology consists of three broad types that vary according to their level of generality: these are *frameworks, theories* and *models.* Frameworks have some of the characteristics of paradigms (Kuhn, 1970) as they refer to a complete system of thinking about a field of inquiry. Paradigms explicitly state assumptions, laws and methods. Frameworks are much looser than paradigms but they are a way of organizing information about a field. Figure 1.3 shows a framework about the main influences on the health of individual human beings. It has been adapted from the work of Dahlgren and Whitehead (1991) and we call this the 'Health Onion'

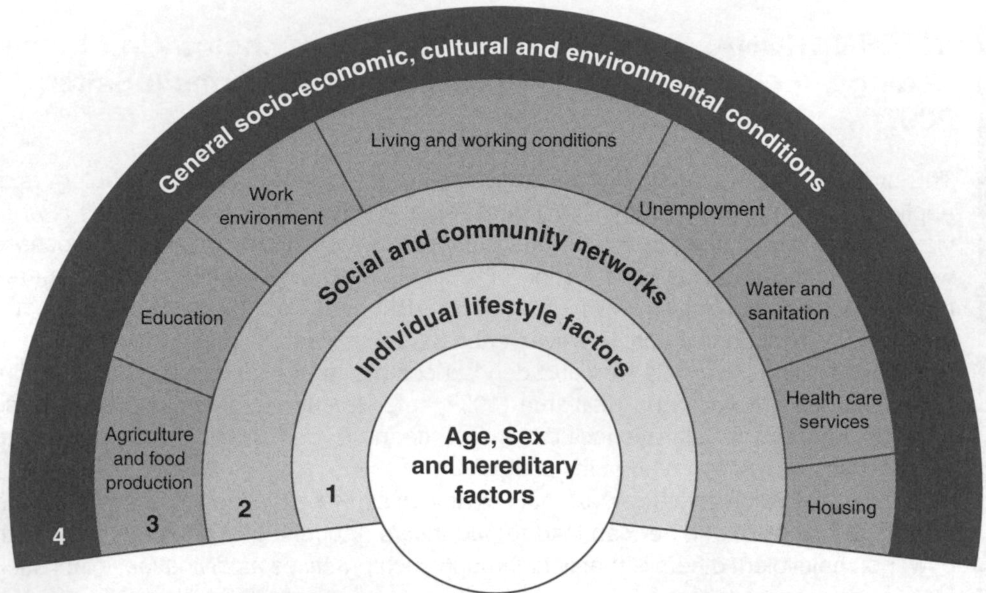

Figure 1.3 A framework for health psychology

Source: Dahlgren & Whitehead, 1991 reproduced with permission

The 'Health Onion' has a multi-layered structure with the individual at its core, surrounded by four layers of influence:

Level 4: general socio-economic, cultural and environmental conditions (covered by Part 1 of this book).
Level 3: living and working conditions (covered by Part 3 of this book).
Level 2: social and community influences (covered throughout this book).
Level 1: individual lifestyle (covered by Part 2 of this book).
Core: age, sex and hereditary factors (covered throughout this book).

The Health Onion has seven characteristics:

1 It is wholistic.
2 It is concerned with all health determinants, not simply with events during the treatment of illness.
3 The individual is at the core with health determinants acting through the community, living and working conditions, and the socio-economic, cultural and physical environment.
4 It places each layer in the context of its neighbours, including possible structural constraints upon change.
5 It has an interdisciplinary flavour that goes beyond a medical or quasi-medical approach.

6 It makes no claim for any one level being more important than others.
7 It acknowledges the complex nature of health determinants.

Different theories are needed for each setting and context. However, there is also a need for a general paradigm for individual health within which specific theories and models can be nested. Such a paradigm should attempt to represent in an explicit, detailed and meaningful way the constraints upon and links between individual well-being, the surrounding community and the health-care system (Marks, 1996). No such general paradigm exists. We are waiting for another Hippocrates, Darwin or Einstein. Or perhaps the sheer diversity of issues and perspectives makes the field non-amenable to a single paradigm.

Box 1.3

Evidence-based practice as a paradigm for knowledge (*Source*: Marks, 2005, 2009)

Some believe we have a paradigm for all of health care in the form of evidence-based medicine or evidence-based practice (EBP). In EBP randomized controlled trials are used to produce conclusions about the effectiveness of different methods and treatments. In theory the approach sounds wonderful. In practice it is far from perfect. Evidence on effectiveness in EBP is assumed to have an objective, inviolable status that reflects 'reality'. It is given an iconic status. In some undefined ways this evidence about 'reality' not only aids decision-making, but also determines it. In truth, evidence is never absolutely certain. It consists of negotiable, value-laden, and contextually dependent items of information. Evidence (= knowledge) for a technique or treatment in health care is not an accident, but the outcome of a series of 'gates' or 'filters' that must be passed before the technique is deemed to be kosher (Marks, 2005).

Consider the sequence of processes from conception to application through which evidence must pass if it is to be considered admissible in EBP. The filtering is so selective that, typically, systematic reviewers will be able to find only a dozen or less of primary studies which fulfil the inclusion criteria from a field of several thousand. Oakley (2001) described a systematic review of peer health promotion for young people that found 5,124 citations of which exactly 12 (0.234 per cent) were judged to have carried out 'sound' outcome evaluations. She compared this search process to 'finding needles in haystacks' (Oakley, 2001: 22–4). Another analogy is making a pot of filter coffee – the stronger the filtering, the less fresh and flavourful the coffee. EBP is somewhat similar – there are no guarantees the end-product will be fit-for-purpose. The filtering process of EBP is illustrated below:

(Continued)

(Continued)

1. Current knowledge, theory and paradigms taught in universities and schools
2. Funding priorities of government, industry and charities
3. Hypotheses considered important by the funders
4. Methodology approved by funders
5. Journal publication
6. Systematic reviews
7. EBP

To be judged 'sound', evidence must pass through all seven of the filters which are disposed towards the preservation of existing practices, traditions and myths. In confirming the 'sound' status of the chosen techniques, which have passed through the filters, the 'unsoundness' of the unfiltered techniques is established by default. Undeniably, this filtering of evidence is systematic and evidence will be considered 'sound' or 'unsound' according to established criteria.

However, EBP is contentious on a number of grounds. Firstly, it is wasteful that so much evidence is 'thrown away'. Many unfiltered techniques are quite possibly as effective as techniques that have been filtered. Secondly, the filtering process gives a high weighting to techniques which conform to beliefs and values of the knowledge establishment. For example, pharmacotherapy will be established ahead of psychological therapies (pharmaceutical industry sponsorship at filters 1-4), quantitative techniques will be preferred to qualitative techniques (filters 5-6), and patient treatment care will be about outputs and outcomes, rather than feeling they have been cared for as human beings (filter 7). Thirdly, innovation may have difficulty breaking through.

In this book we review the results of many studies using the approach of EBP. We also review observational studies *not* based on the assumptions of EBP. Many such studies were situated in settings where EBP would be unethical, impractical or impossible to carry out. We also recognize the contribution of qualitative studies where the information obtained illuminates the psychosocial experience of health and illness.

FUTURE RESEARCH

1 Research is needed at a basic conceptual level to unravel the biopsychosocial model and specify it more clearly so that it can be turned into a genuine theory.
2 Transcultural studies of health, illness and health care are needed to facilitate communication and understanding of systems of healing among different cultural, ethnic and religious groups.
3 Apart from smoking cessation, there is no strong evidence that lifestyle changes cause positive changes to life expectancy and quality of life. That evidence needs to be gathered.
4 Innovative methods of evaluation are needed to provide an alternative to evidence-based practice.

Summary

1. Health is a state of well-being with physical, cultural, psychosocial, economic and spiritual attributes, not simply the absence of illness.
2. To be healthy in body and mind a person's biological needs must be satisfied and also their needs to interconnect with others and to act autonomously.
3. Interests and values condition all health work. A social orientation is necessary if we are to understand health behaviour and experience in context of society and culture. Such an orientation focuses upon health as much as illness, preventive care as much as cure, and considers families, groups and communities as much as individuals.
4. Health psychology consists of the application of psychological knowledge and techniques to health, illness and health care. Its primary purpose is to understand and improve the well-being of individuals and communities.
5. Health psychology is growing rapidly because: (a) there is increasing evidence that much illness and mortality are caused by behaviour; (b) there is increasing awareness of the psychosocial aspects of health and illness.
6. The Health Onion Framework is used in this book as a framework for health and illness. The core is individual health status with particular age, sex and hereditary factors.
7. Four levels of analysis (skins of the Health Onion) consist of individual lifestyle (level 1), social and community influences (level 2), living and working conditions (level 3), and general socio-economic, cultural and environmental conditions (level 4).
8. Health psychology lacks a single paradigm. Two approaches analyse health and illness in different ways: from the perspective of natural science (realism) and from the perspective of human science (constructivism).
9. Concepts about health and disease are embedded in culturally diverse selfways, which manifest significant differences between cultures and places.
10. Theory building in health psychology occurs at three levels of generality: (a) frameworks; (b) theories; (c) models. The evidence base is made up of the outcomes of evidence-based practice and observational methods which may be both qualitative and quantitative.

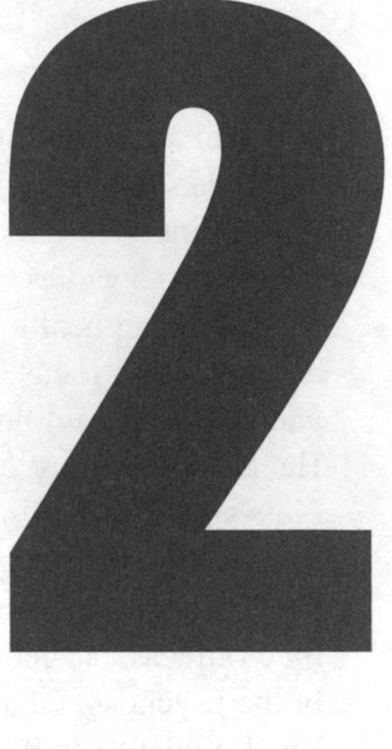

The Macro-Social Environment and Health

As in earlier times, advances in the 21st century will be won by human struggle against divisive values – and against the opposition of entrenched economic and political interests.

Human Development Report, 2000: 6

Outline

In this chapter we use a wide-angle lens to explore the context for health experience internationally. We introduce the demographic, economic and societal factors which impinge upon health experience. Profound population and environmental changes add complexity to the economic and social conditions of human behaviour and health. Population growth, increasing poverty, and lack of resources, especially water, are bringing a worsening of health globally in spite of the advances in medicine. Universal gradients for health experience persist over time and space. Progress in reducing poverty and inequality has been slow. Concerted and meaningful action is required from intergovernmental policymakers and planners.

GLOBAL HEALTH TRENDS

Where a baby is born, the mother's access to water, food, and her education determine whether the baby lives or dies. A baby in Sierra Leone has a 72 per cent chance of making it to age 5. A Japanese baby has a 96 per cent chance of reaching 5. In this chapter we examine why. We review some key factors in the social and economic context for health. Health-care systems need to consider this wider context in developing services, interventions and policies.

It is accepted that health is dependent on a mixture of genetic and environmental influences. The proportionality of these two in any individual case depends upon a person's ancestry, age and gender, and it depends on the specific outcome we are interested in. Our ability to make precise clinical predictions about any individual case using statistical knowledge or epidemiological trends is normally quite limited.

The environment can affect human health in a huge variety of ways. Firstly, devastating 'acts of God' occur in the form of earthquakes, tsunamis, volcanic activity, droughts, famines, floods, hurricanes and tornados. Secondly, epidemics can quickly spread across continents such as the 'Black Death', typhoid, cholera, avian flu, influenza and HIV. Thirdly, human recklessness in our use of fossil fuels is causing global warming, rising sea temperatures, acid rain, coral bleaching, global dimming, ozone depletion, biodiversity loss, and rising water levels which will transform life on this planet as we know it (Flannery, 2006). Global poverty and wars add to the toxic mix that makes life on this planet increasingly fragile.

Political and economic arrangements are not chance affairs but the products of actions and decisions. The laws and policies established by our forebears, together with systems of discrimination, based on race, ethnicity, gender, social classes, castes, religions and cultures create a complex macro-social context for every person on earth. Powerful contextual factors mould all human existence – our aspirations and achievements, literacy, education, employment, beliefs, values and moral codes, as moderated by families, communities and populations. What anybody can do to change his/her life is not simply a matter of making personal choices – such changes are constrained culturally, economically, legally and morally.

In the global economy, everything is inter-connected. Economic factors create the context for everything else that happens, including health, illness and health care. Witness the impact of the 2008 'Credit Crunch' in the USA, which triggered a global financial crisis with banks all over the world going into melt down, leading to many job losses and low interest rates everywhere from the US to China. The US, UK and other European governments injected trillions into financial institutions and increased their regulation of the financial markets to prevent short selling by banks and hedge fund managers. When the Iceland banking system collapsed in 2008, managers of a Wessex children's hospice worried about the future of the hospice, a specialist cancer hospital in Manchester redesigned its research programme, and millions worried about their pensions.

Demographic changes, population growth, and the scourges of poverty, **inequality**, and **inequity** are also putting their fingerprints all over human existence. In attempting to chart the global environment for health, the task is a daunting one. Where to begin? We must

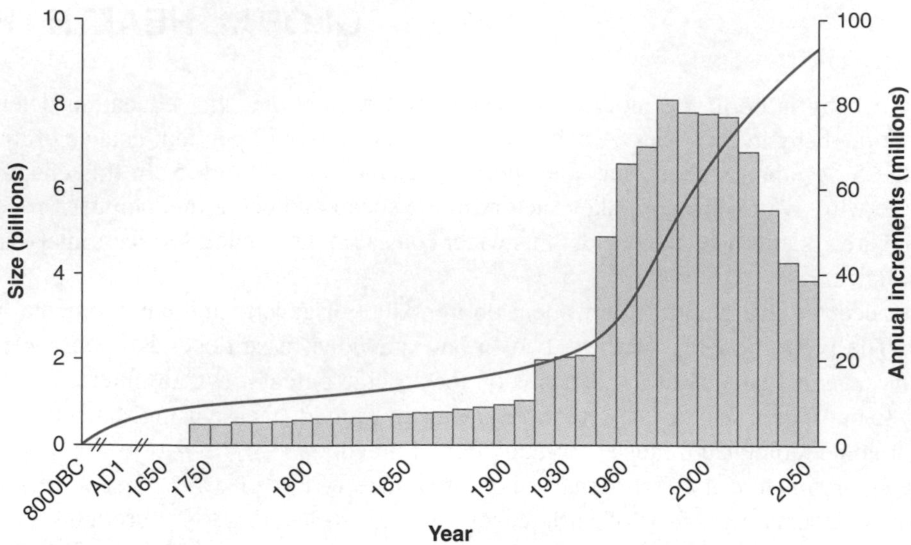

Figure 2.1 World population (line) and annual increments (bars), 8000 BC to 2050 AD
Source: Raleigh, 1999; Reproduced with permission

describe and reflect upon population growth, then consider the poverty epidemic, and then explore inequality, and inequity. These issues set the parameters for everything else in health psychology, and our study needs to reflect this.

POPULATION GROWTH

The US Census Bureau (2008) publishes its best estimate of the world's population on its website daily (www.census.gov/cgi-bin/ipc/popclockw). According to the Bureau, the total population of the World, at 23:10 on 1st July 2010 was 6,853,019,414. It was then being predicted to increase to 9 billion by 2045, an increase of just over 1 per cent per year. As stewards of Planet Earth, we are a privileged and reckless generation, holding the keys to survival in our hands.

The globe can be broken into regions. The most populous region is China. With more than 1.3 billion people in 2008, China accounts for approximately 20 per cent of all people on Earth. The revolutionary Marxist Chinese President, Mao Zedong (1893–1976) was keen to allow the Chinese population to grow to enable a large national defence against future enemies. Later, the population reached almost 25 per cent of the world total while arable land suitable for food production was only 7 per cent of the world total. In 1979 China adopted a one-child policy aimed towards keeping the population at around 1.2 billion in 2000. Family sizes in China are typically smaller in cities than in rural areas where the two-child family is the preferred norm. China's total fertility rate currently is running at around 1.7, i.e., with women giving birth to an average of 1.7 offspring.

China's one-child policy succeeded in reducing family sizes but led to a rising proportion of males, traditionally favoured in Asian cultures, through sex-selection abortion. The reported female/male ratio went from 1.06 in 1979 to 1.17 in 2001 with ratios up to 1.3 in rural Anhui, Guangdong and Qinghai provinces (Hesketh & Xing, 2005). By 2020, China's population is predicted to reach 1.4 billion.

Another 'big player' in the world population stakes is India. India's population will surpass China's in the next few decades, with around 1.5 billion by 2040. Fertility is falling in most of the developing world but there is a huge variation between countries (Raleigh, 1999). In 2005, India's fertility rate was running at 2.8. A large difference in fertility exists between Pakistan, India and Bangladesh. A large generation bulge of future parents already exists so that the population will continue to rise in spite of a reduction in fertility. As a consequence of increasing demand and shortage of supply, increasing numbers of people will live in poverty.

In addition to an uneven spread of resources, religions also influence sexual and reproductive practices. This sensitive issue is difficult to ignore. Consider the position of the Roman Catholic Church as one example. On 25 July 1968, Pope Paul VI's encyclical *Humanae Vitae* ('Of Human Life', subtitled 'On the Regulation of Birth') reinforced the traditional values of the Church by forbidding abortion and artificial contraception. In 2008, Pope Benedict XVI stated: 'What was true yesterday is true also today' (Benedict XVI, international congress, 12 May 2008). The human failure to practice abstinence as the *only* acceptable method for birth control in South America and Africa is adding to population growth, poverty and the spread of HIV/AIDS.

Fertility is highest in Sub-Saharan Africa, not only the poorest region in the world, but where the prevalence of AIDS is at a maximum. This is also the region with the highest growth in numbers of practising (and non-practising) Roman Catholics. According to the *Statistical Yearbook of the Church* (Vatican Publishing House, 2008) over the period 2000–2006, the Catholic presence in the world remained stable at around 17.3 per cent but in Africa numbers increased from 130 million in 2000 to 158.3 million in 2006, an increase of 22 per cent. Yet family planning is cheaper than all other methods of reducing carbon emissions. A report from the London School of Economics (LSE) estimated a \$7 cost of abating a tonne of CO_2 using family planning compared with \$24 for wind power, \$51 for solar and \$57–83 for coal plants with carbon capture and storage (Wire, 2009). Tickell (2008) estimated that each avoided unwanted birth in the USA reduces emissions by 1,500 t CO_2 (based on the per capita annual emissions of 20 t CO_2 and a life expectancy of 75 years). Assuming a health-care cost of \$150, this equates to an abatement cost of \$0.10/t CO_2.

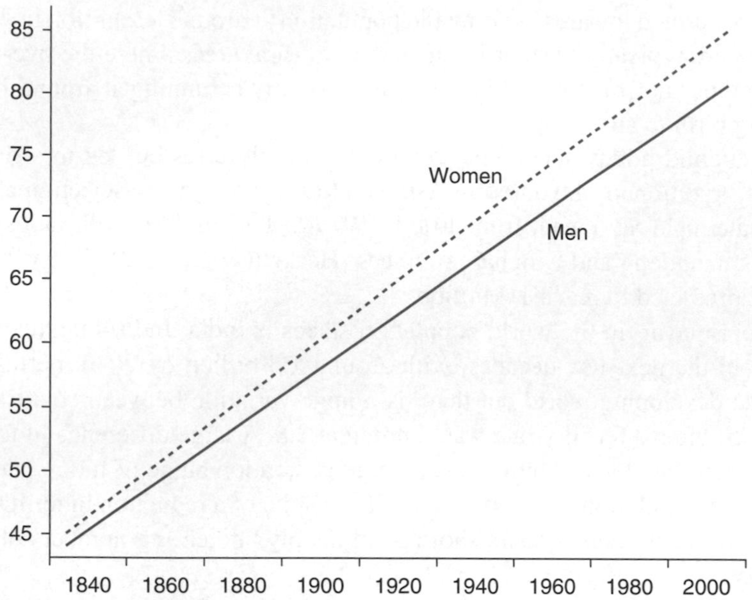

Figure 2.2 The rising longevity of Western populations
Source: Oeppen & Vaupel 2002; Reproduced with permission

INCREASING LIFE EXPECTANCY

Life expectancy has been increasing almost everywhere due to dramatic decreases in infant and adult mortality from infectious diseases. In Britain life expectancy is currently around 75 years for men and 80 years for women. In 2010 in England a working man can expect, on average, about 10 years of pensioned retirement while a working woman can anticipate around 20 years. Recent research suggests that life expectancy will increase in the twenty-first century and that, by 2060, it could reach 100 years (Oeppen & Vaupel, 2002). Life expectancy is said to be increasing three months every year in developed countries (see Figure 2.2). If life expectancy increases to 85, 90 or even 100, social, health and pensions systems will be difficult to maintain in their current form.

The age profile of any population is displayed as a 'population pyramid' in which numbers in each age group are plotted on a vertical axis. In the United Kingdom the number of people older than 85 is increasing dramatically. Figure 2.3 shows the major shift in the demographic profile of the UK population that is expected to occur between 2010 and 2050. Inflows and outflows suggest that, by 2050, the UK will be the largest country in Europe. In 2050, like many other places, the country will be crowded and warm.

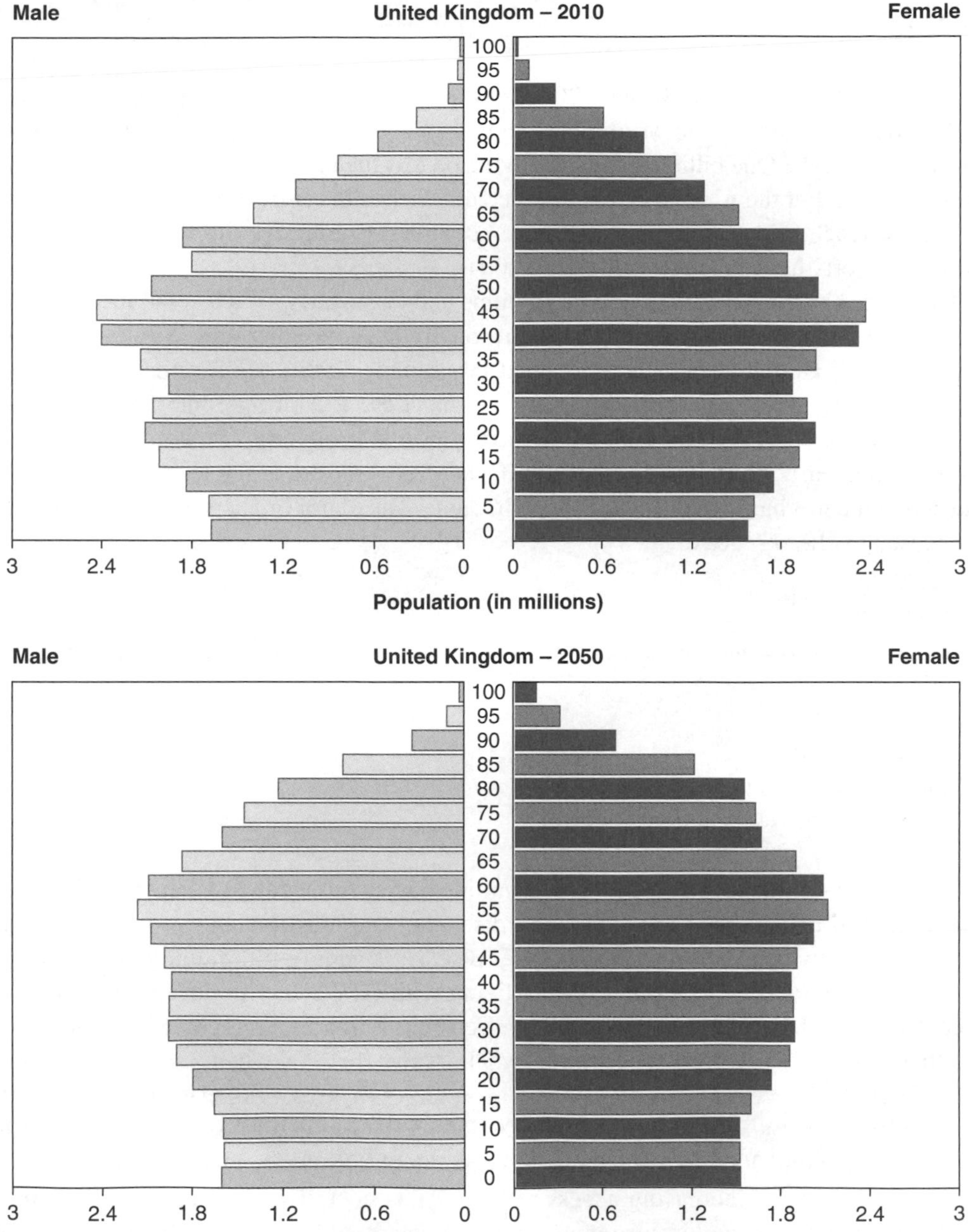

Figure 2.3 Population pyramids for the United Kingdom, 2010 and 2050 showing the changing demographics of the UK population. The proportion of the population over 75 is expected to increase dramatically

Source: US Census Bureau, 2010

POVERTY

Of 6.8 billion people alive in January 2010, approximately 5.5 billion (81 per cent) are living in developing countries. The word 'developing' is a euphemism for poor. World **poverty** is on a massive scale. One billion people are living on less than one dollar per day – one person in every seven. For them, clean drinking water, toilets, health services and modern medicines are out of reach. Many initiatives that have attempted to improve the health of people in extreme poverty have failed (World Bank, 2004).

The United Nations Development Programme defines poverty as 'a level of income below that people cannot afford a minimum, nutritionally adequate diet and essential non-food requirements' (United Nations Development Programme, 1995). Half of the world's population lacks regular access to medical care and most essential drugs. International organizations such as the UN state with some justification that poverty is the greatest cause of ill-health and early mortality. The health effects of poverty are tangible and the biological and economic mechanisms are everywhere the same. The major impacts of poverty on health are caused by the absence of:

- safe water;
- environmental sanitation;
- adequate diet;
- secure housing;
- basic education;
- income generating opportunities;
- access to medication and health care.

These are familiar themes. All were mentioned as basic needs in Chapter 1. The most common health outcomes are infectious diseases, malnutrition and reproductive hazards (Anand & Chen, 1996). A major killer disease is acquired immune deficiency syndrome (AIDS). In 2004, 6 million people living with HIV/AIDS in developing countries urgently needed access to HIV/AIDS antiretroviral treatment (HAART). The World Health Organization (WHO) began the '3 by 5 Initiative' in 2004 when less than 10 per cent of sufferers had access to HAART. WHO set a target of providing HAART to 3 million HIV/AIDS sufferers by the end of 2005. In 2004 WHO hoped to extend this free drugs programme beyond 2005 to reach the 3 million other AIDS victims who also needed help. The major barrier to increasing access to HAART is cost. The pharmaceutical industry holds the patents and would lose huge profits if patent rights are relinquished to enable generic production of HAART medication. Further discussion of HIV/AIDS can be found in Chapters 6 and 20.

Economic growth is the rate of increase in the total production of goods and services within an economy. Such growth increases the capacity of an economy to produce new goods and services allowing more needs and wants to be satisfied. A growing economy increases employment, stimulates business enterprise and innovation. Sustained growth is fundamental to the raising of living standards and to providing greater quality of life. The monetary value of all goods and services produced in a country over a year is defined as the country's **Gross National Income (GNI)**. GNI is a useful indicator for measuring growth.

Poverty reduction is a major priority for many international organizations. At the United Nations in 2000, 189 countries adopted the 'Millennium Development Goals', including halving poverty rates by 2015, reducing child mortality, decelerating the growth of AIDS and educating all children. Greatest progress is being made in China, India and Brazil. It is expected that the world poverty rate of 28 per cent as it was in 1990 will be reduced by half by 2015, a tremendous achievement. However, poverty in sub-Saharan Africa is still getting worse. In September 2008, world leaders pledged to reinvigorate 'global partnership of equals' to end poverty, hunger, underdevelopment in Africa. United Nations Secretary-General Ban Ki-moon asserted that '…the current trends …indicate that no African country will achieve all the Goals by 2015' (http://www.un.org/News/Press/docs/2008/ga10748.doc.htm2008). Much more needs to be done to reduce poverty in Africa.

Case Study

INTERNATIONAL CASE STUDY Reducing poverty in Brazil

The Millennium Development Goal set poverty and hunger targets, to halve, from 2000 to 2015, the proportion of people living on less than a dollar a day and people who suffer from hunger. Brazil is working towards these targets and expects to reach these targets. Doctors at a local health clinic in Brazil observed that their patients who regularly came in with health problems related to poverty were visiting less often. This can be reasonably attributed to a national anti-hunger programme that gives children three meals a day. Children were starting to eat better as a consequence of the national 'Fome Zero' ('Zero Hunger') campaign. The goal is to give every Brazilian at least three meals a day. With one quarter of Brazil's 170 million people currently below the poverty line, this goal is a challenge. The government provided emergency help to 11 million families. However this effort must be sustainable in the long-term to enable families to buy their own food.

If the Millennium Poverty and Hunger Reduction targets are to be met by 2015, this Brazilian success story needs to be replicated all over the world.

Source: Galindo, 2004

The production of good population health requires much more than simply providing doctors, nurses and hospital services. Basic social, educational and economic foundations need to be in place. This means that some fairly dramatic economic changes are needed if we are to see health improvements during the twenty-first century. Among these changes, the cancellation of unpaid debts of the poorest countries and trade justice have good potential to bring health improvements to match those of the last 50 years.

A case can be made that health improvements are a necessary pre-condition of economic growth. This was suggested by the WHO Commission on Macroeconomics and Health. The Commission Report stated: 'in countries where people have poor health and the level of education is low it is more difficult to achieve sustainable economic growth' (WHO, 2002). If current trends continue, health in sub-Saharan Africa will worsen over the next decades. If the Millennium Development Goals are going to have any chance of success in Africa, health must be given a higher priority in development policies. Sub-Saharan Africa contains 34 of the 41 most indebted countries, and the proportion of people living in absolute poverty (on under one dollar per day) is growing. The health of sub-Saharan Africans is among the worst in the world. Consider the following indicators:

- Two-thirds of Africans live in absolute poverty.
- More than half lack safe water.
- 70 per cent are without proper sanitation.
- Forty million children are not in primary school.
- Infant mortality is 55 per cent higher than in other low-income countries.
- Average life expectancy is 51.
- The incidence of malaria and tuberculosis is increasing.

These figures indicate the very large gaps that exist between the Haves and Have-nots on the international stage. International debt is a significant factor in poverty. Rich nations will need to honour pledges they have given to cancel debts and establish fair trade to produce reductions in poverty and hunger in Africa.

INEQUALITIES WITHIN A COUNTRY

Many of the determinants of ill health were identified by Chadwick in his studies of public health in Victorian England: poverty, housing, water, sewerage, the environment, safety and food. In addition, we recognize today that illiteracy, tobacco, AIDS/HIV, immunization, medication and health services are also important.

Recent studies of the social determinants of health have pinpointed various kinds of inequity. The first of these is based on **socio-economic status** – people who are higher up the 'pecking order' of wealth, education and status have better health and live longer than those at the lower end of the scale. Figure 2.4 shows a map of the Jubilee Line, which travels along an East–West axis across London. When you travel eastwards along this tube line from Westminster to Canning Town, the life expectancy of the local population is reduced by one year for every stop.

Health gradients are found in all societies. Wealthier groups always have the best health; poorer groups have the worst health. These differentials occur in both illness and death rates and health gradients are equally dramatic in both rich and poor countries. The majority of studies have been carried out in rich countries.

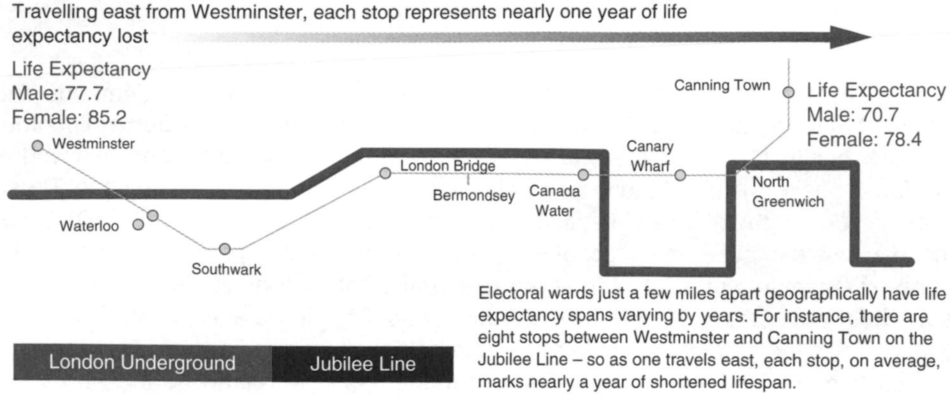

Figure 2.4 Differences in life expectancy within a small area of London. Travelling east from Westminster along the Jubilee line, each stop represents one year of life (Department of Health, 2008)

KEY STUDY The Whitehall Studies

The Whitehall studies were led by Professor Sir Michael Marmot. The objective was to investigate social class, psychosocial factors and life style as determinants of disease. The first Whitehall study of 18,000 men in the Civil Service was set up in the 1960s. The Whitehall I study showed a clear gradient in which men employed in the lowest grades were much more likely to die prematurely than men in the highest grades.

The Whitehall II study started in 1985 with the aim of determining the causes of the social gradient and also included women, including potential psychological mediators. The Whitehall II study invited non-industrial civil servants between 35 and 55 in Central London to a cardiovascular screening at their workplace. 10,308 employees participated in the baseline survey, two-thirds men and one-third women. All participants were sent a self-completion questionnaire about a wide range of topics. This cohort has been followed up over time with medical examinations and surveys. Most participants are now retired or approaching retirement.

There have been seven phases of data collection so far, alternating postal self-completion questionnaires with medical screenings and questionnaires. In phase 6, responses came from 7,770 participants, 75 per cent of the original group. In addition to cardiovascular measures, blood pressure, blood cholesterol, height, weight, and ECGs were taken along with tests of walking, lung function, mental functioning, questions about diet and diabetes screening.

(Continued)

(Continued)

The Whitehall studies have found that it is the imbalance between demands and control that leads to illness. A combination of **high demand** and **low control** contributes to ill health. Control is less when a worker is lower in the hierarchy and so a worker in a lower position is unable to respond effectively if the demands are increased. These findings support the theories of stress proposed by Karasek and Theorell (1990). Other mechanisms can buffer the effect of work stress on mental and physical health: **social support** (Stansfeld et al., 1997), an **effort-reward balance** (Kuper et al., 2002), **job security** (Ferrie et al., 2002), and organizational stability (Ferrie et al., 1998). The figure below shows the gradient of death rates vs. employment grades over a 25-year period in men from the Whitehall studies. The death rate is shown relative to the whole civil service population (reproduced from Ferrie, 2004, with permission).

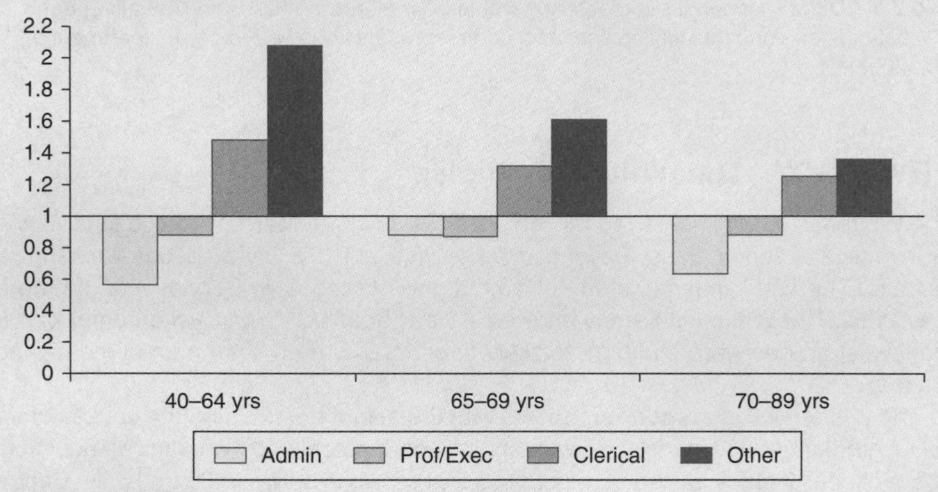

Figure 2.5 Death rates for different employment grades in Whitehall studies
Source: Ferrie, 2004

There are a few studies of health gradients in poor countries. The data are cross-sectional rather than longitudinal, but show a similar pattern to those observed with Whitehall civil servants. The health gradient is a law within health care. Marks (2004) analysed data from the Demographic and Health Surveys (DHS) programme of the World Bank (2002). These are large-scale household sample surveys carried out periodically in 44 countries across Asia, Africa, the Middle East, Latin America and the former Soviet Union. Marks analysed the data from two regions, Sub-Saharan Africa and Latin America. Socio-economic status was evaluated using answers about assets given by the head of each household. The asset score reflected the household's ownership of consumer items ranging from a fan to a television and car, dwelling characteristics such as flooring material, type of drinking water source and toilet facilities used, and other characteristics related to wealth.

Each household was assigned a score for each asset, or, in the case of sleeping arrangements, the number of people per room. The scores were summed for each household, and individuals are ranked according to the total score of the household in which they reside. The sample was divided into population wealth quintiles – five groups with the same number of individuals in each.

The gradient of under-5 mortality rates (U5MRs) for 22 countries in Sub-Saharan Africa are shown collectively in Figure 2.6. The U5MR indicator is the number of deaths

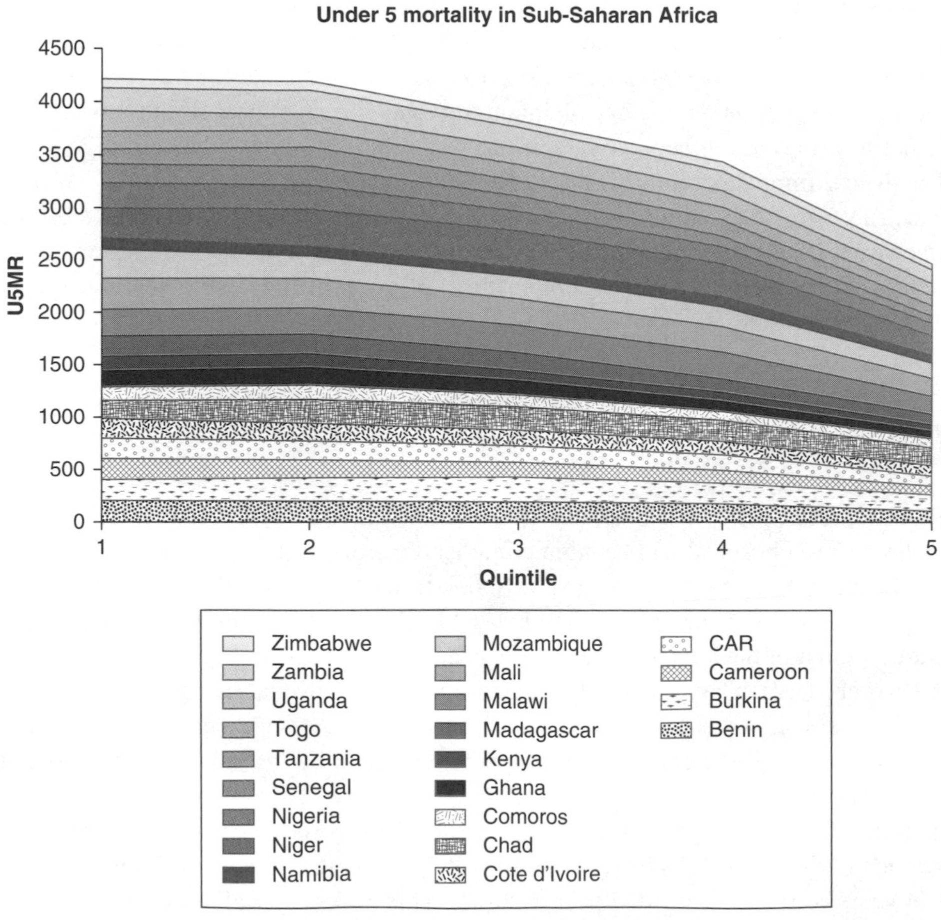

Figure 2.6 Under-5 mortality gradients for Sub-Saharan Africa plotted against asset quintile. The area under each line represents the individual country rates. Quintile 1 has least assets, quintile 5 the most

Source: Marks, 2004

to children under 5 years of age per 1000 live births. This figure shows gradients in all countries. A wide gap in health outcomes exists between the rich and the poor even within these very poor countries. Similar gradients exist for countries in Latin America and the Caribbean and throughout the 44 countries included in the DHS. Infant mortality is halved between quintiles 1 and 5 representing the poorest of the poor and the wealthiest of the poor.

An interesting set of relationships was observed between the U5MRs, literacy and resources (Marks, 2004). The U5MRs in 44 countries were positively correlated with female illiteracy rates (0.69, $p < .0001$) and the proportion of households using bush, field or traditional pit latrines (0.60, $p < .0001$), and negatively correlated with the proportion of households having piped domestic water (–0.65, $p < .0001$), national health service expenditure (–0.33, $p < .01$), the number of doctors per 100,000 people (–0.51, $p < .0001$), the number of nurses per 100,000 people (–0.35, $p < .01$), and immunization rates (–0.27, $p < .05$).

The most important predictors of infant survival are educational and environmental. High literacy among mothers, and access to water supplies and toilets are highly associated with low infant mortality. High numbers of doctors and nurses, immunization rates and health service expenditure are associated with lower mortality rates, but these health service variables are less influential statistically speaking than literacy, domestic water and sanitation. These latter provide the foundations of good health, while health services are the bricks and mortar.

GENDER

Major differences occur in the health of men and women. Recent research has focused on the political, psychosocial and economic implications of gender. Attitudes have changed a little over the last 100 years. A medical textbook from the nineteenth century stated: 'childbearing is essentially necessary to the physical health and long life, the mental happiness, the development of the affections and whole character of women. Woman exists for the sake of the womb' (Holbrook, 1871: 13–14; cited in Gallant, Keita & Royak-Schaler, 1997). Women's health is towards the top of the health agenda. Men's health, unfortunately, is nearer the bottom. These changes were supported in the USA by the Office of Research on Women's Health in 1990.

In industrialized societies today men die earlier than women, but women generally have poorer health than men (Macintyre & Hunt, 1997). In 1996 UK boys had a life expectancy of 74.4 years compared with 79.7 years for girls. This excess mortality of 5.3 years in males in 1996 increased over the course of the twentieth century from only 3.9 years in 1900–1910. However, the evidence suggests that from the Paleolithic period to the industrial revolution men lived longer than women, 40 years as compared to 35. Also, in less developed countries (e.g. India, Bangladesh, Nepal and Afghanistan) men still live longer than women (WHO,

1989). To complicate the picture further, the health gradient is steeper for men than for women, while illness rates, treatment rates, absenteeism and prescription drug use are generally higher for women (Macintyre & Hunt, 1997).Women suffer more non-fatal chronic illnesses and more acute illnesses. They also make more visits to their family physicians and spend more time in hospital. Women suffer more from hypertension, kidney disease and autoimmune diseases such as rheumatoid arthritis and lupus (Litt, 1993). They also suffer twice the rate of depression. Men, on the other hand, have a shorter life expectancy, suffer more injuries, suicides, homicides and heart disease.

Psychosocial and lifestyle differences play a mediating role in gender-linked health differences. In industrialized societies women suffer more from poverty, stress from relationships, childbirth, rape, domestic violence, sexual discrimination, lower status work, concern about weight and the strain of dividing attention between competing roles of parent and worker. Financial barriers may prevent women, more than men, from engaging in healthier lifestyles and desirable behaviour change (O'Leary & Helgeson, 1997). Men are more likely to suffer diseases of the cardiovascular system, more often suffer a violent death and die younger.

Social support derived from friendships, intimate relationships and marriage, although significant, appears to be of less positive value to women than to men. Although physical and mental well-being generally benefit from social support, women often provide more emotional support to their families than they receive. Thus, the loss of a spouse has a longer and more devastating effect on the health of men than on that of women (Stroebe & Stroebe, 1983). The burden of caring for an elderly, infirm or dementing family member also tends to be greater for females in the family than for males, especially daughters (Grafstrom, 1994). Gallant et al. (1997) reviewed psychological, social and behavioural influences on health and health care in women.

While the health of women is a focus for much health care, the health of men has been somewhat neglected. More research is needed on the health of men, why they suffer more from alcoholism and drug dependency, and why they are so reluctant to seek help from professionals.

ETHNICITY

Evidence suggests that the health of minority ethnic groups is generally poorer than that of the majority of the population. This pattern has been consistently observed in the USA between African–Americans (or blacks) and whites for at least 150 years (Krieger, 1987). There has been an increase in income inequality in the USA that has been associated with a leveling off or even a decline in the economic status of African–Americans. The gap in life expectancy between blacks and whites widened between 1980 and 1991 from 6.9 years to 8.3 years for males and from 5.6 years to 5.8 years for females (National Center for Health Statistics, 1994). Under the age of 70, cardiovascular disease, cancer and problems resulting in infant mortality account for 50 per cent of the excess deaths for black males and 63 per cent of the excess deaths for black females (Williams & Collins, 1995). Similar findings exist in other countries. Analyses of three censuses from 1971 to 1991 have shown that people born in South Asia are more likely to die from ischaemic heart disease than the majority of the UK population (Balarajan & Soni Raleigh, 1993).

There are many possible explanations for these persistent health differences between people of different races who live in the same country and are served by the same educational, social, welfare and health-care systems (Williams & Collins, 1995; Williams, Yu, Jackson & Anderson, 1997). First, the practice of **racism** means that minority ethnic groups are the subject of discrimination at a number of different levels. Such discrimination could lead directly or indirectly to health problems additional to any effects related to SES, poverty, unemployment and education. Discrimination in the health-care system exacerbates the impacts of social discrimination through reduced access to the system and poorer levels of communication resulting from language differences.

Second, ethnocentrism in health services and health promotion favours the needs of majority over minority groups. The health needs of members of minority ethnic groups are less likely to be appropriately addressed in health promotion that in turn leads to lower adherence and response rates in comparison to the majority population. These problems are compounded by cultural, lifestyle and language differences. For example, if interpreters are unavailable, the treatment process is likely to be improperly understood or even impaired and patient anxiety levels will be raised. The lack of permanent addresses for minority ethnic group families created by their high mobility makes communication difficult so that screening invitations and appointment letters are unlikely to be received.

Third, health status differences related to race and **culture** are to a large extent mediated by differences in SES. Studies of race and health generally control for SES and race-related differences frequently disappear after adjustment for SES. Race is strongly correlated with SES and is even sometimes used as an indicator of SES (Williams & Collins, 1995; Modood et al., 1997).

Fourth, differences in health-protective behaviour may occur because of different cultural or social norms and expectations. Fifth, differences in readiness to recognize symptoms may occur also as a result of different cultural norms and expectations. Sixth, differences could occur in access to services. There is evidence that differential access to optimal treatment may cause poorer survival outcomes in African–Americans who have cancer in comparison to other ethnic groups (Meyerowitz, Richardson, Hudson & Leedham, 1998). Seventh, members of minority ethnic groups are more likely to inhabit and work in unhealthy environments because of their lower SES. Eighth, there could be genetic differences between groups that lead to a differing incidence of disease and some diseases are inherited. There are several well-recognized examples, including sickle cell disorder affecting people of African–Caribbean descent; thalassaemia, another blood disorder that affects people of the Mediterranean, Middle Eastern and Asian descent; and Tay-Sachs disease that affects Jewish people.

Other possible mechanisms underlying **ethnicity** differences in health are differences in personality, early life conditions, power and control, and stress (Williams & Collins, 1995;

Taylor, Repetti & Seeman, 1997). Research is needed with large community samples so that the influence of the above variables and the possible interactions between them can be determined. Further research is needed to explore the barriers to access to health care that exist for people from different groups.

CONCLUSIONS

There is one set of resources in this world for all to share. Perfect equality will never happen but currently the shares are extremely far from equal. The macro-social conditions will require radically different policies if the health of 5 billion-plus people living in dire poverty is ever to be improved. Changes must occur in global power structures if health for all people is ever going to happen. This seems unlikely in our lifetimes. The next 50 years is a thin slice of time in which the world population is expected to expand by 50 per cent to around nine billion. The lion's share of this expansion will be in the poorest countries. Eleven million homeless children live in India alone. Poverty and AIDS/HIV are not abating in sub-Saharan Africa, and life expectancy will continue to be in decline there for some time to come. Policy changes are necessary if AIDS prevention and poverty reduction are going to be more successful in future than has been achieved to date.

Sadly, the research that fills psychology textbooks is almost all irrelevant to the important social issues of the day. For the Brave New Worlds of 2050 and 2100, will the priorities of psychology academia have changed? Will global warming, population, poverty, ideologies of oppression, survival and suffering be on the agenda? Will concepts such as 'stress', 'coping', 'resilience', 'hardiness' and 'change' be given wider interpretation and meaning? Will theories and research concerned with sustainability, empowerment, altruism, sharing, cooperation, cultural, spiritual and religious understanding be more to the fore? Will new concepts, theories and methods have been created to deal with the social and psychological problems of the day? The answer to all of these questions must be 'Yes!' – but it depends on you.

FUTURE RESEARCH

1. The causes of poverty and interventions to ameliorate poverty should be *the* priority for economic and social research.
2. Studies in psychology and sociology must be designed to understand humanitarian values, altruism, oppression, fear, aggression and cross-cultural issues.
3. Possible mechanisms underlying ethnicity differences in health, such as differences in personality, early life conditions, power and control, and stress must be explored.
4. Research is needed with large community samples so that the influence of the above variables and their possible interactions can be determined.

Summary

1. The world population is increasing dramatically. From 1 billion in 1800 it will reach 9 billion in 2050.
2. As the global population climbs to 9 billion by 2050 the amount of drinkable water available per person will fall by 33 per cent. The increased shortage will affect mainly the poor where the water shortage is already most chronic.
3. The greatest influence on health for the majority of people is poverty. Half of the world's population lacks regular access to treatment of common diseases and most essential drugs. Globally, the burden of death and disease is much heavier for the poor than for the wealthy.
4. In developed countries life expectancy is increasing by three months every year. If this trend continues, life expectancy will approach 100 years by 2060. This will place social, health and pensions systems in a perilous position.
5. Economic growth does not reduce disparities in wealth across a society.
6. Health gradients are a universal feature of the health of populations in both rich and poor countries.
7. The UN Millennium Development Goals on poverty and health require rich countries to allocate more resources to poor countries, cancel debts of the poorest countries, and establish fair trade.
8. Gender differences in health, illness and mortality are significant and show striking interactions with culture, history and SES.
9. The health of minority ethnic groups is generally poorer than that of the majority of the population. Possible explanations include racial discrimination, ethnocentrism, SES differences, behavioural and personality differences, cultural differences and other factors.
10. A critical perspective argues for an agenda relevant to the socio-political struggles of yesterday, today and tomorrow.

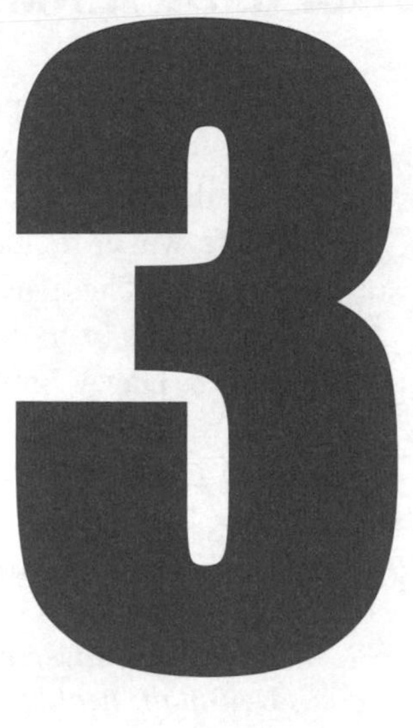

Social Inequalities, Social Justice and Health

Life is unfair.

John F. Kennedy

Outline

There is substantial evidence linking poor social conditions with ill-health. The explanations for this include material, behavioural and psychosocial factors. This chapter considers the extent of social inequalities in health within developed countries, the competing explanations and the role of health psychology in creating a healthier society. The explanation of health inequalities creates many important challenges for theory and research in health psychology.

SOCIAL DETERMINANTS OF HEALTH

One of the earliest reports on the relationship between health and social conditions was by the French physician Villerme (1782–1863) who in the 1820s examined the health of residents in different neighbourhoods of Paris. From a careful review of the data he concluded that there was a relationship between the wealth of the neighbourhood and the health of its residents. Those living in the poorer neighbourhoods had a higher death rate and military conscripts from those neighbourhoods were smaller, had more illnesses and disabilities (Krieger & Davey Smith, 2004).

Shortly afterwards Frederich Engels published his classic *The Condition of the Working Class in England in 1844* (Engels, 1845). This book provided a detailed description of the appalling living and working conditions and the limited health care of working-class residents of Manchester. He wrote:

> *All of these adverse factors combine to undermine the health of the workers. Very few strong, well-built, healthy people are to be found among them. Their weakened bodies are in no condition to withstand illness and whenever infection is abroad they fall victims to it. This is proved by the available statistics of death rates.* (1845/1958: 118–119)

When Engels compared the death rates within the city he found that they were much higher in the poorer districts. Further, he realized the importance of early development and noted: 'common observation shows how the sufferings of childhood are indelibly stamped on the adults' (p. 115).

Although these early researchers realized the importance of the impact of adverse social conditions, interest in the social aspects of health was marginalized with the rise of germ theory and the growth of **Social Darwinism** (Krieger & Davey Smith, 2004). The former theory focused on controlling specific pathogens rather than social reform whereas the second argued that innate inferiority, not social injustice, was the cause of ill-health. However, the growth of social movements in the 1960s rekindled interest in this field.

In 1977 the UK government established a working group to investigate social inequalities in health further. The subsequent **Black Report** (Townsend & Davidson, 1982), named after Sir Douglas Black, the working group's chair, summarized the evidence on the relationship between occupation and health. It showed that those classified as unskilled manual workers (Social class V) consistently had poorer health status compared with those classified as professionals (Social class I). Further, the report graphically portrayed a social gradient in health status. It concluded:

> *present social inequalities in health in a country with substantial resources like Britain are unacceptable and deserve to be so declared by every section of public opinion ... we have*

> *no doubt that greater equality of health must remain one of our foremost national objectives and that in the last two decades of the twentieth century a new attack upon the forces of inequality has regrettably become necessary.* (Townsend & Davidson, 1982: 79)

The report not only clearly documented the link between social position and health but detailed four possible explanations:

- An **artefact**: the relationships between social position are an artefact of the method of measurement.
- Natural and social selection: the social gradient in health is due to those who are already unhealthy falling downwards while those who are healthy rising upwards.
- Materialist and structuralist explanations: emphasize the role of economic and socio-structural factors.
- Cultural and/or behavioural differences: 'often focus on the individual as the unit of analysis emphasizing unthinking, reckless or irresponsible behaviour or incautious life-style as the moving determinant' (p. 23).

While accepting that each explanation may contribute something, the report emphasized the importance of the materialist explanations and developed a range of policy options that could address the inequalities.

Other major reports such as the Acheson Report (1998) and the WHO Commission on the Social Determinants of Health (2008) also appeared. In 2003, the British government made the reduction of health inequalities a priority and set the target of producing a 10 per cent reduction by 2010, as measured by infant mortality and life expectancy at birth (Department of Health, 2003). Unfortunately, this target is going to be missed. It has been reported that, over the 10-year period 1999–2008, the gap increased by 4 per cent in women and 11 per cent in men (House of Commons Health Committee Health Inequalities Report, 2009). The committee suggested some reasons why the gap is failing to narrow:

- Nutrition is much worse among the poorest segment of the population (Chapter 7)
- Tobacco smuggling impacts negatively on the health of the poor (Chapter 9)
- Cheap alcohol with special promotions and lowered prices (Chapter 8)
- Activity such as walking and cycling is discouraged with many supermarkets and hospitals located out-of-town requiring people to drive or use public transport (Chapter 10)
- The Healthy Schools initiative lacked proper targets and evaluation (Chapter 15)

In addition to these easily identifiable '**proximal**' determinants of inequality, more '**distal**' or '**upstream**' factors could also play a role, such as economic determinants that are difficult to change. Some practical and theoretical complexities involved in tackling inequalities are discussed further in the sections below.

SOCIAL INEQUALITY AND HEALTH

Extent of social inequality

Over the past 20 years there has been a steady increase in **social inequality** in many Western societies. In the UK the proportion of individuals living in poverty increased from 15 per cent in 1981 to 24 per cent in 1993/94. There was a slight decline to 22 per cent in 2002/03 but this still represented 12.4 million people (Paxton & Dixon, 2004). Other indicators of social inequality in the UK include:

- The richest people have increased their share of total income. The richest 1 per cent increased their share of income from 6 per cent in 1980 to 13 per cent in 1999.
- The unequal distribution of wealth continues to increase. The percentage of wealth held by the richest 10 per cent of the population increased from 47 per cent in 1990 to 56 per cent in 2001.
- Over the same period, life expectancy increased overall but more rapidly for social class I (best off). than social class V (worst off). (House of Commons Health Committee Health Inequalities Third Report, 2009)

In the US there is also evidence of a continuing increase in social inequality. Using a more restrictive definition of poverty, the US Census Bureau estimated that the proportion of Americans living in poverty increased from 11.3 per cent in 2000 to 12.5 per cent in 2003. In households of single mothers, poverty increased from 25.4 per cent in 2000 to 28 per cent in 2003. The inequality in income between the richest and poorest households increased by 3.6 per cent between 2002 and 2003, the largest increase since figures started to be recorded in the 1960s.

There is now a substantial amount of research evidence from dozens of countries linking social inequalities with health. These studies have consistently shown that the life expectancy of those in the lower social classes is lower than those in the higher social classes. There is also evidence that there is a social gradient in morbidity and mortality such that those one step down the social ladder are unhealthier than those at the top and so on.

This persistent gradient is often referred to as a health gradient. When mortality is the measure, a more apposite term would be 'mortality' or '**death gradient**'. 'Death gradients' have been observed in all human societies in both rich/developed countries and in poor/developing countries (Marks, 2004). Such gradients are normally continuous throughout the range of economic variation. If the gradient were stepped, or flat at one end of the range and steep at the other, it could be inferred that the causative mechanism(s) had a threshold value before any of the 'ill-effects' could appear. However there is no evidence of any such thresholds. For the vast majority of data, the gradient is a continuous one. In reviewing health inequalities in 14 countries, Benzeval, Judge and Whitehead (1995) concluded:

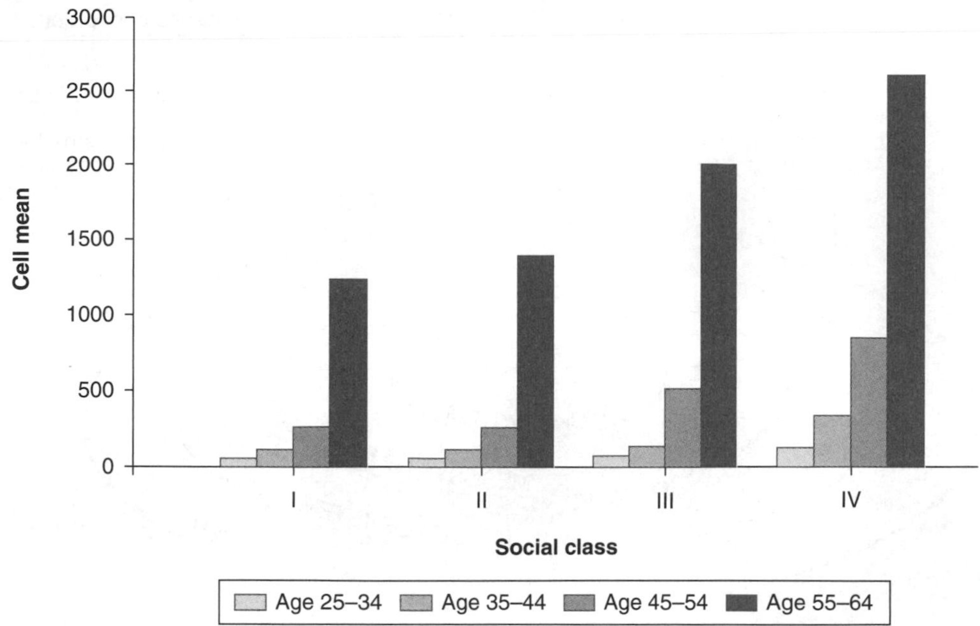

Figure 3.1 Mean annual death rates (all causes) per 100,000 men by age and social: class, 1991–93, for England and Wales (computed from Blane, Bartley & Davey Smith, 1997: Table 1)

> *People who live in disadvantaged circumstances have more illnesses, greater distress, more disablement and shorter lives than those who are more affluent. Such injustice could be prevented, but this requires political will. Health inequalities are endemic characteristics of all modern industrial societies, but the size of the differential varies between countries and over time, indicating that there is nothing fixed or inevitable about having such a health divide.* (1995: xvii)

Socio-economic status

The health variations reflect the social and economic circumstances of individuals. In rich countries one of the most significant factors is **socio-economic status (SES)**. SES is normally defined in terms of occupation, education or income, but it is a complex and multidimensional construct that defies simple definition.

Data from many quantitative studies show that SES is strongly correlated with illness and mortality. The health gradient such as that shown in Figure 3.1 shows continuously increasing poor health as SES changes from high to low. Figure 3.1 shows male all-cause mortality plotted against social class for England and Wales for 1991–93. Similar gradients exist in the USA and throughout industrialized countries.

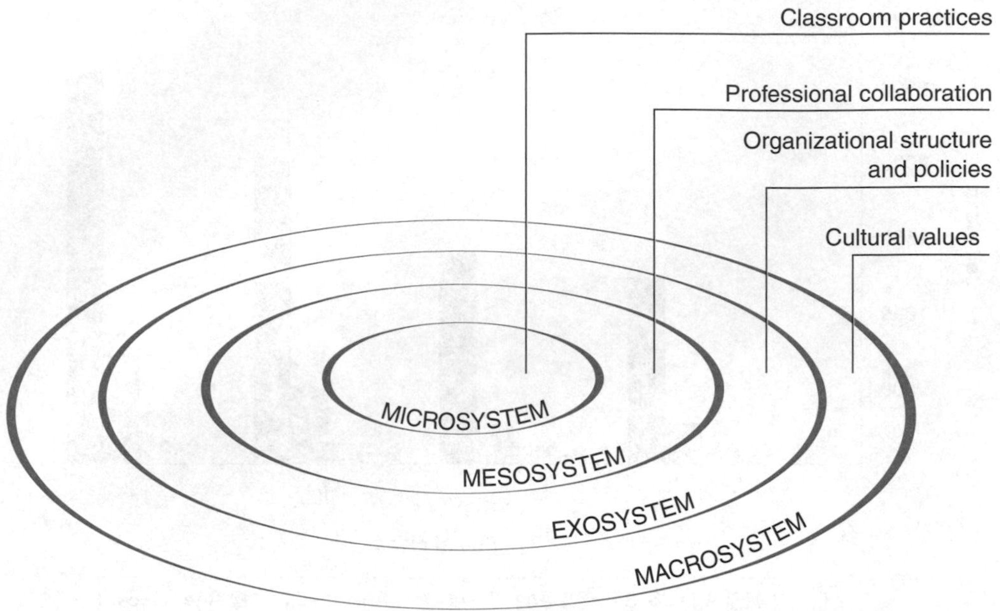

Figure 3.2 Bronfenbrenner's ecological systems model
Source: Odom et al., 1996: 18–30; Reproduced with permission

The mediators of SES effects on health experience are likely to be behavioural and psychosocial. The behavioural factors include diet, exercise and smoking while the psychosocial factors include such processes as self-efficacy, self-esteem and perceived control (Siegrist & Marmot, 2004).

One of the largest studies exploring the relationship between health and occupation has been the Whitehall studies. The original Whitehall study was designed to examine risk factors for coronary heart disease. The Whitehall II study had as its explicit objective the investigation of this social gradient in health status. It collected data on over 10,000 civil servants and related their health to their position in the civil service. Once again it confirmed the social gradient.

Health inequalities can be considered from an **ecological approach** or **systems theory approach**. Bronfenbrenner's (1979) ecological approach conceptualized developmental influences in terms of four nested systems:

- *microsystems*: families, schools, neighbourhoods;
- *mesosystems*: peer groups;
- *exosystems*: parental support systems, parental workplaces;
- *macrosystems*: political philosophy, social policy.

These systems form a nested set, like a set of Russian dolls, microsystems within mesosystems, mesosystems within exosystems and exosystems within macrosystems (see Figure 3.2).

Ecological theory assumes that human development can only be understood in reference to the structural ecosystems. We described a general systems framework for understanding the determinants of health and illness in Chapter 1 (see Figure 1.1). Of key importance is the principle that it is the *perceived environment* and not the so-called 'objective' environment that affects human behaviour and experience.

In Box 3.1 we list some of the characteristics of low SES using Bronfenbrenner's systems approach. The box shows how many different disadvantages there can be across all four systems of the social, physical and economic environment. In addition to these factors, we can add the high levels of perceived injustice that many people with low SES may well feel.

Box 3.1

Behaviours and experiences associated with low socio-economic status

Microsystems: families, schools, neighbourhoods

- low birth weight
- family instability
- poor diet/nutrition
- parental smoking and drinking
- overcrowding
- poor schools and educational outcomes
- poor neighbourhoods

Mesosystems: peer groups

- bullying, gangs and violence
- smoking
- drinking
- drugs
- unprotected sex

Exosystems: parental support systems, parental workplaces

- low personal control
- less social support
- unemployment or unstable employment
- high stress levels
- low self-esteem
- poorer physical and mental health

(Continued)

(Continued)

Macrosystems: political philosophy, social policy

- poverty
- poor housing
- environmental pollution
- unemployment or unstable employment
- occupational hazards
- poorer access to health services
- inadequate social services

Any explanation of the SES-health gradient needs to consider psychosocial systems that structure inequalities across a broad range of life opportunities and outcomes, health, social and educational. As illustrated in Box 3.1, in comparison to someone at the high end of the SES scale, the profile of a low SES person is one of multiple disadvantage. The disadvantages of low SES accumulate across all four ecosystems.

It is this kind of *accumulation* and *clustering* of adverse physical, material, social and psychological effects that could explain the health gradient. While each factor alone can be expected to produce a relatively modest impact on mortality, the combination and interaction of many kinds of ecosystem disadvantage are likely to be sufficiently large to generate the observed gradient.

Studies in many countries have shown that people with lower SES have a higher behavioural risk profile. A study analysed the gradients in behavioural risk factors in 11 European countries using data from the Eurobarometer survey. Inequities between high and low education groups in each country were investigated. A north–south difference in behavioural risk inequalities occurred for heavy smoking and infrequent vegetable consumption in men, with larger inequalities in northern European countries than in southern European countries. This pattern matches the gradients for ischaemic heart disease in men, which also show larger gradients in the north and smaller gradients in the south. The evidence suggests that the behavioural factors of smoking and diet contribute to the SES-related health gradient.

EXPLANATIONS FOR SOCIAL INEQUALITIES IN HEALTH

Much recent work has focused on the relationship between the extent of social inequality in a particular society and the extent of ill-health. Wilkinson (1996) argued that health was poorer in more unequal societies. This research has attracted substantial critique and it would seem that the relationship is not so straightforward as was initially conjectured (Lynch et al., 2004). However, as Lynch and Davey Smith (2002) warn, we should be careful not to throw the 'social inequality baby' out with the 'income inequality bathwater'. Rather there is much more to social inequality than inequality of income. A systematic review by Lynch et al. (2004) reached mixed conclusions and, overall, little support for the hypothesis that income inequality is the determinant of population health within or between rich countries. However the authors concluded that raising the incomes of the most disadvantaged will improve their health, help to reduce inequalities and improve the health of the general population.

Scientific Explanations

Contemporary research into explanations for social inequalities in health has been reviewed by Macinko, Shi, Starfield and Wulu (2003). Their classification extends the fourfold explanation developed in the Black Report and is summarized in Table 3.1.

The **psychosocial explanations** are considered at the more individual (micro) and the more social (macro) level. At the micro level it is argued that 'cognitive processes of comparison', in particular perceived relative deprivation, contribute to heightened levels of stress and subsequent ill-health. At the macro level psychosocial explanations focus on impairment of social bonds and limited civic participation, so-called social capital (see below), that flows from income inequality. These explanations are particularly favoured by Wilkinson (1996) to explain the social gradient in health.

Wilkinson and Pickett (2009) have provided a comprehensive analysis of the empirical association that exists between health/social problems and inequality among rich countries. The same index of health/social problems was found to be only very weakly related to national income but strongly to inequality. Wilkinson and Pickett (2009) hypothesize that the structural inequality in society causes people to become more anxious, stressed, ashamed, untrusting and unhappy.

The neo-material explanations have drawn increased support recently in critiques of the psychosocial approaches (see Macleod & Davey Smith, 2003). They focus on the importance of income and living conditions. At the micro level it is argued that in more unequal societies those worse off have fewer economic resources, leading to increased vulnerability to various health threats. At the macro level high income inequality contributes to less investment in the social and physical environment. Those who favour the neo-material explanations argue that the psychosocial explanations ignore the broad political context within which social and health inequalities are nested.

There are also the artefact and selection explanations of the social inequalities in health. Although these initially attracted attention, there is less support for these arguments today.

Lay Explanations

Recently there has been increasing interest in what ordinary people have to say about social inequalities in health. This literature connects with the broader literature on popular health beliefs (Chapter 4). In an early qualitative study of a sample of women in England, Calnan

Table 3.1 Explanations for the relationship between income inequality and health (Macinko et al., 2003)

Explanation	Synopsis of the argument
Psychosocial (micro): Social status	Income inequality results in 'invidious processes of social comparison' that enforce social hierarchies causing chronic stress leading to poorer health outcomes for those at the bottom.
Psychosocial (macro): Social cohesion	Income inequality erodes social bonds that allow people to work together, decreases social resources, and results in low trust and civic participation, greater crime, and other unhealthy conditions.
Neo-material (micro): Individual income	Income inequality means fewer economic resources among the poorest, resulting in lessened ability to avoid risks, cure injury or disease, and/or prevent illness.
Neo-material (macro): Social disinvestment	Income inequality results in less investment in social and environmental conditions (safe housing, good schools, etc.) necessary for promoting health among the poorest.
Statistical artefact	The poorest in any society are usually the sickest. A society with high levels of income inequality has high numbers of poor and consequently will have more people who are sick.
Health selection	People are not sick because they are poor. Rather, poor health lowers one's income and limits one's earning potential.

(1987) found that working-class women were reluctant to accept that they were less healthy than middle-class people. As one working-class woman said: 'I think as long as they eat the right foods and do have a proper balanced diet, I mean, even the poorest of people can be just as healthy as the others' (p. 76). Those who did accept that wealthy people had better health attributed it to differential access to health care. Conversely, professional women were more likely to accept the existence of a health gradient and attributed the poorer health of working-class people to low job satisfaction, low wages, poor diet and the hazards of the working environment.

The reluctance of working-class people to attribute the cause of social variation in ill-health to structural factors was explored by Blaxter (1997). Her secondary analysis of a large survey of British health and lifestyle found limited evidence of popular discussion about health inequalities. This was especially the case among people from poorer backgrounds.

Chamberlain (1997) reviewed evidence from qualitative research concerning how people from upper and lower SES positions understand health and illness. These studies interviewed small groups of middle-class and working-class women and men classified on the basis of their occupations. Several differences are evident between these two groups.

Working-class people tend to use more physicalistic terminology in their accounts of health and illness while middle-class people are more mentalistic and person-centred.

Contact and communication with professionals can be affected by their class relationship with patients so, not surprisingly, surgeons and doctors are often perceived as 'upper' class by working-class patients, while nurses are seen as more 'down to earth'.

Meanings of health show class-related differences. Working-class men and women see health in a more utilitarian way concerned with an absence of disease, being able to work and get through the day without feeling ill. Middle-class people see health as a value concerned with feeling good and having energy to indulge in leisure activities.

Chamberlain (1997), however, suggests a more complex picture with four differing views of health. The *solitary* view, presented by lower SES participants, sees health as involving only physical components of energy, lack of symptoms and a good diet. The *dualistic* view, held by some lower and higher SES people, sees health as having both physical and mental aspects, which act in parallel and independently of each other. The *complementary* view, presented mainly by upper SES people, sees physical and mental elements as integrated together in an alliance. The *multiple* view, held by higher SES people, sees multiple aspects to health – physical, mental, emotional, social, spiritual – as interdependent, interconnected, in balance in health and out of balance in illness.

Lay explanations about social inequalities in health are apparent from an early age. A study in Scotland (Backett-Milburn, Cunningham-Burley & Davis, 2003) found that children identified social relationships and social life as important as material concerns in explaining health inequalities. This indicated that their direct experiences of relationships and unfairness were important for them in making sense of health inequalities. Further studies are needed to explore the relationship between social positioning and health experience.

CLASS, RACE AND GENDER AND HEALTH INEQUITIES

Much of the research on social inequalities in health has focused on differences in income or wealth. As such it has ignored issues of power and politics. Hofrichter (2003) developed a more inclusive approach by considering inequalities in terms of class, gender and race. Issues of social and material exploitation link these three social groupings. This approach enables the development of a more expansive approach to explaining health inequities in terms not only of income inequality and poverty but also in terms of institutional racism, gender discrimination, corporate globalization, degradation of the environment, destruction of the public sector, dangerous workplace conditions, and neighbourhood characteristics.

An important factor in explaining these processes is the weakening of working-class power and the strengthening of capital over the past generation. It has been found that greater working-class power and political participation is associated with improved community health (Muntaner et al., 2002). Examples of the negative impact of increased corporate power itemized by Hofrichter include:

> *economic disinvestment in poor communities, extensive layoffs, mass firings and restructuring, gentrification, targeting of industrial and toxic waste facilities in communities of colour, elimination of protective regulatory structures, profiteering by drug companies seeking to maintain control of patents, financial speculation, use of dangerous technologies, restricting competition, shifting the tax burden to the less fortunate, tax subsidies to wealthy corporations, and failure to improve living conditions for farm workers.* (2003: 23)

It is these factors that in turn threaten already weakened communities, leading to further stress and ill-health.

An integrative model has been developed by Coburn (2004). In this class/welfare model issues of income inequality and social cohesion are nested within a broader causal chain. This model argues that over the past 20 years the power of business has increased while that of the working class has declined. This has been achieved through the introduction of neo-liberal policies by the ruling class that have increased income inequality and led to poverty and reduced access to services. In those countries with more social democratic rather than neo-liberal governments the power of capital has been resisted and the impact on health has been less. They have achieved this through a combination of both material and psychosocial advantages.

HEALTH AND PLACE

Although the evidence linking ill-health and poverty is clearly established there is also evidence of regional or area variations. This has given rise to a growing programme of research on health and place that has explored how major structural changes, such as those itemized above, lead to ill-health.

Taylor et al. (1997) have described the features of 'healthy' and 'unhealthy' environments:

> *Across multiple environments, unhealthy environments are those that threaten safety, that undermine the creation of social ties, and that are conflictual, abusive or violent. A healthy environment, in contrast, provides safety, opportunities for social integration, and the ability to predict and/or control aspects of that environment.* (Taylor et al., 1997: 411)

Unhealthy environments are associated with chronic stress and 'the lower one is on the SES continuum, the greater the amount of hassle and time needed to address basic tasks of living' (Taylor et al., 1997: 419). Diez Roux et al. (2001) investigated how a person's local neighbourhood can act as an independent predictor of health using data from the Atherosclerosis Risk in Communities Study (ARIC Investigators, 1989). Diez Roux and colleagues investigated the relationship between neighbourhood characteristics and the incidence of coronary heart disease among residents of four localities in the USA. A summary score for the socio-economic environment of each neighbourhood included information about wealth and income, education and occupation.

During a median of 9.1 years of follow-up, 615 coronary events occurred in 13,009 participants. Residents of disadvantaged neighbourhoods (those with lower summary scores) had a higher risk of disease than residents of advantaged neighbourhoods, even after controlling for personal income, education and occupation. These findings show that, even after controlling for personal income, education and occupation, living in a disadvantaged neighbourhood is associated with an increased incidence of coronary heart disease.

In an accompanying editorial, Marmot states:

> *Walk the slums of Dhaka, in Bangladesh, or Accra, in Ghana, and it is not difficult to see how the urban environment of poor countries could be responsible for bad health. Walk north from Manhattan's museum district to Harlem, or east from London's financial district to its old East End, and you will be struck by the contrast between rich and poor, existing cheek by jowl. It is less immediately obvious why there should be health differences between rich and poor areas of the same city. It is even less obvious, from casual inspection of the physical environment, why life expectancy for young black men in Harlem should be less than in Bangladesh.* (2001: 183)

Ethnic variations in health within rich countries are very large. For example, white men in the 10 'healthiest' counties in the US have a life expectancy above 76.4 years while black men in the 10 least healthy counties have a life expectancy of 61 years in Philadelphia, 60 in Baltimore and New York, and 57.9 in the District of Columbia. The main determinants of the excess deaths among Harlem men are circulatory disease, homicide and HIV infection. However the study by Diez Roux et al. (2001) suggests that socio-economic characteristics of communities, in addition to individual characteristics such as income, education and occupation, are related to the incidence of coronary events.

We have to explain not only why the poorest members of rich societies have higher rates of disease, but also why health follows a social gradient. As indicated above, the usual explanation for inequalities in health is lifestyle. There are clear socio-economic differences in smoking and other unhealthy types of behaviour that are risk factors for coronary artery disease. Yet controlling for these factors had little effect on the socio-economic differences in coronary heart disease in the study by Diez Roux et al. Something in addition to smoking, physical activity, hypertension, diabetes, low-density lipoprotein cholesterol, high-density lipoprotein cholesterol, and body-mass index must be responsible for the differences in the incidence of heart disease.

Marmot (2001) states: 'the mind is a crucial gateway through which social influences affect physiology to cause disease. The mind may work through effects on health-related behaviour, such as smoking, eating, drinking, physical activity, or risk taking, or it may act through effects on neuroendocrine or immune mechanisms' (p. 203). The Whitehall II study showed that level of control over one's work was an important predictor of the risk of cardiovascular disease and that it had an important role in accounting for the social gradient in coronary heart disease and depression (Marmot, Shipley, Brunner & Hemmingway, 2001).

People who report feeling low control at home and over life circumstances have an increased risk of depression, especially among women in low-status jobs. The findings of Diez Roux et al. (2001) suggest an important target for intervention: the neighbourhood. This finding is exactly what would be expected from a community perspective to health psychology. The studies reviewed above suggest that behavioural, material and local circumstances vary with SES. It is impossible to decide with the presently available information how much each of these causes is contributing to the gradients in illnesses and deaths. Understanding the material, behavioural and locality-based causes and the interactions between the three is a priority for further research.

Three theoretical approaches to the study of health and place have been identified (Curtis & Rees Jones, 1998):

- Hazard exposure: physical and biological risk factors are spatially distributed. This approach posits a direct pathway between hazard exposure and health risk.
- Social relationships: space and place shapes the character of social relationships and in turn psychosocial and behavioural risk factors.
- Sense of place and subjective meanings: this approach considers the shared social meanings people have of their community.

The second explanation connects with the growing literature on social capital while the third is connected with the literature on community identity and community narratives. We look at this topic again in Chapter 15.

SOCIAL CAPITAL

There is increasing interest in **social capital** as an aid to explaining social variations in health. The concept has been especially promoted by Robert Putnam who used it to characterize civic life in Italy (Putnam, Leonarchi & Nanetti, 1993). He argued that certain communities had higher degrees of civic engagement, levels of interpersonal trust and norms of reciprocity. Together, these characteristics contributed to a region's degree of social capital. Putnam (2000) subsequently explored the extent of social capital in the USA and argued that over the past generation there has been a steady decline in participation in social organizations and thus a steady decline in social capital.

There has been a series of studies investigating social variations in social capital and its connection with health. States with a low degree of income inequality also have low social capital as measured by group membership and social trust. Further, those states with high rates of social mistrust and low rates of membership of voluntary organizations have higher mortality rates.

A qualitative study by Campbell, Wood and Kelly (1999) compared the **sense of community** engagement in two communities near London. They reported evidence that two aspects of social capital (trust and civic engagement and perceived citizen power) were higher in the 'high health' community while two aspects (local identity and local community facilities) were higher in the 'low health' community. They suggested that certain aspects of social capital, in particular perceived trust and civic engagement, are more health enhancing than others. Whereas Putnam emphasized the importance of voluntary associations, Campbell et al. found that these were rare in both communities. However, whereas the 'low health' community made almost no reference to community-level networks in their community, these phenomena (e.g. residents' association) were important in the 'high health' community.

An important distinction that Putnam (2000) makes is that between 'bridging' and 'bonding' social capital. The latter refers to inward looking social ties that bond the community together. Bridging social capital refers to links with diverse groups and provides an opportunity for community members to access power and resources outside their community. Campbell (2004a) stresses that both forms of social capital are essential in building healthy communities.

There has been a wide range of criticisms of social capital as an explanatory concept (e.g. Lynch, Due, Muntaner & Davey Smith, 2000). These include confusion over what exactly the term implies, debates over ways of measuring it, and ignorance of the broader political context. However, an interest in social relations does not preclude acceptance of the importance of political and material factors. However, Baum (2000) emphasizes caution in the use of the concept in that 'there are dangers that the promotion of social capital may be seen as a substitute for economic investment in poor communities particularly by those governments who wish to reduce government spending' (p. 410).

KEY STUDY A Sense of Community Identity (Popay, Bennett, Thomas, Williams, Gatrell & Bostock, 2003)

An alternative to the rather behaviourist assumptions underlying much of the work on social capital is to consider the character of the **sense of community** meaning. The most comprehensive investigation of these processes is the work by Popay and colleagues (Popay et al., 2003). They conducted a detailed ethnographic study of four neighbourhoods in North West England. They found that residents of the more disadvantaged neighbourhoods identified place as the major explanation for health inequalities whereas those in relatively advantaged areas preferred individualistic explanations. However, the residents often suggested a complex interaction of macro-structural, place and lifestyle factors. For example, the residents of the more disadvantaged areas described how macro-structural factors interacted with place-based factors shaping particular lifestyle patterns. The mediating factor linking these factors was often seen as stress.

The way the residents described their communities was categorized into three normative guidelines:

(Continued)

(Continued)

- Relationships: this guideline emphasized the importance of supportive social relationships with neighbours, trust and respect between people, and respect for property.
- Physical dimensions: this guideline referred to aspects of safety, appropriateness, convenience and cleanliness.
- Ontological identity: this guideline is concerned with the relationship between one's sense of identity and place.

These guidelines helped to distinguish between 'good' and 'bad' neighbourhoods. It was not simply the material disadvantage of the neighbourhood but rather the community dynamics and the extent to which the residents could identify with it. The residents of more disadvantaged areas reported more problems with their neighbours and less safety. These residents were also less likely to identify with their neighbourhood.

An important component of this research is the emphasis on the importance of community narratives (Williams, 2003). Attention to these narratives enables the researcher to understand the lived experience of people's lives, of the connections between social and political change and everyday life.

REDUCING INEQUALITIES

If inequalities can be reduced at all, the evidence suggests that this will only happen by adopting a thoroughly multi-layered approach. Dahlgren and Whitehead (1991) identified four different levels for tackling health inequalities:

1 Strengthening individuals.
2 Strengthening communities.
3 Improving access to essential facilities and services.
4 Encouraging macroeconomic and cultural change.

These four levels correspond to the four layers of influence in Whitehead's 'onion model' of the determinants of health outlined in Chapter 1 (see Figure 1.3). Extra microsystem and mesosystem levels as in Bronfenbrenner's model could perhaps be added to Whitehead's list. Psychologists do not usually talk quite so simplistically about 'strengthening' individuals; we analyse the personal characteristics and skills associated with positive health (e.g. self-efficacy, hardiness, sense of coherence, social skills). Developing interventions aimed at individual health beliefs and behaviours is a core feature of psychological theory, research and practice.

Interventions aimed at tackling inequalities at an individual level have shown mixed results. There are four possible reasons. First, people living and working in disadvantaged circumstances have fewer resources (time, space, money) with which to manage the process of change. Second, health-threatening behaviours such as smoking tend to increase in difficult or stressful circumstances as they provide a means of coping. Third, there may have been a lack of sensitivity to the difficult circumstances in which people work and live that constrain the competence to change. Fourth, there has been a tendency to blame the victim. For example, cancer sufferers may be blamed for the disease if they are smokers on the grounds that they are responsible for the habit that caused it.

Overall, efforts directed at the individual level have been inconclusive and small scale. Because many health determinants are beyond the control of the individual, psychological interventions aimed at individuals are likely to have limited impact on public health problems when considered on a wider scale. This suggests that there is a need for psychologists to work beyond the individual level, with families, communities, work sites and community groups.

STIGMA

Humans have an innate tendency to categorize and stereotype individuals on the basis of differences between them. This process provides a kind of shorthand for what to expect from another person and how to react towards them. However, categories have a tendency to coalesce into dichotomies, so that people are labelled as male or female, black or white, gay or straight, young or old, healthy or ill, able or disabled (Gordon & Rosenblum, 2001). Such dichotomization implicitly involves judgements about which differences are socially valued, desired and accepted and which are devalued, feared and objectionable and therefore stigmatized.

'Stigma' refers to unfavourable reactions towards people when they are perceived to possess attributes that are denigrated. Stigmatization is universal, found in all cultures throughout history. The majority of people will experience it at some time, as both the young and the elderly are stigmatized groups. In addition people can be multiply stigmatized, as in the case of HIV/AIDS, which is associated with certain highly stigmatized groups (e.g. homosexuals, sex workers, intravenous drug users) and adds a further source of stigma as well as intensifying existing stigma(s). Stigma involves a pattern of discrediting, discounting, degradation and discrimination, directed at stigmatized people and extending to their significant others, close associates and social groups.

Stigmatization devalues the whole person, ascribing them a negative identity that persists (Miles, 1981), even when the basis of the stigma disappears (e.g. when someone recovers from mental illness they remain characterized forever as a person who had mental health problems). It is a form of social oppression and operates to disqualify and marginalize stigmatized individuals from full social acceptance and participation. Health-care professionals are as likely to stigmatize as any other group, influencing their behaviour and decision-making in the provision of health care. The consequences of stigma include physical and psychological abuse, denial of economic and employment opportunities, non-seeking or restricted access to services and social ostracism. It is not surprising then that individuals frequently expend considerable effort to combat stigmatization and manage their identities, including passing (acting as if they do not have the stigmatized attribute), covering (de-emphasizing difference), resistance (e.g. speaking out against discrimination) and withdrawal. They may also internalize the stigmatization, feeling considerable guilt and shame and devaluing themselves.

The pervasive Western idealization of physical perfection, independence and beauty may play an important role in the constant devaluation of disabled people and people who are ill. Particular characteristics of illness or disablement increase stigmatization including perceptions that the condition is the person's own fault (e.g. obesity), incurable and/or degenerative (e.g. Alzheimer's disease), intrusive, compromises mobility, contagious (e.g. HIV/AIDS) and highly visible. Goffman (1963) distinguished between discredited and discreditable categories of stigma. Discredited refers to conditions that are self-evident, in which the stigma is visible. Discreditable conditions relate to conditions where the stigma is not visible but may be discovered, at which point they would become stigmatized. Stigma is also increased when it is perceived to be threatening or disruptive (Neuberg, Smith & Asher, 2000), which may account for the high level of stigma associated with mental illness, intellectual disabilities and HIV/AIDS.

The lower value placed on the lives of disabled people can be seen in the way disabled people are segregated from the general population including education, housing, employment and transportation. It is also apparent in the way crimes against disabled people are minimized (e.g. discourses of abuse rather than theft/fraud/rape, acquittals and light sentences in cases of 'acceptable' euthanasia). For both disabled people and those with severe or terminal illness, stigma may be central to debates around suicide/euthanasia and abortion (see below). Stigma is a powerful determinant of social control and exclusion. By devaluing certain individuals and groups, society can excuse itself for making decisions about the rationing of resources (e.g. HIV antiretroviral drugs), services (e.g. health insurance exclusions), research funding/efforts and care (e.g. denying operations to individuals who are obese) to these groups. In terms of the social model of disablement, stigmatization may be the main issue concerning disablement.

Multidisciplinary research is needed to further explore how stigma is related to health, disablement and social justice. Why is recognition of the similarities between stigmatized and non-stigmatized individuals over-ridden and obscured by perceived differences that are devalued? How do different stigmas, particularly health-related stigmas, interact? How is stigma manifested by health-care professionals and what interventions might mitigate the negative effects of stigma?

LIVES WORTH LIVING VERSUS THE RIGHT-TO-DIE

The pervasive devaluation of disabled people with disabilities, and the negative assumptions about their lower quality of life, are central to the current debates about abortion of impaired foetuses and legalization of assisted suicide/euthanasia or the right-to-die. Disablement rights organizations champion the argument that abortion decisions should not be made on the basis of foetal impairment indicators whereas they challenge the 'right-to-die' rhetoric on the basis of disablement.

The disablement movement argues against abortion on the grounds of potential impairment due to the eugenic implications of such a practice (Sharpe & Earle, 2002). The reason for their concern is encapsulated in Singer's quote: 'the killing of a defective infant is not morally equivalent to the killing of a person; very often it is not morally wrong at all' (1993: 184). The new genetic testing and selection technologies allow the identification of suspected foetal impairment during pregnancy and subsequent foetal termination. Shakespeare (1998: 669) argues that such technologies operate as a weak form of eugenics 'via non-coercive individual choices' based on the assumed unacceptable quality of life of disabled people. The rationales for screening and termination include assumptions that people with disabilities are more costly to society, that the lives of disabled children with disabilities are harmful to their families and that some impairments involve a level of suffering and misery that makes life not worth living.

The way professionals describe test results and the influence of the advice they give is also a concern. There is substantial evidence that the advice given, while often subtle, most frequently encourages termination in response to potential impairment results and most testing takes place within a plan-to-abort context. There is a tension between this argument and the feminist position that women have a categorical right to make decisions about their own bodies including the decision to terminate an unwanted pregnancy. However, the disablement movement position is not against abortion itself, rather it revolves around the bases upon which the decision is made. Aborting a specific foetus on the basis of a devalued attribute is different from aborting any foetus on the basis of not wanting to have a child at that time (Fine & Asch, 1982). It is unlikely that a woman would be encouraged to terminate a pregnancy because a test indicated the child is likely to have ginger hair; however, the same is not true when a test suggests a possibility of impairment. It is this difference that makes it an issue of discrimination. The disablement movement also asserts the rights of disabled women to have children. This fundamental human right is denied to many women, particularly those with cognitive and emotional impairments, as the additional support and resources that they need to allow them to raise a child are often not available. In some countries, forced sterilization still occurs, including Australia, Spain and Japan.

The right-to-die debate revolves around the argument that people with severe or terminal illness and disabled people have the right to end their lives when they feel they have become unbearable, and that assisting them to do so should not be illegal. The taken-for-granted assumption that underlies this argument is the belief that the quality of life for such individuals is so severely reduced that it makes it unendurable and is bound up with a rhetoric of the moral imperative to relieve suffering. Such assumptions underlie the decisions of many health-care professionals concerning assisted dying.

A review by Gill (2000) challenges this assumption. In general, disabled people have rated their quality of life as good to excellent. Lower quality of life ratings may relate more to socio-demographic factors (e.g. poverty, exclusion, lack of social support) than disablement *per se*. Consistently, research has failed to show an association between diminishing quality of life and increasing severity of physical impairment. Many factors mediate quality of life. Overall the research indicates that disabled people derive life satisfaction through performing expected social roles, enjoying reciprocal relationships and a sense of living in a reciprocal social world. Despite no empirical basis suggesting compromised quality of life, health-care professionals consistently and significantly underestimate it in disabled people. The negative attitudes of these professionals inform their own decision-making and are communicated, directly and indirectly, to their patients and patients' families. Negative attitudes about disabled people include underestimating quality of life, underestimating future capabilities (especially for children), overestimating depression, viewing it as a normal and inevitable response (therefore not treating it) and underestimating the functional ability to commit suicide. Health-care professionals have to make explicit decisions about whether to assist a patient who asks for help to die. They also have to make less explicit decisions around provision of life-sustaining treatment (e.g. whether to withhold heart operations for Down Syndrome children). Professionals who most underestimate quality of life also appear to be most likely not to support life-saving treatment. Life-sustaining efforts are often less rigorously applied to infants with severe impairments.

More importantly, the entrenched disablement prejudices held by health-care professionals result in unsupported assumptions that the quality of life of disabled people is diminished in such a way that it makes it more unendurable, more hopeless and more limited than that of people for whom other factors have diminished their quality of life (e.g. someone whose family have been killed and finds life unbearable without them). In addition, assisting certain disabled people to die would not be countenanced. For example, it is unlikely that assisting the survivors of genocide to die would be countenanced, despite them enduring extreme suffering, pain, disablement and distress. There are a number of forms of 'assisted-dying' including a person ending their own life by their choice using a tool supplied by someone else, someone else ending a person's life with their consent, someone else ending a person's life without their consent and withholding life-sustaining treatment (with or without that person's consent). All of these forms of 'assisted-dying' have been applied to disabled people. That 'assisted-dying' can refer to the act without the consent of the person who dies is particularly worrying. It has been suggested that many disabled people fear that episodes of illness may be viewed as an opportunity to 'allow' them 'merciful' release (D. Marks, 1999), and there may be some basis for this. In the

Netherlands, assisted suicide has been legalized and people with physical and psychiatric disabilities have been helped to die with their consent.

The argument against the right-to-die lobby, although implicitly anti-suicide, is not necessarily about whether suicide *per se* is right or wrong. It should be viewed as being about the differential treatment of the issue for disabled or severely ill people as opposed to 'healthy' people. Morally sanctioning assisting people with incurable terminal or non-terminal conditions to end their lives or withholding life-sustaining treatment/support, while morally opposing the right of suicidal 'healthy' individuals to end their lives (and offering them suicide prevention interventions), equates to a severe form of discrimination based on stigmatization of these individuals.

The two debates discussed above are about the differential value placed on the lives of people disabled versus the able-bodied. Stigmatized individuals are regarded as flawed, compromised, less than fully human (Heatherton, Kleck, Hebl & Hull, 2000) and, in the case of disabled people, may be thought of as worthless. Being judged as having a life not worth living may represent the most fundamental claim to injustice and inequality on a slippery slope with the genocide of the Holocaust.

SOCIAL JUSTICE AND HEALTH

Critics of the research into social inequalities in health often charge that social inequalities are both an inevitable part of life and also are necessary for social progress. An alternative perspective is to consider not simply inequalities *per se* but inequities in health. According to Dahlgren and Whitehead (1991) health inequalities can be considered as inequities when they are avoidable, unnecessary and unfair. The issue of fairness leads us to consider the issue of **social justice** and health.

A useful starting point is the theory of 'justice as fairness' developed by the moral philosopher John Rawls (1999). He identified certain underlying principles of a just society, as follows:

- Assure people equal basic liberties including guaranteeing the right of political participation.
- Provide a robust form of equal opportunity.
- Limit inequalities to those that benefit the least advantaged.

When these principles are met citizens can be confident that they are respected by others and can acquire a sense of self-worth.

Daniels, Kennedy and Kawachi (2000) argue that adhering to these principles would address the basic social inequalities in health. They detail a series of implications for social organization that flow from the acceptance of these principles. First, assuring people equal basic liberties implies that everyone has an equal right to fully participate in politics. This will in turn contribute to improvements in health since according to social capital theory political participation is an important social determinant of health.

Second, providing active measures to promote equal opportunities implies the introduction of measures to reduce socio-economic inequalities and other social obstacles to equal opportunities. Such measures would include comprehensive childcare and childhood interventions to combat any disadvantages of family background (Daniels et al., 2000). They would also include comprehensive health care for all including support services for the disabled.

Finally, a just society would allow only those inequalities in income and wealth that would benefit the least advantaged. This requires direct challenge to the contemporary neo-liberal philosophy that promotes the maximization of profit and increasing the extent of social inequality.

Increasingly psychologists have recognized the link between poor social conditions and physical and mental health. In 2000 the American Psychological Association passed a landmark resolution on Poverty and Socioeconomic Status. This resolution called for a programme of research on the causes and impact of poverty, negative attitudes towards people living in poverty, strategies to reduce poverty, and the evaluation of anti-poverty programmes. This resolution has been followed by a number of initiatives.

Bullock and Lott (2001) developed a research and advocacy agenda on issues of economic justice. Such an agenda is not just concerned with describing the impact of poverty and inequality on health and well-being but also with advocating for social and economic justice.

This agenda includes challenging the victim-blaming ideology that is often adopted in psychological approaches to the study of health and illness. It also includes defining health psychology as a resource for social change (Murray & Campbell, 2003). This can involve a variety of strategies. This leads to a more politically engaged health psychology such as the one championed by Martín-Baró (1994) who challenged psychologists to adopt a 'preferential option for the poor'.

Three approaches have been suggested by Fine and Barreras (2001):

- Public policy: documenting the impact of regressive social policies and agitating against such policies.
- Popular education: challenging popular victim-blaming beliefs ('common-sense') about the causes of ill-health.
- Community organizing: working with marginalized communities and agitating for social change.

The success of such a strategy requires building alliances with social groups most negatively impacted by social inequalities. These can range from patient-rights groups to trade unions and other activist groups (Steinitz & Mishler, 2001). As Martín-Baró stressed: 'the concern of the social scientist should not be so much to explain the world as to transform it' (1994: 19).

FUTURE RESEARCH

1. There is a need to clarify the character of the psychosocial explanations for the social inequalities in health.
2. Research on social inequalities needs to be combined with further research on ethnic and gender inequalities in health. Qualitative studies of the health experiences of people from different socio-economic backgrounds are of particular importance to our understanding of the psychological mechanisms underlying health variations. Further qualitative studies are also needed to explore the relationship between social positioning and health experience.
3. Forms of research on social inequalities in health need to explicitly consider how they can contribute to reducing them.
4. An essential aspect of future research is to consider the social and psychological obstacles to movements to alleviate social inequalities in health.

Summary

1. Health and illness are determined by social conditions.
2. There is a clear relationship between income and health leading to the development of a social gradient.
3. Psychosocial explanations of these social variations include perceived inequality, stress, lack of control and less social connection.
4. Material explanations of the social gradient in health include reduced income and reduced access to services.
5. Political factors connect both psychosocial and material explanations in a broader causal chain.
6. Lay explanations of social inequalities in health include people's immediate social and physical environment.
7. Social environment includes the character of people's social relationships and their connection with the community.
8. Social justice is concerned with providing equal opportunities for all citizens. Socio-economic status (SES) and wealth are strongly related to health, illness and mortality. These gradients may be a consequence of differences in social cohesion, stress and personal control.
9. A health psychology committed to social justice needs to orient itself to address the needs of the most disadvantaged in society.

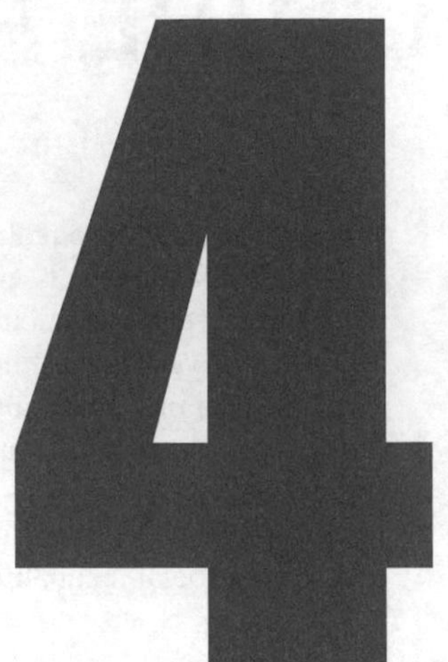

Culture and Health

There is no such thing as human nature independent of culture.

Clifford Geertz, 1973

Outline

The way people think about health, become ill and react to illness is rooted in their broader health belief systems that are in turn immersed in culture. This chapter provides some examples from the work of historians and anthropologists who have investigated how health belief systems vary across time and space. We consider some of the different expert health belief systems that have existed historically in Western society and contemporary popular belief systems. We also consider several non-Western health belief systems and discuss some of the issues related with the rapid cultural changes in today's modern society and the interpenetration of cultural groups and belief systems.

WHAT IS CULTURE?

We are cultural beings and an understanding of health beliefs and practices requires an understanding of the cultural, historical and social context within which we live. It is impossible to extract humans from the context that gives them meaning. Culture is all around us and pervades our very being. An inclusive definition of **culture** has been provided by Corin who defines it as:

> *...a system of meanings and symbols. This system shapes every area of life, defines a world view that gives meaning to personal and collective experience, and frames the way people locate themselves within the world, perceive the world, and believe in it. Every aspect of reality is seen as embedded within webs of meaning that define a certain world view and that cannot be studied or understood apart from this collective frame.* (1995: 273)

An understanding of people's reactions to illness requires an understanding of these culturally specific health belief systems.

HEALTH BELIEF SYSTEMS

As societies evolved they have developed various **health belief systems**, knowledge of which is sometimes confined to those who undergo specialized training. This has given rise to the separation of what have become known as *expert* or technical belief systems as opposed to the *traditional folk* or indigenous systems. These systems are not discrete but interact and are in a process of constant evolution. Although the majority of people in any society organize their world through indigenous belief systems the character of these is connected in some form with the expert belief system. Kleinman (1980) distinguished between three overlapping sectors of any health-care system:

1 The *popular sector* refers to the lay cultural arena where illness is first defined and health care activities initiated;
2 The *professional sector* refers to the organized healing professions, their representations and actions; and
3 The *folk sector* refers to the non-professional, non-bureaucratic, specialist sector that shades into the other two sectors.

In view of the central role of health in our self-definition, these different health sectors both reflect and contribute to broader worldviews. Although this threefold division is widely cited, other researchers (e.g. Blumhagen, 1980) have preferred a simpler two-fold division into professional and popular realms. 'Systematicity, coherence and interdependence are aspects of the professional belief systems' (Blumhagen, 1980: 200). Conversely, the lay health belief system can appear disconnected. This broad classification avoids an accusation that certain specialized health belief systems are classified as folk when they have limited status in society although they may have an extensive codification of health complaints and treatments. These two broad belief systems interact such that the lay person can draw upon more specialized knowledge but also the specialist will make use of more popular knowledge. Further, both ways of thinking about health draw upon a more general worldview and are located within a particular local and political context. Blumhagen (1980) also argues that these two health belief systems should be considered distinct from the individual belief system that the individual uses to understand their personal experience of illness. An understanding of popular health beliefs requires an understanding of the dominant expert health belief systems.

Western Health Belief Systems

Classical views of health

The classical view of health and illness in the West is derived from the Graeco-Arabic medical system. **Galenic medicine** provided an expert system developed from the Greeks, in particular the work of Hippocrates and his colleagues. As discussed in Chapter 1, the central concept in Galen's formulation was the *balance* of four bodily fluids or humours: bile, phlegm, blood and black bile. Balance was equated with health and imbalance implied ill-health. These fluids have been linked with the *four seasons* (e.g. an excess of phlegm was common in the winter leading to colds, while an excess of bile led to summer diarrhoea); the *four primary conditions* (i.e. hot, cold, wet and dry); and the *four elements* (i.e. air, fire, earth and water). Medieval scholars also added *four temperaments* (i.e. choleric, sanguine, melancholic and phlegmatic). Figure 4.1 shows a plan of the Hippocratic humoral system (see also Table 1.1).

Besides a focus on understanding natural processes, the Galenic tradition also placed responsibility on individuals to look after themselves. Ill-health was a consequence of natural processes, not a result of divine intervention. In many ways Galen's ideas not only prefigured but also continue to influence much of contemporary health beliefs.

Christian ideas

Galenic ideas dominated the expert system of medicine in Europe for almost two millennia. However, during the Middle Ages in Europe, Galen's work became confined more to the learned few and other ideas based upon religion became more commonplace. Illness was often seen as punishment for humankind's sinfulness. The Church's *seven deadly sins* even came to be associated with pathological conditions of the body. For example, pride

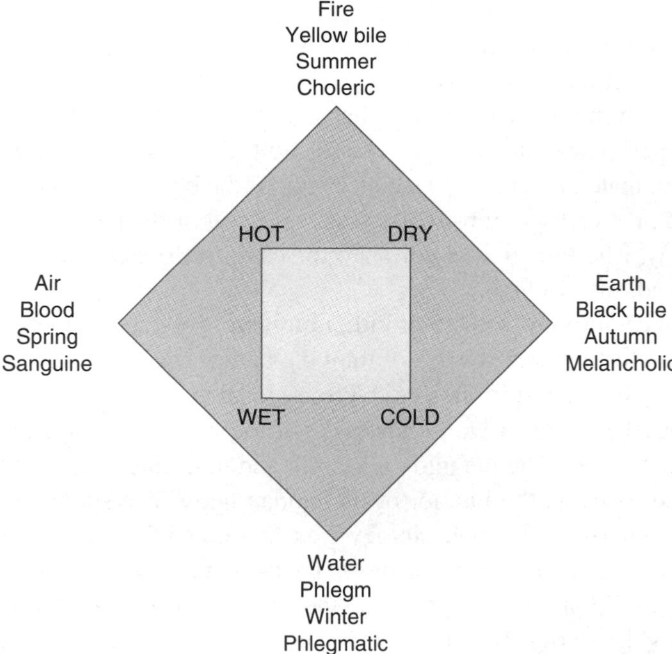

Figure 4.1 Hippocratic system of humours

was symbolized by tumours and inflammations while sloth led to dead flesh and palsy (Thomas, 1979).

Christianity drew upon different traditions. The *ascetic tradition* scorned concern for the body and instead promoted acts such as fasting and physical suffering, which supposedly led to spirituality. With the *Protestant Reformation* this belief was replaced with the idea that the body had been given to humans by God. It was the individual's religious duty to look after and care for the body. Illness was seen as a sign of weakness and neglect. To honour God required living a healthy life and abstaining from excess, especially in terms of sex and diet. Wear (1985) noted that religious writers frequently made reference to the body. For example, Robert Horne described the body as the 'Temple of God' and that it was necessary to keep it pure and clean. These ideas were widely promulgated in the new Protestant Reformation. The way to heaven was through attention to health behaviour and was also linked to a social morality. The poor were expected to take responsibility for their condition while at the same time the rich were wrong to indulge themselves while there was so much poverty and suffering.

Despite the authority of the Church, these religious interpretations began to decline with the growth of medical science. While in terms of the expert belief system there has been increasing acceptance of a naturalistic view of disease, the moral basis of health continues to underlie much of contemporary health belief.

Biomedicine

Two streams of thought in knowing the world dominated during the Enlightenment. The first was the acceptance of the distinction between superstition and reason. The second was the emergence of **positivism** that emphasized that science based upon direct observation, measurement and experimentation gave direct access to the real world. This approach concentrated attention on material reality and a conception of the body as distinct from the mind. A central figure was Descartes (1596–1650) who conceived of the human being as composed of mind and body. The former was not open to scientific investigation whereas the latter could be conceived as a machine.

The eighteenth century saw the rise of **individualism** in Western society. In previous eras the group or collective organized ways of thinking and acting, which in turn was interconnected with the physical and spiritual world. Professional understanding of health and illness became more closely entwined with knowledge of the individual physical body. Foucault (1976) described how between the mid-eighteenth and mid-nineteenth centuries the 'medical gaze' came to focus on the interior of the human body. The symptoms of illness now became signs of underlying pathophysiology. Foucault noted that the change in perspective of the physician was illustrated in the change in the patient query from 'How do you feel?' to 'Where does it hurt?'. For this new physician the stethoscope became the symbol of having insight into the bodily interior. Treatment centred on changing the character of this physiology either by medical or surgical means.

This approach to the study of health and illness has become known as **biomedicine**, cosmopolitan or allopathic medicine (Leslie, 1976). It came to dominance for several reasons, including the fact that it was in accord with a broader view of humans, its alliance with physical science and the steady improvement in the health of the population that was attributed to medical intervention. The focus on the body is in accord with the Western emphasis on the individual. Further, the separation of mind and body 'offers a subtle articulation of the person's alienation from the body in Western society, but this alienation is found, as well, in every sphere of economic and political life' (Benoist & Cathebras, 1993: 858). Biomedicine separates the person from the body.

Friedson (1970) described how the coming to dominance of the biological approach was not without resistance. It required strong political action to organize the profession of medicine and to take legal action against other health practitioners. Throughout there was the dismissal of alternative perspectives and the assertion that biomedicine was the central force that had led to the substantial improvements in society's health. Biomedicine was based upon a positivist epistemology that supposedly gave it access to an outside reality. Only this approach was the true approach. All other approaches could be disparaged.

The biopsychosocial model of health

The dominance of this biomedical system has come in for substantial challenge both from the scientific establishment and the public. Initially, this was reflected in a call for more attention to the psychological and social aspects of health. This led to the development of the **biopsychosocial** model of health and illness (Engel, 1977). According to Engel (1980) the various aspects of health and illness can be organized in a hierarchy from the biosphere and society down through the individual's level of experience and behaviour to the cellular and subatomic level. All of these levels interact and need to be considered if we are to understand health and illness. With varying degrees of enthusiasm this model has in some respects replaced the basic biomedical model (see Chapter 1 for further discussion of this point).

In addition, the increasing evidence of the link between social and behavioural factors and health has led to the promulgation of a health promotion ethic by the medical establishment with an emphasis on personal responsibility for health. Crawford (1980: 365) argued that 'in an increasingly "healthist" culture, healthy behaviour has become a moral duty and illness an individual moral failing'. Admittedly, the adoption of a more biopsychosocial approach to health care, especially by general practitioners, is sometimes met with hostility by patients who have accepted the basic biomedical model. This might explain why some people feel concerned that their physician is becoming too involved in their psychosocial problems.

Criticisms of the biomedical model also led the World Health Organization to propose an extensive definition of health as a state of complete physical, mental and social well-being, not the mere absence of disease or infirmity. This definition widened the scope of health care to consider not only the well-being of the individual but also of the community. In Chapter 1 an even wider definition was offered, encompassing the economic, political and spiritual domains. Currently, much of health care in Western society is attempting to shift from a concern with bodily processes to concern with the wider concept of quality of life.

Popular views of health in the West

Evidence from a series of studies of popular beliefs about health and illness in Western society illustrates the interaction of what can be described as the classic, the religious, the biomedical and the lifestyle approaches to health and illness. Probably the most influential study of Western lay health beliefs was carried out by Herzlich (1973). She conducted interviews with a sample of French adults and concluded that health was conceived as an attribute of the individual – a state of harmony or balance. Illness was attributed to outside forces in our society or way of life. Laypeople also referred to illness in terms of both organic and psychosocial factors. On their own organic changes did not constitute illness. Rather, for the layperson 'physical facts, symptoms and dysfunctions have, of course, an existence of their own, but they only combine to form an illness in so far as they transform a patient's life'. The ability to participate in everyday life constitutes health, whereas inactivity is considered the true criterion of illness. Herzlich's study was seminal because it provoked further research into popular health beliefs.

For example, Blaxter (1990) analysed the definitions of health provided by over 9000 British adults in the health and lifestyles survey. She classified the responses into nine categories:

1 Health as not-ill (the absence of physical symptoms)
2 Health despite disease
3 Health as reserve (the presence of personal resources)
4 Health as behaviour (the extent of healthy behaviour)
5 Health as physical fitness
6 Health as vitality
7 Health as psychosocial well-being
8 Health as social relationships
9 Health as function

In analysing the responses across social classes, Blaxter (1990) noted considerable agreement in the emphasis on behavioural factors as a cause of illness. She commented on the limited reference to structural or environmental factors, especially among those from working-class backgrounds. Williams and Calnan (1996) suggest that the growth of the self-help consumer movement in health care is another symbol of popular opposition to the passive patient model of biomedicine. They noted that this opposition 'can be located within the broader socio-cultural and political framework of self-determination and a reclaiming of control over the body, self and wider environment' (1996: 1617).

However, health beliefs go beyond descriptive dimensions to consider underlying etiology. In a discussion of **social representation theory**, Moscovici (1984) suggested that people rarely confine their definition of concepts to the descriptive level. Rather, lay descriptions often include reference to explanations. This is apparent in a study of lay descriptions of health and illness by Stainton-Rogers (1991) who used Q-sort methodology to identify the concepts used by a sample of British adults to explain health. Seven different accounts of health and illness have been identified (see Table 4.1)

Lay perceptions of health and illness can be rooted in the social experience of people, in particular sub-cultures. A study of East and West German workers found similar findings to that of Herzlich but with an added emphasis on health as lifestyle (Flick, 1998). Similarly,

Table 4.1 Popular explanations of health (Stainton-Rogers, 1991)

Accounts	Explanations
Body as machine	Illness is naturally occurring and 'real' with biomedicine considered the main form of treatment.
Body under siege	Illness is a result of external influences such as germs or stress.
Inequality of access	Emphasized the unequal access to modern medicine.
Cultural critique	Based upon a sociological worldview of exploitation and oppression.
Health promotion	Recognized both individual and collective responsibility for ill-health.
Robust individualism	Concerned with every individual's right to a satisfying life.
Willpower account	Defined health in terms of the individual's ability to exert control.

in a study of Canadian baby-boomers Murray, Pullman and Heath Rodgers (2003) found a very activity-orientated conception of health. They defined health in terms of lifestyle, functionality, social engagement and attitude as well as reserve and also in a vacuum. It was suggested that this conception reflected a greater self-responsibility for health that is promoted in Canadian culture. However, there was also evidence of a certain resistance to this stance among those from working-class backgrounds.

In Western society the metaphor that is associated with health is that of *self-control*. This metaphor is in turn infused with moral connotations such that to become ill is not to take care of oneself (Crawford, 1980). Admittedly, health is a contested arena since release from certain controls, or even the rejection of them, can be considered a sign of good health. Conversely, the person who abides by certain controls can be perceived as unhealthy. In her study of laypeople's views of health and illness Crossley (2003) found that for some to transgress the moral imperative to health was perceived as good. A study comparing the health beliefs and practices of adults living in Japan with adults, from Japanese and Caucasian heritage, resident in Hawaii found that the Japanese residents had less concern about their health and were less likely to believe that they had control over their health (Gotay, Shimizu, Muraoka, Ishihara, Tsuboi & Ogawa, 2004). These findings illustrate the close interweaving of health beliefs and practices with culture.

Non-Western Views of Health

Chinese views of health

Chinese medicine is greatly influenced by the religion and philosophy of *Taoism*. According to this view the universe is a vast and indivisible entity and each being has a definite function within it. The balance of the two basic powers of yin and yang governs the whole universe including human beings. *Yang* is considered to represent the male, positive energy that produces light and fullness, whereas the *yin* is considered the female, negative force that leads to darkness and emptiness. A disharmony in *yin* and *yang* leads to illness. A variety of methods including *acupuncture* and the use of *herbal medicines* can be used to restore this harmony.

Confucianism is also influential in the traditional Chinese views on health. Within this culture, human suffering is traditionally explained as the result of destiny or *ming*. Cheng (1997) quotes the Confucian teacher Master Meng: 'A man worries about neither untimely death nor long life but cultivates his personal character and waits for its natural development; this is to stand in accord with Fate. All things are determined by Fate, and one should accept what is conferred' (1997: 740). An important part of your destiny depends upon your horoscope or *pa-tzu*. During an individual's life, his or her *pa-tzu* is paired with the timing of nature. Over time these pairings change and create the individual's luck or *yun*.

Buddhist beliefs are also reflected in Chinese medical belief systems. Good deeds and charitable donations for example are promoted. Heavenly retribution is expected for those who commit wrongs. This retribution may not be immediate but it will be inevitable. An important concept in this respect is *pao* that has two types: 1) reciprocity and 2) retribution (Cheng, 1997). In mutual relationships reciprocity is expected. When this does not occur some form of retribution will take place.

These influences are not only codified within Chinese medicine but influence everyday lay beliefs about health and illness both in China and in Chinese communities around the world. For example, Chen et al. (2009) discussed how these three philosophical foundations influence Chinese patients' perspectives on cancer pain and its management (see Table 4.2).

Table 4.2 Chinese perspectives on cancer pain and management (Chen et al., 2009)

	What is pain?	In practice
Taoist philosophy	Blockage in the Qi (blood circulation)	To relieve pain, blockage needs to be removed and the person needs to maintain harmony with the universe
Confucian philosophy	An essential element of life, like a 'trial' or 'sacrifice'	Since pain is a part of life, a person in pain might rather endure it and not report to a clinician until it becomes unbearable
Buddhist philosophy	A form of unwanted but existing power that came from 1) a barrier in the past life; 2) the objective world; 3) the person's own sensation; or 4) from other people, animals and materials	To end pain, the person needs to follow the eight right ways (i.e. right view, intention, speech, action, livelihood, effort, mindfulness and concentration)

These lay belief systems remain strong within immigrant communities. In a qualitative study on social representations, Jovchelovitch and Grevais (1999) showed that despite differences related to age and degrees of acculturation, Chinese people in England share common representational systems relating to health and illness which is still based on the notions of 'balance' and 'harmony' of the yin and yang. Similarly, in a quantitative study examining cultural health beliefs held by older Chinese in Canada, Lai and Surood (2009) reported that their health beliefs are loaded onto factors related with traditional health practices, beliefs about traditional Chinese medicine and beliefs about preventive diet.

Ayurvedic medicine

The **Ayurvedic** system of medicine is based upon the Sanskrit words *ayus* (life) and *veda* (science). This system remains extremely extensive in India. It is estimated that 70 per cent of the population of India and hundreds of millions of people throughout the world use Ayurvedic medicine (Schober, 1997). According to this system that is based on Hindu philosophy both the cosmos and each human being consists of a female component, *Prakrti*, which forms the body, and a male component, *Purusa*, which forms the soul. While the Purusa is constant, the Prakrti is subject to change. The body is defined in terms of the flow of substances through channels. Each substance has its own channel. Sickness occurs when a channel is blocked and the flow is diverted into another channel. When all channels are blocked the flow of substances is not possible and death occurs. At this stage the soul is liberated from its bodily prison. The task of Ayurvedic medicine is to identify the blockages and to get the various essences moving again. The different forms of imbalance can be corrected through both preventive and therapeutic interventions based on diet, yoga, breathwork, bodywork, meditation and/or herbs (Schober, 1997).

As with the Chinese medical system, the Ayurvedic system pervades much of popular beliefs about health and illness throughout the Indian sub-continent and among Indian communities in other parts of the world. However, Ayurvedic medicine has not gained the hegemony of Western biomedicine, even within India. There is a variety of other competing health belief systems that has led to the development of a pluralistic health culture made up of several different systems. In an interview study of a community in Northern India, Morinis and Brilliant (1981) found evidence not only of Ayurvedic beliefs, but also 'unami' (another indigenous health system), allopathic, homeopathic, massage, herbalist, folk, astrologic and religious systems. They note that while these systems may formally seem to conflict, in their study participants could draw on some or all of them to help explain different health problems. Further, the strength of these beliefs is related to the immediate social situation and the roles and expectations of the community. For example, for women in some parts of Pakistan, the health belief system is a mixture of biomedicine and 'unami' medicine that is a version of Galenic medicine.

African health beliefs

A wide range of traditional medical systems continues to flourish in Africa. These include a mixture of herbal and physical remedies intertwined with various religious belief systems. As Porter (1997) notes, belief systems that attribute sickness to 'ill-will, to malevolent spirits, sorcery, witchcraft and diabolical or divine intervention still pervade the tribal communities of Africa, the Amazon basin and the Pacific' (1997: 9). In a more developed assessment Chalmers (1996) summarized the African view as reflecting 'a belief in an integrated, independent, totality of all things animate and inanimate, past and present' (1996: 3). As with other traditional health systems a central concept is balance: 'Disturbances in the equilibrium, be they emotional, spiritual or interpersonal, may manifest in discordance at any level of functioning' (Chalmers, 1996: 3).

Two dimensions are paramount in understanding **African health beliefs**: *spiritual influences* and a *communal orientation*. It is common to attribute illness to the work of ancestors or to supernatural forces. Inadequate respect for ancestors can supposedly lead to illness. In addition, magical influences can be both negative and positive, contemporary and historical. Thus, illness can be attributed to the work of some malign living person. The role of the spiritual healer is to identify the source of the malign influence. Rather than the individualistic orientation of Western society, African culture has a communal orientation. Thus, the malign influence of certain supernatural forces can be felt not just by an individual but also by other members of his or her family or community. Thus intervention may be aimed not only at the sense of balance of the individual but also of the family and the community.

Mulatu (1999) investigated the illness causal beliefs of a large sample of adults from Ethiopia. Four dimensions have been identified: 1) psychological stressors; 2) supernatural retribution; 3) biomedical defects; and 4) social disadvantage. Psychological stressors and supernatural retribution were considered more important causes of psychological than of physical illnesses. A relationship between these causal beliefs and treatment choices, attitude to patients and demographic characteristics has also been found. For example, belief in supernatural retribution is associated with use of religious prayer, holy water, consulting traditional healers and both traditional and modern medicine. There is also a relationship between education and causal beliefs such that the less educated placed more emphasis on supernatural causes. This reflects the extent of acculturation to the Western biomedical model of illness.

As with other medical systems, immigrant communities have brought their health beliefs to their new countries of residence. Landrine (1997) criticized studies of North American health beliefs that have largely ignored the distinctive culture of black Americans. African slaves maintained their pre-slavery health beliefs, practices and indigenous healers. When they gained emancipation African–Americans found they were denied access to medical care. As a consequence they relied on their indigenous healers and over time developed a unique African–American folk medicine. She suggests that in contemporary North America many people from African backgrounds are returning to this medical system as they feel rejected or excluded by what they perceive as the racism of white American health care.

Indigenous health

As with other non-Western health belief systems, **indigenous health** belief systems are typically characterised by 'a combination of practices and knowledge about the human body, and coexistence with other human beings, with nature, and with spiritual beings' (Cunningham, 2009: 157). The United Nations (2009) adopts Martinez Cobo's (1987) definition of indigenous communities as:

> *...peoples and nations which, having a historical continuity with pre-invasion and pre-colonial societies that developed on their territories, consider themselves distinct from other sectors of the societies now prevailing on those territories, or parts of them. They form at present non-dominant sectors of society and are determined to preserve, develop and transmit to future generations their ancestral territories, and their ethnic identity, as the basis of their continued existence as peoples, in accordance with their own cultural patterns, social institutions and legal system.* (2009: 4)

There are almost 400 million indigenous people coming from thousands of different cultures worldwide (Gracey & King, 2009). Unfortunately many of these communities experience some of the lowest standards of health. Generally, indigenous people tend to have poorer health outcomes than their non-indigenous counterparts (Stephens et al., 2005). They have lower life expectancies and have higher mortality rates for specific diseases such as heart disease, cancer, respiratory disease, stroke and diabetes (Horton, 2006). Even after adjustment for stage at diagnosis, treatment and comorbidity, non-indigenous cancer patients survive longer than indigenous ones (Valery et al., 2006). Indigenous populations are also six times more likely to die from injuries (Desapriya et al., 2006); and have worse access to health services and education (Horton, 2006; Stephens et al., 2006). This is reflected among indigenous communities in Australia, New Zealand and the Pacific (Anderson et al., 2006); Latin America and the Caribbean (Montenegro & Stephens, 2006); and Africa (Ohenjo et al., 2006). Some of the persistent problems and areas of deterioration for these communities are summarized in Table 4.3 below.

Table 4.3 Persistent problems and areas of deterioration on indigenous health (Gracey & King, 2009)

Persistent problems	• Shortened life expectancy • Infant and child malnutrition, growth failure, high infant and young child mortality • Maternal ill-health and high mortality • Chronic ill-health and disabilities • Poverty, hunger, environmental contamination, frequent infections and parasites • Widespread prejudice about perceived inadequacies of indigenous people • Insufficient chances for indigenous people to be trained and take part in their health care • Poor understanding of the complexities of indigenous health by health professionals • Government preoccupation with sickness services rather than wellness strategies and false expectations that medical strategies alone can overcome indigenous health problems • Government indifference, ignorance, neglect and denial about the poor state of indigenous health • Bureaucratic mishandling of culturally sensitive matters beyond their rigid protocols • Inadequate systematic data to allow surveillance and improvement of indigenous health care
Areas of deterioration	• Erosion of the authority of indigenous elders • Illnesses associated with overcrowding and environmental contamination in squatter settlements, urban slums and disaster situations • The rapid upsurge of lifestyle diseases • Respiratory and peripheral vascular disease associated with cigarette smoking • Diseases and social problems associated with misuse of alcohol and other drugs • Emotional, mental and psychiatric illnesses • Interpersonal and family violence, including child abuse, homicide and suicide • Motor vehicle and other accidents and poisonings • Sexually transmissible diseases, including HIV/AIDS

While efforts are being made to address inequalities that disadvantage indigenous communities, Stephens and her colleagues (2005) pointed out that interventions that target indigenous communities often fail to recognize the difference between Western models of health and the holistic notion of health among indigenous peoples. Thus, there is a need to actively involve community members themselves in generating the knowledge base to effectively inform interventions aimed to address key issues that are relevant to them.

CHANGING CULTURES AND HEALTH

Our modern world is a world of rapid change and interpenetration of cultural groups and belief systems. There is increasing evidence that laypeople are mixing and matching their use of health systems which can lead to confusion among health professionals. Health psychology needs to recognize this complexity rather than assuming that health belief systems are fixed (MacLachlan, 2000). It is important to recognize that culture goes far beyond our health belief systems to include an understanding of our changing world. A typology to integrate many of the various ideas around culture and health has been developed by MacLachlan (2004) (see Table 4.4).

Table 4.4 A typology of themes relating culture, empowerment and health (MacLachlan, 2004)

Theme	Explanations
Cultural colonialism	Comparisons of the superior 'us' with the inferior 'them' with the aim of managing 'them' in the interests of the elites
Cultural sensitivity	Awareness of the 'them' who now live among 'us' with the aim of making 'our' health care accessible to 'them'
Cultural migration	Awareness of the broad impact of migration on the health and well-being of individuals and communities
Cultural alternativism	Acceptance of different approaches to health care
Cultural empowerment	Empowerment of oppressed groups through cultural reawakening
Cultural globalization	Oppression of indigenous cultures in the interests of the dominant culture/class
Cultural evolution	Impact of the loosening of cultural connections on identities and health

In the remaining sections of this chapter, we will discuss three areas of concern that relate to the changing trends in culture and health: 1) complementary and alternative medicine; 2) racism and health; and 3) the need for **culturally competent health-care systems**.

Complementary and alternative medicine

The biomedical perspective has come to a position of dominance throughout the world, reflecting the imperialistic expansion of Western society more generally. Alternative health-care systems have tended to be disparaged by biomedicine. Being based upon a positivist perspective, the practitioners of biomedicine believe that they have access to a reality that is independent of the patient's effort to understand and control the situation. As such, alternative perspectives are seen as basically wrong. However, alternative professional systems of health care continue to exist in large parts of the world, especially in Asia. Further, as migrants have moved to other countries they have taken their health beliefs with them. In the major Western metropolitan centres there is now extensive availability of health-care systems other than biomedicine. This has led to a feedback into Western ways of thinking about health and illness, especially among those who are disenchanted with biomedicine. Increasingly, **complementary and alternative medicine** (CAM) is gaining popularity and respectability in Western health care. Examples of CAM are listed in Box 4.1.

Box 4.1

Examples of complementary and alternative medicine

Acupuncture
Alexander technique
Aromatherapy
Art therapy
Autogenic training
Ayurvedic medicine
Biofeedback
Breathing techniques
Chiropractic
Dietary and nutritional therapies
Herbal medicine
Homeopathy
Hypnosis
Massage
Meditation
Mindfulness-based stress reduction (MBSR)
Music therapy
Naturopathy
Osteopathy
Qi gong
Reflexology
Reiki
Relaxation techniques
Shiatsu
Tai chi
Therapeutic touch
Traditional Chinese medicine (TCM)
Yoga

In a systematic review of beliefs involved in the use of CAM, Bishop et al. (2007) found that beliefs related to control and participation, perceptions of illness, holism and natural treatments, and general philosophies in life predict CAM use when controlling for demographic and clinical factors. Evidence suggests however that established health professions are very apprehensive at the growth of CAM and are insisting that it meets positivist scientific standards of safety and efficacy (Kelner, Wellman, Boon & Welsh, 2003). Thus in the UK, an evidence base is being developed and maintained by the NHS to provide access to good quality, up-to-date, and relevant information on CAM. This database went live on the Internet on April 2009 at www.evidence.nhs.uk (see Box 4.2).

Box 4.2

NHS evidence – Complementary and alternative medicine, formerly a specialist library of the National Library for Health

Aim: to make good quality, relevant information on complementary and alternative medicine (CAM) available to health professionals and patients.

Target Audience

- General clinicians
- Specialist clinicians
- Other health care professionals (e.g. health care services managers)
- Commissioners and policy makers
- CAM practitioners
- Researchers
- Patients
- General public

Working Definition of CAM Adopted by the Group

> Complementary medicine includes all such practices and ideas which are outside the domain of conventional medicine in several countries and defined by its users as preventing or treating illness, or promoting health and well being. These practices complement mainstream medicine by 1) contributing to a common whole, 2) satisfying a demand not met by conventional practices, and 3) diversifying the conceptual framework of medicine. (Berman, 2006)

Types of Information Included in the Collection

The content of the CAM specialist collection focuses on high quality evidence-based information and includes additional information useful to the CAM community as well as to health care professionals and patients. The following information types will be included:

- Cochrane Reviews (protocols of ongoing reviews will also be included)
- DARE structured abstracts of systematic reviews and DARE provisional records
- Other systematic reviews
- Health Technology Assessment (HTA) reports
- Cost-effectiveness studies from the NHS Economic Evaluation Database
- National and selected international guidelines and guidance
  Guidelines focusing on specific CAM therapies will be included as well as guidelines with a focus on a particular medical condition, which cover CAM therapies. *The latter will be included when it is possible to add a paragraph the resource description pointing to the CAM relevant content.*
- Reference materials (e.g., e-books, online CAM information resources, electronic journals; journals with full text availability from Core Content sources; other relevant publications – subject to evaluation and editorial review)
- Patient information (subject to evaluation and editorial review)
- News and events items (subject to evaluation and editorial review)
- Selected recent large-scale surveys on CAM usage (subject to editorial review)
- Large-scale randomised controlled trials (RCTs) will be included as part of the content for Annual Evidence Updates

Source: http://www.library.nhs.uk/cam

Racism and Health

It is well-established that **racism** contributes to poor health among migrants, ethnic minority groups and indigenous peoples. A review of recent literature (2005–2007) carried out by Williams and Mohammed (2009) continues to show the relationship between discrimination and ill-health. Everyday experiences of discrimination were shown to contribute to stress which could potentially lead to chronic illnesses (Gee et al., 2007). There were also strong associations between racial discrimination and common mental health problems (Schulz et al., 2006). Interpersonal racism and perceived racism in the wider society were also shown to increase the risk of developing psychiatric disorders, after controlling for demographic factors (Karlson et al., 2005). There are various factors that influence racism and discrimination against various communities and cultural groups. One such factor is the media's contribution to this process through the way they portray particular communities in society (Nairn, Peaga, McCreanor, Rankine & Barnes, 2006). A recent open-peer commentary in the *Journal of Health Psychology* raised a debate concerning the issue of racist humour in the media and the role of health psychologists in challenging such oppressive social practices (see Box 4.3).

Box 4.3

Open-peer commentary on racist humour, the media and health

This debate was sparked by the controversial airing of the BBC comedy show 'Harry and Paul' which portrayed a Filipino domestic worker as a sex object. Outraged members of the Filipino community in London demanded for an apology from the BBC and the producers of the show for inciting racial discrimination (see Figure 4.2). It has been argued that the sketch in question insensitively touched on social issues that are widely experienced by vulnerable migrant communities such as human rights abuses against domestic workers and third world poverty and labour migration (Estacio, 2009). Although it was generally acknowledged that racist humour in the media is unacceptable, Hodgetts and Stolte (2009) highlighted the complexity of media content which can contain both racist and anti-racist social representations and warned health psychologists not to overstate the negative influence of the media on racism in society. Nonetheless, it was agreed in these discussions that health psychologists need to take a more active stance in challenging social oppression and its consequences on health by prioritizing 'concrete', real-world social issues (Cornish, 2009) and by carrying out research at micro (McVittie & Goodall, 2009), community (Stephens, 2009), and macro levels (MacLachlan, 2009).

WE WANT
PUBLIC APOLO
FROM THE BB
& PRODUCERS
HARRY & PAU
STOP
RACIST COMED

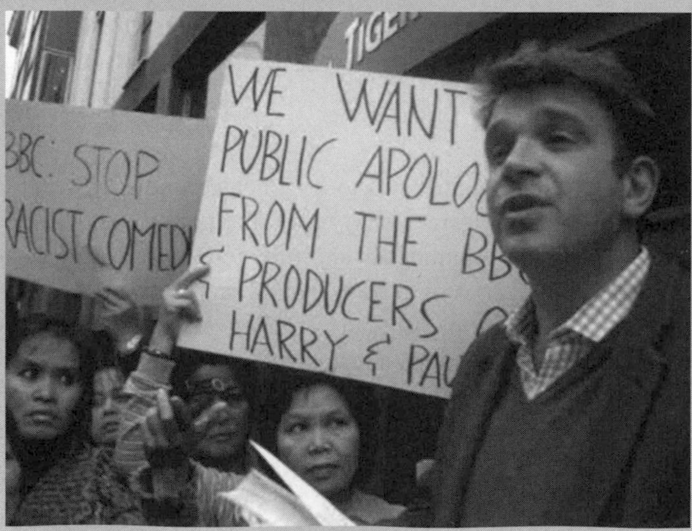

Figure 4.2 Tiger Aspect Productions apologizes for the offence caused by the 'Harry and Paul' show (www.onephilippines.co.uk)

Source: *Journal of Health Psychology*, 2009

Culturally Competent Health-care Systems

There is a need for health-care systems to be culturally competent and to be able to adapt accordingly to the ever changing demographic and cultural trends in today's society. Anderson et al. (2003) provided a conceptual model on how cultural competence can potentially reduce racial and ethnic disparities in health (see Figure 4.3).

The underlying argument for this model asserts the importance of clients and providers being able to clearly communicate and understand each other. As the authors argued, 'when

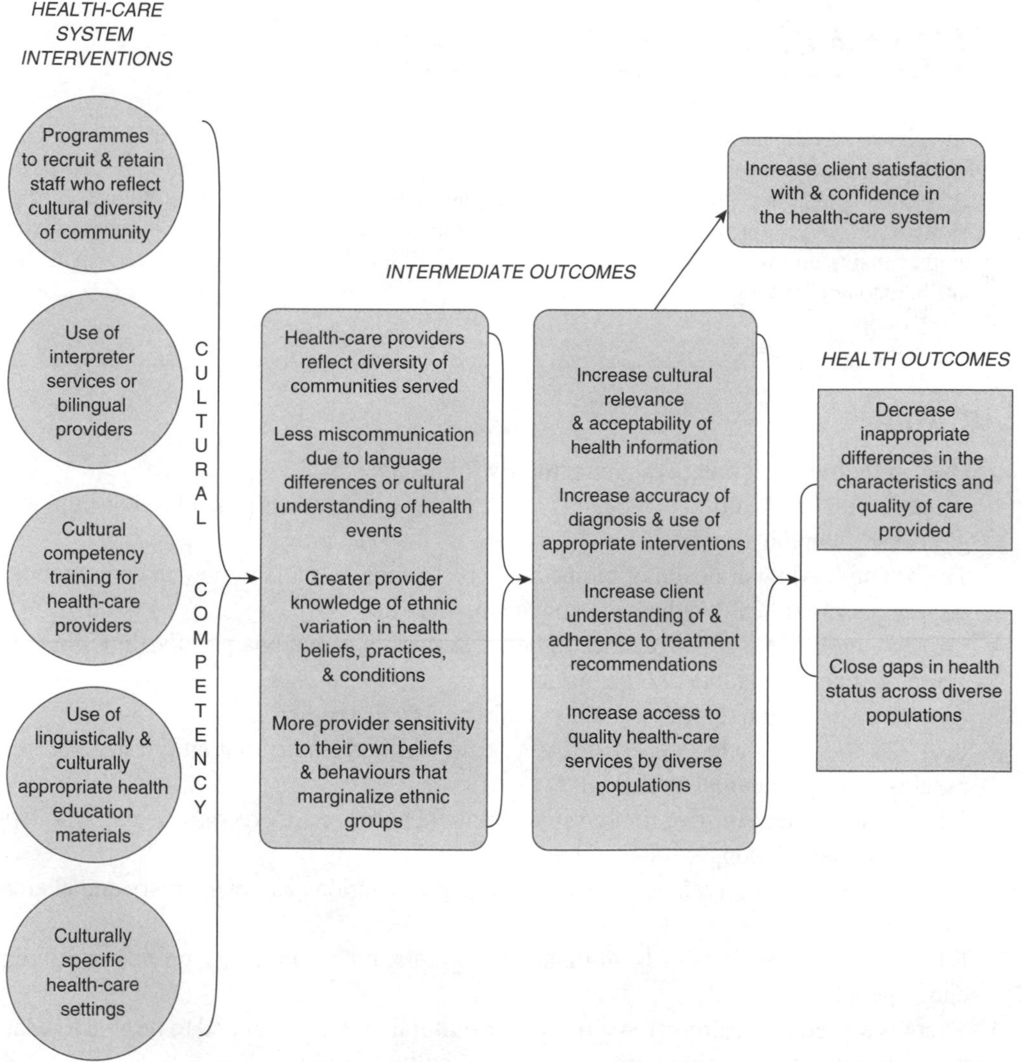

Figure 4.3 Conceptual model on cultural competence in health-care

Source: Anderson et al., 2003: 72; reproduced with permission

clients do not understand what their health-care providers are telling them, and providers either do not speak the client's language or are insecure to cultural differences, then the quality of health care can be compromised' (Anderson et al., 2003: 68). This resonates key ideas of effective communication (see Chapter 11) and the role of **health literacy** in health promotion (see Chapter 14). Beagan and Kumas-Tan (2009) also advocated *self-reflection* among practitioners and the acknowledgement of how both their and their patients' individual and socio-cultural influences contribute to the experience of health and health care.

FUTURE RESEARCH

1 Through access to historical documents, psychologists can assist in expanding our understanding of the evolution of contemporary health beliefs.
2 Understanding of popular health beliefs requires an understanding of their social and cultural context.
3 The increasing development of alternative health care in Western society requires ongoing research.
4 Comprehensive and accurate measurement of perceived discrimination and its mechanisms that contribute to poor health.

Summary

1 Human thought and practices are culturally immersed.
2 Western view of health has moved through various stages from the classic to the religious and then the scientific.
3 The scientific view of health or biomedicine is the most dominant view in contemporary society but other health belief systems remain popular.
4 Chinese medicine is an expert health belief system that remains popular in China and among Chinese migrants in other societies.
5 Ayurvedic medicine remains popular in other parts of Southern Asia.
6 In Africa there is a wide variety of other health belief systems that emphasize spiritual aspects and a communal orientation.
7 Interventions that aim to promote indigenous health need to recognize the wholistic notion of health among these communities.
8 In contemporary society there is increasing interest in various complementary and alternative therapies.
9 Racism contributes to poor health among migrants, ethnic minority groups and indigenous peoples.
10 There is a need for health-care systems to be culturally competent and to be able to adapt accordingly to the changing demographic and cultural trends.

5

A–Z of Research Methods in Health Psychology

Outline

This chapter presents a basic A–Z of research and methods within health psychology. Not all letters have a method, but those that do generally fall into one of three categories: *quantitative*, *qualitative* and *action research*. Quantitative research designs place emphasis on reliable and valid measurement in controlled experiments, trials and surveys. Qualitative methods use interviews, focus groups, narratives or texts to explore health and illness concepts and experience. Action research enables change processes to directly feed back into improvement, empowerment and emancipation.

INTRODUCTION

Health psychology generates a diversity of research questions and requires a wide range of methods to answer them. As the field develops, the role of theory and model development is crucial. However, methodology is of equal importance in testing theories and models, putting theory into practice, and evaluating the consequences of doing so. In applying health psychology principles and practice in health work by making interventions or taking concerted actions to produce change, it is necessary to be evidence based. Interest in action research and methods of evaluation is increasing.

Many of psychology's traditional methods and research designs are quantitative in nature, placing emphasis on reliable and valid measurement in controlled investigations with experiments, trials and surveys. Multiple sources of such evidence can be synthesized using systematic reviews and meta-analysis. Case studies are more suited to unique, one-off situations that require investigation. Qualitative methods use interviews, focus groups, narratives or texts to explore health and illness concepts and experience. Action research enables change processes to feed back into plans for improvement, empowerment and emancipation. These three different kinds of method complement each other, and all are necessary in painting a complete picture of psychology and health.

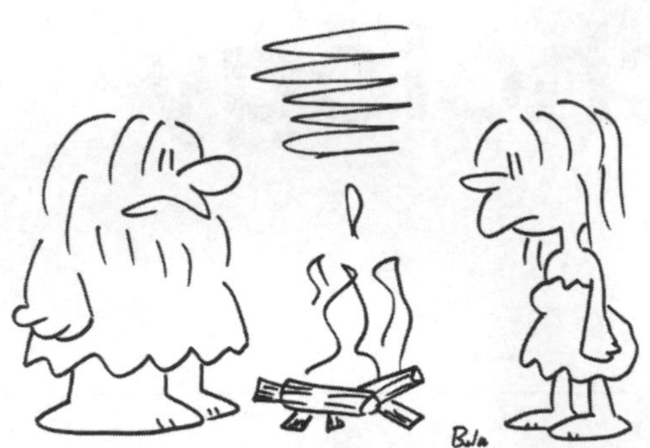

"I was just rubbing sticks together for fun — I didn't realize I was doing basic research."

Reprinted by permission of www.cartoonstock.com

No method is essentially 'better' or 'worse' than any other. A method that suits one purpose will not suit another. Which method is appropriate in any given situation depends entirely upon the question being asked and the context. The sections below present an A–Z of the most commonly used methods for data collection and analysis in health psychology. The majority of studies in health psychology have used the methods or designs described below. Progress in health psychology follows a creative problem-solving approach by many different individuals and groups using a multiplicity of skills and expertise of which implementation of sound methodology is but one. Rigour in methodology needs to be appropriately matched by rigour in theory and practice.

The most basic human curiosity to understand how things work remains a primary motive for carrying out research.

ACTION RESEARCH

Action research is concerned with the process of change and what is decided upon to stimulate change. The investigator acts as a facilitator/collaborator/agent-of-change who works with the stakeholders in a community or organization to help a situation to develop or make a change of direction. The aim is to bring about change in partnership with the community or organization concerned. Action research is particularly suited to organizational and consultancy work when a system or service requires improvements. In a community context it aims to be emancipatory, helping participants to go through an empowering process of increasing agency, control and self-determination.

Action research stems from Kurt Lewin's studies of the 1940s (Lewin, 1947, 1948). The Lewinian perspective on social change is sometimes viewed as 'unscientific' because it does not use control groups or random samples. However this is a misunderstanding of the approach. Lewin wrote about what he called 'Feedback problems of social diagnosis and action' (1947: 147–53) and presented a diagram (p. 149) of his method (see Figure 5.1 below).

Figure 5.1 shows a series of feedback loops in which changes to plans might result from the preliminary results of initial actions. Disciples of Lewin (e.g. Argyris, 1975) interpret Lewin in terms

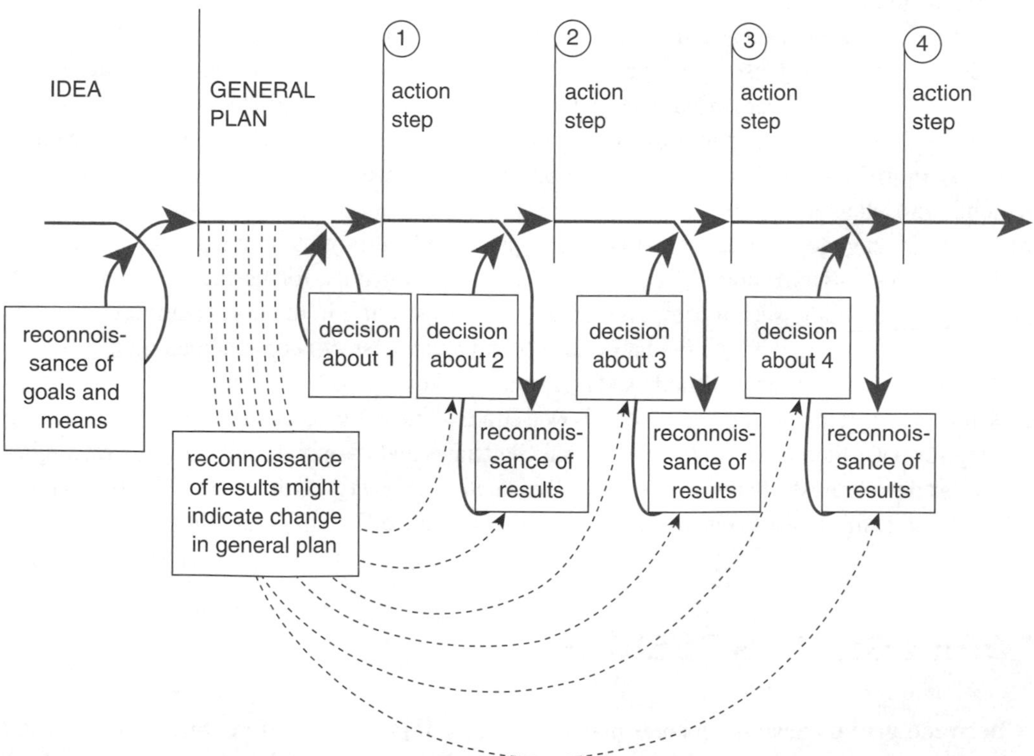

Figure 5.1 Planning, fact-finding and execution as described by Kurt Lewin (1947)

of increasing participation and collaboration of community members, stakeholders and researchers in the design and interpretation of the study. Feedback of the early results to the participants often can lead to redesigning methods or theory in light of consultation meetings about the findings.

As yet the various forms of action research have not been used extensively within health psychology. However, there is growing evidence of a certain resistance among communities and individuals at what can be characterized as research surveillance. This is reflected in the increased demand that researchers deliberately demonstrate the relevance of their work to participants and actively share with them their findings. This can be considered a weak form of action research. Simultaneously there has been an increasing recognition of the limitations of traditional didactic approaches to health promotion (see Chapter 11 and Campbell, 2004b).

Many PAR researchers have used the arts as a vehicle for promoting change. A particularly effective example is the use of photo-novella (Wang, Burris & Xiang, 1996a; Lykes, 2001) whereby community residents were offered the opportunity to reflect on their own community and to consider broader health issues through photography. Through the process of taking and displaying photographs the community members became more aware of themselves and were able to mobilize around particular local issues to campaign for greater resources. (For an in-depth discussion of the use of photo-novella within PAR, see Lykes (2000), which is Reading 25 in Marks (2002a).)

Drama can also be used as a means of creating community awareness. A study of accidents in a fishing community used this approach (Murray & Tilley, 2004). In this study interviews and group discussions were initially held with fish harvesters. Local artists then used this material to develop a variety of compositions including a song and a play. Gray and his colleagues (Gray, Ivonoffski & Sinding, 2001; Gray & Sinding, 2002) transformed interviews with cancer patients into plays that were subsequently performed to support groups. Participatory action research can engage in direct social action to promote health-related change. An example is assisting in the organization of housing campaigns with groups for homeless people. Yeich (1996) described how such a campaign could involve assisting in the organization of demonstrations and working with the media to raise broad awareness of people's housing needs.

Action research is often a method that takes time and requires collaboration with different agencies. It is also an approach that does not follow a straight line but proceeds in a much more halting zig-zag format. Often there are many personal challenges and disappointments for the researcher who must devote substantial emotional as well as intellectual energy to the project (Brydon-Miller, 2004). Despite this it also offers much promise for a revitalized health psychology.

BETWEEN GROUPS DESIGNS

A **between groups design** allocates matched groups of people to different treatments. If the measures are taken at one time this is sometimes called a **cross-sectional design**, in contrast to a **longitudinal design** where the groups are tested at two or more time-points.

When we are comparing only treatment groups, a failure to find a difference between them on the outcome measure(s) might be for one of three reasons: they are equally effective; they are equally ineffective; they are equally harmful. For this reason, one of the groups should be a **control group** that will enable us to discover whether the treatment(s) shows a different effect from no treatment.

Ethical issues arise over the use of control groups. Not treating someone in need of treatment is unacceptable. However, if there is genuine uncertainty about what works best, it is better to compare the treatments with a control condition than to continue for ever applying a treatment that may be less effective than another. Once we have determined which therapy *is* the most effective, this should be offered to the control group and to all future patients (see Clark-Carter & Marks, 2004).

The choice of the control condition is important. The group should receive the same amount of attention as those in the treatment condition(s). This type of control is known as a **placebo control** (see below) as treatment itself could have a non-specific effect to 'please' the client and enhance his/her well-being.

If all of the various groups' responses are measured only after an intervention, then we haven't really measured change. All groups, including the control group, could have changed but from different starting positions, and failing to find a difference between the groups after the treatment could miss this. We can help to deal with this problem by using a mixed design when we measure all groups before and after the treatment. However, we would be introducing some of the difficulties mentioned above for a cross-over or within-subjects design (see Clark-Carter, 1997).

CASE STUDIES

The term 'case study' is used to describe a detailed descriptive account of an individual, group or collective. The purpose of such **case studies** is to provide a 'thick description' (Geertz, 1973) of a phenomenon that would not be obtained by the usual quantitative or qualitative approaches. It requires the researcher to be expansive in the type of data collected with a deliberate aim to link the person with the context, e.g. the sick person in the family.

In developing the case study the researcher usually attempts to provide a chronological account of the evolution of the phenomenon from the perspective of the central character. A challenge for the researcher is in establishing the boundaries of the case. These need to be flexible to ensure that all information germane to the case under investigation is collected.

The major strength of the case study is the integration of actor and context and the developmental perspective. Thus the phenomenon under investigation is not dissected but rather maintains its integrity or wholeness and it is possible to map its changes over time.

There are several different types of case study. The empirical case study is grounded in the data. The aim of this type of case study is to see the general in the particular. Thus the researcher tries to move from the specific to the general in an inductive manner. The theoretical case is an exemplar for a process that has already been clarified. The latter case is the one often used in clinical teaching. These clinical cases will be selected to provide the best examples of a particular phenomenon. The case histories provided by Freud are classic examples of this form. Often the researcher will move back and forward in his/her research identifying certain patterns in a particular case and then confirming and extending his/her understanding in another case.

The researcher can use a variety of techniques to collect information for the case study. Thus the researcher can conduct interviews, or repeat interviews and observe the case in different settings.

The process of analysis can be considered the process of shaping the case. Thus the researcher selects certain pieces of information and discards others so as to present a more integrated case. This is a challenge since at this stage the creative role of the researcher assumes importance.

CONFIDENCE INTERVAL

A **confidence interval** (CI) is the interval around the mean of a sample that one can state with a known probability contains the mean of the population. A population parameter is always estimated using a sample. The reliability of the estimate varies according to sample size. A confidence interval specifies a range of values within which a parameter is estimated to lie. The narrower the interval, the more reliable the estimate. Typically the 95 per cent or 99 per cent CI is stated in the results of a study which has obtained a representative sample of values, e.g. the mean heart rate for a sample might be 75.0 with a 95 per cent CI of 72.6–77.4. Confidence intervals are normally reported in tables or graphs along with point estimates of the parameters, to indicate the reliability of the estimates.

CROSS-OVER OR WITHIN-PARTICIPANTS DESIGNS

The **cross-over or within-participants design** is used when the same people provide measures at more than one time and differences between the measures at the different times are recorded. An example would be a measure taken before an intervention (pre-treatment) and again after the intervention (post-treatment). Such a design minimizes the effect of individual differences as each person acts as his or her own control.

There are a number of problems with this design. Any change in the measure may be due to other factors having changed. For example, you may have introduced an intervention that is designed to improve quality of life (QoL) among patients in a particular long-stay ward of a hospital but the hospital has also introduced other changes, for example, a new set of menus introduced by the catering department. In addition, the difference may be due to some aspect of the measuring instrument. If the same measure is being taken on both occasions, the fact that it has been taken twice may be the reason that the result has changed. If, to get around this problem, a different version of the measure is used then the difference might be due to the difference in the nature of the measures and not the efficacy of the intervention.

Another issue is that failure to find a difference between the two occasions doesn't tell you much; in a worsening situation the intervention still might have been effective in preventing things from worsening more than they have already. Additionally, if you use a cross-over design to compare two or more treatments, the particular results could be an **artefact** of the order in which the treatments were given. Perhaps there is a carry-over effect so that later trials show improvement as a result of practice or later trials could demonstrate poorer performance as a result of fatigue and these effects would have happened even if the treatment had remained the same. To counter such order effects one can use a baseline or 'washout period' before and after treatment periods. Also one can randomly assign people to different orders or, if one is interested in seeing whether order does have an effect then a more systematic allocation of participants to different orders can be employed: e.g. if there are only two conditions participants could be alternately placed in the two possible orders, or if there are more than two conditions a Latin square design could be employed. Such systematic allocations of participants allow us to test formally whether there is an effect of order (see Clark-Carter and Marks, 2004 for further details).

CROSS-SECTIONAL STUDIES

Cross-sectional studies obtain responses from respondents on one occasion only. With appropriate randomized sampling methods, the sample can be assumed to be a representative cross-section of the population(s) under study and it is possible to make comparisons between sub-groups (e.g. males versus females, older versus younger people, etc.). Cross-sectional designs are quite common because they are relatively inexpensive in time and resources. However, there are problems of interpretation whenever there is doubt about the randomness/representativeness of the samples. Also cause and effect can never be inferred between one variable and another and it is impossible to say whether the associations that may be observed are caused by a third variable not measured in the study. Examples of cross-sectional studies and the associated problems of interpretation may be found in Chapter 12.

DIARY TECHNIQUES

In health research diaries (**diary techniques**) have been frequently used as a method for collecting information about temporal changes in health status. These diaries can be prepared

Table 5.1 The applicability of a diary to psychological research (Reid et al., 2003)

Diary uses	Description of use	Example of population used	References
Gold standard	Possible to validate use of questionnaires examining the same behavioural change or psychological characteristics as recorded in diary.	Chronic headache sufferers	Stewart, Lipton, Simon, Liberman and Von Korff (1999)
Reflective practice/medical documentation	Traditional use of diary to note observations and thoughts regarding illness/treatment/ research.	Health care provider	Heath (1998)
Communication device	Provides a voice for the patient and an insight into how the patient interprets illness and treatment.	Patients with longstanding illness	Stensland and Malterud (1999)
Evolving methodology	Provides an opportunity to gain qualitative data that can inform hypothesis generation and testing.	ICU patients and families	Berghom, Svensson, Berggren and Kamsula (1999)
Tracking/time series	Psychological, behavioural and physiological data can be collected to map changes over time.	Sleep/wake times	Eissa, Poffenbarger and Portman (2001)
Efficacy of treatment	Outcome measure.	Behavioural therapy for irritable bowel syndrome	Heyman-Monnikes, Arnold, Florin, Herda, Melfsen and Monnikes (2000)

by either the researcher or participant or both, and they can be quantitative or qualitative or both. They can be compared to the time charts that have been used by health professionals for generations to track changes in the health status of individuals.

A useful summary of the current uses of the diary in health research has been prepared by Reid, Asbury, McDonald and Serpell (2003) and is reproduced in Table 5.1.

Diaries have been especially used as an aid to the evaluation of particular interventions. The more detailed the diary records the more detailed the evaluation. However, a major challenge is convincing the research participant to complete the diary entry on a regular basis. Often, they will be completed at irregular intervals or alternatively several entries may be completed at the same time. It is essential that the participant see the value in completing the diary.

Evidence suggests that diary keeping can have benefits for the participant irrespective of the researcher. Works by Pennebaker (1995) and others have confirmed that writing can be psychologically beneficial. A series of empirical studies have provided evidence that journal writing can lead to reduction in illness symptoms and in the use of health services (e.g. Smyth,

Stone, Hurewitz & Kaell, 1999). There are a number of explanations for this including release of emotional energy, cognitive processing and assistance with narrative restructuring.

DIRECT OBSERVATION

The simplest kind of study involves directly observing behaviour in a relevant setting, for example, patients waiting for treatment in a doctor's surgery or clinic. The observation may be accompanied by recordings in written, oral, auditory or visual form. Several investigators may observe the same events and reliability checks conducted. **Direct observation** includes casual observation, formal observation and participant observation. However, ethical issues are raised by planned formal observational studies of people who have not consented to such observations.

DISCOURSE ANALYSIS

Discourse analysis is a set of procedures for analysing language as used in speech or texts. It focuses on the language and how it is used to construct versions of 'social reality' and what is gained by constructing events using the particular terms being used. It has links with ethnomethodology, conversation analysis and the study of meaning (semiology).

Two forms of discourse analysis have evolved over the past decade. The former, now termed *discursive psychology*, evolved from the work of Potter and Wetherell (1987) and is particularly concerned with the conversational context of the discourse. According to this approach language is 'a medium of social action rather than a mode for representing thoughts and ideas' (Edwards, 1997: 84). Discursive psychology is concerned with the discursive strategies people use to further particular actions in social situations, including accounting for their own behaviour or thoughts. These strategies are not considered evidence of participants' insincerity or of impression management but rather part of the social construction of identity in everyday conversation. This approach has been used to explore the character of patient talk and the character of doctor–patient interactions. There is a particular preference for naturally occurring conversations, e.g. mealtime talk (Wiggins, Potter & Wildsmith, 2001).

The other approach is known as critical or *Foucauldian discourse analysis* (FDA). This approach has been especially developed by Ian Parker (1997) who criticizes the previous approach as evading issues of power and politics. FDA aims to identify the broader discursive resources that people in a particular culture draw upon in their everyday lives. These resources not only shape the way we interpret and act in the world but also how we define ourselves. This approach has been used to explore such health issues as smoking (Gillies & Willig, 1997) and anorexia nervosa (Benveniste et al., 1999). They each are concerned with how the discourse resources that are drawn upon in turn position people in certain ways.

EFFECT SIZE

An **effect size** is the strength of the association between study variables and outcome as measured by an observed difference or correlation. Cohen's *d* and Pearson's *r* are the most popular indices of effect size in psychological studies. The effect size is a measure of the importance of an effect rather than its statistical significance. Effect sizes are used in meta-analysis as a means of measuring the magnitude of the results obtained over different studies. Effect size is related to the power of a study to detect a difference that really exists. A weak study cannot detect a real difference because it has samples that are too small relative to the magnitude of the difference that exists, a common problem in psychology. It has been estimated that approximately 60–70 per cent of published studies in psychology journals lack sufficient power to obtain statistical significance.

ETHNOGRAPHIC METHODS

Ethnographic methods seek to build a systematic understanding of a culture from the viewpoint of the insider. Ethnographic methods are multiple attempts to describe the shared beliefs, practices, artefacts, knowledge and behaviours of an intact cultural group. They attempt to represent the totality of a phenomenon in its complete context in its naturalistic setting.

Detailed observation is an important part of ethnographic fieldwork. The observation can be either overt or covert. In the overt case the researcher does not attempt to disguise his/her identity but rather is unobstrusive such that the phenomenon under investigation is not disturbed. In this case the researcher can take detailed notes, in either a prearranged or discursive format.

In certain cases the researcher may decide that his/her presence may disturb the field. In this case two forms of covert observation may be used. In one form the focus of observation is not aware at all of the presence of the researcher. Thus the researcher may observe the person from behind a screen or record conversation unobstrusively using an audio or video-recorder. An alternative approach is when the person observed may be aware of the researcher's presence but is unaware that he/she is a researcher. To achieve this covert form of observation the researcher becomes a participant observer by which he/she engages in complementary activities to that of the case. In both of these forms the researcher needs to consider the ethics of deception.

A form of participant observation that is not covert is when the researcher accompanies the person but tries not to interfere with the performance of everyday tasks. A classic example of this is Willis' (1977) study of the entry of working-class boys into the workplace. In this study Willis sat in during classes in school and accompanied the boys during their first weeks at work. He also conducted individual and group interviews with the boys, their teachers and parents. In addition, he considered other material such as careers brochures and other printed material available to the boys. At all times the boys were aware of Willis but gradually accepted him as part of the background. To be accepted the researcher usually has to show some empathy with the study participants. Again, the researcher needs to consider the broader ethical issues of apparently espousing certain beliefs and engaging in certain activities.

FOCUS GROUPS

Focus groups comprise one or more group discussions in which participants 'focus' collectively upon a topic or issue usually presented to them as a group of questions, although sometimes as a film, a collection of advertisements, cards to sort, a game to play, or a vignette to discuss. The distinctive feature of the focus group method is its generation of interactive data (Wilkinson, 1998).

Focus groups were initially largely used in marketing research. As its title implied they had a focus that was to clarify the participants' views on a particular product. Thus from the outset the researcher had set the parameters of the discussion and as it proceeded he/she deliberately guided the discussion such that its focus remained limited.

More recent use of the focus group has been much more expansive. In many cases the term *discussion group* is preferred to give an indication of this greater latitude. This approach was originally developed by Willis (1977) to explore working-class boys' views on life and work. In this case the participants have a much greater say on the direction of the group conversation and so it can be considered more naturalistic.

The role of the researcher in the focus group is to act as the moderator for the discussion. The researcher can follow similar guidelines as those with an interview by using a guide, except that the discussion should be allowed to flow freely and not constrained too much by the investigator's agenda. The researcher needs to ensure that all the group participants have opportunity to express their viewpoints.

At the beginning of the discussion the researcher should follow the usual guidelines. It is important that the group is briefed on the basic principles of confidentiality and respect for different opinions. It is useful for them to know each others' first names and to have name badges. This facilitates greater interaction. It is also useful to have some refreshments available.

Although it is usual for the moderator to introduce some themes for discussion, this can be supplemented with a short video extract or pictures relevant to the topic being investigated. As the discussion proceeds, the researcher can often take a background role, but ensuring that the discussion does not deviate too far from the focus of the research and that all the participants have an opportunity to express their views.

It is useful to have an assistant or a colleague participate in focus group research. This person can help completing consent forms, providing name-tags, organizing refreshments, keeping notes on who is talking (this is useful for transcription), and monitoring the recording equipment. The focus group recording should be transcribed as soon as possible afterwards since it is often difficult to distinguish speakers.

GROUNDED THEORY ANALYSIS

Grounded theory analysis is a term used to describe a set of guidelines for conducting qualitative data analysis. It was originally developed by Glaser and Strauss (1967) and has subsequently gone through various revisions.

In its original form qualitative researchers were asked to dispense with theoretical assumptions when they began their research. Rather they were encouraged to adopt a stance of *disciplined naivety*. As the research progresses certain theoretical concepts are discovered and then tested in an iterative fashion. In the case of the qualitative interview, the researcher is encouraged to begin the analysis at a very early stage, even as the interview is progressing. Through a process of *abduction* the researcher begins to develop certain theoretical hypotheses. These hypotheses are then integrated into a tentative theoretical model that is tested as more data is collected.

This process follows a series of steps beginning with generating data. At this stage the researcher may have some general ideas about the topic but this should not restrict the talk of the participant. From the very initial stages the researcher is sifting through the ideas presented and seeking more information about what are considered to be emerging themes. From a more positivist perspective it is argued that the themes emerge from the data and that the researcher has simply to look for them. This approach is often associated with Glaser (1992). From a more social constructionist perspective, certain theoretical concepts of the researcher will guide both the data collection and analysis. This approach is more associated with the symbolic interactionist tradition (Strauss, 1987; Charmaz, 2008).

Having collected some data the researcher conducts a detailed coding of it followed by the generation of bigger categories. Throughout the coding the researcher follows the process of *constant comparative analysis*. This involves making comparison of codes within and between interview transcripts. This is followed by the stage of *memo-writing* which requires the researcher to begin to expand upon the meaning of the broader conceptual categories. This in turn can lead to further data generation through *theoretical sampling*. This is the process whereby the researcher deliberately selects certain participants or certain research themes to explore further because of the data already analysed. At this stage the researcher is both testing and strengthening the emergent theory. At a certain stage in this iterative process the researcher feels that he/she has reached the stage of *data saturation* – no new concepts are emerging and it is considered fruitless to continue with data collection.

HISTORICAL ANALYSIS

Health and illness are socially and historically located phenomena. As such psychologists have much to gain by detailed historical research (**historical analysis**) on the development of health beliefs and practices. They can work closely with medical or health historians to explore the evolution of scientific and popular beliefs about health and illness or they can work independently (see Chapter 3).

An excellent example is the work of Herzlich and Pierret (1987). Their work involved the detailed analysis of a variety of textual sources such as scientific medical writings but also popular autobiographical and fictional accounts of the experience of illness. They noted the particular value of literary works because of their important contribution to shaping public discourse. Such textual analysis needs to be guided by an understanding of the political and philosophical ideas of the period.

All societies have ways of interpreting the world and defining health and illness. For example, historically people in Western society attributed illness to various supernatural forces. However, with the scientific revolution ideas about illness were increasingly located within the physical body. More recently we have increased concern about a wider definition of health encompassing quality of life. An understanding of these changing ideas requires connecting them to the changing historical periods (e.g. Porter, 1997; Flick, 2002).

Health psychologists need also to be reflexive about the history of their own discipline. It arose at a particular historical period sometimes described as late modernity. Initially it was seen as providing a complement to the excessive physical focus of biomedicine. Now some see it as part of the broader lifestyle movement.

There are different approaches to the writing of history. There are those who can be broadly characterized as descriptive and who often provide a listing of the growth of the discipline in laudatory terms (e.g. Stone, Weiss, Matarazzo, Miller & Rodin, 1987). Conversely there are those who adopt a more critical approach and attempt to dissect the underlying reasons for the development of the discipline. Within health psychology, this latter approach is still in its early stages (e.g. Stam, 2004).

Such writings can be complemented with interviews with elderly people about their health problems and their experiences with health services in their youth. This oral historical research connects with ageing and narrative research. This work can enable the researcher to identify the changing character of health beliefs and practices. In turn, this work can be connected to forms of action research.

INTERPRETATIVE PHENOMENOLOGICAL ANALYSIS

Phenomenological research is concerned with exploring the lived experience of health, illness and disability. Its aim is to understand these phenomena from the perspective of the particular participant. A challenge for the researcher is how, as it were, to get inside the head of the person being investigated through what the person has to say about the experience. This in turn has to be interpreted by the researcher. A technique that addresses this challenge is **interpretative phenomenological analysis (IPA)** (Smith, 2004).

IPA focuses on the cognitive processing of the participant. Smith (2004) argues that it accords with the original direction of cognitive psychology being concerned with exploring meaning-making rather than information-processing. IPA also accepts that what the study participants have to say has to be interpreted by the researcher since their perceptions and interpretations are not directly accessible.

IPA provides a guide to conducting this interpretation. It begins by accessing the participant's perceptions through the conduct of an interview or series of interviews with a homogeneous sample of individuals. The interview is semi-structured and focuses on the particular issue of concern.

The actual data analysis suggested in IPA goes through a number of stages. Initially the researcher reads through the interview transcripts and annotates it identifying any feature of interest in the text. The researcher then re-reads the text and develops a higher order thematic analysis. The skill at this stage is to develop these more abstract categories that are clearly rooted in the text and that can be connected across cases. Having identified the key themes or categories the researcher then proceeds to look for connections between them by identifying clusters. At this stage the researcher is drawing upon her broader understanding to make sense of what has been said. Once the researcher has finished the analysis of one case he/she can proceed to conduct an analysis of the next case in a similar manner. Alternatively, the researcher can begin to apply the analytic scheme developed in the previous case. The challenge is to identify repeating patterns but also to be alert to new patterns. Further details of this form of analysis are available in Smith, Jarman and Osborn (1999) and Smith and Osborn (2008).

INTERVENTIONS

Interventions are deliberate attempts to facilitate improvements to health. The idea for the intervention can come from a theory or model, from discussions with those who are knowledgeable about the condition or situation that needs to be changed, or from 'out of the blue'. A key aspect of designing, and/or implementing any intervention is evaluation – attempting to prove whether or not the intervention is effective or efficacious. In health psychology there is lack of power in published studies. This lack of power is caused by study samples being too small to permit definite conclusions. Furthermore, reports of intervention studies are typically brief, opaque descriptions of what can often be complex interventions. There is no meaningful method of relating the practice of behaviour change to any single theory or taxonomy. This means that the researcher does not know how to label what they have done in a way that communicates this in any precise manner to others (Marks, 2009). A key criterion for the reporting of an intervention must be *transparency*. Can another person or group repeat the study in his/her/their own setting with his/her/their own participants? The need to be concise in publishing studies means that the level of detail required for successful replication may often be missing. It is, therefore, almost impossible for new investigators to repeat a published intervention with any exactitude in their own settings.

CONSORT guidelines for randomized controlled trials (Moher, Schultz & Altman, 2001) and the TREND statement for non-randomized studies (Des Jarlais, Lyles & Crepaz, 2004) were intended to bridge the gap between intervention descriptions and intended replications. These guidelines have driven efforts to improve the transparency of reports of intervention studies. Davidson and colleagues (2003) expanded the CONSORT guidelines by proposing that authors should report: (1) the content or elements of the intervention; (2) characteristics of those delivering the intervention; (3) characteristics of the recipients; (4) the setting; (5) the mode of delivery; (6) the intensity; (7) the duration; and (8) adherence to delivery protocols/manuals.

INTERVIEWS (SEMI-STRUCTURED)

Semi-structured interviews are designed to explore the participant's view of things with the minimal amount of assumptions from the interviewer. Open-ended questions are useful in this kind of interview. They have several advantages over closed-ended questions. The answers will not be biased by the researcher's preconceptions as much as closed-ended questions can be. The respondents are able to express their opinions, thoughts and feelings freely using their own words in ways that are less constrained by the particular wordings of the question. The respondents may have responses that the structured interview designer has overlooked. They may have in-depth comments that they wish to make about your study and the topics that it is covering that would not be picked up using the standard questions in a structured interview.

In preparing for the interview the researcher should develop an interview guide. This can include a combination of primary and supplementary questions. Alternatively, the researcher may prefer to have a list of themes to be explored. However, it is important that the researcher does not formally follow these in the same order but rather introduces them at the appropriate time in the interview. Prior to the interview, the researcher should review these themes and order them from the least invasive to the more personal.

Some general guides to promote discussion in the interview have been suggested by Wilkinson, Joffe and Yardley (2004):

- Be a good listener: the researcher should show a strong interest in what the participant has to say.
- Be empathetic, not judgemental: the participant can easily be discouraged by any evidence that their viewpoint is not accepted.

- Allow the participant's worldview to develop: encourage the participant to express herself fully in her own words.
- Allow expression of feelings: the participant may be happy, sad or angry about certain experiences. The researcher should not be disturbed by this expression of feelings. It is important to remember that the focus of the interview is research, not psychotherapy, and the researcher should maintain those boundaries. If the interview becomes strained then the researcher and the interviewer should negotiate its continuation.

As with all qualitative research, preparation is essential. Thus the researcher should ensure that the participant knows what the research is about in general terms prior to the interview. Novice interviewers should always liaise closely with their mentors to ensure personal safety and to debrief fully afterwards. This will enable them to refine their interview techniques and possibly review the questions and themes they have used.

INTERVIEWS (STRUCTURED)

A **structured interview** schedule is a prepared, standard set of questions that are asked in person, or perhaps by telephone, of a person or group concerning a particular research issue. A semi-structured interview is more open ended and allows the interviewee to address issues that he/she feels relevant to the topics raised by the investigator.

LONGITUDINAL DESIGNS

These designs involve measuring responses of a single sample on more than one occasion. The measurements may be *prospective* or *retrospective*. Prospective longitudinal designs allow greater control over the sample, the variables measured and the times when the measurements take place. Such designs are superior to cross-sectional designs because one is more able to investigate hypotheses of causation when the associations between variables are measured over time. **Longitudinal designs** are among the most powerful designs available for the evaluation of treatments and of theories about human experience and behaviour, but they are also the most costly in labour, time and money.

META-ANALYSIS

Meta-analysis is the use of statistical techniques to combine the results of primary studies addressing the same question into a single pooled measure of effect size, with a confidence interval. The analysis is often based on the calculation of a weighted mean effect size in which each primary study is weighted according to the number of participants. A meta-analysis follows a series of steps as follows:

1 *Develop a research question*: A concise, clear question is most likely to lead to a clear, unambiguous answer, e.g. Does cognitive behaviour therapy offer a more cost-effective approach to smoking cessation than pharmacotherapy? Or: Does music therapy reduce experienced pain? Or: Does doctor's advice to reduce alcohol consumption lead to reduced drinking?
2 *Identify all relevant studies*: The literature has to be trawled exhaustively for all relevant studies. It is customary practice to consult all major review articles, reference lists, and abstracts in databases such as PsycInfo, Dissertation Abstracts, and PubMed, using Boolean combinations of keywords. At this stage it is not uncommon that several hundred, or even a few thousand, items will be examined. It is essential to examine unpublished theses and dissertations as well as published papers and to include both randomized and nonrandomized studies. Comprehensiveness at this stage is important. Relying on published papers only tends to overestimate the true effect size because there is a publication bias towards publishing only statistically significant findings.
3 *Select studies on the basis of the issue being addressed and methodological criteria*: A clear and precise set of inclusion and exclusion criteria are used to select studies for the analysis. (1) The intervention must be precisely described and defined within the relevant category to address the research question; (2) The sample must fall within the relevant range, e.g. adults over 18; (3) The study design must be suitable and appropriate, for example, a between-groups design in which the treatment is compared to a no-treatment control group or to an alternate treatment group; (4) The report should contain empirical data, provide the necessary information to compute an effect size; fit the appropriate time scale, e.g. between January 1970 and December 2009; and, be reported in the working language(s) of the research team, typically English and/or Spanish and/or French. When a list of such criteria are applied, the selection of studies is normally reduced to around 5–10 per cent of the original total number of items.
4 *Decide which dependent variables or summary measures are allowed*: Treatment outcomes must be assessed to fit appropriate criteria regarding *when, what, and how* the outcome is measured. This criterion will again reduce the selected studies by another factor of perhaps, 50–75 per cent.
5 *Calculate a summary effect*: This will be carried out using one of the recognized indices of effect size, e.g. Cohen's *d* or Pearson's *r*. In some cases a diagram may be produced showing the cumulative effect size as different studies are aggregated to a single summary effect.
6 *Reach a conclusion in answer to the original research question*. The conclusion will follow directly from the summary effect size obtained.

NARRATIVE APPROACHES

This approach is concerned with the desire to seek insight and meaning about health and illness through the acquisition of data in the form of stories concerning personal experiences. These **narrative approaches** assume that human beings are natural storytellers and that the principle task of the psychologist is to explore the different stories being told (Murray, 2008).

The most popular source of material for the narrative researcher is the interview. The focus of the narrative interview is the elicitation of narrative accounts from the interviewee. This can take various forms. The life-story interview is the most extended form of the narrative interview. As its name implies, the life-story interview seeks to obtain an extended account of the person's life. The primary aim is to make the participant at ease and encourage him/her to tell their story at length.

More frequently, the health psychologist is interested in a particular health and illness experience such as what it is like to live with a chronic illness. In this case the focus will be more on the actual lived experience of the illness but bearing in mind that illness exists within a certain social world and cannot be extracted from it.

A particular version of the narrative interview is the episodic interview in which the researcher encourages the participant to speak on a variety of particular experiences (Flick, 2002). This approach assumes that experiences are often stored in memory in narrative-episodes and that the challenge is to reveal these without integrating them into a larger narrative. Throughout the interview the role of the interviewer is to encourage sustained narrative accounting. This can be achieved through a variety of supportive remarks. The researcher can deliberately encourage the participant to expand upon remarks about particular issues.

Narrative analysis (NA) can take various forms. It begins with a repeated reading of the text to identify the story or stories within it. The primary focus is on maintaining the narrative integrity of the account. The researcher may develop a summary of the narrative account that will help identify the structure of the narrative, its tone and the central characters. It may be useful to engage in a certain amount of thematic analysis to identify some underlying themes. But this does not equate with narrative analysis. NA involves trying to see the interconnections between events rather than separating them. Having analysed one case the researcher can then proceed to the next, identifying similarities and differences in the structure and content of the narratives.

This inductive form of analysis does not connect with the theoretical assumptions guiding the researcher. This requires deliberately identifying particular psychological processes underlying the narrative. An example of this is the work of Hollway and Jefferson (2000) who explored the unconscious defences against anxiety underlying narrative accounts of crime. Alternatively, the researcher can connect with personal narrative with the broader cultural narrative (e.g. Crossley, 1999).

OBSERVATIONAL STUDIES

The term **observational studies** is used to describe research carried out to evaluate the effect of an intervention or treatment which does not have the advantages of a control group. A single group of patients are observed at various points before, during and after the treatment in an attempt to ascertain the changes that occur as a result of the treatment. There are strict limitations on the conclusions that can be reached as a consequence of the lack of control group (e.g. see Randomized Controlled Trials). However, there are occasions when a randomized controlled trial is impossible to carry out because of ethical or operational difficulties.

ODDS RATIO

The **odds ratio** (OR) compares the probability of a certain event in two groups. The odds for an event are calculated by using the probability of an event happening and the probability of it not happening. So if I think the probability of rain in a given place on a given date and time is 75 per cent, I am saying that rain at that place and time has an odds of .75/.25 = 3.0, which can otherwise be stated as 3:1. A similar reasoning can be applied to the probabilities of outcomes of various categories in a study. If there is no significant difference in the outcome, then the probability of the outcome will be the same in two different groups of conditions and the odds ratio will be 1.0. An odds ratio of 1.0 implies that the outcome is equally likely in both groups. An odds ratio greater than one implies that the event is more likely in the first group than in the second group. An odds ratio less than one implies that the event is less likely in the first group than in the second group.

Table 5.2 Smoking status by group: 12-month abstinence rates

	CBT group	Control group	Totals
Abstinent	23 (A)	6 (B)	29
Smoking	93 (C)	98 (D)	191
Totals	116	104	220

The data in Table 5.2 are from a randomized controlled trial on smoking cessation that compared abstinence rates for a cognitive behaviour therapy for smokers and a control group receiving standard care at 12-months follow-up (Marks & Sykes, 2002). The two possible outcomes concern smoking status as ‘abstinence’ or ‘smoking’.

The odds of being abstinent relative to being a smoker in the CBT group was 23/93 (A/C). In the control group the odds of being abstinent relative to being a smoker was 6/98 (B/D). The odds ratio, OR, for abstinence in the CBT group versus the control group was $(23 \times 98)/(93 \times 6)$ or $(A \times D)/(C \times B) = 4.039$. Thus CBT was four times more effective than the control condition in producing abstinence at 12 months following the intervention. The 95 per cent confidence interval (see above) for this OR value is 1.57–10.36 (computed in SPSS). As this confidence interval does not include 1.00, there is a statistically significant difference in the OR between the two conditions.

PARTICIPATORY ACTION RESEARCH

Participatory action research (PAR) is a version of action research that deliberately seeks to provoke some form of social or community change (see Box 5.2). The researcher works with the organization or community before defining an issue or research question. The researcher then works with the community in exploring the question and in seeking a solution to the problem. Together the researcher and the community begin to understand the issue and the solution through the very process of action.

Historically, this form of research has been used with socially disadvantaged or marginalized groups. It deliberately links popular education, community-based research and social action (Brydon-Miller, 2004). This focus reflects its broader political commitment to social change. Thus, while the immediate focus of concern may be a particular community issue the PAR researcher does not lose sight of the broader social inequalities within which the community is nested (Campbell & Murray, 2004).

Theoretically PAR draws much inspiration from the work of the Brazilian educator Paulo Freire (1979/1993). Freire's work was especially developed around promoting literacy among impoverished communities in Brazil. Through this work he developed a critique of traditional education. He characterized this as a form of banking in which the teacher is the depositor and the students are the depositories. To this he counterposed the concept of *conscientization*, the process of developing a critical understanding among community members about the broader socio-political contradictions and ways of taking action against oppressive elements.

PAR is also connected with a more generalized liberation psychology. This form of psychology begins with a broad political critique of the injustices in society and locates psychology as a potential agent for change. Martin-Baro (1994) stressed that psychology should start by taking a stand alongside those most oppressed in society: 'We have to redesign our theoretical and practical tools, but redesign them from the standpoint of the lives of our own people: from their sufferings, their aspirations, and their struggles' (1994: 25). PAR involves collaboration between the researcher and the community with a common aim to 'identify an area of concern to that community, generate knowledge about that issue, and plan and carry out actions meant to address the issue in some substantive way' (Brydon-Miller, 2004: 188).

Box 5.2

Example of Participant Action Research

'Health Inequity and Social Injustice for the Aytas in the Philippines: Critical Psychology in Action' (Estacio & Marks, 2007)

This study was a collaborative effort involving an Ayta community, health psychologists, NGOs and the local government in Floridablanca, Philippines. The Aytas were the earliest inhabitants of the archipelago having occupied the territory for approximately 30,000 years. Having the violent eruption of Mount Pinatubo in June 1991, the traditional Ayta way of life is in danger.

The Ayta concept of health incorporates economic, psychosocial, environmental, and spiritual attributes. For the Aytas, achieving health is a process whereby livelihood stability, good social relations, cleanliness, and spiritual wellness are viewed as essential components of a good and decent way of living. Household income averaged at approximately US$1 to $2 a day for a family of five. A day's wage is spent almost instantaneously to buy food and provisions.

Estacio and Marks (2007) worked with a small Ayta community in an effort to improve the health of the community. Consultation and dialogue with key players was divided into seven stages: 1) establishing rapport and planning, 2) knowledge generation, 3) data validation, 4) recommendations for action, 5) planning for action, 6) implementation, and 7) evaluation and follow-up.

Four barriers to health were highlighted: (i) economic exploitation due to unfair trade relations with lowlanders; (ii) inaccessibility of government services restricts the Aytas' fundamental right to health and education; (iii) persisting culture of discrimination; (iv) lack of security of tenure.

Illiteracy and economic exploitation are the main forces that keep the Aytas impoverished, unhappy, and unhealthy. Within the current social structure, they recognized that they are poor and are kept poor by those in power because they are being robbed of their natural wealth, perseverance, and hard work. They are unable to protect themselves from such an injustice since they cannot read, write, or count. Furthermore, since they have been denied their right to education, they have not been given the same opportunity to develop their fullest human potential. The Aytas are feeling hopeless because they are witnessing how poverty, discrimination, and ill health are being passed from one generation to the next.

Although this research was within one small community of 15 households, this group of Aytas is a microcosm of global poverty. The key issue is inequity which is 'those inequalities in health that are deemed to be unfair or stemming from some form of injustice' (Kawachi, Subramanian and Almeida-Filho, 2002, p.647).

Researchers engaged in PAR acknowledge that those living within the community hold the expert knowledge about their situation.

In relation to improving the health/well-being of marginalized communities, empowerment – or the process of increasing people's control over the determinants of health – has been recognized as a key component towards health promotion (World Health Organization, 1986). The process requires the strengthening of skills and capabilities of individuals, communities and social groups. This can be achieved by creating favourable social conditions from micro to macro levels, ensuring equal opportunities for all, and mediating between all sectors of society (Nutbeam, 1999). Within this context, addressing inequalities in health through health promotion becomes a social and political endeavour.

PAR is more an approach rather than a single method. As such it can use both quantitative and qualitative methods so long as they contribute to the overall goal of increasing understanding and promoting social change. It is through the process of social change that the participants begin to understand themselves and the limitations on their social progress.

PLACEBO CONTROL

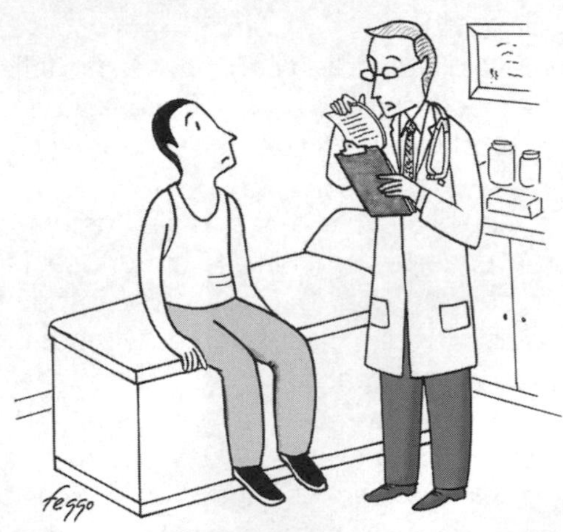

"Apparently your health insurance only covers placebos."

QUESTIONNAIRES

Many constructs are measured using **questionnaires** consisting of a standard set of items with accompanying instructions. Ideally a questionnaire will have been demonstrated to be both a reliable and a valid measure of the construct(s) it purports to measure.

Questionnaires vary in objectives, content, especially in their generic versus specific content, question format, the number of items, and *sensitivity* or *responsiveness* to change. Questionnaires may be employed in cross-sectional and longitudinal studies. In prospective studies the same measures are taken from a number of groups of participants on a number of occasions and the principal objective will be to evaluate the differences that occur between groups across time. When looking for changes over time, the responsiveness of a questionnaire to clinical and subjective changes is a crucial feature. A questionnaire's content, sensitivity and extent, together with its reliability and validity, influence a questionnaire's selection.

Guides are available to advise users on making a choice that contains the appropriate generic measure, domain or disease of interest (e.g. Bowling, 2001, 2004). These guides are extremely useful as they include details on content, scoring, validity and reliability of dozens of questionnaires for measuring all of the major aspects of psychological well-being and quality of life, including disease-specific and domain-specific questionnaires and more generic measures.

There are hundreds of questionnaires available, measuring almost every imaginable aspect of health behaviour and clinical experience. There are some essential characteristics that should be considered in selecting or designing a questionnaire: your objectives, type of respondents, the content, question format, number of items, reliability, validity and sensitivity to change.

The investigator must ask: What is it that I want to know? The answer will dictate the selection of the most relevant and useful questionnaire. The most important aspect of questionnaire selection is therefore to *match the objective of the study with the objective of the questionnaire*. For example, are you interested in a disease-specific or broad ranging research question? When this question is settled, you need to decide whether there is anything else that your research objective will require you to know. Usually the researcher needs to develop a specific block of questions that will seek vital information concerning the respondents' socio-demographic characteristics that can be placed at the beginning or the end of the main questionnaire.

Questionnaire content may vary from the highly generic (e.g. 'How has your health been over the last few weeks: Excellent, Good, Fair, Poor, Very Bad?') to the highly specific (e.g. 'Have you had any arguments with people at work in the last two weeks?'). The items may all be different ways of trying to measure the same thing, or there may be a variety of scales and sub-scales for measuring different dimensions or variables within a single instrument.

Questionnaires vary greatly in the number of items that are used to assess the variable(s) of interest. Single-item measures use a single question, rating or item to measure the concept or variable of interest. For example, the now popular single verbal item to evaluate health status, 'During the past 4 weeks how would you rate your health in general? Excellent, Very good, Good, Fair, Poor'. Single items have the obvious advantages of being simple, direct and brief.

KEY STUDY Self-rated health and mortality: A review of 27 community studies (Idler & Banyamini, 1997)

Traditionally, medical researchers evaluated the health of a population or group by measuring mortality rates (deaths) and illness rates (morbidity). Critics have pointed out that death and illness rates are rather 'blunt instruments' for making an assessment of the overall well-being of people. This led researchers to wonder whether a simple one-item question about how well a person has been might provide a more valid and direct measure of the experience of well-being. A single self-assessed item such as 'How has your health been over the last few weeks: Excellent, Good, Fair, Poor, Very Bad?' has been used for this purpose.

Since 1972, there have been at least 6500 studies which have used self-rated health as a measure of well-being. Idler and Banyamini (1997) reviewed studies of survey respondents' global self-ratings of health as predictors of mortality in longitudinal studies of representative community samples. The review indicated that, until that date, there had been 27 studies in US and international journals which had showed 'impressively consistent findings'. The authors concluded that: 'Global self-rated health is an independent predictor of mortality in nearly all of the studies, despite the inclusion of numerous specific health status indicators and other relevant covariates known to predict mortality' (Idler & Banyamini, 1997, p. 21).

This review shows the value of a person's self assessment of their own health. Questionnaires, even as simple as a single item, can often reveal more than a host of so-called objective measurements about a person's health. In the end, it is how a person feels about their own health that will determine whether they seek help and advice from the health-care system. Many symptoms which are crucial to accurate diagnosis such as pain, dizziness and fatigue can only be reported by the patient. Without this information, a health-care professional is often unable to act.

RANDOMIZED CONTROLLED TRIALS

Randomized controlled trials (RCTs) involve the systematic comparison of interventions using a fully controlled application of one or more 'treatments' with a random allocation of participants to the different treatment groups. This design is the 'gold standard' to which much research in psychology and health care aspires. Participants are allocated randomly to one or more intervention conditions and to a control condition. The statistical tests that are available have as one of their assumptions that participants have been randomly assigned to conditions. However, when researchers move beyond the laboratory setting to real world clinical and health research, it soon becomes evident that the so-called 'gold standard' cannot always be achieved, in practice, and, in fact, may not be desirable for ethical reasons.

We are frequently forced to study existing groups that are being treated differently rather than have the luxury of being able to allocate people to conditions. Thus, we may in effect be comparing the health policies and services of a number of different hospitals and clinics. Such a design is sometimes described as '**quasi-experimental design**' in that we are comparing treatments in as controlled a manner as possible, but we have been unable for practical reasons to manipulate the independent variable, the policies, or allocate the participants ourselves.

The advantage of a randomized controlled trial is that differences in the outcome measure between the participants treated in the different ways can be attributed with more confidence to the manipulations of the researchers, because individual differences are likely to be spread in a random way between the different treatments. As soon as that basis for allocation of participants is lost, then questions arise over the ability to identify causes of changes or differences between the groups; in other words, the **internal validity** of the design is in question.

SINGLE CASE EXPERIMENTAL DESIGNS

Single case experimental designs are investigations of a series of experimental manipulations with a single research participant.

SURVEYS

Surveys are systematic methods for determining how a sample of participants respond to a set of standard questions attempting to assess their feelings, attitudes, beliefs or knowledge at one or more times. For example, we may want to know how drug users' perceptions of themselves and their families differ from those of non-users, or to better understand the experiences of patients receiving specific kinds of treatment, how health and social services are perceived by informal carers of people with dementia, Parkinson's, multiple sclerosis (MS) or other chronic conditions, or learn more about how people recovering from a disease such as coronary heart disease feel about their rehabilitation. The survey method will be the method of choice in many of these types of study.

The survey method, whether using interviews, questionnaires, or some combination of the two, is versatile, and can be applied equally well to research with individuals, groups, organizations, communities or populations to inform our understanding of a host of very different types of research issues and questions. Normally a survey is conducted on a sample of the study population of interest (e.g. people aged 70+; women aged 20–44; teenagers who smoke; carers of people with dementia, etc.). Issues of key importance in conducting a survey are: the objective(s); the mode of administration; the method of sampling; the sample size; the preparation of the data for analysis.

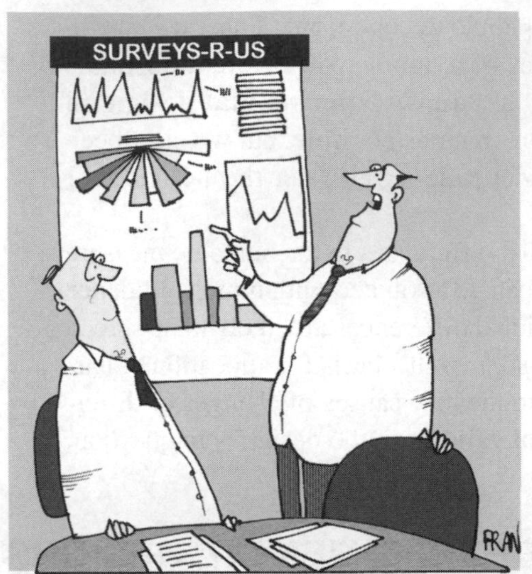

87% OF THE 56% WHO COMPLETED MORE THAN 23% OF THE SURVEY THOUGHT IT WAS A WASTE OF TIME

Reprinted by permission of www.cartoonstock.com

In running a survey it is essential to have a clear idea in mind about the objective before starting it. We must have a very clear idea about *why* we are doing our study (the theory or policy behind the research), *what* we are looking for (the research question), and *where* we intend to look (the setting or domain). We must also decide *who* will be in the sample (the study sample), and *how* to use the tools we have at our disposal (the specific procedures for applying the research methods). We have to be cautious that our procedures do not generate any self-fulfilling prophecies. *Lack of clarity about purposes and objectives* is one of the main stumbling blocks for the novice investigator to overcome. This is particularly the case when carrying out a survey, especially in a team of investigators who may have varying agendas with regard to the *why*, *what*, *who*, *where* and *how*? questions that must be answered before the survey can begin.

The main modes of administration are: face-to-face interview, telephone interview, group self-completion and postal self-completion. These modes may also be used in combination.

Next you need to decide *who* will be the sample for your survey and also *where* you will carry it out. The first issue that needs to be addressed is who are your study population? In other words, which population of people is your research question about? And how specific can you be about the definition of this population?

The sample for any survey should represent the study population as closely as possible. In some cases, the sample can consist of the entire study population, e.g. every pupil in a school; every student at a university; every patient in a hospital. More usually however, the sample will be a random selection of a proportion of the members of a population, e.g. every tenth person in a community, or every fourth patient admitted into a hospital. This method is called simple random sampling (SRS).

A variation on SRS is systematic sampling. In this case the first person in the sampling frame is chosen at random and then every *n*th person on the list from there on, where *n* is the sample fraction being used.

In stratified sampling the population is divided into groups or 'strata' and the groups are randomly sampled, but in different proportions so that the overall sample sizes of the groups can be made equal, even though they are not equal in the population (e.g. the 40–59, 60–79 and 80–99 age groups in a community sample, or men and women in a clinical sample). These groups will therefore be equally represented in the data. Other methods include non-probability sampling of six kinds: convenience samples, most similar/dissimilar samples, typical case samples, critical case samples, snowball samples and quota samples.

All such sampling methods are biased; in fact there is no perfect method of sampling because there will always be a category of people that any sampling method under-represents.

In any survey it is necessary to maximize the proportion of selected people who are recruited. If a large proportion of people refuse to participate, the sample will not represent the population, but be biased in unknown ways. As a general principle, surveys that recruit at least 70 per cent of those invited to participate are considered representative. The sample size is a key issue. The variability of scores obtained from the sampling diminishes as the sample size increases. So the bigger the sample, the more precise will be the estimates of the population scores, but the more the survey will cost.

SYSTEMATIC REVIEW

A **systematic review** is an integration of evidence about an effect or intervention involving the summary and integration of evidence from all relevant and usable primary sources. What counts as 'relevant and usable' is a matter for debate and judgement. Rules and criteria for selection of studies and for data extraction can be agreed by those carrying out the review. Publishing these rules and criteria along with the review enables such reviews to be replicable and transparent. Proponents of the systematic review therefore see the systematic review as a way of integrating research that limits bias. Traditionally the method has been applied to quantitative data. Recently, researchers have begun to investigate ways and means to synthesize qualitative studies also.

The synthesis of research evidence has been discussed in psychology since the mid-1970s when Glass (1976) coined the term 'meta-analysis'. From the late 1980s, research synthesis was discussed in the medical sciences (Mulrow, 1987; Oxman & Guyatt, 1988). The foundation of the Cochrane Collaboration in the 1990s, an organization that prepares and updates systematic reviews, was pivotal in establishing the systematic review as the method of choice for synthesizing research in health care. The use of systematic reviews is now widespread and strongly linked to 'evidence-based practice'. Systematic reviews of randomized controlled trials (RCTs) are seen as the 'gold standard' for determining 'evidence-based practice'.

Knowing how to carry out a systematic review and how to critically interpret a systematic review report are skills that health psychologists need to acquire. They are competences that enable the psychologist to integrate and implement research findings in making improvements in clinical and health care.

Inevitably systematic reviews act like a sieve, selecting some evidence but rejecting other evidence. To retain the visual metaphor, the reviewers act as a filter or lens; what they see and report depends on how the selection process is operated. Whenever there is ambiguity in evidence, the selection process may well tend to operate in confirmatory mode, seeking positive support for a position, model or theory rather than seeking disconfirmation. It is essential to be critical and cautious in interpreting and analysing systematic reviews of biomedical and related topics. Over time systematic reviews have the potential to influence clinical and health psychology practice in many different ways. However, the criteria for the selection of studies determine the outcome of the review, and so different criteria may well lead to different outcomes.

If we want to implement new practice as a direct consequence of such reviews, we had better make certain that the findings are solid and not a mirage. This is why the study of the method itself is so important. However seductive the view that systematic reviews can produce evidence that is bias-free, systematic reviews of the same topic can produce significantly different results, indicating that bias is difficult to control. Like all forms of knowledge, the results of a systematic review are the consequences of a process of negotiation about rules and criteria, and cannot be accepted without criticism and debate. We shall see later in this book how systematic reviews of evidence may cause controversy (e.g. Chapter 17).

FUTURE RESEARCH

1. The heavy focus on quantitative research in health psychology needs to be broadened to encompass more studies using qualitative and action research methods.
2. More research is needed on the health experiences and behaviour of children, ethnic minority groups, disabled people and older people.
3. The evidence base on efficacy and effectiveness of psychosocial interventions needs to be strengthened by larger-scale randomized controlled trials.
4. Collaboration with health economists is necessary to carry out cost-effectiveness studies of psychosocial interventions.
5. Policy-oriented research within health psychology is relatively under-developed. If health psychology is to achieve its full potential as an agent of change, policy-relevant research must be publicized and more widely disseminated through the media.

Summary

1. The principal research methods of health psychology fall into three categories: quantitative, qualitative and action research.
2. Quantitative research designs emphasize reliable and valid measurement in controlled experiments, trials and surveys.
3. Qualitative methods use interviews, focus groups, narratives, diaries or texts to explore health and illness concepts and experience.
4. Action research enables change processes to feed back into plans for improvement, empowerment and emancipation.
5. Evaluation research to assess the effectiveness and efficacy of interventions is generally on too small a scale and of insufficient quality. These is a need for much larger scale studies which are methodologically rigorous.
6. Multiple sources of evidence may be synthesized in systematic reviews and meta-analyses.
7. Health psychology research of the highest quality should be widely disseminated at all levels of society.

Part 2

Health Behaviour and Experience

In Part 2 we review research and interventions focusing on health behaviour and experience. Chapter 6 reviews sexually risky behaviour leading to STIs and HIV infections. We review the principal theories and models about health-related behaviours, with particular reference to sexual health. Individual-level theories are based on constructs, intended to be universally applicable, concerning how behaviours are adopted, maintained and changed. We summarize findings from studies that have tested the models in the arena of sexual health interventions. We critique the approach and suggest lines for future inquiry.

In Chapter 7 we examine the part played by food and eating in the changing patterns of illnesses and deaths. In particular, we focus on obesification, the increasing prevalence of obesity. Changes in Western lifestyles and the built environment have led to a toxic ecology for food production, distribution and consumption. Improvements in eating habits could reduce the prevalence of obesity, diabetes, cardiovascular diseases, cancers, osteoporosis and dental disease. We discuss the ecological, social and psychological factors associated with food choices and diet in modern times. We review the evidence on the effectiveness of interventions.

Chapter 8 discusses theories and research concerned with alcohol consumption and the causes, prevention and treatment of drinking problems. It begins with a discussion of the ambivalent attitudes to alcohol that have characterized many cultures from the distant past to the present day. An analysis of the physical and psychosocial dangers of drinking is followed by an examination of contrasting theories about the causes of excessive drinking. The chapter concludes with a discussion of the relative merits of different approaches to the prevention and treatment of drinking problems.

Chapter 9 reviews research on smoking prevention and cessation. With the accumulation of evidence on the negative aspects of smoking, Western governments have promoted measures to reduce the prevalence. These measures have met with substantial success, in spite of attempts by the tobacco industry to deliberately misinform the public. Smoking prevalence is increasing throughout the developing world and many people continue to smoke in the industrialized world. This chapter documents the extent of smoking, its major health impacts, and factors that help to explain its continued popularity. Smoking is a complex practice involving a mixture of biopsychosocial processes. Three main theories, the biological, psychological and social, are outlined. The primary methods to assist smokers to quit are reviewed together with the results of evaluation studies. Methodological issues with placebos and vested interests of industry suggest caution in interpreting studies funded by the pharmaceutical industry.

Chapter 10 reviews studies of physical activity. Recent years have seen an increased official concern at the apparent widespread decline in the participation of people in all types of physical activity. This chapter reviews the evidence for this and for its potential impact on health. It also considers the social and psychological factors associated with participation. It then considers the varying meanings of different forms of physical activity and the strategies that have been used to promote greater participation.

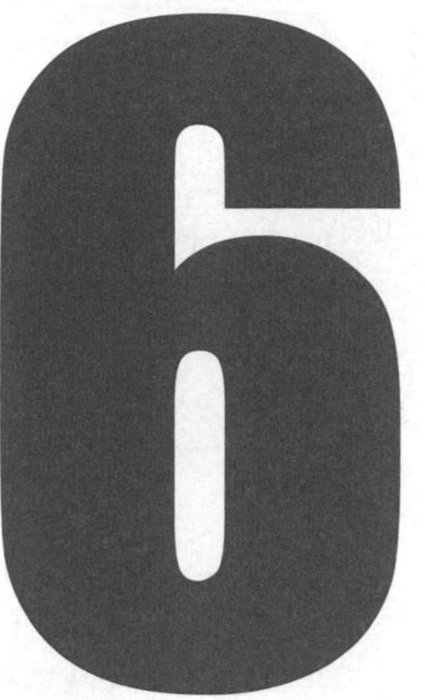

Theories, Models and Interventions Applied to Sexual Health

WE WILL HAVE DELIVERED IF…we stop the rise in STI rates over the next two years and then see a fall, and we reduce the 'under 18 conception rate by 50 per cent by 2010 as part of a broader strategy to improve sexual health'.

2004 UK Government target

In 2009, the Office of National Statistics reported that the rates of STI and under-18 conception were still rising indicating that the government target had not been reached.

Outline

This chapter focuses on sexually risky behaviour leading to STIs and HIV infections. We review the principal theories and models about health-related behaviours, with particular reference to sexual health. Individual-level theories are based on constructs, intended to be universally applicable, concerning how behaviours are adopted, maintained and changed. We summarize findings from studies that have tested the models in the arena of sexual health interventions. We critique the approach and suggest lines for future inquiry.

Sexual behaviour is any activity that arouses sexual arousal for pleasure or procreation. Sexual behaviour often leads to an exchange of bodily fluids. It may leave other physical or emotional traces. Individuals induce sexual arousal by mutual or self-stimulation or masturbation. Sexual attraction is a focus for flirtation, fantasy and fun, but sexual encounters may have serious consequences: pregnancy, **HIV**, and sexually transmitted infections (STIs). The latter cause serious medical complications including chronic illness, infertility, disability and death. This chapter will focus on sexually risky behaviour leading to STIs and HIV infection. The most important issue is the prevention of STIs and HIV infections.

INCIDENCE AND PREVALENCE OF STIS, HIV AND AIDS

Sexually transmitted infections (STIs) are passed on through intimate sexual contact. They can be passed on during vaginal, anal and oral sex, as well as through genital contact with an infected partner. Common STIs are chlamydia, genital warts and gonorrhoea. Two of the most serious, but fortunately more rare STIs, are syphilis and HIV. The greatest affected age group for the common STIs is young people aged 16–24 years. Even though they account for just 12 per cent of the population, more than half of all STIs diagnosed in the UK occur in young people. This includes 65 per cent of new chlamydia cases and 55 per cent of new genital warts cases. In the UK, the incidence of STIs has been rising steadily since the 1990s. Between 2007 and 2008, the Health Protection Agency (HPA) reported a 0.5 per cent increase in the number of diagnosed STIs, with a total of 399,738 new cases reported in 2008. Since 1999, in the UK, numbers of diagnoses in genito-urinary medicine (GUM) clinics of uncomplicated **chlamydia** infections, infectious **syphilis**, genital warts (first attack) and genital herpes (first attack) increased considerably (Health Protection Agency, 2009: Table 6.1). The **incidence**, the numbers of new diagnoses in one year, of **gonorrhoea**, and more recently infectious syphilis, were slightly in decline.

Table 6.1 The number of new diagnoses of STIs in Genito-Urinary Medicine (GUM) clinics in the UK in 2008

		% change	**% change**
	2008	2007–2008	1999–2008
Chlamydia	123,018	1 %	116 %
Genital warts	92,525	3 %	29 %
Genital herpes	28,957	10 %	65 %
Gonorrhoea	16,629	–11 %	1 %
Syphilis	2,524	–4 %	1 %

The UK Office for National Statistics (2009) showed 41.9 conceptions per 1000 15 to 17 year olds in 2007 – up from 40.9 in 2006. The under-16 conception rates also increased from 7.8 per 1000 to 8.3, nearly 8200 pregnancies. Teenage girls in the North East, where there is high poverty and unemployment, were the most likely in England to become pregnant, with 52.9 pregnancies per thousand girls aged 15–17 – more than one in twenty.

Until 2009, over 102,000 people in Britain had been diagnosed as HIV+, including 4200 children and teenagers. Some 10,391 20- to 24-year-olds have been infected, according to figures released by the Health Protection Agency. The Health Protection Agency report in November 2009 indicated that the number of people living with HIV in the UK was continuing to rise, with an estimated 83,000 infected at the end of 2008, of whom over a quarter (27 per cent) were unaware of their infection. During 2008, there were 7298 new diagnoses of HIV in the UK, a slight decline on previous years. New HIV diagnoses among those who acquired their infection heterosexually within the UK had risen, from 740 in 2004 to 1130 in 2008. The report estimated that: 'Preventing the 3,550 HIV infections that were probably acquired in the UK, and subsequently diagnosed in 2008, would have reduced future HIV-related costs by more than £1.1 billion' (Health Protection Agency, 2009).

US statistics are similar. The Centers for Disease Control (CDC, 2009) reported that teenage pregnancies and syphilis rose sharply among US school girls under the Bush administration when they were urged to avoid sex before marriage. According to the CDC, birth rates among teenagers aged 15 or older had been in decline since 1991 but were up sharply in more than half of American states since 2005. The study also revealed that the number of teenage females with syphilis has risen by nearly half after a significant decrease while a two-decade fall in the gonorrhea infection rate was being reversed. The number of AIDS cases in adolescent boys also nearly doubled. The CDC stated that Southern states, where there is a greatest emphasis on abstinence and religion, tended to have the highest rates of teenage pregnancy and STIs. In addition, about 16,000 pregnancies were reported among 10- to 14-year-old girls in 2004 and a similar number of young people in the age group reported having a STI. **Prevalence** of HIV across the globe has been rising steadily with the majority (67 per cent) in sub-Saharan Africa (see Figure 6.1).

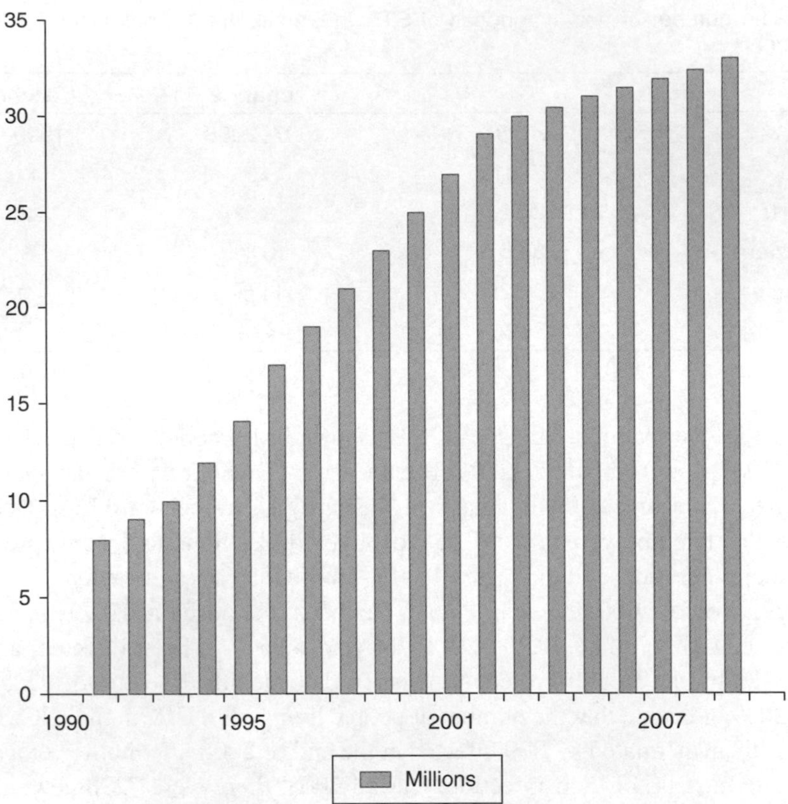

Figure 6.1 The number of people living with HIV has risen from around 8 million in 1990 to 33 million today, and is still growing

Source: UNAIDS epidemic update report, 2009; http://www.unaids.org/en/KnowledgeCentre/HIVData/Epidemiology/2009_epislides.asp

The statistics show that sexual behaviour is leading to a considerable health-care burden of HIV/AIDS, STIs and unwanted pregnancies. The figures for developing countries are high, and the high cost of medicines prohibits the most effective forms of treatment. Much of the limited funds that exist for HIV and STI prevention programmes are committed to poster campaigns for which there is little solid evidence of effectiveness.

KNOWLEDGE, AWARENESS AND CONDOM USE

In spite of decades of health education about STIs and HIV, there is still widespread ignorance about these diseases. The National AIDS Trust's (2008) *Public Attitudes Towards HIV*

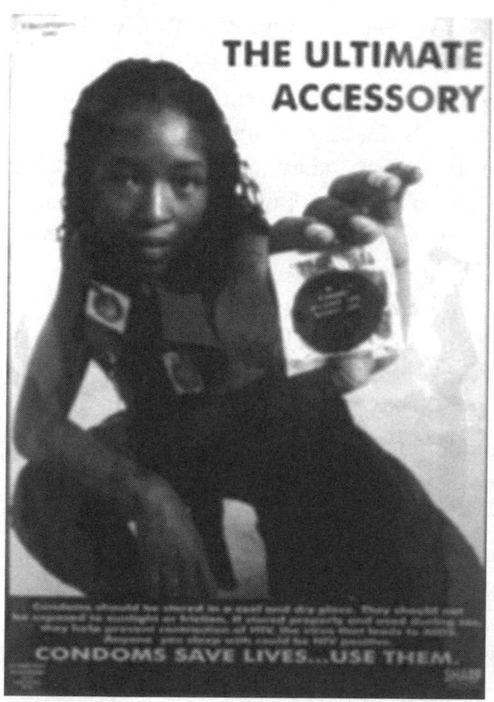

Figure 6.2 This South African HIV/AIDS poster is both eye-catching and impressive. It is aimed at the at-risk younger sexually active population

Source: University of Cape Town; Reproduced with permission

Survey showed more than 1 out of 5 people in the UK could not identify the main ways in which HIV is transmitted. The survey also revealed *fewer* people in 2007 were able to identify the correct ways in which HIV is transmitted than in 2000. Over a fifth (21 per cent) did not understand that unprotected sex between a man and a woman is a way of contracting HIV. Also, 26 per cent of British people did not know that unprotected sex between two men is a way of contracting HIV and 31 per cent of people did not know that sharing a syringe when injecting drugs carries a risk of HIV. However, the survey found an increase in the percentage of people who would only stop using condoms in a relationship 'once we've both been tested for STIs and HIV', up from 12 per cent in 2005 to 24 per cent in 2007. However 24 per cent stated they sometimes, rarely or never used a condom with a new sexual partner.

A research survey involving 1566 young people from 99 countries was carried out by the student organisation AIESEC International (2009) in collaboration with Standard Chartered Bank. A press release on 12 August 2009 announced that: 'Half the world's teenagers admit to being dangerously ignorant about HIV risks – and many do not use condoms.' The report stated that one in three youngsters apparently do not believe using protection stops the spread of sexually transmitted diseases. Yet half of the world's new HIV infections are among 15- to 24-year-olds. In south-east Asia 57 per cent of youngsters admit to knowing little about HIV or AIDS as compared to 74.3 per cent of young Africans, sub-Saharan Africa having the world's highest **AIDS** rate (AIESEC International, 2009).

Risky sexual behaviour has been studied in relation to social and educational status, and to habits such as drinking alcohol and taking drugs. Health risks are often associated, e.g. smoking, drinking, drugs and alcohol. Sexual risk taking has been associated with poorer academic performance. Poor academic performance at high school predicts risky sexual behaviour post-high school (Bailey, Fleming, Henson, Catalano & Haggerty, 2008). Bogart, Collins, Ellickson and Klein (2006) found that poor grades in high school predicted health risk behaviour in adulthood, including high risk sexual behaviour. The reasons for the association between academic performance and sexual risk behaviour remains unclear. A possible mediator is alcohol and drug use.

Hittner and Kryzanowski (2010) investigated academic performance, residential status, class rank and gender as predictors of risky sexual behaviour under two different substance use contexts, being 'drunk or high' and 'not drunk or high'. Results indicated that gender moderated the association between residential status and risky sex, such that males living on-campus engaged in more frequent casual sex than males living off-campus. The data for females did not differ on- or off-campus, possibly resulting from the under-reporting of sexual behaviour by females. All studies on sexual behaviour using self-reports tend to find disparities between the males' and females' reports in line with gender stereotypes in which it has traditionally been 'macho' to report plenty of encounters and 'feminine' to report few.

Cleland, Ali and Shah (2006) studied trends in protective behaviour among single vs. married young women in Sub-Saharan Africa. The authors reported an increase of 1.4 per cent per year in condom usage by single women for pregnancy prevention in 18 countries. However, only a modest increase occurred for married or cohabiting women despite the fact that more than 50 per cent of HIV infections in Southern and East Africa occur in this group.

Randrianasolo et al. (2008) studied barriers to the use of diaphragms and implications for woman-controlled prevention of sexually transmitted infections in Madagascar. The researchers approached women seeking care for vaginal discharge at a public health clinic for a semi-structured interview or focus group discussion. Of 46 participating women, while 70 per cent reported occasional use of male condoms, only 14 per cent reported using hormonal contraception. Three barriers to using modern contraceptives were: gaps in knowledge; misinformation and negative perceptions; concern about social opposition from male partners.

One group receiving a lot of research attention is college students. The majority have multiple sex partners and yet report inconsistent condom use (Lewis, Miguez-Burbano & Malow, 2009). The American College Health Association (2005) found 52 per cent of college students had vaginal intercourse at least once in the past 30 days with 63 per cent reporting inconsistent condom use. Alcohol and drug use prior to sexual activity is a predictor of unsafe sex (Hittner & Kennington, 2008; Lewis et al., 2009) because it compromises sexual decision-making (Wechsler et al., 1994) and increases unsafe sexual contact (Bon, Hittner & Lawandales, 2001). Negative psychological consequences, guilt and reduced self-esteem, tend to follow unplanned sexual activity (Paul, McManus & Hayes, 2000). Ma et al. (2009) investigated behavioural and psychosocial predictors of condom use among students in Eastern China using a questionnaire survey. Among 1850 sexually active participants, frequent condom use was reported by about only 40 per cent of men and women. Given the strict laws on procreation in China, these data illustrate the low adoption of condom use among students in eastern as well as western countries.

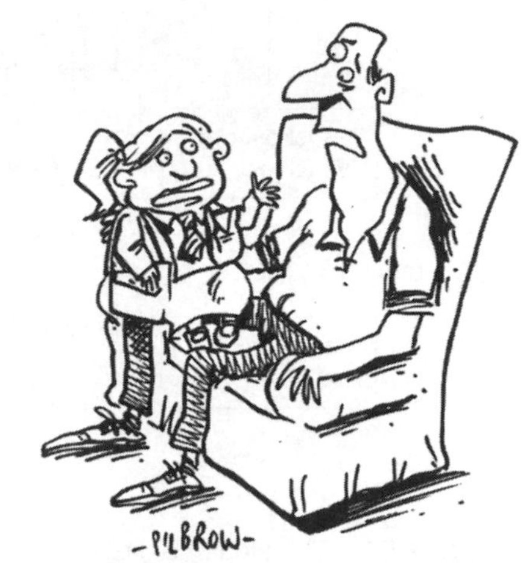

"Is this birds and bees chat going to take long? I'm late for my pre-natal class."

Reprinted by permission of www.cartoonstock.com

Low condom usage, and its consequences for STIs and unwanted pregnancies, is not simply caused by lack of awareness or knowledge. Motivational and emotional factors play a very significant role, as does culture. Explaining and reducing sexual risk taking is therefore a significant challenge for theories and models in health psychology. The need to put theory into practice has never been greater. In the rest of this chapter we explore the main theoretical approaches and evaluate their success with data from controlled studies and meta-analyses.

INDIVIDUAL-LEVEL THEORIES AND MODELS

Individual-level approaches use theoretical concepts and models as a basic for studying people's actions and choices. Because interventions using this approach are based on preconceived theoretical ideas, they may aptly be described as **'top-down'**. The interventions using this approach are constructed without any involvement of the intended participants. The psychologist decides what makes people behave the way that they do using internalized concepts and then tests the theory to see if it fits controlled data. Many theories and models have been applied to the study of contraceptive use and safer sex practices. In this section, we outline the eight main theories which have informed interventions targeted at individual sexual risk taking: the Health Belief Model, Protection Motivation Theory, the Theory of Reasoned Action, the Theory of Planned Behaviour, the Information-Motivation-Behavioural Skills Model, the Common Sense Model or Self-Regulation Theory, the Transtheoretical or Stages of Change Model and Social Cognitive Theory. In each case, recent data are briefly summarized before moving on to the results of meta-analyses.

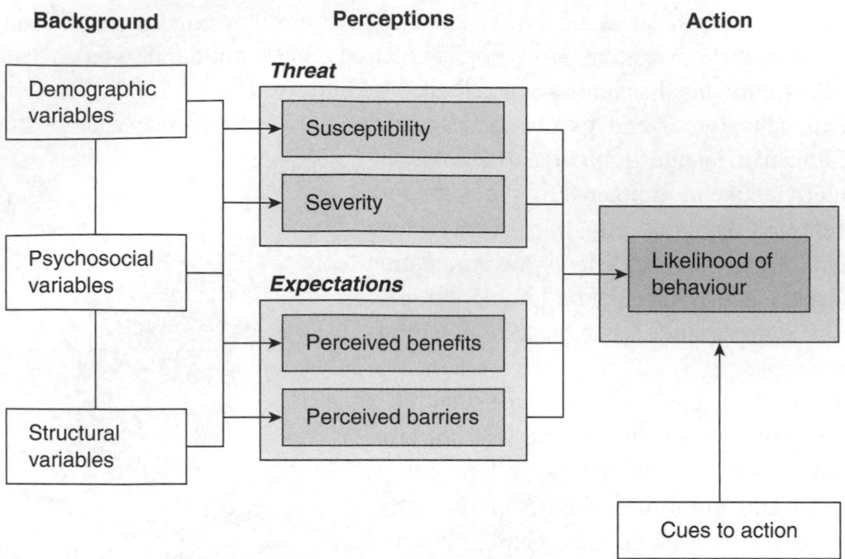

Figure 6.3 The Health Belief Model

The Health Belief Model

The Health Belief Model (HBM), developed by Rosenstock (1966), is an example of a cognition model which examines the predictors and precursors to health behaviour. The HBM contains four constructs:

1. **Perceived susceptibility** (an individual's assessment of their risk of getting the condition)
2. **Perceived severity** (an individual's assessment of the seriousness of the condition, and its potential consequences)
3. **Perceived barriers** (an individual's assessment of the influences that facilitate or discourage adoption of the promoted behaviour)
4. **Perceived benefits** (an individual's assessment of the positive consequences of adopting the behaviour).

The likelihood of a behaviour is influenced also by *cues to action* which are reminders or prompts to take action consistent with an intention. These cues to action can be *internal* (e.g. feeling fatigued can trigger actions to take time out or relax) or *external* (e.g. seeing health promotion leaflets/posters, personal communication from health professionals, family members, peers, etc.)

The HBM takes these factors into account to predict the likelihood of implementing health-related behaviour. The HBM has been developed over the years and additional factors have been included in the model (Becker, 1974; Rosenstock, Strecher & Becker, 1988). For example, demographic factors (e.g. age, sex and socio-economic background), psychosocial factors (e.g. personality traits, peer influence, family, etc.) and structural factors (e.g. knowledge of the health condition or previous contact to the disease) have been added into the model.

The HBM has been tested in several studies of sexual health. A few examples follow, showing inconsistent results. Lollis, Johnson and Antoni (1997) investigated the efficacy of the Health Belief Model for predicting condom usage and risky sexual practices in 122 white heterosexual college students (aged 17 to 33 years). The findings suggested that HBM did not significantly explain condom usage in the 58 men and 64 women surveyed and only partially explained the variance in sexual risk behaviours. The HBM explained 9 per cent of the variance in the likelihood of women being intoxicated or high during sex and 18 per cent of the variance in the number of sexual risk behaviours endorsed by women. These authors concluded that the HBM had limited utility for predicting sexual practices in university students suggesting the need for more comprehensive models of behaviour change.

Maguen, Armistead and Kalichman (2000) studied predictors of HIV antibody testing among gay, lesbian and bisexual youth. Data were collected at a conference for gay youth and at a Gay and Lesbian Community Center in Southeastern US. Variables related to the Health Belief Model were evaluated together with self-reported demographics, risk behaviours and HIV testing data. About one third of participants reported engaging in anal and vaginal sex without a condom while 25 per cent reported at least one other HIV risk factor. Of those engaging in sexual risk behaviours, only two thirds had tested for HIV antibodies. Drug use was reported by 61 per cent of the youth, of whom only 57 per cent had been tested. Regression analyses revealed that unprotected anal sex and the Health Belief Model variables predicted having been tested for HIV. The final model explained 42 per cent of the variance in HIV testing, a moderately positive outcome for the model.

Adolescents, students and men who have sex with men have been the focus of most research attention. Davis, Duncan, Turner and Young (2001) studied perceptions of HIV and STI risk among low-income heterosexual adults, a somewhat neglected group. The Health Belief Model guided the survey instrument. The findings suggested that respondents perceived their vulnerability to infection declining with increasing age and decreasing frequency of coitus. Condom use significantly declined with increasing age.

Wiggers, De Wit, Gras, Coutinho and Van Den Hoek (2003) investigated social-cognitive determinants of condom use among ethnic minority communities in Amsterdam. Wiggers et al. tested the predictive utility of the Health Belief Model and the Theory of Planned Behaviour (TPB, see below) with a sample of 537 Surinamese, Antillean and sub-Saharan African heterosexual men and women. Participants were interviewed and donated saliva for HIV testing. Consistent condom use was reported in only 23 per cent of primary partnerships and in 77 per cent of the casual partnerships. Controlling for socio-demographic and behavioural factors, analyses showed that perceived behavioural control and subjective norms regarding condom use were the main social-cognitive determinants of consistent condom use, confirming the TPB. However, perceived susceptibility and severity of HIV infection, perceived benefits of condom use, and cues to action, did not help to explain condom use, disconfirming the HBM in this sample.

Downing-Matibag and Geisinger (2009) studied how 'hooking up' with friends, strangers and acquaintances enables students to experience sexual intimacy without committing to a romantic relationship, preferably not even exchanging names. 'Hooking up' often involves risky behaviours because it frequently occurs in situations in which prophylactics are unavailable or judgement is impaired through drinks or drugs. The authors carried out 71 semi-structured interviews with students about their experiences of hooking-up. The authors found the Health Belief Model a useful framework for understanding sexual risk taking, and sexual risk-prevention programmes on college campuses. The findings showed that students' self-assessments of susceptibility to STIs are often misinformed, enabling situational characteristics, such as spontaneity, to their students' sexual self-efficacy.

Protection Motivation Theory

Protection Motivation Theory (PMT) was developed by Rogers (1983) to describe coping with a health threat in light of two appraisal processes, threat appraisal and coping appraisal. According to PMT the appraisal of the health threat and the possible coping response results in an intention, or 'protection motivation', to perform either an adaptive response or a maladaptive response, which will place an individual at health risk. According to PMT, behaviour change is best achieved by appealing to an individual's fears. The PMT proposes four constructs, which are said to influence the intention to protect oneself against a health threat:

1 The perceived *severity* of a threatened event (e.g., HIV infection)
2 The perceived probability of the occurrence, or *vulnerability* (e.g. the perceived vulnerability of the person to HIV)
3 The efficacy of the recommended preventive behaviour (i.e. how effective is the wearing of a condom)
4 The perceived *self-efficacy* (e.g., the person's confidence in putting a condom in place) (see Figure 6.4).

This theory takes account of both costs and benefits of behaviour in predicting the likelihood of change. PMT assumes that protection motivation is maximized when:

- the threat to health is severe
- the individual feels vulnerable
- the adaptive response is believed to be an effective means for averting the threat
- the person is confident in his or her abilities to complete successfully the adaptive response
- the rewards associated with the maladaptive behaviour are small
- the costs associated with the adaptive response are small

Such factors produce protection motivation and, subsequently, the enactment of the adaptive, or coping, response.

Li et al. (2004) studied HIV/STD risk behaviours and perceptions among 2153 sexually active rural-to-urban migrants in China. Migration often places individuals at increased risk for HIV and STI. The applicability of the constructs of the PMT to the study population was evaluated. The authors measured migrant mobility, sexual risk and the seven constructs of the PMT. The data confirmed that the high mobility among the rural-to-urban migrant population was associated with increased sexual risk (see Figure 6.5). The PMT constructs were found to be applicable in identifying perceptions and attitudes associated with sexual risk behaviours in this population. Increased sexual risk was associated with increased perceptions of extrinsic rewards, intrinsic rewards and response cost. Also consistent with PMT, increased sexual risk was associated with perceptions of decreased severity, vulnerability, response efficacy and self-efficacy. After controlling for a number of confounding factors, all seven PMT constructs were found to be associated with sexual risk in the manner posited by the theory. The association between mobility and sexual risk emphasizes the importance of having effective HIV/STD prevention efforts among this

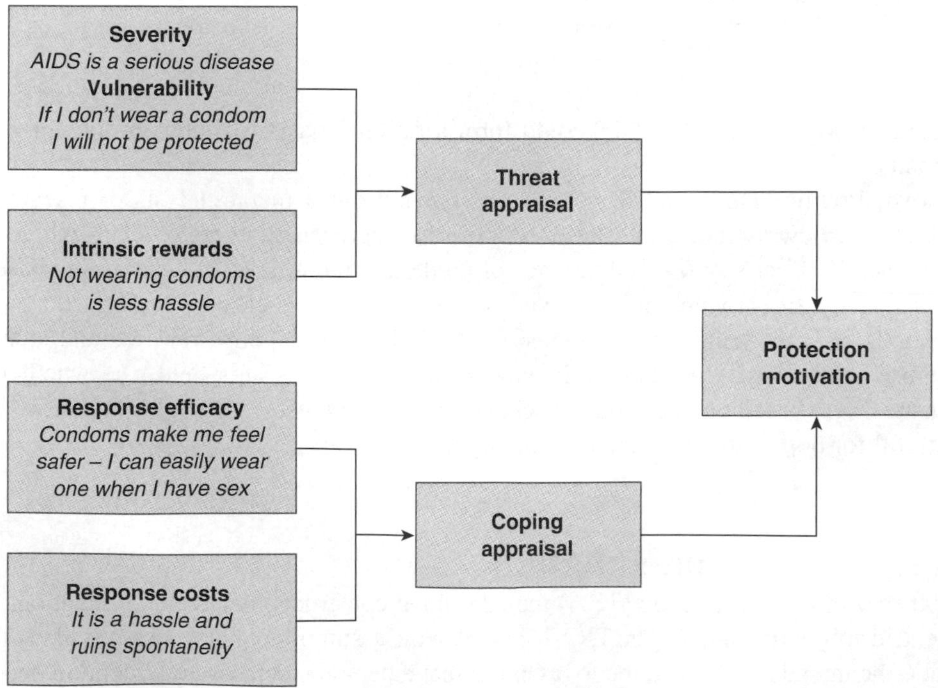

Figure 6.4 The four constructs and the two appraisal processes which result in protection motivation

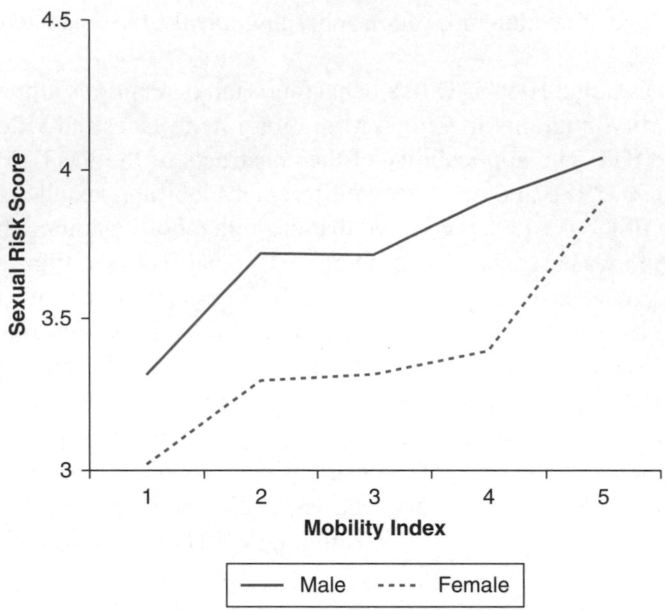

Figure 6.5 Sexual risk scores for Chinese rural-to-urban migrants for different levels of mobility
Source: Li et al., 2004; Retrieved 23 November 2009, from Academic Search Premier database

vulnerable population. The PMT could form a rational basis for interventions targeting migrants.

Floyd, Prentice-Dunn and Rogers (2000) carried out a meta-analysis of research on PMT. The review included 65 relevant studies that represented over 20 health issues. The mean overall effect size ($d+ = 0.52$) was of moderate magnitude. In general, increases in threat severity, threat vulnerability, response efficacy and self-efficacy facilitated adaptive intentions or behaviours while decreases in maladaptive response rewards and adaptive response costs increased adaptive intentions or behaviours. This held true whether the measures were based on intentions or behaviours, and suggests that PMT components may be useful for both individual and community interventions.

Theory of Reasoned Action

The theory of reasoned action (TRA) includes three constructs: behavioural intention, **attitude**, and **subjective norm**. The TRA is based on the assumption that a person is likely to do what (s)he intends to do. The theory assumes that a person's behavioural intention depends on the person's attitude about the behaviour and subjective norms. The model is illustrated in Figure 6.6.

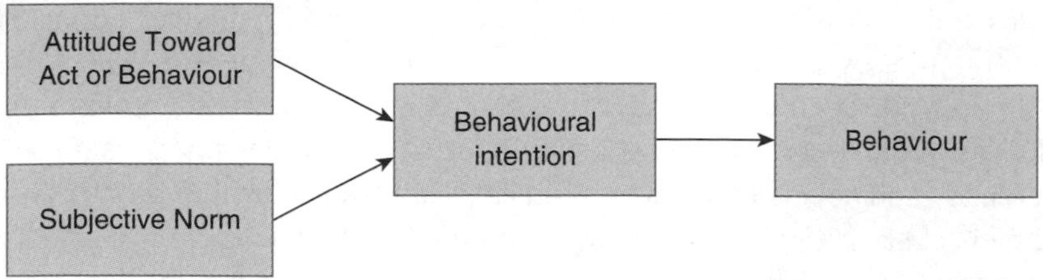

Figure 6.6 The Theory of Reasoned Action
Source: Fishbein and Ajzen, 1975

Recent studies of the TRA include:

1 Patterson, Semple, Fraga, Bucardo, Davila-Fraga and Strathdee (2005) developed an HIV-prevention intervention for sex workers in Tijuana, Mexico.
2 Koniak-Griffin and Stein (2006) used TRA predictors of sexual risk behaviours among adolescent mothers in a human immunodeficiency virus prevention programme.
3 Randolph et al. (2009) developed an STI-prevention for seriously mentally ill women using the theory of reasoned action.

The Theory of Planned Behaviour

Not all behaviours are under volitional control as implied by the TRA. Smoking, eating healthily and drinking alcohol are examples of behaviour that people have difficulty controlling in a free and voluntary way. Ajzen (1985) added the variable of *perceived behavioural control* to produce the Theory of Planned Behaviour (TPB) (see Figure 6.7). Perceived behavioural control refers to one's perception of control over the behaviour and reflects

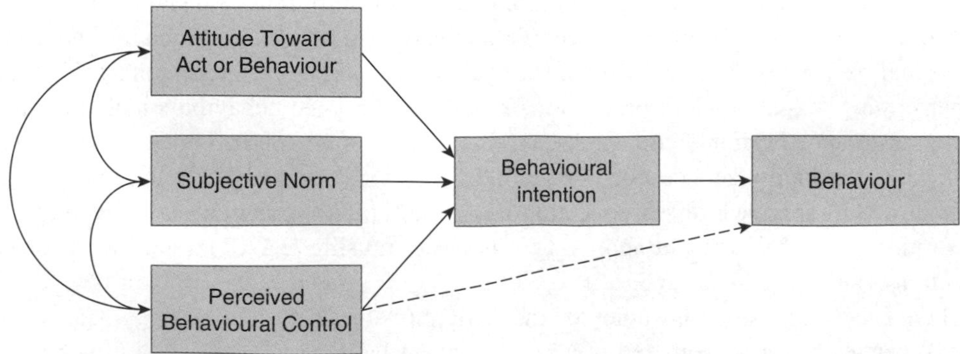

Figure 6.7 The Theory of Planned Behaviour
Source: Ajzen (1991)

the obstacles and successes encountered in past experience with this behaviour. There were more than 50 studies using the TPB in the sexual health arena in the five-year period 2005–9. The TPB proposes that perceived behavioural control can influence intentions and behaviour directly. For example, in the college student population, attitudes toward safe sex, condom use, self-efficacy and beliefs about peer norms have all been shown to predict unsafe sexual activity (Lewis et al., 2009; Hittner & Kryzanowski, 2010). The success of the TPB in predicting safer sexual behaviour has been reviewed in a meta-analysis published by Albarracín, Johnson, Fishbein and Muellerleile (2001) (see below).

Important factors are missing from the TPB, for example, culture and religion. Sinha, Curtis, Jayakody, Viner and Roberts (2007) studied sexual behaviour and relationships amongst Black and minority ethnic (BME) teenagers in East London. The authors wanted to learn how these relationships are shaped by culture, gender, peer norms and religion. They collected data from 126 young people, aged 15–18, mainly using focus groups in the London boroughs of Hackney, Newham and Tower Hamlets. The findings suggested that sexual behaviour is mediated by gender, religion and youth in multiple ways not included in the TPB.

The Information-Motivation-Behavioural Skills Model

The Information-Motivation-Behavioural Skills (IMB) model was proposed by Fisher and Fisher (1992, 2000). The IMB model focuses on informational, motivational and behavioural skills factors that are found to be associated with sex-related problem-prevention and wellness-promotion behaviours. According to the IMB model, the learning of sexuality-related information is a prerequisite to action in these areas. HIV-related information is likely to include facts about HIV (e.g., 'Oral sex is safer than vaginal or anal sex') that could facilitate preventive behaviour performance. The IMB model assumes that having the motivation to practise specific sex-related behaviours is necessary for the production of problem-prevention or wellness promotion. Finally, sexuality-related behavioural skills are a third fundamental determinant of acting effectively to avoid sexual problems and achieving sexual well-being. The behavioural skills construct focuses on the person's self-efficacy in performing sexual problem-prevention or well-being related behaviours including insisting on abstinence from intercourse, discussing and practising contraceptive use, and sexual behaviours that optimize a couple's sexual pleasure. Barak and Fisher (2001) proposed an Internet-driven approach to sex education using the Internet based on the IMB model. An illustration of the IMB model applied to adherence in using HAART medication for HIV infection is shown in Figure 6.8.

There have been several studies of the IMB model in different settings. Carey et al. (2000) carried out a randomized clinical trial of an IMB-based intervention using information, motivational enhancement and skills training to reduce the risk of HIV infection for low-income urban women in Syracuse, New York. The 102 participants, who ranged in age from 17 to 46, were predominantly African–American (88 per cent). Ninety-three

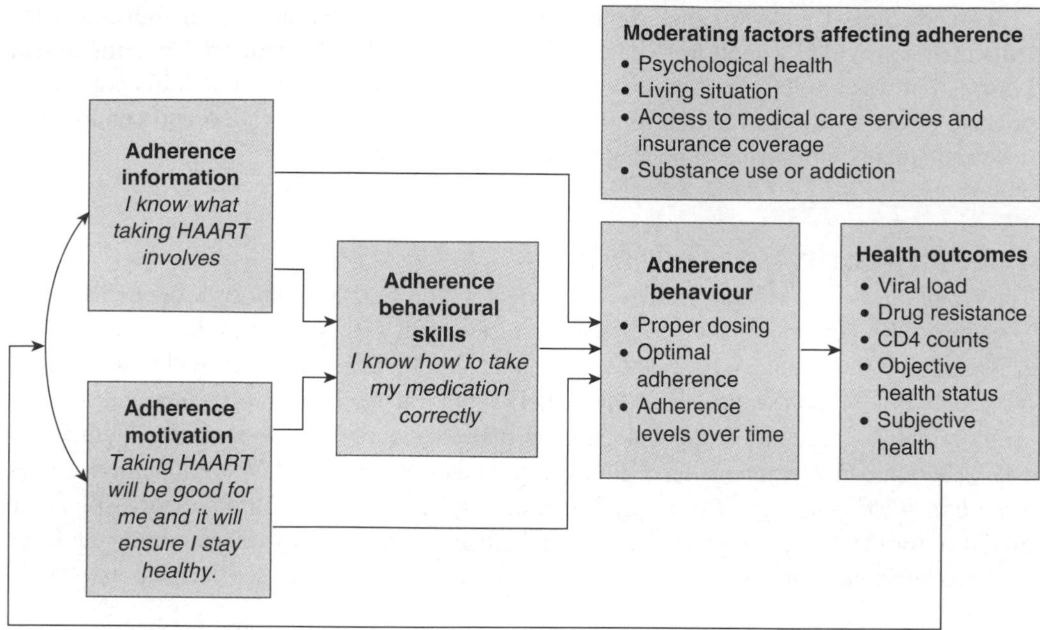

Figure 6.8 The Information-Motivation-Behavioural Skills Model applied to adherence in using HAART medication

Source: Fisher et al., 2006

per cent reported a family income of less than $12,000 per year. Risk markers in the past year included a non-monogamous partner (82 per cent), more than one partner (62 per cent), sex trading (32 per cent), an STI (24 per cent), a bisexual partner (23 per cent), and a partner who had injected drugs (5 per cent); only 1 per cent reported needle-sharing. Participants completed a questionnaire on their demographics, HIV-related information, motivation (risk perception, behavioural intentions), and risk-related behaviour. Carey et al. offered two interventions randomly to the participants: (i) The HIV-Risk Reduction (HIV-RR) intervention was designed to reduce HIV-related risk behaviours by first enhancing motivation for behaviour change by using motivational interviewing strategies (Miller & Rollnick, 1991). **Motivational interviewing** (MI) is a widely used strategy for building up a person's drive to change their behaviour in accordance with their decision to make a change. Following motivational sessions, women were offered the opportunity to increase their HIV-related knowledge and sharpen the interpersonal skills needed to adopt safer sexual practices; (ii) The Health Promotion (HP) intervention served as an 'attention control', and targeted stress, anger, nutrition and breast health. The findings indicated that women in the HIV-RR programme had enhanced their knowledge and strengthened their risk reduction intentions relative to the HP controls. HIV-RR women who expressed 'imperfect' intentions were found to have increased their condom use, talked more with partners about condom use and HIV testing, and were more likely to have refused unprotected sex.

Scott-Sheldon, Carey, Vanable, Senn, Coury-Doniger and Urban (2010) found that the IMB model provided a good fit to data collected from 1474 STD patients. They found that information was unrelated to condom use but motivation and behavioural skills both had a positive effect on condom use. Stronger associations between motivation and condom use occurred among participants reporting no prior STD treatment.

The Common Sense Model

The Common Sense Model (CSM), also known as the Self-Regulatory Model (SRM), or Leventhal's Model, was developed by Howard Leventhal and colleagues (Leventhal, Meyer & Nerenz, 1980; Leventhal, Brissette & Leventhal, 2003). A key construct within the CSM is the idea of illness representations or 'lay' beliefs about illness. These representations integrate with normative guidelines that people hold, to make sense of their symptoms and guide any coping actions. Five components of illness representations in the CSM are: *Identity*; *Cause*; *Time-line*; *Consequences*; *Curability/controllability*. The self-regulation theory offers no guidance for the design of interventions and there are no meta-analyses examining evidence for the effectiveness of this theory. For further discussion of the CSM, see Chapter 16 (p. 367).

The Transtheoretical Model or Stages of Change Model

This Transtheoretical Model (TTM), otherwise known as the Stages of Change Model, was developed by Prochaska and DiClemente (1983). It has been highly influential in the literature on health behaviour change. The TTM hypothesizes six discrete stages of change, which people are alleged to progress through in making a change:

1 *Precontemplation* – a person is not intending to take action in the foreseeable future, usually measured as the next 6 months
2 *Contemplation* – a person is intending to change in the next 6 months
3 *Preparation* – a person is intending to take action in the immediate future, usually measured as the next month
4 *Action* – a person is making specific overt modifications in his/her lifestyle within the past 6 months
5 *Maintenance* – a person is working to prevent relapse, a stage which is estimated to last from 6 months to about 5 years
6 EITHER *Termination* – an individual has zero temptation and 100 per cent self-efficacy, OR, *Relapse* – an individual reverts to the original behaviour.

The TTM has been tested in multiple studies with mixed results. For example, Velasquez, von Sternberg, Johnson, Green, Carbonari and Parsons (2009) carried out a trial designed to reduce sexual risk behaviours and alcohol use among HIV-positive men who have sex with men. They used a Stages of Change-based intervention and also the technique of motivational

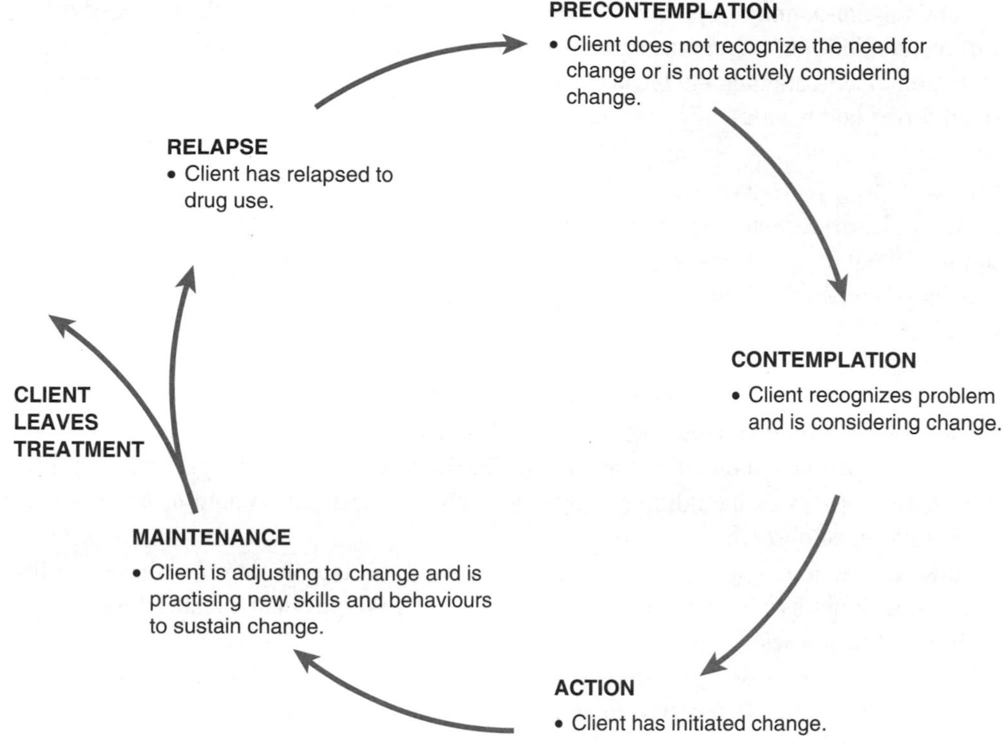

Figure 6.9 The Transtheoretical or Stages of Change Model
Source: Prochaska & DiClemente, 1982

interviewing (MI). Valasquez et al. found reductions in the number of drinks per 30-day period, number of heavy drinking days per 30-day period and the number of days on which both heavy drinking and unprotected sex occurred. Chacko et al. (2010) tested the efficacy of a motivational/behavioural intervention to promote chlamydia and gonorrhea screening in young women, which is critical to reduction of asymptomatic cervicitis and its complications. Three hundred and seventy-six sexually active, young women were randomized to two groups: intervention plus standard care or standard care alone. The intervention used the Transtheoretical Model of Change and MI. However, no significant differences occurred between the two groups. A meta-analysis by Noar, Black and Pierce (2009) indicated that interventions using the Stages of Change model were relatively effective (see below).

Social Cognitive Theory

Bandura's (1986) Social Cognitive Theory (SCT) examines the social origins of behaviour in addition to the cognitive thought processes that influence human behaviour and functioning.

Bandura's social-cognitive approach proposes that learning can occur in the absence of direct reinforcement through observation of models in the absence of any overt reinforcement. The acquisition of skill and knowledge have an intrinsic reinforcement value independent of biological drives and needs. Basic constructs within SCT include the following:

Observational learning

People can learn by watching or observing others, by reading about what people do, and by making general observations of the world. This learning may or may not be demonstrated in the form of behaviour. Bandura proposed a four step conceptual scheme for observational learning:

1 Attentional processes including certain model characteristics which may increase the likelihood of the behaviour being attended to and the observer characteristics such as sensory capacities, motivation and arousal levels, perceptual set and past reinforcement.
2 Retention processes including the observer's ability to remember and to make sense of what has been observed.
3 Motor reproduction processes including the capabilities that the observer has to perform the behaviours being observed. Specific factors include physical capabilities and availability of responses.
4 Motivational processes including external reinforcement, vicarious reinforcement and self-reinforcement. If a behaviour is to be imitated, an observer must be motivated to perform that behaviour.

Self-efficacy

Bandura (1994) defined the concept of 'perceived self-efficacy' as: 'People's beliefs about their capabilities to produce designated levels of performance that exercise influence over events that affect their lives. Self-efficacy beliefs determine how people feel, think, motivate themselves and behave. Such beliefs produce these diverse effects through four major processes. They include cognitive, motivational, affective and selection processes' (p. 71). Self-efficacy is a person's belief that they have behavioural competence in a particular situation. Self-efficacy is related to whether or not an individual will undertake particular goal-directed activities, the amount of energy that he or she will put into their effort, and the length of time that the individual will persist in striving to achieve a particular goal. Among the sources of self-efficacy are:

1 Performance accomplishments: past experiences of success and failure
2 Vicarious experience: witnessing others' successes and failures
3 Verbal persuasion: being told by others that one can or cannot competently perform a particular behaviour
4 Emotional arousal: when engaging in a particular behaviour in a specific situation.

The concept has been widely applied in studies of, and interventions for, health protecting behaviours. The concept mirrors the self-help literature of the Dale Carnegie kind founded on the principal that people can achieve great things by believing that they can do so – so-called 'positive thinking'. Carnegie (1913) was an erudite scholar of the art of rhetoric who believed that reading yielded priceless knowledge. There can be little doubt that ideas about positive thinking and self-efficacy are very prevalent in popular culture. Bandura has made some extremely important observations about human learning and thought. Observational learning and self-efficacy are invaluable concepts. However, critics argue that the relationship between the concepts is not clear.

Applying social cognitive theory in mass communication

Bandura's (1986) theory of vicarious learning has been applied to the use of role models in the mass media as a method for shaping cultural attitudes and behaviour. Of particular interest are the use of serial melodramas, 'telenovelas' and 'soaps' using the methodology developed by Sabido (1981) in Mexico which aim to reinforce social values through the use of drama. Ryerson's (2010) Population Media Centre has been actively promoting reproductive health in many different countries. Research is carried out prior to the development of TV programmes to measure audience attitudes and norms. Characters for the soaps are developed to reflect the interests of the audience. Through the evolution of characters as they respond to problems that many audience members are also facing, soap operas can show the adoption of new, non-traditional behaviours in a way that generates no negative response and little resistance from the audience. Audience members form bonds with soap characters, and adopt them as role models. Evaluation of these methods has shown excellent results (Ryerson, 2010).

Galavotti, Pappas-DeLuca and Lansky (2001) describe a successful approach to prevent HIV/AIDS using Modeling and Reinforcement to Combat HIV (MARCH). This approach combines individual behaviour change with efforts to change social norms by using entertainment as a vehicle for education (long-running serialized dramas on radio or television portray role models evolving toward the adoption of positive behaviours) and interpersonal reinforcement at the community level (support from friends, family members and others can help people initiate behaviour changes; support through changes in social norms is necessary for behavioural effects to be sustained over time). Galavotti et al. argue that media and interpersonal intervention activities should be linked to existing community resources and, wherever possible, provide increased access to preventive services, supplies and other supporting elements.

A recent evaluation by Kuhlmann, Kraft, Galavotti, Creek, Mooki and Ntumy (2008) examined the use of radio role models for the prevention of mother-to-child transmission of HIV and HIV testing among pregnant women in Botswana. A programme for the prevention of mother-to-child-transmission of HIV (PMTCT) suffered from low uptake. Using 2003 survey data from 504 pregnant and post-partum women, Kuhlmann et al.

Table 6.2 Key features of successful behavioural interventions

Feature	Contribution to behaviour change
Use of role models	Provides examples of how to change. Increases confidence in ability to change behaviour. Persuades audience of positive benefits of change.
Affective impact	Affective/emotional responses encourage attention to and retention of information. Emotions create opportunities for identification.
Links to social and cultural narratives	Information can be easily integrated into social expectations, norms, values, and political and economic culture of affected audience. Intervention is applicable to audience's everyday lives. Intervention is presented in a narrative form familiar to audience.
Personalization	Message is reinforced interpersonally. Attention is individualized. Messages are developed with issues and concerns of affected population in mind.
Cognizance of impediments and facilitators	Links programme to services or supplies. Reflects infrastructure accurately. Capitalizes on formal and informal supporting norms and structures.

Source: Galavotti et al., 2001

assessed associations between exposure to a long-running radio serial drama that encourages use of the PMTCT programme and HIV testing during pregnancy. Controlling for demographic, pregnancy and other variables, women who spontaneously named a PMTCT character in the serial drama as their *favourite* character were nearly twice as likely to test for HIV during pregnancy as those who did not. The authors concluded that identification with characters in the radio serial drama is associated with testing during pregnancy. Coupled with other supporting elements, serial dramas could contribute to HIV prevention, treatment and care initiatives. We discuss the use of modelling in mass communication further in Chapter 15.

Meta-Analyses

Munro, Lewin, Swart and Volmink (2007) provided a summary of meta-analyses carried out until February 2005 concerned with long-term medication adherence. The effects were modest and highly variable with theoretical constructs accounting for anywhere between 0 and 25 per cent of the variance in behaviour. This means that the theoretical models left anything between 75 and 100 per cent of the variations in medication adherence behaviour unaccounted for, a rather depressing conclusion. Is the outcome of meta-analyses of sexual health behaviour any more encouraging?

Albarracín and colleagues (2001) meta-analysed data on the ability of the TRA and TPB to predict condom use. In total, 96 data sets with over 22,000 participants were analysed. Consistent with the TRA: (a) condom use correlated with intentions with a mean coefficient, r, of 0.45; (b) intentions were based on attitudes (r = 0.58) and subjective norms (r = 0.39); (c) attitudes were correlated with behavioural beliefs (r = 0.56) and norms were correlated with normative beliefs (r = 0.46). Consistent with the TPB: perceived behavioural control was related to condom use intentions (r = 0.45) and condom use (r = 0.25), but, contrary to the TPB, it did not correlate significantly to condom use. However, the strength of these associations was influenced by the consideration of past behaviour. It must be borne in mind that the correlation coefficient needs to be squared to compute the variance explained by a variable. Thus the strongest relationship observed by Albarracín et al. (2001), the correlation of 0.58 between attitudes and subjective norms, accounted for 0.58 × 0.58 or 34 per cent of the variance, certainly no cause for celebration. In fact, one might be excused a certain degree of surprise at how weak this relationship actually is.

Noar and colleagues (2009) carried out a meta-analysis of the efficacy of computer technology-based HIV prevention interventions aimed at increasing condom use among at-risk populations. The overall effect size for condom use was moderate (d = 0.259) but indicated a statistically significant impact of the interventions. The findings showed that interventions were more efficacious when directed at single sex groups (men or women) rather than mixed sex groups, with individualized tailoring, using the Stages of Change model. On the basis of these data, HIV prevention using computer technology may have similar efficacy to traditional human-delivered interventions, which, if true, leaves one wondering what possible role is left for the therapist.

KEY STUDY What works best in HIV-prevention? (Albarracín et al., 2005)

In the largest meta-analysis of HIV-prevention strategies ever conducted, Albarracín et al. (2005) tested the main theoretical assumptions in models of behaviour change in contrasting 'passive' and 'active' HIV-prevention interventions. The investigators compared the effectiveness of different intervention strategies and attempted to look at the sequence of psychological change that different interventions produce, e.g., behavioural skills training should first increase behavioural skills that promote condom use. Another objective was to investigate the generalizability of different intervention strategies to different populations. They reviewed 194 research reports from 1985 to 2003, the most comprehensive review to date.

(Continued)

(Continued)

Albarracín et al. (2005) studied the impact of interventions to increase condom use on (a) attitudes, (b) norms, (c) control perceptions, (d) intentions, (e) HIV knowledge, (f) behavioural skills, (g) perceived severity of HIV, (h) perceived susceptibility to HIV, and ultimately (i) condom use. They also compared 'passive' and 'active' interventions. Passive interventions involve minimal participation by using messages to (a) induce pro-condom attitudes, (b) induce pro-condom norms, (c) increase relevant knowledge, (d) to verbally model skills that promote condom use, and (e) increase perceived threat. Active interventions include client-tailored counselling, HIV testing, or activities to increase behavioural skills, such as role-playing of behaviours related to condom use.

There were 2 main conclusions from this extensive review. First, the most effective interventions were those that contained attitudinal arguments, educational information, behavioural skills arguments, and behavioural skills training. The least effective were those that attempted to induce fear of HIV. The impact of the interventions and the different strategies behind them was found to vary according to gender, age, ethnicity, risk group, and past condom use.

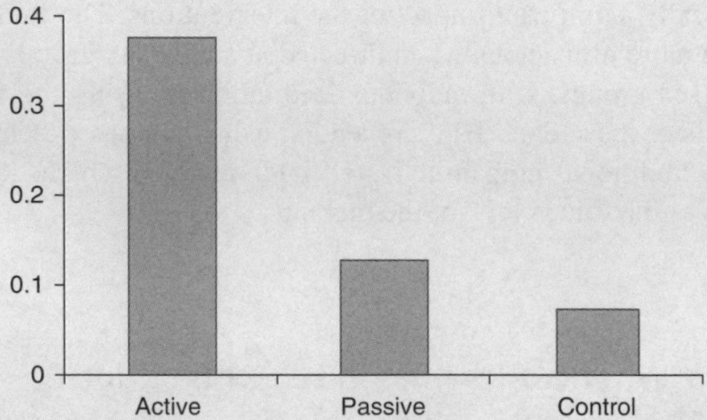

Figure 6.10 Mean behaviour change for active interventions, passive interventions and control groups (adapted from Albarracín et al., 2005: Figure 1)

The difference between active and passive interventions was highly significant ($p < .001$).

The overall outcome of meta-analyses of theory testing suggests that, unfortunately, current psychological theories of sexual health do not provide a viable foundation for effective interventions. We analyse the reasons for this in the next section. Alternative approaches are necessary if we are to make significant progress in stemming the tide of STIs, HIV and unwanted pregnancies.

Critique of Individual-Level Approaches

Individualistic bias

The individual-level approaches of traditional health psychology fall under the umbrella of individualism which we discussed in Chapter 1. The processes of choice and responsibility are internalized inside each individual's head as a set of processes operating on information similar to a computer. The processes are assumed to be universal and rational, following a fixed set of formulae as defined by the models. Along with the individualism comes the positivism of a purely quantitative empirical approach. Yet even within its own terms, the programme of model testing and confirmation is failing to meet the goals it has set for itself.

Lack of ecological validity and questionable statistical methods

Thousands of published studies – and an imponderable number unpublished – have used null hypothesis testing with small samples of college students or smaller samples of patients. The power, ecological validity and generalizability of these studies is questionable, yet we do not really know their true merit because of the uncertainties about representativeness, sampling, and statistical assumptions (Marks, 2006). Rarely are alternative, and arguably superior, approaches to theory testing utilized, for example, by using Bayesian statistics, and power analyses carried out to assess the *importance* of the effects rather than their *statistical significance* (Cohen, 1994).

Neglect of culture, religion and gender

Key factors such as religion, culture and gender are not included in the SCMs. We have seen above that studies of sexual behaviour (e.g. Sinha et al., 2007) show the importance of these factors and yet the models neglect them. The theories and models aim at a universal application that is unwarranted and implausible.

Tautological and unfalsifiable

Critics of social cognition models have suggested that they are **tautological** and, therefore, irrefutable (Smedslund, 2000; Ogden, 2003). A tautology is a statement that is redundant, repetitious or necessarily true, e.g. 'Jill will either stop or not stop smoking'. Whatever data we obtain about Jill's smoking, the statement will always be true, a very safe prediction. Smedslund (2000) further deduced that, if tautological theories are disconfirmed or only partially supported by empirical studies, then the studies themselves must be flawed for not 'discovering' what must be the case. Others have argued that behavioural beliefs (attitudes) and normative beliefs are basically the same thing. Ogden (2003) analysed empirical articles published between 1997 and 2001 from four health psychology journals that tested or applied one or more social cognition models (theory of reasoned action, theory of planned behaviour, health belief model and protection motivation theory). Ogden concluded that the models do not enable the generation and testing of hypotheses because their constructs are unspecific. Echoing Smedslund (2000), she suggested that the models focus on analytic truths which must be true by definition.

However, not all theorists agree that SCMs are tautological and/or unfalsifiable. Trafimow (2009) claims to have demonstrated that the TRA and TPB are falsifiable because these theories make risky predictions. He furthermore claims to have falsified one of the assumptions of the TPB, namely, that perceived control is a worse predictor of behavioural intentions than perceived difficulty (Trafimow, Sheeran, Conner & Finlay, 2002). Yet perceived behavioural control is usually measured by items evaluating control and items evaluating difficulty. If empirical falsification of the TPB has actually occurred then the theory must, *ipso facto*, be falsifiable, and one of the main criticisms has been eliminated.

Unsupported assumptions

The Transtheoretical Model has received particular criticism. Sutton (2005) argued that the stage definitions are logically flawed, and that the time periods assigned to each stage are arbitrary. Herzog (2008) suggested that, when applied to smoking cessation, the TTM does not satisfy the criteria required of a valid stage model and that the proposed stages of change 'are not qualitatively distinct categories'.

Procedural issues

French, Cooke, Mclean, Williams and Sutton (2007) investigated what people think about when they answer TPB questionnaires using the 'think aloud' technique. French et al. found problems relating to information retrieval and to participants answering different questions from those intended and they concluded that: 'The standard procedure for developing TPB questionnaires may systematically produce problematic questions' (p. 672).

Neglect of motivation

Another common complaint about the SCMs is that they do not adequately address the motivational issues about risky behaviours. Surely it is their very riskiness that in part is responsible for their adoption? Willig (2008) questioned the assumption that lies behind much of health and sex education 'that psychological health is commensurate with maintaining physical safety, and that risking one's health and physical safety is necessarily a sign of psychopathology' (p. 690). Flowers, Hart and Marriott (1999) studied gay men's concept of 'risk' in the context of public sex environments (parks) using semi-structured, in-depth interviews. Flowers et al. reported that: 'Risk reduction, danger and safety figured frequently in men's accounts of sex and sexual decision-making. However, the risks men reported related more directly to the threat of attack or arrest rather than the avoidance of sexually transmitted infections. Indeed, danger itself was occasionally something to be sought and enjoyed' (p. 483). If risk taking is actually a key part of the excitement in having sex, then theories that assume risk taking is a deterrent, are doomed to failure. The failure of theories of sexual behaviour to deal adequately with the multiple contexts and manners in which people have sex and construct sexuality is a major shortcoming. On the basis of current evidence, grand theories intended to have universal application are futile.

Other criticisms

> *Studies measuring social cognitions about sexual practices rely upon questionnaires which presuppose that cognitions are stable entities residing in people's heads. They do not allow for contextual variables which may influence social cognitions. For example, an individual's attitude towards condom use may well depend upon the sexual partner with whom they anticipate having sexual contact. It may depend upon the time, place, relationship and physiological state (e.g. intoxication) within which sex takes place. As a result, the attempt to predict actual behaviour from decontextualized attitude measures is unlikely to succeed. In addition, it can be argued that sexual intercourse, which is a joint activity, is less likely to be shaped by individual cognitions than solitary health behaviours such as flossing or exercising … the vast majority of social cognition studies of sexual behaviour has focused upon young heterosexual people and gay men, who are perceived to be most vulnerable to HIV infection. However, Johnson et al. (1994) found that people who are divorced, widowed or separated report higher rates of risky sexual practices than those who are single. Also, most heterosexual women in the USA suffering from STI infections have become infected by a partner with whom they have had a long-term involvement (Reiss, 1991). Thus, there is a need for studies of older and/or cohabiting/married heterosexuals' sexual decision-making. (Marks et al., 2005: xx–yy.)*

Weinstein (1993: 324) summarized the state of health behaviour research as follows: ' … despite a large empirical literature, there is still no consensus that certain models of health behaviour are more accurate than others, that certain variables are more influential than others, or that certain behaviours or situations are understood better than others'. Unfortunately, there has been little improvement since then. The traditional individual-level approach to health interventions focuses on theoretical models, piloting, testing and running randomized controlled trials to demonstrate efficacy. It has been estimated that the time from conception to funding and completing the process of demonstrated effectiveness can take 17 years (Clark, 2008). The meta-analyses, reviewed above, suggest that the 'proof of the pudding' in the form of truly effective individual-level interventions is yet to materialize. Alternative means of creating interventions for at risk communities are urgently needed. We review studies and interventions using an alternative community level approach in Chapter 15.

FUTURE RESEARCH

1. Large-scale international studies are necessary to evaluate the cost-effectiveness of the main approaches using systematic trials.
2. It is essential to carry out cross-cultural comparisons of theories and models to determine whether theoretical constructs and assumptions are universal or mono-cultural.

3 Efforts are needed to improve the effectiveness of interventions in ways that are transferable across time and space.
4 Reports of interventions must use transparent systems of classification or typologies to facilitate replication.

Summary

1 Sexual activity, whether for pleasure or procreation, is associated with risks in the form of STIs and HIV infections.
2 In spite of efforts by health authorities at global, national and local levels, the incidence and prevalence of STIs and HIV is increasing in most regions of the world.
3 Individual-level theories and models are based on universal constructs concerning behavioural adoption, maintenance and change. These theories and models assume a set of processes that may or may not be applicable in any given situation.
4 Thousands of studies and many meta-analyses have tested individual-level theories and models with mixed success. Relatively modest amounts of variation in intentions and behaviour are accounted for using this approach.
5 Critics have suggested that individual-level theories and models are fundamentally flawed, or may be un-falsifiable or even tautological.
6 An alternative approach is the community level of analysis, which is **bottom-up**, flexible, and involves the participants in the design of interventions.
7 The community-level approach is difficult to evaluate using traditional evaluation methods and designs. Key constructs such as 'empowerment' have been critiques and need to be analysed.
8 Future research is necessary to evaluate the cost-effectiveness of the two main approaches in systematic trials, to carry out cross-cultural comparisons, and to improve the effectiveness of interventions in ways that are transferable and transparent.

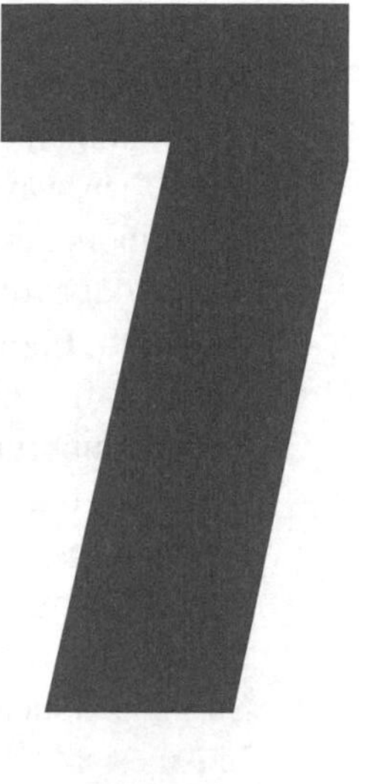

Food, Eating and the Environment

our greatest power is in our ability to change what people consider to be normal behavior.

William N. Ryerson, President,
Population Media Center

Outline

We examine the part played by food and eating in the changing patterns of illnesses and deaths and, in particular, to obesification, the increasing prevalence of obesity. Changes in Western lifestyles and the built environment have led to a toxic ecology for food production, distribution and consumption. Improvements in eating habits could reduce the prevalence of obesity, diabetes, cardiovascular diseases, cancers, osteoporosis and dental disease. We discuss the ecological, social and psychological factors associated with food choices and diet in modern times. We review the evidence on the effectiveness of interventions.

EATING AND OBESITY

From the cradle to the grave, many of the most significant, social and pleasurable activities in human experience are centred on eating and drinking. Eating and drinking are much more than ways of satisfying hunger and thirst, they are also social activities that are rich in symbolic, moral and cultural meanings. Changes in diet, lifestyle and social organization during our evolutionary history have produced a mixture of beneficial and deleterious effects on health. Eating the 'right' balance of foods and setting the 'right' balance between energy input from eating and drinking and energy expenditure through activity and exercise are of critical importance. Eating preferences and habits are influenced by a complex interaction of processes that include conditioning, customs and culture. A fourth crucial factor is the environment, especially climate change. The World Health Organization predicts there will be 2.3 billion overweight adults in the world by 2015 and more than 700 million of them will be obese. This rapidly increasing prevalence of **obesity** is a primary focus for concern. The US Surgeon General has claimed that: 'Obesity is the fastest growing cause of disease and death in America' (Carmona, 2003: paragraph 5). Obesity among young people has risen fast over the past 30 years, with the percentage of US children and adolescents overweight or at risk of becoming overweight tripling to 37 per cent and 34 per cent, respectively (Ogden et al., 2006). In the Middle East and North Africa, Eastern Europe and Latin America, the prevalence of overweight and obesity in women is similar to, or exceeds, that of the USA (Chopra & Darnton-Hill, 2004). There appears to be widespread agreement that the overweight and obesity epidemic requires concerted effort at all levels of health action but especially at the level of policy and regulation (e.g. Kumanyika, Jeffrey, Morabia, Ritenbaugh & Antipatis, 2002; Rossner, 2002; Wadden, Brownell & Foster, 2002; Hu, 2003; Chamberlain, 2004). As with alcohol and tobacco control (Chapters 8 and 9), voluntary agreements with industry have proved completely ineffective.

Like other 'diseases of affluence', obesity has multiple causes that include genetic predisposition, culture, diet and inactivity. Total calorie intake has increased as food has become more processed and more energy dense (Chopra & Darnton-Hill, 2004). In North America, fat and sugar provide over half of total energy intake. This obesogenic diet is becoming common in poor countries. In developing countries, the per capita supply of beef, mutton, goat, pork, poultry, eggs and milk rose by 50 per cent between 1973 and 1996. **Obesification** is also occurring at lower income levels generally. Small changes at a population level can have an immense impact on obesity prevalence levels. The rise in obesity in the United States during 1980–94 can be explained by an average daily increase in consumption of only 3.7 kilocalories (kcal) above maintenance energy requirement for 35-year-old men and 12.7 kcal for 35-year-old women (Khan & Bowman, 1999).

In the USA, 170,000 fast-food restaurants and 3 million soft drink vending machines have encouraged people to eat and drink out of their homes (Chopra & Darnton-Hill, 2004). Wadden et al. refer to 'a toxic environment that implicitly discourages physical activity while explicitly encouraging the consumption of supersized portions of high-fat, high-sugar foods' (2002: 510). A survey reported by Gardner and Halweil (2000) found that only 38 per cent of meals eaten were home made, and many people have never cooked a meal themselves using raw ingredients. Dumanovsky, Nonas, Huang, Silver and Bassett (2009) measured New Yorkers' lunchtime calorie intake in 2007. Receipts were collected from lunchtime customers, at randomly selected fast-food chains. Lunchtime purchases for 7750 customers averaged 827 calories and were lowest for sandwich chains (734 calories) and highest for chicken chains (931 calories). One-third of purchases were over 1000 calories, predominantly at hamburger chains and chicken chains with sandwich chains the lowest. Dumanovsky et al. (2009) concluded that menu calorie posting may help raise awareness, but reducing portion sizes and changing popular combination meals to include lower calorie options could significantly reduce the average calorie content of purchases.

In the United States the food industry spends over $30 billion per annum on promotion – more than any other industry. The challenge for multinational corporations is to continue to generate growth when the market for food is already saturated in developed countries. The food supply already contains 15.9 megajoules (MJ) (3800 kcal) for every adult and child in the US – nearly twice the daily requirement (Chopra & Darnton-Hill, 2004). The foods industry uses several strategies to maintain their profits:

- Persuading people to consume even more food, especially highly energy dense foods, through advertising and outlets.
- Increasing serving size and adding price inducements to order the larger sizes.
- Opening up markets in transitional and developing countries.
- Substituting agricultural products with efficient artificial foods, e.g. margarine as a substitute for butter.
- Adding sugar, salt, fats, oils and artificial flavourings and dyes to enhance flavour, look and competitiveness.

One part of the explanation is that people are significantly less active than was previously the case (see Chapter 10). Another factor is income. Income is strongly associated with dietary quality (Low Income Project Team, 1996). This is because in low-income households the food budget often acts as a reserve when demands for other items including alcohol, tobacco or bills must be met. Yet another factor is stress. In a study of London schoolchildren, Cartwight Wardle, Steggles, Simon, Croker and Jarvis (2003) found that higher stress was associated with more fatty food intake, less fruit and vegetable intake, more snacking and a reduced likelihood of eating breakfast. This is a similar trend to that existing for smoking and drinking.

A recent concern is a linking of eating habits to climate change as the Earth becomes warmer due to Greenhouse Gas (GHG) emissions into the atmosphere. It has been estimated that 18 per cent of global GHG emissions is generated by livestock, approximately half of food's impacts (Food and Agriculture Organization, 2006). The same study estimated that the demand for milk and meat will almost double between 2000 and 2050, which is unsustainable. In the UK, food travels a total 30 billion kilometres each year. This includes imports by boat and air and transport by lorries and cars. Food transport in the UK adds nearly 19 million tonnes of carbon dioxide (CO_2) to the atmosphere each year. Over 2 million tonnes of CO_2 is produced simply by cars travelling to and from shops (Food Climate Research Network, 2008).

Biological influences on body fat levels include age, sex, hormonal factors and genetics. Recent interest has been shown in a so-called 'fat gene'. A 'melanocortin-4 receptor' (*MC4R*) gene is alleged to play a role in regulating food intake and energy balance. Recent studies have found an *MC4R* variant that appears to be related to obesity and insulin resistance. Qi, Kraft, Hunter and Hu (2008) measured the associations of this gene with dietary intakes, weight change and diabetes risk in 5724 women (1533 with type 2 diabetes) from a prospective cohort. Qi et al. reported that the *MC4R* gene was significantly associated with higher intakes of total energy, dietary fat, greater long-term weight change and increased risk of diabetes in women.

Genetic predisposition to obesity, however, cannot explain the increased prevalence in obesity over the last 50 years which must be environmental. Also genetic predisposition to obesity can provide little consolation to those who are affected unless some form of treatment becomes possible in the future. The body uses chemicals and hormones in a complex way to protect its stores of fat, and no drug treatment is available to inhibit the tendency to protect this well endowed fat storage mechanism. Although the development of an effective drug can never be ruled out, anti-obesity drugs are unlikely to be a practical long-term solution for obesity. They are also potentially unsafe. An appetite suppressant, sibutramine (Reductil), is no longer being prescribed in Europe as the increased risks of heart attacks and strokes outweigh the benefits. We turn now to consider evolutionary and environmental determinants of obesity.

AN EVOLUTIONARY PERSPECTIVE

The study of human evolution and pre-history provides a perspective on contemporary ways of life, especially aspects related to food, eating and energy. Early humans can be traced to sites in Africa dating approximately 3.4 million years BP (before the present) when the tool-making *Australopithecus afarensis* lived in Ethiopia. The early hominids were hunter–gatherers, killing and processing their food with weapons and tools fashioned from pieces of volcanic obsidian (McPherron et al. 2010). They may have communicated using an early form of speech. Early hominids evolved at a time when the temperature of the earth was cooling and the northern hemisphere was becoming increasingly glaciated. The ice sheets have advanced and retracted several times during the last million years when the earth's surface temperature has shifted dramatically by up to an average of 10 degrees Centigrade every few thousand years (Lamb & Sington, 1998).

Allowing 25 years for each generation, 100,000 generations of humans separate contemporary *Homo sapiens* from our hominid ancestors *Homo habilis*. In evolutionary terms, this is not very many generations for changes to occur. Another species of hominids, *Homo erectus,* is dated from about 1.8 million years BP and contemporary *Homo sapiens* from about 130–100,000 years BP. The survival of the genus *Homo* over the last 2.5 million years can be attributed to a very high adaptability to geological and climatic variations. An efficient body temperature control system, the ability to hunt, fish, gather and process foods throughout the entire earthly terrain, a communication system and social organization to support the nomadic way of life must have all aided human survival.

For 99.5 per cent of evolutionary history, members of genus *Homo* lived as nomadic 'hunter–gatherers'. At the start of the Holocene 10,000 years ago, following the last Ice Age 18,000 years ago (Lamb & Sington, 1998), groups of humans began permanent settlements as agricultural communities and the 'agricultural revolution' had begun. Because phylogenetic evolution is slow, the genetic make-up of contemporary humans remains adapted to a nomadic existence of gathering and hunting (Powles, 1992). In essence humans are urban hunter–gatherers; our afflictions and diseases reflect that. Contemporary humans are not fitted to the lifestyle and forms of social organization that exist in today's post-agricultural, post-industrial societies. The ecological niches to which genus *Homo* became adapted over 2.4 million years are found today in only a few inaccessible places where wheat fields, supermarkets and televisions are nowhere to be seen.

The vast majority of humans live in cities, towns and villages. However, the toxic ecology of urban lifestyles is generating ill-health and disease on a massive scale. The hypothesis of urban hunter–gatherers receives support from a variety of observations.

HUNTER–GATHERERS PAST AND PRESENT

The hunter–gatherer hypothesis can be evaluated in the light of studies of contemporary hunter–gatherers. Four groups have been studied: Australian aboriginals; the San (or 'Bushmen') of the Kalahari Desert, especially of the !Kung language group; pygmies in the Congo Basin; and the Hadza of East Africa (Powles, 1992). There have also been studies of nomadic peoples in Siberia, Lapland and Greenland. Hunter–gatherers typically lived in bands of 10 to 50 persons with an average band size of perhaps 25. Band composition was fluid. Temporary shelters were built near water and, when food and water supplies were abundant, a band would remain in settlement for several months. A number of bands or 'tribes' of perhaps 500 to 5000 individuals would speak a common language. Population density was below one person per square kilometre. Property had to be carried manually and so, except for a few essential clothes, utensils and weapons, hunter–gatherers would retain few permanent personal possessions. Horses, camels or reindeer transported milk, meat and skins. When fire was discovered, enabling heating and cooking of raw foods, remains uncertain. Ownership, territory and associated issues, were irrelevant to hunter–gatherers. The evidence suggests they lived in an egalitarian manner.

It is believed that early hunter–gatherers spent less time working, building shelters and obtaining food than most humans after the agricultural revolution. The !Kung San typically spend 2.0 hours per day collecting food and the Arnhem Land Aborigines about 4.5 hours per day. It appears likely that about 75 per cent of food energy would have been gathered from vegetable sources by women and the remaining 25 per cent from hunting of animals mainly by men. Powles (1992) estimated the average daily **energy expenditure** for four different historical periods. These estimates suggest that the average daily energy expenditure for a 65 kg male in post-industrial society is 3.5 megajoules (MJ) compared to 4.4 MJ among hunter–gatherers, a difference of more than 25 per cent. In comparison to the 9.3 MJ expended by a labourer in industrial society, however, the difference is much larger at 62 per cent. Yet, the evidence suggests that nomadic, or even early post-industrial, levels of obesity were nothing like those of today.

Even larger differences in energy expenditure may have existed for women – traditionally the principal food gatherers, water collectors, cooks, cleaners, child rearers and child carriers. In most societies nearly all aspects of food getting show differential gender involvement with women being responsible for the majority of food-related activities (Fieldhouse, 1996). In pre-literate societies, three-quarters of over 200 food-related situations were the exclusive province of women. Hunting and fishing tended to be done by males while grinding grain and fetching water were done predominantly by women (Murdock, 1937). In contemporary Africa, women are responsible for 75 per cent of agricultural production, 30 per cent of the ploughing, 50 per cent of planting, 50 per cent of livestock care, 60 per cent of harvesting, 70 per cent of weeding, 85 per cent of food processing, and 95 per cent of domestic work (Fieldhouse, 1996).

A study among !Kung Bushmen, reviewed by Powles, observed that a child is carried by its mother for a distance of 2400 km each year in the first two years of life, 1800 km in year three, and 1200 km in year four, giving a total of 7800 km (4900 miles) over four years. These exceed average activity levels among contemporary adult western women by a wide margin. Reductions in energy expenditure in women may have exceeded that of men; this is consistent with the observation that obesity is generally more common in women than in men (Webb, 1995).

In addition to possible differences in energy expenditure there are differences in diet. Natural ecosystems provide a diet of wild foods that is both varied and plentiful. For example, North American Indians used hundreds of plants in their diets including stinging nettle, common purslane, milkweed, clover, pond-lily, dandelions and fiddleheads (Fieldhouse, 1996). Over 13,000 insects have been classified as edible. In 1950, the Groote Eylandt Aborigines ate 19 large land animals, 76 birds, 97 fish, 39 crustaceans and 82 plants. This diet is adequate both in quality of nutrients and quantity of energy supplied. The evidence suggests that protein, mineral and vitamin intake among hunter–gatherers would have been generally above 'recommended levels'.

For hundreds of thousands of years of human evolution, the capacity to store fat easily was advantageous for survival. Ice Age hunter–gatherers needed to store fat to survive the winters and long journeys in search of food. When the ice retracted and temperatures increased, foods became more accessible and activity levels declined. Thus a metabolic feature promoting survival became a risk factor for diseases that rarely existed in history but which are commonplace today.

Tataranni et al. (2003) measured the body weight gain in 92 free-living Pima Indians to evaluate the effect of energy intake vs. expenditure. Pima Indians living in Southwestern Arizona are one of the most obese populations in the world. Changes in body weight over a follow-up period of about 6 months were available in 74 participants. Tataranni et al. found that a high-energy intake is a risk factor for obesity in humans. They also confirmed that a low resting metabolic rate is a risk factor for weight gain in the Pima population.

Recent studies have explored the role of leptin in human obesity. **Leptin** is a hormone produced by adipose cells, that inhibits food intake and increases energy expenditure in rodents (Ravussin et al., 1997). In humans, plasma leptin concentrations correlate with the amount of adipose tissue. However, there are individual differences in plasma leptin concentrations at any degree of fatness. Ravussin et al. (1997) investigated whether individuals prone to weight gain are hypoleptinemic, i.e. they produce too little leptin. They measured fasting plasma leptin concentrations in two groups of weight-matched nondiabetic Pima Indians who were followed for approximately 3 years, 19 of whom subsequently gained weight and 17 of whom maintained their weight. After adjusting for initial per cent body fat, the mean plasma leptin concentration was found to be lower in Indians who gained weight than in those whose weight was stable. The results suggest that relatively low plasma leptin concentrations may play a role in the development of obesity in Pima Indians.

THE AGRICULTURAL REVOLUTION

The agricultural revolution is dated at about 10,000 years BP when humans in the Middle East began settlements in fertile valleys and river deltas. This development meant that humans lived for the first time in densely populated villages and towns. Wheat, barley and other cereals were cultivated and sheep and goats were kept in captivity and slaughtered to provide a ready supply of meat. For the first time people acquired and retained ownership of property and land. The revolution spread through Europe, reaching Britain about 5000 years ago. Population density increased dramatically from less than four persons per square kilometre to 100 or more persons per square kilometre. In fertile river valleys, densities would have increased several hundredfold. Settlement made it easier for individuals to survive protracted or severe bouts of illness or disability. New forms of social organizations could be established to promote health and provide aid to the sick. However, with the stabilizing influence of settlement and civilization came a number of adverse consequences:

- Food supplies were more dependent on local weather conditions and hazards, e.g. floods, droughts, earthquakes and volcanoes.
- The diet became less varied and balanced.
- Malnutrition, anaemia and osteoporosis become more prevalent.
- Average levels of activity and energy expenditure decreased.
- The prevalence of bowel and respiratory infections increased.
- New pathogens and epidemics were possible.
- The birth rate increased.
- Warring over territory became more likely.
- Social problems related to population density and ownership became more prevalent.
- Psychosocial and socio-economic stress related to population density, property, status and self-esteem became more significant.

A study in Burkina Faso found that the agriculturalist Mossi people were more stressed and marginalized than the pastoralist Fulani people (Van Haaften & Van de Vijver, 1996). Further studies with actual hunter–gatherers and matched sedentary control groups could determine how such differences translate into illness and mortality rates. Unfortunately numbers of true hunter–gatherers are dwindling as their forest abodes are destroyed to plant crops. The impact of deforestation on local animal populations such as orang utans, and on rising levels of GHG emissions, is immense.

THE INDUSTRIAL REVOLUTION

About 200 years ago the next stepping stone in human social evolution was laid – the industrial revolution which came with the steam engine. Later, with the electric motor, light bulb, telephone, computer and Internet, we can now do almost everything we need to live within the comfort of four walls without moving anywhere. The internal combustion and jet engines permit one to travel everywhere on earth with minimum energy expenditure. These new systems of communication and transportation have had radical effects on lifestyles.

The Digital era of television, computers, satellites, mobile phones and the Internet is bringing benefits to working efficiency and communication. Labour-saving products in the form of washing machines, dryers, microwave ovens and dishwashers have brought further reductions in energy expenditure in tasks of daily living. Food is produced ready for the supermarket. The availability of Ready Meals, instant desserts and snacks designed for consumption during a steady 9–5 schedule of sedentary work and television viewing means that food preparation and cooking are being moved from the domestic kitchen to the food-processing industry. The contribution of the industry to the quality of food and eating is ever more critical. Industry generally is slow to make improvements voluntarily. Health only becomes a higher priority than profit when there is a heavy consumer demand backed by policy and legislation. Current legislation lacks teeth as the industry has colonized governmental organizations with the powers to set policy.

AN ECOLOGICAL MODEL

In this section we consider the contemporary ecology of food and eating. A primary focus will be **adiposity**, the fat content of the body, and *'fattiness'*, the fat content of foods, and the relationship between the two. DeMattia and Denney (2008) used the Ecological Systems Theory of Bronfenbrenner (1986) as a framework to discuss ecological considerations in childhood obesity. The principal systems involved in children's eating habits are: (i) the individual child's genetic environment; (ii) the family environment; (iii) the larger community in which the child lives. An ecological approach shows the necessity of community-scale interventions in addition to an approach based on the individual's '**will-power**' to change their behaviour.

Fat and feeling fat

A pan-European survey asked a sample of 15,239 people representative of the population to indicate which of nine figures best described their current and ideal body image. An underweight body image was chosen by 55 per cent as their ideal, in comparison to only 37 per cent who felt that their body image was in the underweight category. The disparity between ideal and current body image was generally greater for females than males (European Commission, 1999). The high value placed on thinness in contemporary affluent societies is not evident in Africa or the Pacific Basin, nor was it seen in previous eras when a fulsome figure was seen as attractive or a symbol of power and status.

The obesity debate has focused on two main subjects: high **fat** foods and overweight people. In most western countries the proportion of food energy derived from fat is close to 40 per cent as compared to a recommended level of 30–35 per cent. **Triglyceride** is the main component of dietary fats and oils and the principal form in which fat is stored in the body. Triglyceride is composed of three fatty acids attached to a glycerol molecule. These acids are saturated (S), monounsaturated (M) and polyunsaturated (P). The proportions of these three acids varies across different fats and oils, butter having 64 per cent, 33 per cent and 3 per cent, olive oil having 15 per cent, 73 per cent and 13 per cent, and rape seed oil (canola) having 7 per cent, 60 per cent and 33 per cent respectively. The P:S ratio is therefore approximately 0.05 for butter and almost 5.00 for canola.

Keys, Anderson and Grande (1959) measured total serum **cholesterol** levels in two groups of men who were given diets that varied in the degree of saturation of fat but matched for total fat content. Diet A that had a P:S ratio of 0.16 produced a much higher serum cholesterol level than diet B with a P:S ratio of 2.79. Cholesterol has been implicated as a causal factor in **coronary heart disease** (Brown & Goldstein, 1984). The findings of Keys et al. led many to conclude that fats and oils with a low P:S ratio like butter or coconut oil were high risk food items while olive oil and rape seed oil were lower risk. This analysis led to a negative health image for food items containing high amounts of saturated fat (Webb, 1995) triggering health promotion campaigns with the aim of reducing saturated fat in western diets. However, it is important to distinguish between two different fractions of cholesterol that are low-density lipoprotein **(LDL)** or 'bad' cholesterol and high-density lipoprotein **(HDL)** or 'good' cholesterol. High levels of LDL are positively associated with cardiovascular disease while high levels of HDL are negatively associated with cardiovascular disease. The different types of fatty acids have a complex set of effects on raising or lowering LDL and HDL. This complicates the issue and presents a considerable challenge to nutritional health promotion. Statins are commonly used to lower levels of LDL cholestrol because a high level of 'bad' cholesterol in the blood – **hypercholesterolemia** – is a risk factor for coronary heart disease.

A second focus has been the characteristics of people who are classified overweight or obese. The excess weight of obese individuals is due mainly to **adipose tissue** mass of which 85 per cent is fat. Models of obesity have placed the cause at one of two levels: (1) individual overweight and obese people have been blamed for their 'sloth' and 'gluttony'; (2) overweight and obese people are assumed to have a genetic predisposition to lowered metabolic rate (Webb, 1995). The first of these causes is seen as potentially controllable, but only in those people who possess 'strong will power' or high 'self-efficacy' (Bandura, 1977). In attributing responsibility to individuals, one must take into account biological, social, ecological and psychological barriers to change. Working with obese people at an individual level is the primary activity of organizations such as Weight Watchers and has been an active area of research in clinical psychology. A second approach considers the toxic environment.

The toxic environment

The ecological approach to obesity sees obesity in the context of the individual's relationship to the surrounding environment. Essentially it attributes obesity as much to the environment as to the obese individuals themselves. Egger and Swinburn (1997) proposed three main influences on equilibrium levels of body fat – biological, behavioural and environmental. Obesity is seen not as a disorder of individuals requiring treatment but an expected consequence of living in an environment that is designed to produce obesity. Contemporary society is said to be **obesogenic** because it generates too high an equilibrium level of fatness across the whole population relative to average activity levels. In this approach, the solution to the increasing prevalence of obesity lies with the structural characteristics of the environment, not at the level of the individual. This ecological theory is based on the **fat balance equation** that states:

Rate of change of fat stores in the body = Rate of fat intake – Rate of fat oxidation (Swinburn and Ravussin, 1993)

Total energy is the mediator of weight gain that, under contemporary conditions, is interchangeable with fat energy. The intake of fat is a significant component of total energy intake while total energy expenditure is the main determinant of fat oxidation. A reduction of dietary fat within an otherwise varied diet leads to weight loss. However, weight loss tends to be associated with rebound weight gain due to physiological defences against weight loss. In an environment that promotes obesity, there is also a high equilibrium point of fat stores.

Although the proportion of energy from fats and oils has decreased in western countries since the 1960s, this reduction is attributed mainly to reductions in food **energy intake** rather than a shift to a lower fat diet (Webb, 1995). However, the average level of energy intake is falling more slowly than the average level of energy output. This imbalance has caused increases in average weight levels and prevalence of obesity.

If the prevalence of obesity is to be successfully tackled, the average energy expenditure of the human population needs to be significantly increased while the average energy intake is reduced. Without intervention at a policy level, the currently high prevalence of obese and overweight people is likely to remain evident for some considerable time.

ENVIRONMENTAL INFLUENCES ON FOOD CHOICES

A vast range of environmental influences affect what and how much is eaten, by whom and under which circumstances. As Egger and Swinburn (1997) point out, these influences are frequently underrated. Influences fall into the 'macro' and 'micro' level categories. Those at the macro level are the consequence of policy, laws and regulations at a societal level. Micro level influences are at a family or individual level. The influences are also divisible into physical, economic and socio-economic categories.

Remick, Polivy and Pliner (2009) argued that variety, how many different foods are accessible and available, is a key factor in determining food intake. These authors consider how different moderators, which can be internal or external in nature, may influence the variety effect in different ways. They suggest that internal moderators such as gender, weight and dietary restraint, do not moderate the variety effect, except possibly old age. On the other hand, external moderators, such as the particular properties of food and the eater's perception of the situation, affect the strength of the variety effect on intake to some degree. Remick et al. (2009) suggest that an evolutionary hypothesis may account for the roles that internal and external variables play in moderating the variety effect.

Variety of foods in the school environment certainly appear to play a key role in children's food choices. Celebrity chef, Jamie Oliver, revealed that only 37 pence was being spent on ingredients in school dinners in South London (Channel 4, 2005). Oliver attempted to improve school dinners by introducing more fresh fruit and vegetables with mixed results. However, as a consequence of Jamie Oliver's direct actions using the powerful medium of television, the British government implemented measures to raise nutritional standards of school meals.

Access to healthy food is a primary environmental factor at both macro and micro levels. Studies have focused on the access people have to grocery, convenience stores and fast foods. Neighbourhoods without grocery stores generally have a reduced access to fresh fruits and vegetables. Baker, Schootman, Barnidge and Kelly (2006) carried out a study of the upper Midwest portion of the US which indicated that neighbourhoods with a mixture of races or high poverty whites had fewer stores selling fresh fruits and vegetables, compared with higher income neighbourhoods. African–American areas had less access to fruits and vegetables. A study in New York by Kwate, Yau, Loh and Williams (2009) found inequalities in the exposure to obesogenic environments created by fast-food restaurants. The density of fast-food restaurants in New York City was found to be significantly higher in predominantly Black areas than in predominantly White areas. High-income Black areas and low-income Black areas had similar exposures. The authors suggest that policy level interventions need to address disparities in food environments if obesity prevention is to be effective. Morland, Diez Roux and Wing (2006) described a large-scale study of more than 10,000 adults. People with access to supermarkets had a lower prevalence of obesity, while those with more access to convenience stores had a higher prevalence of obesity. Programmes to make buying fruits and vegetables more convenient are being organized at both government and grassroots levels.

DeMattia and Denney (2008) describe a programme organized by Governor Ed Rendell of Pennsylvania to form public–private partnerships that improve access to healthy foods. Supermarket development is encouraged in low-income areas by awarding grants and loans to organizations willing to invest into these areas (Robert Wood Johnson Foundation, 2006). Also, in 2005 Nevada passed Senate Bill 229 into law which gave a temporary tax incentive for locating or expanding grocery stores in the southern part of the state (Robert Wood Johnson Foundation, 2006). An interesting Case Study of a community intervention promoting healthy eating is shown below (see p. 164).

A core factor in traditional family life has been eating a family meal together. However, in modern times, this tradition is weakening as families are eating more outside their homes, spending almost 50 per cent of total food dollars at restaurants and on fast food (Institute of Medicine, 2004). Bowman, Gortmaker, Ebbeling, Pereira and Ludwig (2004) reported that 30 per cent of 4–19 year old children were consuming at least one fast-food meal per day with a total calorie increase of 187 kcal/day. New York City and Seattle have passed regulations requiring chain restaurants to label menus with calorie information. This is a trend that will spread as legislators take on the food industry with more determination.

Working in Liverpool, England, Hackett, Boddy, Boothby, Dummer, Johnson and Stratton (2008) mapped the dietary habits of children in an investigation of factors that determine their food choice. They were interested in the idea that 'food deserts' are a barrier to making healthier food choices. Hackett et al. conducted a cross-sectional survey of the dietary habits of 1535 9–10-year-old children from 90 primary schools. Two areas containing individuals with the 'best' and 'worst' food choices with very similar socio-economic profiles were mapped.

Visual inspection indicated that the contrast in the physical environments was 'striking'. No evidence was found to support the concept that poor eaters lived in so-called food deserts. The area with the worst food choices had many shops selling food, whereas the area with best food choices had no shops in evidence but had more space, wider streets, and more trees, parks and greenery (Hackett et al., 2008; see Figure 7.1).

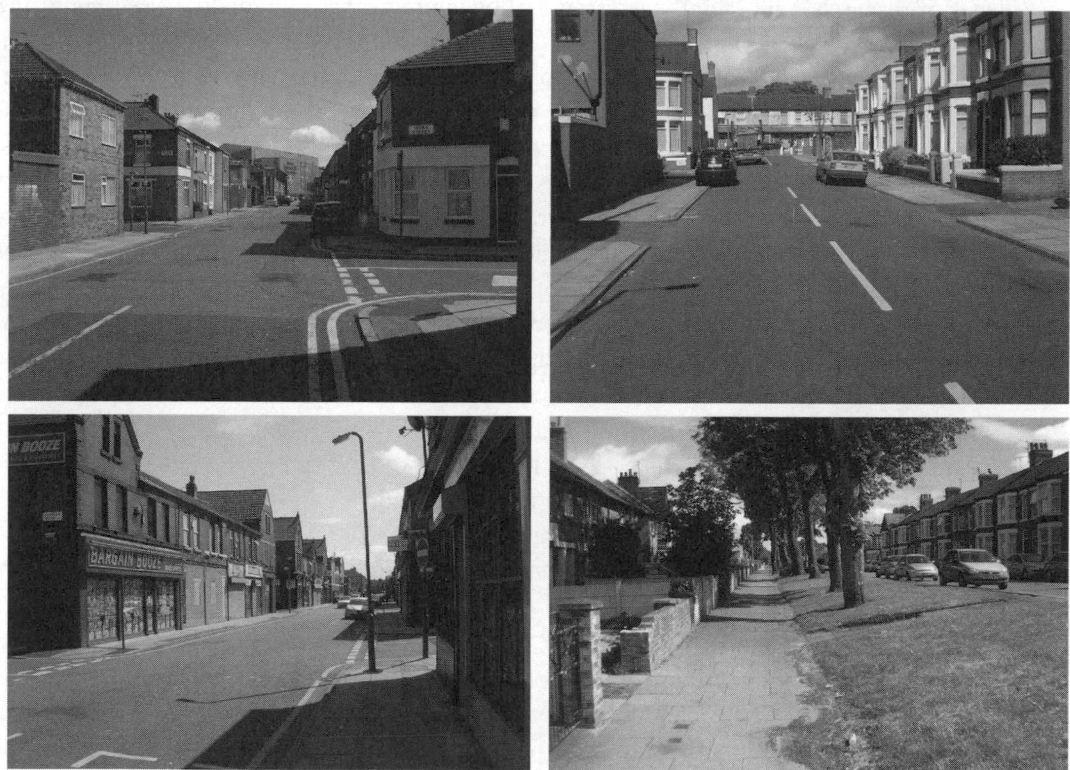

Figure 7.1 Neighbouring areas in Liverpool with unhealthy (on left) and healthy dietary habits
Source: Hackett et al., 2008; Reproduced with permission

FOOD PROMOTION/ADVERTISING INFLUENCES ON CHILDREN

A primary influence in creating an environment that is toxic is food advertising. Every day in the US, children view an average of 15 TV food advertisements (Federal Trade Commission, 2007) with an overwhelming majority (98 per cent) promoting high fat, sugar, and/or sodium products (Powell, Szczpka, Chaloupka & Braunschweig, 2007). High exposure to food advertising is a leading cause of unhealthy consumption (Brownell & Horgen, 2004; Institute of Medicine, 2006). Food advertising typically shows unhealthy eating behaviours such as snacking at non-meal times which occurred in 58 per cent of food ads during children's programming (Harrison & Marske, 2005). In addition to their enjoyable taste, products are depicted as 'fun' and 'cool' (Harrison & Marske, 2005; Folta, Goldberg, Economos, Bell & Meltzer, 2006).

The Food Standards Agency (2003) published a systematic review examining how foods promoted to children are linked to children's eating patterns. 29,946 potentially relevant pieces of research were initially assessed. Following relevance and quality assessment, 118 research papers describing a total of 101 studies passed the authors' methodological criteria. The report found that advertising targeted at children has an effect on their preferences, purchases and consumption. These effects occur not for brands but food types. The review report found that food promotion to children is dominated by television advertising of the 'Big Four': pre-sugared breakfast cereals, soft-drinks, confectionary and savoury snacks. However, fast-food chains have rapidly become more dominant, making a 'Big Five'. Advertised foods are promoted for fun, fantasy and taste, not health and nutrition. The review found a link between the amount of television viewing and diet, obesity and cholesterol levels. However, it could not be determined whether it is the advertising itself, or the sedentary nature of television viewing or the snacking that often takes place while viewing, that is major cause of this problem. To summarize, the reviewers found that:

- There is a lot of food advertising to children.
- The advertised diet is less healthy than recommended.
- Children enjoy and engage with food promotion.
- Food promotion influences children's preferences, purchase behaviour and consumption.

Dixon, Scully, Wakefield, White and Crawford (2007) surveyed children's TV viewing habits and associated these with food-related attitudes and behaviour. The survey showed that greater TV use and more frequent commercial TV viewing were independently associated with positive attitudes toward junk food. TV use was also associated with higher junk food consumption. Dixon et al. also conducted an experiment to assess the impact of differing combinations of TV ads for unhealthy and healthy foods on children's dietary knowledge, attitudes and intentions – 919 grade five and six students from schools in Melbourne, Australia, were participants. Ads for nutritious foods promoted positive attitudes and beliefs concerning these types of foods. Dixon et al. concluded that changing the food-advertising environment on children's TV towards more nutritious foods would help to normalize and reinforce healthy eating. These findings confirm what has been suspected for some time. The study increases understanding of how children's choices and eating habits are being moulded by large corporate interests. Action is needed to limit the power of industry, to bring about improvements in eating habits in young people.

KEY STUDY 'Priming effects of television food advertising on eating behavior' (Harris, Bargh & Brownell, 2009)

This study experimentally tested whether TV food advertising is capable of priming an increase in snack food consumption. The authors predicted that advertising that conveys snacking and fun automatically cues eating behaviour among adults as well as children and also that advertising will affect consumption of any available foods, not only those advertised.

These experiments replicated conditions in which people are exposed to food advertising on TV. Advertisements were embedded within a TV programme during commercial breaks at a typical regularity that applies in everyday life. Experiments 1a and 1b utilized common types of children's food advertisements and measured effects on snack food consumed by children while watching TV. Experiment 2 investigated the impact of snack- and nutrition-focused food advertising on adult consumption of a range of snack foods. The advertisements were not related to the brands or types of foods to be consumed by participants, in an effort to minimize the participants' awareness of the experimental hypotheses.

Following parental consent, the children met with the experimenter individually at their school or camp for approximately 30 minutes in an unoccupied classroom or conference room. The children watched a 14-minute episode of 'Disney's Recess,' a cartoon typically viewed by 7- to 11-year-olds. In this episode, the class goes on a field trip to a science museum. One-half of the children were randomly assigned to watch a version that included four 30-second food commercials inserted during two advertising breaks. The commercials promoted snack and breakfast foods of poor nutritional quality using a fun and happiness message (a high-sugar cereal, waffle sticks with syrup, fruit roll-ups, and potato chips). The other half watched the same cartoon with four non-food commercials (games and entertainment products).

Children received a bowl of cheddar cheese 'goldfish' crackers (150 gr.) and a glass of water and were told that they could snack while watching. Advertising for goldfish crackers was not presented during the cartoon. The experimenter left the room, returned after the cartoon was finished, and asked the children when they had last eaten prior to the experiment. After the children left, the experimenter weighed the remaining goldfish crackers and recorded the amount consumed.

Harris et al. found that children who saw food advertising ate 8.8 g. more during the 14 minutes of TV viewing. The authors concluded that: 'at this rate, snacking while watching commercial TV with food advertisements for only 30 minutes per day would lead to 94 additional kcal. consumed and a weight gain of almost 10 pounds per year, if not compensated by reduced consumption of other foods or increased physical activity' (Harris et al., 2009: 409).

(Continued)

(Continued)

In a second experiment adult participants were not provided with a snack while watching but were invited into a 'second experiment' when they tasted snack foods that varied in perceived nutritional value. Participants were 98 university students between 18 and 24 years old. A 16-minute version of a comedy TV programme ('Whose Line is it Anyway?') was shown with 11 commercials (4 minute total), inserted during two commercial breaks. Three versions were created; each version included seven of the same non-food commercials. One version included four commercials for food and beverages with a snacking message that emphasized fun and excitement (two fast-food products, candy bar, and cola soft drink); another included four food and beverage commercials with a nutrition message (granola bar, orange juice, oatmeal, and an 'instant breakfast' beverage); and the control included four additional non-food commercials. The advertising message had a significant effect on the amount consumed for individual foods (controlling for taste ratings) as shown in Figure 7.2.

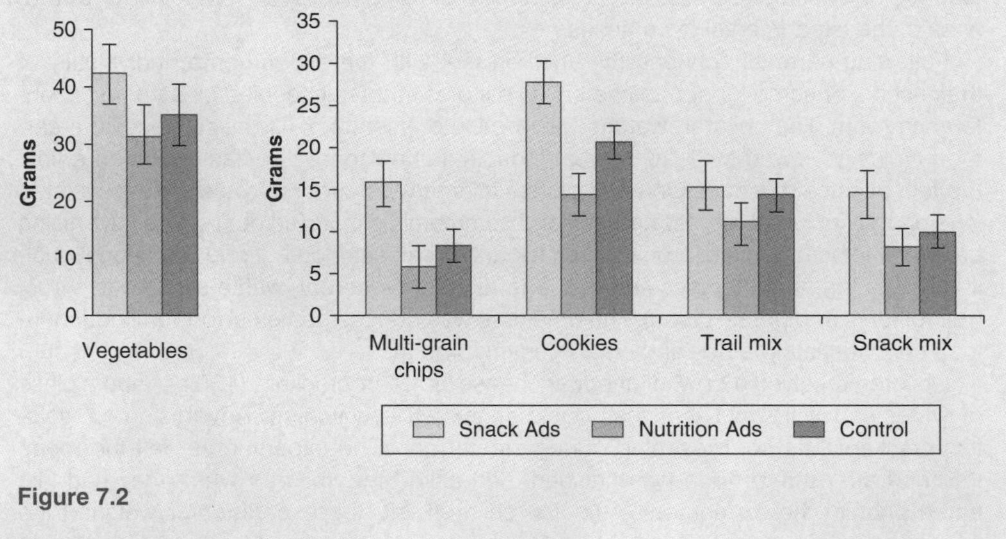

Figure 7.2

For further discussion of the ecological approach to obesity, see Egger & Swinburn (1997), Reading 12 in Marks (2002a).

CONTENT AND FLAVOUR OF FOODS

Fat and fibre

A major focus for epidemiological research has been dietary fat and fibre in the form of meat, cereals, fruit and vegetables. Animal-derived foods are high in fat but contain almost no fibre. Fruit and vegetables contain high amounts of fibre but no fat. One approach to study the impact of contrasting amounts of fat and fibre in the diet is to compare the mortality and illness rates of meat eaters and non-meat eaters. Although meat consumption increases the risk of cancers of the colorectum, breast and prostate, until recently the evidence of reduced illness and mortality among vegetarians has not been conclusive.

NEWS
NEW STUDIES SHOW ALL FOODS BAD FOR YOU
ED FISCHER

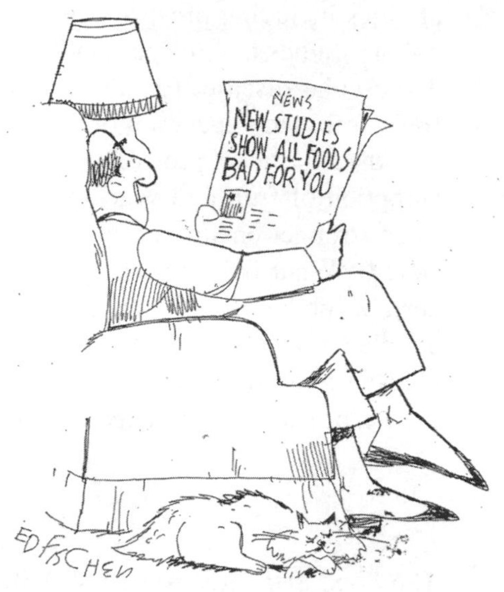

Key et al. (1998) compared the mortality rates of vegetarians and non-vegetarians among 76,000 men and women who had participated in five prospective studies. This meta-analysis collated the entire body of evidence collected in prospective studies in western countries from 1960 to 1981. The original studies were conducted in California (2), Britain (2) and Germany (1) and provided data concerning 16- to 89-year-olds for whom diet and smoking status information was available. The results were adjusted for age, sex and smoking. Vegetarians were defined as those who did not eat any meat or fish (n = 27,808). Participants were followed for an average of 10.6 years when 8330 deaths occurred. The results showed that vegetarians as a group contained a lower proportion of smokers and current alcohol drinkers, a higher proportion of high exercisers and had a consistently lower **body mass index (BMI)**.

The death rate ratio for ischaemic heart disease for vegetarians versus non-vegetarians across the five studies was 0.76 (95 per cent CI 0.62–0.94). The all cause mortality ratio was 0.95 (95 per cent CI 0.82–1.11). The reduction in mortality among vegetarians varied significantly with age at death, younger ages at death being associated with much lower rate ratios: 0.55 for deaths under 65; 0.69 for deaths between 65 and 79; 0.92 for deaths between 80 and 89. When non-vegetarians were subdivided into regular meat eaters and semi-vegetarians who ate fish only or ate meat less than once a week, there was evidence of a significant dose-response. The death rate ratio for ischaemic heart disease, caused by a narrowing of the arteries, for semi-vegetarians and vegetarians compared to regular meat eaters was 0.78 and 0.66 respectively. These data suggest that vegetarians have a lower risk of dying from ischaemic heart disease than non-vegetarians. Like any epidemiological study, this study could not control for all relevant factors and could be subject to confounding. For example, vegetarians may differ from carnivores in many ways that could not be controlled for (e.g. in exercise levels, use of drugs, religious beliefs and health values).

Other studies have found an association between diet and cancer. Block, Patterson and Subar (1992) reviewed the role of fruit and vegetables in cancer prevention and concluded that 132 of 170 studies indicated a significant protective effect for cancers at all sites including prostate. Ness and Powles (1997) reviewed ecological, **case-control**, cohort studies and unconfounded trials in humans concerning fruit, vegetables and cardiovascular disease from the period 1966 to 1995. All studies in the review reported on fresh fruit and vegetables or a nutrient that could serve as a proxy. Many of the studies found a significant protective association for coronary heart disease and stroke with consumption of fruit and vegetables or surrogate nutrients. The protective effect appeared to be stronger on stroke than on coronary heart disease. Cummings and Bingham (1998) stated: 'What is remarkable about the diet–cancer story is the consistency with which certain foods emerge as important in reducing risk across the range of cancers.' They concluded that vegetables and fruit are protective for almost all of the major cancers. Consumption of meat, especially red meat and processed meat, is linked with bowel, breast, prostate and pancreatic cancer.

Salt

The Food Standards Agency (2010) stated that 26 million adults in the UK eat too much salt with about 75 per cent of that salt already in the food that they buy. Salt (sodium chloride) has long been associated with essential hypertension. Ecological studies suggest that populations with low salt intake such as the Kalahari Bushmen have low incidence of hypertension in comparison to societies such as the UK and USA where salt intake and hypertension incidence are both high (Webb, 1995). However, there are many confounding variables in these ecological studies that could explain this link: high physical activity, low levels of obesity, low alcohol and tobacco use and high potassium intake in those groups with low salt diets.

In a controlled study, Law, Frost and Wald (1991) correlated blood pressure and salt intake from 24 populations and found a highly significant relationship that increased with age and baseline levels. Populations with lower mean salt intake generally have a lower blood pressure and a less steep rise of blood pressure with age. Much of the salt in Western diets, perhaps 80 per cent, comes from processed food. There is a need to restrict the salt content of processed foods requiring regulation of the food industry.

Viera, Kshirsagar and Hinderliter (2007) examined variations in reports of receipt of lifestyle modification advice in 28,457 hypertensive individuals. Exercise advice was reported most frequently (75 per cent), followed by advice to reduce salt intake (69 per cent), change eating habits (62 per cent), and reduce alcohol intake (44 per cent). Eighteen to 39 year-olds were more likely to report receipt of advice than adults aged 60 years or older (odds ratio, 1.42; 95 CI, 1.11–1.81). Overweight people (OR, 1.64; 95 CI, 1.40–1.93) and obese people (OR, 2.75; 95 CI, 2.28–3.31) were also more likely to report receipt of advice. Persons receiving antihypertensive medication were also more likely to report receiving advice (OR, 2.35; 95 CI, 1.98–2.81). As in many fields of behaviour change, the advice received by people depends on their personal characteristics. In this case, if a person is 'slim' and/or older, s/he is not seen as needing any such advice.

Sugar

Sugar or sucrose appeared in the West in the eighth century (Mintz, 1997). Sugar is a disaccharide composed of one unit of glucose and one of fructose, which is found in fruits and vegetables, particularly sugar beet and sugar cane, from which it is extracted and purified to make white sugar, brown sugar, treacle or syrup. It is used as a sweetener and preservative by food processors. It has been strongly linked with the development of obesity, maturity onset diabetes and the rotting of teeth (dental caries). Increasing obesity rates can be attributed in part to the prominence in our diet of the 'empty' calories of sugar that carry no nutritional value.

Cust et al. (2009) assessed the total dietary intake of carbohydrate, sugar, starch and fibre intakes in ten European countries as a part of the European Prospective Investigation into Cancer and Nutrition. From 1995 to 2000, 36,034 people between 35–74 years completed a standardized, 24-hour dietary recall. Intakes (gm/day) of carbohydrate, sugars, starch and fibre were estimated. Carbohydrate intakes were highest in Italy and in the UK health-conscious cohort, and were lowest in Spain, Greece and France. Bread contributed the highest proportion of carbohydrates (mainly starches) in every centre. Fruit contributed a greater proportion of total carbohydrates (mainly sugar) in women than men, and in southern compared to northern places. Bread, fruits and vegetables were the largest sources of fibre, but these sources varied from place to place. Carbohydrate intakes were higher among the physically active, never-smokers or non-drinkers. O'Connor, Jones, Conner, McMillan and Ferguson (2008) studied the effects of daily hassles and eating style on eating behaviour in a naturalistic setting using a multilevel diary design. Daily diary reports of between-meal snacking, fruit and vegetable consumption and variations in food intake were monitored. In accord with anecdotal evidence, increased snacking on high fat or sugar items, with a proportionate reduction in main meals and vegetable consumption, occurred on days with high numbers of hassles. The authors concluded that 'emotional eating' was the moderator of the hassles–snacking relationship indicative of a pathway through which stress can influence risks to health.

Caffeine

Caffeine is the most popular drug on earth with more than 80 per cent of the world's population consuming it daily (James, 1997). It is consumed in coffee, tea, drinking chocolate, cocoa and cola drinks providing a slight psychoactive effect on arousal and mood. Coffee has achieved symbolic status as a recreational and exotic beverage. Consumption varies across countries with four of the highest consumers being the UK, Sweden, Canada and the USA with average daily levels of 444, 425, 238 and 211 mg (Gilbert, 1984).

Because of its widespread usage even small increases in relative risk for heart disease or cancers could have large absolute effects. James (1997) reviews evidence from hundreds of studies concerning caffeine's psychopharmacological and epidemiological effects. James suggests that caffeine use *could* account for 9–14 per cent of cases of coronary heart disease, 17–24 per cent of stroke cases and could contribute to adverse reproductive outcomes when used in pregnancy. However, these estimates require further research.

Learning Food Preferences

Following Pavlov's (1927) studies of conditioned reflexes, learning and conditioning became the main focus of research on food preferences and aversions. Although experience generally determines food choices, sweet tastes and possibly fatty tastes are innately attractive while bitter tastes are innately avoided. Capaldi (1996) suggests that preferences for foods are modifiable in four ways:

1. *Mere exposure*.
2. *Flavour–flavour learning*: flavours that are repeatedly associated with an already preferred flavour such as saccharin will themselves become preferred. A sweetener produces liking in almost any other food with which it is mixed.
3. *Flavour–nutrient learning*: flavours that are repeatedly associated with a nutrient such as a protein become preferred.
4. *Taste aversion learning*: this occurs when a novel taste solution (the conditioned stimulus or CS) is followed by an unpleasant stimulus (the unconditioned stimulus or UCS) that produces transient gastrointestinal illness or vomiting (the unconditioned response or UR) (Garcia, Ervin & Koelling, 1966). This type of learning is adaptive in animals that need to learn rapidly to differentiate between positive and toxic foods. However, taste and food aversions are also quite common in humans, for example, with specific types of alcohol (gin or whisky) as a result of nausea caused by over-imbibing on the first occasion of use.

The flavour of food is conveyed by the senses of taste, smell and chemical irritation. The foetus receives its first nutrients in the amniotic fluid that is a potential carrier of flavour and odour (Mennella & Beauchamp, 1996). By term the human foetus has swallowed quite large amounts of amniotic fluid (200–760 ml daily) and has been exposed to glucose, fructose, lactic acid, pyruvic acid, citric acid, fatty acids, phospholipids, creatinine, urea, uric acid, amino acids, proteins and salts (Mennella & Beauchamp, 1996). The amniotic fluid and mother's milk are both primed by a maternal diet that is unique and so may have similar aromatic profiles providing a 'thread of chemical continuity between the pre- and postnatal niches' (Schaal & Orgeur, 1992). Studies of foetal swallowing and of preterm infant sucking even suggest that a preference for sweet flavours is evident before birth (Tatzer, Schubert, Timischi & Simbruner, 1985). This evidence suggests that preferences for flavour and smell are influenced very early in life. In fact the earliest and most emotional life events revolve around eating and drinking and the taking and giving of food are, from initiation, 'exquisitely social' (Rozin, 1996: 235).

INTERVENTIONS

Individual-Level Interventions

A variety of interventions have been tried at the individual level of influence. The quality of the research used to evaluate the interventions is of varied quality but mostly rather poor. Sample sizes are small, power analyses are rarely if ever carried out, and designs are overall rather poor. Recent systematic reviews on effectiveness will be briefly summarized to illustrate the near crisis situation that exists in dealing with the obesity problem.

Campbell, Waters, O'Meara, Kelly and Summerbell (2002) systematically reviewed interventions for preventing obesity in children. The objective was to assess the effectiveness of educational, health promotion and/or psychological/counselling interventions that focused on diet, physical activity and/or lifestyle and social support which were designed to prevent obesity in childhood. Randomized controlled trials (RCTs) and non-RCTs were included where observations were taken for a minimum of three months. The preferred interval of 12 months yielded only seven acceptable studies. By going to three months a total of 10 studies could be included. The seven accepted 12-month studies were carried out during the period 1986–2001. The results were non-significant overall. However, one long-term study and two short-term studies focusing on physical activity resulted in a slightly greater reduction in overweight.

A second systematic review evaluated interventions for treating obesity in children (Summerbell, Ashton, Campbell, Edmunds, Kelly & Waters, 2004). Eighteen RCTs with 975 participants that used a minimum six-month period for the follow-up were studied. Five studies with 245 participants investigated changes in physical activity and sedentary behaviour; two studies with 107 participants compared problem-solving with usual care or behaviour therapy. Nine studies with 399 participants compared behavioural therapy at varying degrees of family involvement with no treatment or usual care. Finally two studies with 224 participants compared CBT with relaxation. The authors state that most of the studies were 'too small to have the power to detect the effects of the treatment'. They were unable to carry out a meta-analysis because so few of the trials included the same comparisons and outcomes. Therefore a narrative synthesis only was used and no direct conclusions could be confidently made.

A third systematic review assessed the evidence on advice on low-fat diets for obesity (Pirozzo, Summerbell, Cameron & Glasziou, 2004). Twelve RCTs were selected with varying periods of follow-up: four with six-months follow-up; five with 12-months follow-up; three with 18-months follow-up. No significant differences were evident at any of these three periods. The authors concluded that low fat diets do no better than low calorie diets in terms of long-term weight loss.

A fourth systematic review was carried out by Powell, Calvin and Calvin (2007) who were interested in sustained weight change capable of influencing clinical endpoints with minimal risks. Powell et al. reviewed methodologically rigorous trials on lifestyle change, drug therapy and surgical interventions. They only considered trials that provided evaluations for at least two years from the intervention. The authors found that both lifestyle and drug interventions are capable of producing 'modest but clinically significant sustained change in weight with minimal risks'. However only 20–40 per cent of patients given lifestyle or drug interventions sustain weight loss targets for two or more years. Such approaches have produced a modest average net loss of 7 lb (3.2 kg) between treated and control participants which is clinically significant for diabetes and hypertension.

A fifth systematic review by Spring et al. (2009) reviewed behavioural interventions to promote smoking cessation and prevent weight gain. The authors asked whether behavioural weight control interventions provided an effective way to reduce post-cessation weight gain. Of 35 relevant RCTs, 10 met the authors' criteria for the meta-analysis. Patients who received smoking and weight treatment showed increased abstinence and reduced weight gain in the short term (<3 months) compared to patients who received smoking treatment alone. However differences in abstinence and weight control were not significant in the long term (>6 months).

Bariatric Surgery

Bariatric or weight loss surgery reduces the size of the stomach with an implanted device (gastric banding) or by removal of a portion of the stomach or by resecting and re-routing the small intestines to a small stomach pouch (gastric bypass surgery). Such procedures are capable of producing significant long-term loss of weight, recovery from diabetes, improvement in cardiovascular risk factors, and a reduction in mortality of 23 per cent to 40 per cent (Robinson, 2009). Bariatric surgery is offered to people with a body mass index (BMI) of 40 plus, and for people with a BMI of 35 and serious coexisting medical conditions such as diabetes. There are three main types of procedure: malabsorptive, restrictive and mixed. The most commonly used procedure is restrictive surgery through the insertion of a gastric band. This is illustrated in Figure 7.3.

In the UK, the NHS is rationing the treatment to those with a BMI of 50 or even 60. Access to NHS weight-loss surgery is said to be 'inconsistent, unethical and completely dependent on geographical location' according to a statement by the Royal College of Surgeons of

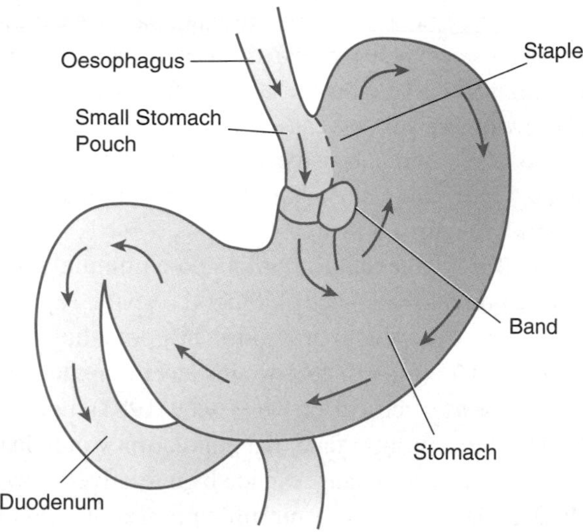

Figure 7.3 Vertical banded gastroplasty

Source: US National Institute of Diabetes and Digestive and Kidney Disease, National Institutes of Health; Reproduced with permission

England (2010). Around one million people in the UK are eligible, with around a quarter of them wanting to go ahead with surgery, but only 4300 operations were carried out in England in 2009.

Community-Level Approaches

The poor results obtained from small-scale individual level interventions suggest the need for large-scale approaches to obesity prevention in communities and populations. These use legislation to control promotion of unhealthy foods and health education to better inform consumers. Diets are influenced by a food industry that is continually promoting increased demand for unhealthy, cheaply manufactured foods. Food industry tactics are similar to those used by the tobacco industry – supplying misinformation, publication of supposedly conflicting evidence and hiding negative data. Chopra and Darnton-Hill (2004) suggest that tactics used in tobacco control have relevance for the fight against unhealthy diets because the experience of using voluntary codes of conduct with the food industry has not worked. They suggest that international standards on marketing unhealthy food products, restrictions on the advertising and availability of unhealthy products in schools, standard packaging and labelling of food products, or potential price or tax measures to reduce the demand for unhealthy products should all be considered.

Effective methods of health promotion and behaviour change are needed at a population level. Such initiatives need to be created using building blocks from psychology, nutrition and epidemiology. It is necessary to build these interventions on a solid foundation which acknowledges the powerful influences of evolution, history and culture. Explanatory accounts of eating and diet in purely behavioural terms cannot be expected to succeed if these contextual factors are ignored. Evolution, history and culture are significant contextual determinants of why we eat what we eat and when and how we eat it.

DeMattia and Denney (2008) note that a coordinated community approach is often missing from interventions designed to influence childhood obesity. A population or community approach to disease prevention and health promotion has potential to be more effective than individual-level approaches. Community approaches have a higher impact, provide a more efficient use of funds and are more cost effective (Tolley, 1985). For example, a small reduction in dietary fat made by a large proportion of the population would lead to greater improvements in population health than large changes made by a relatively few people (Rose, 1992). Boyle and Morris (1999) review community nutrition programmes in the USA. Winett, King and Altman (1989) and Bennett and Murphy (1997) discuss community health promotion from a psychological perspective. In the case study below, we outline a community market gardening project based in Milwaukee and Chicago called 'Growing Power'.

Case Study

INTERNATIONAL CASE STUDY A community, national and global sustainable foods project

In 1993, Growing Power started as an organization with teenagers who needed a place to work. Will Allen was a farmer with land. Will designed a programme that offered teens an opportunity to work at his store and renovate the greenhouses to grow food for their community. What started as a simple partnership to change the landscape of the north side of Milwaukee has blossomed into a national and global commitment to sustainable food systems. Will Allen, Chief Executive Officer, believes: 'If people can grow safe, healthy, affordable food, if they have access to land and clean water, this is transformative on every level in a community. I believe we cannot have healthy communities without a healthy food system.' Growing Power has served as a 'living museum' or 'idea factory' for the young, the elderly, farmers, producers and other professionals ranging from USDA personnel to urban planners. Growing Power's projects fall into three essential areas:

- Grow – Growing Power demonstrates easy to replicate growing methods through on-site workshops and hands-on demonstrations. There are farms in Milwaukee and Merton, Wisconsin, and in Chicago, Illinois. Growing Power has also established satellite-training sites in Arkansas, Georgia, Kentucky, Massachusetts and Mississippi.

Case Study

- Bloom – Education and Technical Assistance: Growing Power educates people through local national, and international outreach for farmers and communities. They also run multiple youth programmes, have an active volunteer base, and actively work on policy initiatives regarding agriculture.
- Thrive – Food Production and Distribution. Food production occurs in demonstration greenhouses, at the rural farm site in Merton, and at urban farms in Milwaukee and Chicago.

Source: http//www.growingpower.org/

FUTURE RESEARCH

1 The hunter–gatherer hypothesis could be tested by investigating the health of groups and communities who belong to similar cultures but differ with respect to hunter–gatherer characteristics, e.g. agriculturalists versus pastoralists.
2 More study is needed at a policy level to explore the best ways of working with the food industry, both manufacturing and retail, to improve the quality of food at affordable prices.
3 Evaluation research of the impact of community sustainable food projects such as Growing Power are needed.

Summary

1 Acquiring, preparing and eating are symbolic, moral and cultural activities binding people in families and collectives.
2 Human beings spent 99.5 per cent of evolutionary history as hunter–gatherers. The genetic make up of humans is adapted to a nomadic existence of hunting and gathering.
3 The agricultural revolution brought deleterious changes to diet and lifestyle. Diets became less varied and balanced; fat consumption increased; average levels of activity and energy expenditure decreased.
4 Eating a balanced diet and setting an optimum balance between energy input and energy expenditure are key aspects of health.

(Continued)

(Continued)

5. Four leading causes of death – cancer, coronary heart disease, stroke, and obesity – are associated with Western diets.
6. Obesity has multiple causes including heredity, culture, diet and lifestyle, with inactivity playing a key role.
7. Food preferences are influenced very early in life. The earliest and most emotional life events revolve around eating and drinking.
8. An ecological approach analyses eating in the context of the surrounding environment. Obesity is the end-product of a toxic, 'obesogenic' environment.
9. A diet high in fruit, vegetables and cereals and low in meat and fat is protective against cancer. This diet helps to prevent chronic diseases, including coronary heart disease, hypertension and obesity. Further health benefits accrue from consumption of less sugar, salt and caffeine.
10. Community and population approaches to healthy eating have the potential for high impact and cost effectiveness.

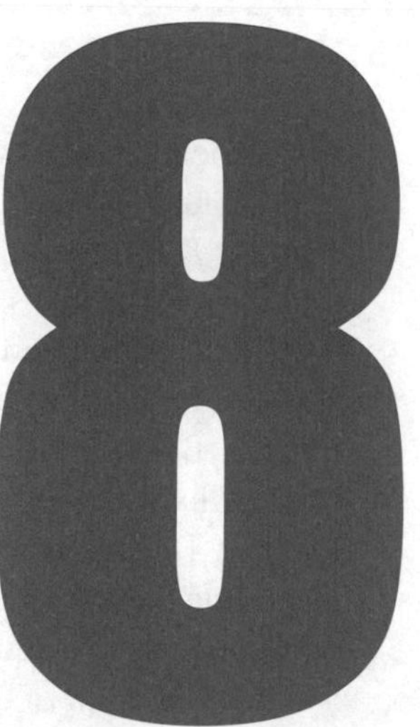

Alcohol and Drinking

Dionysus discovered and bestowed on men the service of drink, the juice that streams from the wine-clusters; men have but to take their fill of wine, and the sufferings of an unhappy race are banished, each day's troubles are forgotten in sleep – indeed this is our only cure for the weariness of life.

Euripides, *The Bacchae*, trans. P. Vellacott, 1954

Outline

This chapter discusses theories and research concerned with alcohol consumption and the causes, prevention and treatment of drinking problems. It begins with a discussion of the ambivalent attitudes to alcohol that have characterized many cultures from the distant past to the present day. An analysis of the physical and psychosocial dangers of drinking is followed by an examination of contrasting theories about the causes of excessive drinking. The chapter concludes with a discussion of the relative merits of different approaches to the prevention and treatment of drinking problems.

THE BLESSING AND CURSE OF ALCOHOL: PAST AND PRESENT ATTITUDES

Ambivalence towards alcohol is characteristic of many past civilizations and is illustrated in Euripides' tragedy, *The Bacchae*, written in 414 BC and quoted at the beginning of this chapter. The tragedy revolves around the conflict between the stern killjoy attitude of the protagonist Pentheus and the wild abandon of the Bacchic women, a conflict orchestrated by Dionysus, the god of wine. Modern views on alcohol as a social problem can be traced back to the eighteenth century when distilled spirits became available for the first time in Europe. Because of their relative cheapness, they were popular with the English working class. This was the subject of much concern, at least among the educated middle classes. William Hogarth's 1751 prints, *Beer Street* and *Gin Lane* (see Figure 8.1), illustrate the prevailing view by contrasting the pleasant and supposedly harmless effects of drinking beer with the dire consequences of drinking spirits. Notice the general sense of industriousness and well-being in Beer Street; many people are working and the only shop that is boarded up is the pawnbrokers. In Gin Lane nobody is working except the busy pawnbroker and there is a grim depiction of emaciation, death and the neglect of children.

Since the early nineteenth century popular beliefs about the dangers of alcohol have been shaped by organizations known as **temperance societies**. Beginning with the formation of the American Temperance Society in 1826 and then spreading to many other countries, their

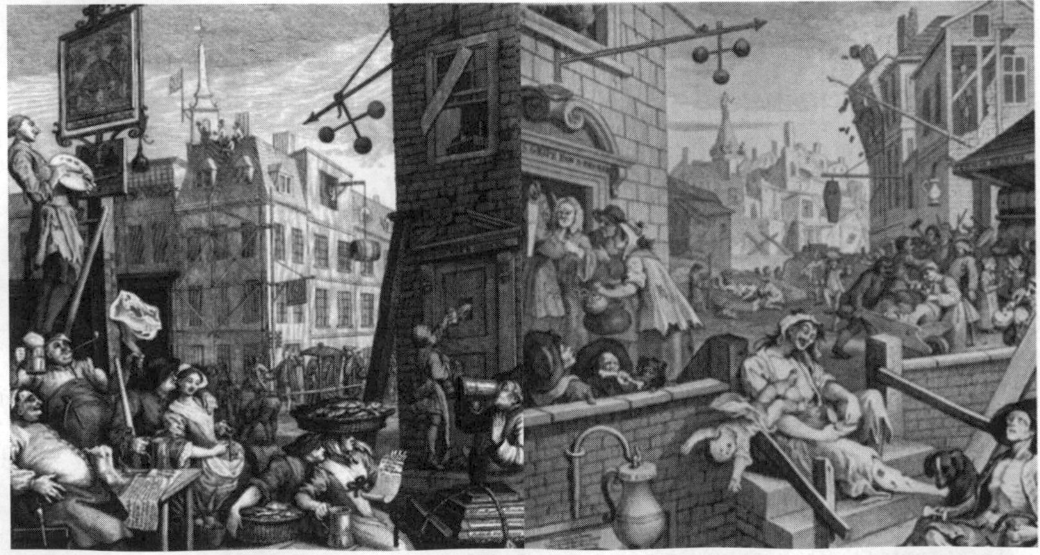

Figure 8.1 Hogarth's Beer Street and Gin Lane
(© The British Museum; Reproduced with permission)

influence has been enormous not only in bringing about the era of prohibition in the USA from 1920 to 1934 but also in helping to establish as received medical opinion the belief that alcoholics can never return to moderate drinking but can only be cured by remaining abstinent for the rest of their lives. A range of sometimes conflicting views can be found among different temperance societies, some simply preaching moderation and the avoidance of excess; some taking the view that spirits are intrinsically dangerous while weaker alcoholic drinks are harmless; some believing that alcohol is highly addictive for everyone; others that it only presents dangers for a small minority of individuals with a predisposition to become addicted. Of particular historical importance were the Washingtonians in the USA in the 1840s, self-help associations running regular meetings along the lines of religious revivalist groups with an emphasis on the confessions of the repentant sinner and an appeal to a 'Higher Power' for support. This particular tradition remains strong today in Alcoholics Anonymous which has branches in almost every North American and British town of any size and in many other countries.

With the exception of some countries with majority Muslim populations, alcohol is legally obtainable nowadays in most parts of the world. The predominant view seems to be that it is 'all right in moderation, harmful in excess'. We will review the evidence for this view in the next section. For the time being we will focus on the undisputed harm that occurs as a consequence of regular heavy drinking and of 'binge drinking', both now seen as major problems in many countries. In 2007 the World Health Organization estimated that 3.7 per cent of global mortality and 4.4 per cent of disease was attributable to alcohol, noting also that this does not include social harm such as family and interpersonal problems, work problems, violence and other crimes (WHO, 2007). Room, Babor and Rehm (2005) estimated the global burden of disease attributable to alcohol as 4 per cent varying from 1.3 per cent in the poorest countries with low consumption to 12.1 per cent in the former socialist countries. Reviewing the situation in the European Union, Anderson and Baumberg (2006) point out that, among young people (aged 15 to 29), 25 per cent of male mortality and 10 per cent of female mortality is attributable to alcohol.

Alcohol problems and approaches to prevention and treatment vary greatly from country to country. The example of India, described briefly in the case study below, illustrates the extent to which specific cultural and historical circumstances need to be taken into account. In Britain at present the major source of concern is binge drinking, with many city centres on weekend evenings notorious for the presence of large numbers of extremely drunk and disorderly young people (Raistrick, 2005; Plant & Plant, 2006). The British government has been much criticized for contributing to this by liberalizing the drinking laws under the influence of the Portman Group, a drinks industry public relations organization, while ignoring medical and other professional opinion opposed to liberalization. The drinks industry has also been criticized for doing nothing to discourage all-you-can-drink, 'happy hour', and other similar promotions offered by many city centre pubs and bars, which are fuelling the problem. While Britain's youth certainly lead the way when it comes to binge drinking, it now seems that Spain is not far behind; the equivalent phenomenon is known as the 'Botellón', literally 'big bottle', where young people gather in large numbers in public places at the weekends until the small hours, listening to music and drinking to intoxication. Gual (2006) comments 'Spain is becoming famous for its unending weekend nights where people can buy drinks all night long, and can drink both in bars and off premises'.

Case Study

INTERNATIONAL CASE STUDY Alcohol consumption in India

It is misleading to characterize India as a 'dry' or 'abstaining' culture. Prior to British colonial rule, a relaxed attitude to alcohol prevailed. British attempts to profit from the production and sale of alcohol led to opposition. Gandhi and the nationalist movement campaigned against alcohol as a symbol of colonial oppression and demands for prohibition were associated with the desire for the ritual purity of the Indian nation. In practice, since independence, alcohol policy has varied from state to state and, although there have been periods of national prohibition, currently most states permit the sale of alcohol, and in fact derive 15 to 20 per cent of their income from alcohol tax. Although alcohol is stigmatized in many sectors of society, an ambivalent attitude can be seen from the fact that many states stimulate the production of alcohol by demanding that increasing sales quotas be met by manufacturers as a condition of renewing licences. The drinks industry in turn seeks to influence government by making contributions to political parties.

The majority of Indians abstain from alcohol; currently it is estimated that 21 per cent of men and less than 5 per cent of women drink. However, of those that do drink, half drink at levels known to be hazardous. The drinks industry is increasingly seeking to make drinking more popular among women by lifestyle advertising and the types of drink they produce. Local manufacturers are also being taken over by multinationals who view India as a key target for expansion. Attempts to control levels of consumption by increased taxation tend to have a weak effect because illegal production and smuggling are rife. There is also opposition to the publication of 'safe' drinking advice, because it is felt that this may prove counterproductive by encouraging consumption in the currently abstinent majority.

Source: Benegal, 2005

Babor and Winstanley (2008) reviewed papers on the alcohol experiences of 18 countries commissioned for the journal *Addiction* from 2004–7. One problem already mentioned is the high level of consumption currently prevalent in the former socialist countries. In Russia, during the Gorbachev era from 1985, public health initiatives led to a 25 per cent reduction in consumption followed by dramatic increases in male life expectancy. These reforms were subsequently abandoned and consumption increased again with concomitant increases in health problems. A problem confronting many countries wishing to address alcohol problems is the powerful influence of international drinks companies. Babor and Winstanley note that potentially expanding markets such as India, Nigeria, China and Brazil are being targeted with 'highly sophisticated western marketing techniques'. At the same time, the papers which they reviewed mention specifically that the drinks industry is an obstacle to effective alcohol policy in India, Nigeria, the United Kingdom, Thailand, South Africa and Mexico. We will examine approaches to prevention and treatment for alcohol problems later in this chapter.

THE DANGERS OF DRINKING ALCOHOL

In this section we will consider evidence of the health risks associated with the consumption of alcohol as well as the possible health benefits. A brief summary of the major risk factors is given in Box 8.1.

Box 8.1

Risks incurred by the consumption of alcohol

Risks that can be incurred on any single occasion of heavy drinking

- Driving, industrial and household accidents; falls, fires, drowning.
- Domestic and other forms of violence as perpetrator.
- Domestic and other forms of violence as victim.
- Unwanted pregnancies; HIV or other sexually transmitted diseases following unprotected sexual exposure.

Risks incurred by regular heavy drinking

- Death from liver cirrhosis and acute pancreatitis.
- Irreversible neurological damage.
- Increased risk of cardiovascular disease and certain cancers.
- Problems caused by alcohol dependence.
- Exacerbation of pre-existing difficulties such as depression and family problems.
- Loss of employment, reduced career prospects.

Risks incurred by women who drink during pregnancy

- Fetal alcohol syndrome.
- Spontaneous abortion.
- Low birth weight babies.

Physical Health

An analysis of the research findings on the health hazards of drinking is considerably more complicated than is the case for smoking. Whereas smoking is dangerous even for low levels of consumption, and increasingly so for heavy smokers, the dangers to health of alcohol consumption are not always found for light and moderate drinkers, who may even experience health benefits compared with non-drinkers. We will therefore examine the evidence for risk associated with heavy drinking, and go on to consider the possible benefits of light and moderate drinking.

To begin with, it is necessary to be a little more precise about what is meant by 'light', 'moderate' and 'heavy' drinking. We will adopt the British system of informal measurement in which one 'unit' is assumed to equal 8 gm of alcohol or one glass of wine of average strength, half a pint (250cc) of normal strength beer, and a single measure (25 ml) of spirits. It is important to bear in mind that strong wines and beers may contain up to twice this amount of alcohol. We will consider moderate drinking to be at the average level of 3/2 units a day for men/women; less than half of that level will be regarded as light drinking and anything over 7/5 regular daily units will be regarded as heavy drinking.

Prolonged heavy drinking is known to be the main cause of **liver cirrhosis**, a serious condition that frequently results in death. Using figures provided by the British Department of Health, the Academy of Medical Sciences (2004) noted a four- to five-fold increase in deaths from chronic liver disease in the UK from 1970 to 2000, with over nine-fold increases among young men and women. Using more recent figures the UK Office for National Statistics estimated that mortality from liver disease had doubled from 1991 to 2007 (ONS, 2008). While some of these changes are attributable to increased rates of hepatitis C infection, effects that are themselves exacerbated by alcohol consumption, the main reason for the changes are increases in levels of heavy drinking. Although it receives much less publicity than liver cirrhosis, acute pancreatitis is another frequently fatal disease that is often caused by heavy drinking. Goldacre and Roberts (2004) surveyed hospital admissions for this disease in England from 1963 to 1998, noting that they have more than doubled over the 35-year period, with particularly large increases among the younger age groups. These changes closely parallel the patterns of increased alcohol consumption over this period of time.

The evidence linking alcohol consumption to cancer has been reviewed in detail by Bagnardi, Blangiardo, La Vecchia and Corrao (2001). They considered the evidence for three levels of consumption, 14, 21 and 28 units a week, and found associations increasing at each level for cancers of the oral cavity and pharynx, larynx, breast, liver, colo-rectum and stomach. The association with breast cancer is of particular importance because this is the one of the most common causes of premature death in women. Hamajima et al. (2002) conducted a detailed re-analysis of data from 53 studies with a total sample size of over 150,000. They found that there was a clear relationship with risk increasing steadily from teetotallers through to those drinking more than five units a day. However, the level of risk is quite modest and the authors note that it needs to be interpreted in the context of the possible beneficial effects of moderate alcohol consumption; but they conclude that alcohol could be the cause of about 4 per cent of deaths from breast cancer.

Drinking during pregnancy has been shown to be associated with a significant risk of damage to the unborn child. Heavy drinking is the main cause of **fetal alcohol syndrome**, in which the child suffers from a particular type of facial abnormality as well as mental impairment and stunted growth. Drinking has also been linked to below average birth weight and an increased risk of spontaneous abortion. There has been considerable controversy as to whether there is any risk of these outcomes for light drinkers; in some countries medical authorities recommend that pregnant women should not drink at all throughout pregnancy, while in others the usual recommendation is that light drinking does no harm. In a recent report for the British Department of Health, Gray and Henderson (2006) reviewed research on the fetal effects of low-to-moderate alcohol consumption and binge drinking, concluding that, for most outcomes, there was no consistent evidence of adverse effects from low alcohol consumption. However they also state that the evidence is probably not strong enough to rule out any risk. There was also some evidence of adverse effects on neurodevelopment of binge drinking during pregnancy.

The possible benefits of light to moderate drinking have been the subject of considerable controversy. Here we will concentrate on large prospective epidemiological studies and meta-analyses published within the last 10 years. The main focus of attention has been coronary heart disease, where a number of studies have reported a J-shaped function, with light and moderate drinkers having substantially lower risk than both abstainers and heavy drinkers (Murray et al., 2002; Britton & Marmot, 2004; Corrao, Bagnardi, Zambon & La Vecchia 2004; Mukamal, Chiuve & Rimm, 2006; Tolstrup, Jensen, Tjønneland, Overvad, Mukamal & Grønbæk, 2006; Dorn et al., 2007). It should be emphasized that some of these studies have also reported substantially increased rates of coronary heart disease for binge drinkers (Murray et al., 2002; Dorn et al., 2007) and for very heavy drinkers (Corrao et al., 2004). In the case of strokes, Berger et al. (1999) found that light and moderate drinkers had a reduced risk compared with abstainers, while Hart, Davey Smith, Hole and Hawthorne (1999) and Mukamal et al. (2005) found little difference, both of these studies concurring in finding a substantially increased risk among heavy drinkers. Two further lines of enquiry have also yielded J-shaped functions with light drinkers at lower risk than either abstainers or heavier drinkers. Ruitenberg et al. (2002) found this for dementia in a study of men and women aged over 55, and similar findings for mild cognitive decline in older people have been reported by Antilla et al. (2004) and Ganguli, Vander Bilt, Saxton, Shen and Dodge (2005).

The results of these and other studies are not entirely consistent with each other, especially for the purpose of establishing upper limits for safe drinking, but they are at least consistent with the statement that men and women who drink moderately are not taking any significant risk with their physical health. The additional claim that light to moderate drinking is actually beneficial to health is more open to doubt. Although non-drinkers do have higher mortality rates than drinkers, this may be only because the category of non-drinkers includes a substantial number of individuals who have given up drinking because of poor health. This is a useful illustration of the statistician's dictum that 'correlation does not entail causation'.

It could be that not drinking is a cause of poorer health but, equally well, it could be that poor health is a cause of not drinking. The latter view was first analysed in detail by Shaper, Wannamethee and Walker (1988), using data from 7000 middle-aged men, confirming that those who suffered from health problems cut down or abstained from drinking. It has since been developed by a number of other critics, notably Fillmore and her associates (Fillmore, Stockwell, Chikritzhs, Bostrom & Kerr, 2007).

Accidents and Psychosocial Problems

The importance of drink-driving as a cause of road traffic accidents, and the deaths of drivers, passengers and pedestrians, is universally acknowledged. The risk begins even at the lowest blood-alcohol levels and increases proportionately thereafter (Anderson & Baumberg, 2006). Legislation lowering the maximum permitted level of blood-alcohol, increasing the amount of police attention paid to drink driving and the introduction of random breath testing are all measures which have been shown to reduce fatalities (Room et al., 2005).

Alcohol consumption has also been shown to be a factor in many other kinds of injuries, including deaths from falls, fires, industrial accidents and drowning. In a 16-year follow-up study of Finnish men, Paljärvi, Mäkelä and Poikolainen (2005) found that heavy drinking was associated with an increased frequency of fatal injury, the risk being highest among those who reported the largest annual number of heavy drinking occasions. In a study of 11,536 patients with non-fatal injuries attending 28 emergency departments in 16 countries, Borges et al. (2006) found the relative risk to be considerably greater among those who had been drinking within 6 hours of injury.

Anderson and Baumberg (2006) reviewed an extensive range of studies from many countries demonstrating an association between heavy drinking and many personal and social problems, including violent assaults and homicide, marital violence and marital breakdown, child abuse, impaired work performance, depression and suicide. To what extent is alcohol to blame? This raises all of the usual chicken-and-egg problems of interpreting statistical correlations. For example, does drinking incite people to commit crimes or do criminals drink to reduce their fear before carrying out the crimes which they have already decided to commit? Do people take to drink in an effort to ameliorate their psychological problems, or are these problems caused by heavy drinking? Probably the most sensible response that can be made to this latter question at the present time is to reiterate the well-known health education slogan: 'If you drink because you have a problem, then you will end up with two problems.'

THE CAUSES OF ALCOHOL DEPENDENCE

To understand the motivation for drinking and problems of dependence it is best to begin by considering the psychological effects of alcohol. These effects are much influenced by culture and by people's expectations about potential benefits, including enjoyment, stress reduction and increased sociability (Anderson & Baumberg, 2006). This explains why it is consumed in social gatherings such as parties and weddings, when people wish to interact in a much more relaxed and informal way than they might otherwise, and also why heavy drinking is common among people with psychological problems. Alcohol dependence is particularly common among people suffering from anxiety disorders, and the use of alcohol to induce sleep is also known to aggravate sleep disorders, because it leads to increased wakefulness and arousal a few hours later (Anderson & Baumberg, 2006).

Let us now look more closely at the question of why some people develop drinking problems while others do not. Here a number of contrasting theoretical perspectives need to be considered. They are not mutually exclusive in the sense that this can sometimes be said of theories in the natural sciences. The discerning reader will notice various ways in which elements of each can be consistent with elements of the others. They are best thought of as reference points that are useful aids to thinking about the issues. A brief summary of the main theoretical views is given in Table 8.1.

Table 8.1 Theories of problem drinking

Type of theory	Causes of problem drinking
Genetic theories	DNA variations possibly associated with the metabolism of alcohol mean that certain individuals are much more likely than most to develop alcohol problems if they drink.
Addiction, disease and dependence theories	Individuals who drink heavily may develop a physiological addiction and psychological dependence which can only be effectively treated by lifelong abstinence.
Learning theories	Mechanisms of conditioning and social learning can explain the development of excessive consumption, and the phenomena of dependence, craving, increased tolerance and withdrawal symptoms.

Genetic Theories

Genetic theories propose that some people have an inherited predisposition to develop drinking problems. Those who are convinced of the overwhelming importance of heredity believe that certain people are 'born alcoholics', destined to succumb to alcoholism almost as soon as they take their first drink. Perhaps surprisingly, this 'biological determinist' view is also attractive to manufacturers of alcoholic drinks. They can argue that the born alcoholic is bound to have a drink and become alcoholic sooner or later, however much the availability of drink is restricted. The rest of us can drink as we wish without running the risk of becoming alcoholic.

While it is certainly true that alcohol problems tend to run in families, this is not in itself enough to prove the existence of genetic influences. Drinking habits can be passed on from parents to children as the result of upbringing and imitation just as much as they may be passed on through genes. The most widely cited evidence for genetic influences comes from twin and adoption studies. Twin studies are based on comparisons of the concordance rates for drinking patterns in *monozygotic* (MZ, identical) and *dizygotic* (DZ, fraternal) *twins*. The theory behind this is that both types of twin grow up in the same family environment, so that a greater concordance for the 100 per cent genetically similar MZ twins than for the 50 per cent similar DZ twins is evidence of genetic effects. Adoption studies examine whether adopted children grow up to acquire similar drinking habits to their biological parents, or whether they are more influenced by their adopting parents.

Twin and adoption studies have been used to estimate 'heritability', a statistical assessment of the relative importance of hereditary and environmental influences which can take values from 100 per cent for fully inherited characteristics to 0 per cent for those which are purely environmentally determined. In practice heritability estimates for drinking patterns have varied greatly from study to study, partly as the result of methodological problems which are difficult to overcome, and partly because the estimates vary as a function of what is measured. The highest estimates have sometimes been found for 'chronic alcoholism' and sometimes for 'teetotalism'; some have found greater heritability for males than females, and some the exact opposite (see, for example, Heather & Robertson, 1997). Insofar as generalizations have been made about the heritability of alcohol problems, figures of 50–60 per cent have sometimes been suggested (Anderson & Baumberg, 2006); however Walters (2002) carried out a meta-analysis of 50 studies and concluded that heritability was quite low, unlikely to be higher than 30–36 per cent.

Given the current vogue for DNA-based research, it is not surprising that there have been a number of recent attempts to demonstrate specific genetic loci for alcohol problems, but these have only met with modest success (Cook & Gurling, 2001; Anderson & Baumberg, 2006). As with other forms of human behaviour, there are likely to be a multitude of complex genetic routes that may make some individuals more likely than others to become problem drinkers. For example, there may be inheritable differences in the way that alcohol is metabolized, so that some people find its effects pleasant, others unpleasant; some find it takes more alcohol, others less, to achieve the same effect. There may be differences in genetic predisposition to experience anxiety, so that some are predisposed to drink more than others on discovering that it temporarily suppresses anxiety.

On the basis of existing research evidence, there is certainly no reason to suppose that some people are 'born alcoholics'. Although there is enough evidence to show that there is some degree of genetic predisposition towards different patterns of drinking, it seems unlikely that this is as important an influence as environmental factors. To appreciate what this means, take as an analogy the fact that some people may have an inherited proneness to develop heart disease, but whether or not they will do so still depends on whether they smoke, eat fatty foods, avoid exercise and so on. The risks are just greater for some people than for others. Similarly, there could be many environmental reasons why drinking problems develop in those who have an inherited predisposition and also in those who do not.

Addiction, Disease and Dependence Theories

The history of these theories has been examined in a broad social and historical context by Thom (2001). **Addiction theories** can be traced back to the classic works of Benjamin Rush of Philadelphia and Thomas Trotter of Edinburgh, published respectively in 1785 and 1804. Rush and Trotter replaced the traditional view of habitual drunkards as moral degenerates by one in which they are victims of an addiction. Once the addiction is established, the victims lose all voluntary control over their drinking. They have become incapable of resisting their craving for the 'demon drink'. Rush and Trotter succeeded in popularizing their belief that alcohol is a highly addictive substance 70 years before the case was made for opium.

Later **disease theories** focused increasingly on the at-risk individual who has a predisposition to become alcoholic once he or she starts drinking. Although a predisposition to become alcoholic does not have to be hereditary (we have already mentioned that it may be the result of upbringing), nevertheless the concept of the born alcoholic proved attractive to disease theorists. In common with earlier addiction theories, disease theories emphasized craving and loss of control. The difference was that, for the later disease theorists, alcohol is only highly addictive for a small number of people. The rest of us can drink with impunity. This change of emphasis proved attractive, especially to a North American society that had abandoned prohibition, embraced personal liberty and responsibility and has a powerful drinks industry.

From the mid-1970s, the disease theory was being revised and extended, notably by Griffith Edwards and Milton Gross, to become the **alcohol dependence syndrome**. In this new conceptualization, the sharp distinction which had previously been made between physical addiction and psychological dependence was abolished and the syndrome was viewed instead as a psycho-physiological disorder. The descriptions given by Edwards and Gross are not always very clear and tend to change from one publication to another. Box 8.2 lists the main aspects of Edwards' more recent accounts as summarized by Sayette (2007).

The concept of the alcohol dependence syndrome has been much criticized, originally by Shaw (1979) who pointed out that much woolly thinking lies behind it. Most people, on reading the list of symptoms in Box 8.2, would conclude that anyone who drinks regularly would exhibit one or more of them to some degree. As a list, it seems consistent with the idea that, rather than being a disease, alcohol dependence is an arbitrary point that can be chosen on a continuum from the light social drinker to the homeless street drinker. Yet proponents of the syndrome insist that it is a clinical entity, admittedly with somewhat varying symptomatology, which only applies to a relatively small number out of all the people who drink heavily.

Box 8.2

Symptoms of alcohol dependence syndrome

According to Griffith Edwards, this includes some or all of the following symptoms:

- Tolerance: a diminished effect of alcohol, usually accompanied by increased consumption.
- Withdrawal symptoms following reduced consumption.
- Consumption of larger amounts or for a longer time period than was intended.
- Persistent desire or unsuccessful efforts to cut down or control drinking.
- Excessive time spent obtaining, consuming or recovering from the effects of alcohol.
- Reduction of important activities due to drinking.
- Continued drinking despite knowing that it is causing or exacerbating a physical or psychological problem.

Source: Sayette, 2007

One should not, of course, 'throw out the baby with the bath water'. No theory of alcohol use can afford to neglect the phenomena of physical dependence associated with prolonged heavy drinking and most clearly manifested in the spectacular withdrawal symptoms that can occur following sudden abstinence. These include some of the most unpleasant to be found among all types of drug withdrawal, including tremors ('the shakes'), sweating, nausea, vomiting, hallucinations ('pink elephants') and convulsions. Indeed, Lerner and Fallon (1985) note that, in a significant number of cases, sudden withdrawal can actually prove fatal. The phenomena of psychological dependence also need to be addressed by any theory of alcohol use. While alcohol dependence syndrome may be poorly defined as a clinical entity, the psychological problems that are often associated with heavy drinking certainly need to be explained.

Learning Theories

Learning theorists consider drinking problems to develop as a result of the same learning mechanisms that are at work in establishing patterns of 'normal drinking'. They argue that the reasons why some people become problem drinkers and others do not lie in their particular personal histories of learning to drink, their present social environment insofar as it provides opportunities and encouragement to drink, and in physiological variables that may make the effects of alcohol more pleasurable or positively reinforcing for some people than others.

Operant conditioning is the type of learning that occurs when animals are trained to respond in a particular way to a stimulus by providing rewards after they make the appropriate response. In the classic experiment, hungry rats were confined in small boxes and trained to press a bar in order to obtain food pellets. This phenomenon, which was of course well known to animal trainers, pet owners and the parents of small children long before it was 'discovered' by psychologists, has some applicability to the understanding of problem drinking. Of particular importance is the **gradient of reinforcement**, the fact that reinforcement which occurs rapidly after the response is much more effective in producing learning than delayed reinforcement. In the case of drinking alcohol, a small amount of positive reinforcement, such as reduced anxiety, that occurs fairly soon after drinking, may cause a strong habit to develop in spite of the counterbalancing effect of a large amount of punishment (hangover, divorce, loss of employment) that occurs much later.

Drinking, eating, smoking, drug and sexual addictions all have the 'irrational' characteristic that the total amount of pleasure gained from the addiction seems much less than the suffering caused by it. According to learning theorists, the reason for this lies in the nature of the gradient of reinforcement. Addictive behaviours are typically those in which pleasurable effects occur rapidly while unpleasant consequences occur after a delay. The simple mechanism of operant conditioning and the gradient of reinforcement functions, as it were, to overpower the mind's capacity for rational calculation. Bigelow (2001) discusses the applicability of operant conditioning principles to the understanding and treatment of alcohol problems. He concludes that they have considerable relevance but notes that there has been little interest in them in the alcohol field in recent years, in contrast to the field of illegal substance use where they continue to play quite a dominant role.

Classical conditioning refers to the process whereby a response that occurs as a natural reflex to a particular stimulus can be conditioned to occur to a new stimulus. In Pavlov's early experiments a bell was rung shortly before food was placed in a dog's mouth, thereby eliciting salivation as a physiological reflex. After a number of pairings of bell and food Pavlov found that the dog salivated when the bell was rung unaccompanied by food.

A number of interesting models have been developed by applying classical conditioning principles to addictions, and Drummond, Tiffany, Glautier and Remington (1995) provide a useful survey of this highly technical subject. One interesting application to explain the phenomena of drug dependence, tolerance and withdrawal is the **compensatory conditioned response model**. Initially, when a drug is taken, a physiological 'homeostatic' mechanism comes into operation to counteract its effects. In the case of alcohol, which has a depressing effect, the homeostatic mechanism activates the nervous system in order to maintain the normal level of activation. In the regular drinker this gradually produces tolerance so that increasingly large quantities of alcohol are required to produce the same effect. Furthermore, the homeostatic response of nervous activation may become conditioned to stimuli normally associated with drinking, such as situations where drinking has frequently taken place in the past. If conditioned drinkers avoid alcohol in these situations, the conditioned response of nervous activation will not be balanced by the effects of alcohol and the resultant unpleasant state of excessive activation is what is known as a withdrawal state. In this way classical conditioning can account for the close connection observed between the phenomena of tolerance and withdrawal.

The compensatory conditioned response model has considerable intuitive plausibility but there is a lack of convincing evidence for its applicability to problem drinking. Drobes, Saladin and Tiffany (2001) discuss this model and a range of alternative classical conditioning models with specific reference to alcohol dependence and they conclude that, in all cases, there is a lack of empirical evidence to support the approach.

Social learning theorists argue that classical and operant conditioning provide incomplete explanations of human learning, which also frequently depends on observation and imitation. Bandura (1977) has been particularly influential in emphasizing the importance of learning by imitation and linking it to his concept of **self-efficacy**, a personality trait consisting of having confidence in one's ability to carry out one's plans successfully. People with low self-efficacy are much more likely to imitate undesirable behaviour than those with high self-efficacy. Collins and Bradizza (2001) reviewed applications of social learning theory to drinking, noting that the evidence points to parents having the strongest influence on the initiation of adolescent alcohol use while peers are most influential in determining subsequent frequency of use.

Freud's concept of 'secondary gain' can also be usefully applied to alcohol problems as an extension of the learning theory perspective. Just as hypochondriacs are often seen to be using their condition to avoid work and to get people at their beck and call, so can it be seen that sufferers from many kinds of neurosis often exploit their condition in order to gain attention, avoid things that they do not wish to do and generally manipulate people around them. It is easy to see how patterns of drinking can function in this way, and not only in the regular heavy drinker: 'It's your fault for getting me drunk' or 'I only did it because I was drunk' can provide a convenient way of evading responsibility for the person who commits a sexual indiscretion or beats their partner. Here alcohol has the double function of releasing the inhibitions that might otherwise prevent the impulse from being acted on, while simultaneously being held to blame as if it were the drink that performed the action rather than the drinker. In the case of the alcoholic, it is possible to see here some dangers in adopting the medical or disease model. If alcoholics think of themselves as victims of a disease over which they have no control, not only will they avoid taking responsibility for actions carried out while under the influence of drink, but they will also avoid taking responsibility for drinking, which may make it difficult or impossible to help them.

Box 8.3

The controlled drinking controversy

Can individuals with severe drinking problems ever resume moderate levels of drinking, or is total abstinence their only realistic goal? Because they regard heavy drinking as essentially a habit rather than a disease, learning theorists have taken the view that a return to moderate drinking can, at least in some cases, be a viable objective. Disease theorists, on the other hand, believe that lifelong abstinence is the only realistic goal for the alcoholic. This issue has been the subject of intense controversy over the last 50 years (see, for example, Heather and Robertson, 1997).

In a significant contribution to the debate Miller, Walters and Bennett (2001) analysed data from seven large studies looking at how people fare during the year after treatment for alcoholism. Their findings were:

1 1 in 4 clients were abstinent
2 1 in 10 used alcohol moderately without problems
3 The remaining two thirds made significant improvements reducing their overall alcohol consumption by 87 per cent on average

They conclude that 'This substantial level of improvement in "unremitted" clients tends to be overlooked when outcomes are dichotomized as successful or relapsed.'

PREVENTION AND TREATMENT OF ALCOHOL PROBLEMS

Prevention

Approaches to the prevention of alcohol problems have been the subject of intense controversy in recent years. On the one hand, specialists in this field are generally in favour of measures to reduce overall levels of consumption by increasing prices and imposing restrictions on advertising, promotions and general availability; on the other hand, the drinks industry campaigns against all these approaches and in favour of educational initiatives and self regulation. The main issues are summarized in Box 8.4. Here we will briefly review the evidence in support of the 'population-based approach', and also consider the position of the drinks industry and its influence on government policies.

Box 8.4

Population-based prevention – expert opinion versus the drinks industry

- Specialists on the prevention of alcohol problems are almost unanimous in their support for the population-based approach, which incorporates the principle that the most effective policies for reducing alcohol problems are those which reduce overall levels of consumption. These policies include higher levels of taxation on alcoholic drinks, restrictions on advertising and sponsorship, limiting opening hours for bars and imposing tight controls on which shops can sell alcohol and the hours during which they can do so.
- The population-based approach is opposed by the drinks industry because reduced overall consumption means smaller profits. They propose that 'sensible drinking' can be encouraged by self-regulation of the drinks industry and educational initiatives. They argue that the population-based approach penalizes the majority of sensible drinkers in order to discourage the minority of irresponsible drinkers.
- Critics of the drinks industry suggest that the drinks industry claims are disingenuous because it has been clearly shown that educational initiatives are ineffective at curbing heavy drinking, and also because the drinks industry makes most of its profit from the minority of drinkers who consume well above recommended limits.
- In many countries the drinks industry has been much more successful than the alcohol experts at influencing government policies. This may be because governments do not wish to risk unpopularity by adopting population-based policies.

Sources: Babor et al. (2003); Academy of Medical Sciences (2004); Anderson & Baumberg (2006); WHO (2007)

The detailed reviews of the evidence cited at the foot of Box 8.4 were variously commissioned by the World Health Organization, the European Commission and the British Academy of Medical Sciences and published between 2003 and 2007. These reports concur in finding much evidence that overall levels of consumption in populations are closely associated with the extent of alcohol problems. Earlier in this chapter we indicated some evidence for this coming from the dramatic impact of changes which occurred in Russia during the Gorbachev era. We also noted the huge increase in deaths from chronic liver disease in the UK tracking increases in levels of alcohol consumption in the period from 1970 to 2007. More generally, comparisons of different countries and of changes occurring within countries over lengthy periods of time all arrive at the same result. The WHO (2007) note that half of the world's consumption of alcohol is by the 10 per cent of heaviest drinkers and that 75 per cent of the variation across different regions in the extent of alcohol dependence can be predicted from overall levels of consumption. Much as this must disappoint the drinks industry, there are no examples of countries which have managed to maintain population levels of consumption while at the same time reducing alcohol problems.

Probably the most effective measure for reducing population levels of consumption is increased taxation. This is a policy which requires careful analysis and attention to the specific conditions of individual countries, particularly poor countries where large increases in taxation may lead to increases in the production of illicit and potentially lethal distilled liquor. But in relatively wealthy countries increases in taxation generally lead to proportionate decreases in consumption. The WHO (2007) note that young people's drinking is particularly sensitive to increases in price, which can therefore reduce under-age drinking as well as the extent of binge drinking among teenagers. Furthermore, and contrary to widespread belief, price increases have also been shown to have an impact on the amount consumed among older frequent and heavy drinkers.

Anderson and Baumberg (2006) examined the impact of restrictions on the sale of alcohol including increases in the minimum legal age for purchase and measures to restrict number of outlets and days and hours where sale is permitted. These measures have all been shown to reduce the extent of alcohol problems in a number of countries.

Each of the reports referred to in Box 8.4 also note that the global drinks industry is deploying sophisticated modern marketing techniques aimed at young people including lifestyle advertising, promotions involving sporting teams and events, rock concerts and festivals, fashion shows and carnivals, as well as the development of new products specifically aimed at young people, such as 'alcopops' and 'pre-mix cocktails'. Agostinelli and Grube (2002) reviewed alcohol counter-advertising, including warnings on alcoholic products, with a number of interesting proposals. Unfortunately research to date has been mainly concerned with participants' assessments of the impact of this type of advertising rather than its effectiveness in reducing misuse. It can also be argued that such efforts are a drop in the ocean in comparison with the amount of money that the drinks industry spends on product promotion. An alternative approach, deeply unpopular with the drinks industry, is the introduction of bans on advertising and sponsorship. Although earlier research had indicated that bans have little or no effect on overall consumption, Saffer and Dave (2002) argue that this research is flawed. They used an economic model to analyse pooled data from 20 countries over 26 years and conclude that there is a significant effect that indicates that bans can reduce overall consumption by 5 to 8 per cent. They note that increases in levels of consumption often stimulate the introduction of bans, but that reductions in consumption often lead to the rescinding of bans, as has happened in recent years in Canada, Denmark, New Zealand and Finland.

One area of legislation to control the dangers of alcohol use, which more and more countries are adopting, is strictly enforced drink-driving laws with severe penalties for offenders. It is now almost universally agreed that this has played an important role in reducing traffic fatalities. It even commands the support of the drinks industry which, in view of the high level of public support for the laws, would be foolish to oppose it.

The other main preventive measures that have been much analysed are health education initiatives with the aim of preventing alcohol misuse. Unfortunately, the evidence indicates that they are not very effective. Health education generally appears to improve knowledge about the effects of alcohol and attitudes to it, but has no effect on the amounts actually consumed. Midford and McBride (2001) reviewed alcohol education programmes in schools, noting that, in the USA, efforts have been hampered by excessive emphasis on abstinence, while in Europe and Australasia the emphasis has been on 'sensible drinking'. Although they detect a few promising signs in recent developments, the general finding is that these programmes have either failed to achieve any effects or, at best, have produced very small effects. Foxcroft, Ireland, Lister-Sharp, Lowe and Breen (2003) reviewed reports of 56 interventions aimed at young people aged 25 or under with substantially similar conclusions.

The ineffectiveness of educational campaigns designed to encourage sensible drinking perhaps explains why the drinks industry is happy to support them and even participate in them. Although this may seem an unnecessarily cynical view, there are some reasons for taking it seriously. Heather and Robertson (1997) point out that the drinks industry derives a good part of its profits from very heavy drinkers. In a 1978 survey of Scottish drinking habits, it was estimated that 3 per cent of the population were responsible for 30 per cent of total alcohol consumption. The loss of this source of profits would be crippling to the drinks industry. Hence the continued profitability of the industry requires the existence of a substantial percentage of very heavy drinkers. This provides another salient example of a conflict of interest between good public health and profits in industry.

In considering international perspectives at the beginning of this chapter we noted that the drinks industry is often mentioned as an obstacle to effective alcohol policy. A good example is provided by the UK in recent years. Heather and Robertson (1997) describe attempts by the Portman Group, an organization funded by the British drinks industry, to influence academic debate on alcohol policy by financial offers. The Institute of Alcohol Studies (2003) has commented on the influence of the Portman Group on the recent decision of the British government to extend permitted drinking hours in England and Wales. The British drinks industry apparently has had much more influence than any other organization on another key alcohol policy proposal, the Alcohol Harm Reduction Strategy for England (Cabinet Office, Prime Minister's Strategy Unit, 2004). This document is replete with positive references to the drinks industry and the Portman Group, emphasizing the value of educational programmes and other drinks industry initiatives, while rejecting any increases in taxation or legislation to control advertising and availability. Its main proposed action is to reduce the 'further increase in alcohol related harms in England'. As Plant (2004) points out, given the existing levels of problems, a policy that does not even set out to reduce them substantially is depressing. Certainly it is not a strategy that is likely to cause too much concern to the drinks industry.

In another recent development in the UK, widely reported in the press on 16 March 2009, Chief Medical Officer Sir Liam Donaldson proposed in his annual report that the government should introduce a minimum price policy for alcohol, stating that 'Implementing this minimum price-per-unit policy would save an estimated £1 billion every year, impact high-risk drinkers more than others and eliminate cheap supermarket drink that young people binge on.' (HMSO, 2009). The Prime Minister Gordon Brown promptly rejected this proposal, saying it is important to protect the interests of 'the sensible majority of moderate drinkers', a comment that accords perfectly with the views of the British drinks industry.

Paralleling the activities of the Portman Group in the UK, Heather (2001) draws our attention to those of the International Center for Alcohol Policies (ICAP), funded by the international drinks industry and established in the USA in 1995. Among its publications are *Alcohol and Pleasure: A Health Perspective* (Peele & Grant, 1999), a book that emphasizes the pleasurable and beneficial effects of alcohol against attempts to undermine this view by the 'vast literature on health and social problems associated with alcohol abuse'. The activities of the ICAP have been criticized by McCreanor, Caswell and Hill (2000) on the grounds that they are basically designed to influence public policy in directions that will increase drinks industry profits, especially in the developing world, while having a negative impact on health.

Treatment

A brief synopsis of alternative approaches to treatment is given in Table 8.2.

One of the most striking features of the treatment of alcohol problems is the contrasting approaches taken in different countries. In the USA and Canada, treatment is usually aimed at total abstinence, while in Britain most agencies regard a return to moderate drinking as a legitimate treatment goal for some clients, mainly those with lower levels of dependence. North American programmes are often based on specialist treatment centres with a strong medical orientation. In Finland, on the other hand, alcohol problems are regarded as essentially social problems and dealt with primarily by social workers. These differences have been shaped by social forces and, until recently, have rarely involved any serious critical analysis of the evidence for the efficacy of the approaches.

Table 8.2 Alternative approaches to the treatment of problem drinking

Type of treatment	Approach to treatment
In-patient treatment	'Drying out centres' and private clinics which focus on the alleviation of withdrawal symptoms followed by counselling and therapy to maintain abstinence following discharge.
Alcoholics Anonymous	Self-help groups run by ex-alcoholics using the 'twelve step facilitation programme' to maintain lifelong abstinence. May receive individuals on discharge from in-patient treatments.
Counselling and psychotherapy	Encompasses many approaches deriving from alternative psychotherapeutic models with the shared aim of helping clients to achieve insight into the causes and effects of problem drinking, seen as an essential basis for change.
Cognitive behavioural therapies	Based on learning theories and sometimes aiming to reduce levels of drinking rather than promoting abstinence as the treatment objective. Motivational interviewing is currently the most popular approach.
Brief interventions	Advice on reducing consumption given by general practitioners and other health professionals, including 'opportunistic interventions' given to individuals who have attended for other reasons, such as for screening programmes.

Miller and Wilbourne (2002) provide an extensive review of the amount and quality of the evidence concerning the efficacy of different treatment programmes. They examined studies of 48 different types of treatment, rating each study for its methodological adequacy and then placing the treatments in rank order. The rather surprising result is that brief interventions, often consisting of advice given by general practitioners and at hospital emergency departments, are particularly well supported by the evidence. This finding, which was based on a large number of studies (see the Key Study below for an important example), was confirmed in a further review by Whitlock, Polen, Green, Orleans and Klein (2004) who also note that reductions in amount consumed and in the proportion of participants who reduced their drinking to moderate or safe levels, were maintained up to 4 years after the interventions. Bertholet, Daeppen, Wietlisbach, Fleming and Burnard (2005) reviewed **opportunistic interventions**, brief treatments given at primary care facilities to individuals attending for reasons other than alcohol-related problems. After examining 19 trials that included 5639 individuals, they conclude that these interventions were effective in reducing alcohol consumption measured at 6 and 12 months after the interventions.

KEY STUDY Brief treatments: Project MATCH

In a large five-year study in the USA, known as Project MATCH, 1726 people with drinking problems were divided into three groups receiving respectively: (a) a treatment based on the 'twelve-step facilitation programme' of Alcoholics Anonymous; (b) coping skills therapy based on social learning theory; (c) motivation enhancement therapy, based on the techniques of motivational interviewing which are described below. Motivation enhancement therapy proved just as effective as the other two, although it consisted of only four as against 12 sessions over a 12-week period. This finding applied equally across clients with problems of relatively high and low degrees of severity.

Developed by Miller and his associates over the last 25 years (see Miller & Rollnick, 2002), the motivational interviewing (MI) approach is in direct contrast to the confrontational tactics traditionally adopted by therapists treating addictions, in which every effort is made to overcome the client's supposed resistance to acknowledging that he or she has a problem, aggressively to challenge any dishonesty and to break down his or her defences. Instead, the motivational therapist tries to create a warm empathic relationship with the client and uses a gentle and indirect approach in order to elicit, rather than impose, an increase in motivation to change behaviour, improve self-esteem and develop the feeling of self-efficacy for putting changes into practice.

The successful use of MI in Project MATCH is consistent with the findings of meta-analyses indicating its effectiveness (e.g. Lundahl & Burke, 2009).

Source: Project MATCH Research Group, 1997

Because brief interventions are effective as well as being much less expensive than other forms of treatment, they are becoming increasingly popular. The main problem that has been identified by researchers is the difficulty that has been experienced in persuading general practitioners to undertake them. After discussing the problem Roche and Freeman (2004) propose as a solution that practice nurses could take over the function of general practitioners. However, it remains to be seen whether this is equally effective. For example, it could be that the high status of general practitioners and doctors in hospital clinics is a key reason for the effectiveness of brief interventions.

Of the other types of treatment reviewed by Miller and Wilbourne, there is a considerable quantity of evidence for the effectiveness of **motivational interviewing**. None of the remaining 46 types of treatment considered by Miller and Wilbourne receive much support from outcome studies, although **cognitive behavioural therapies** (CBT) appear to be more effective than psychotherapeutic approaches. Furthermore, and in spite of its enduring popularity, there are few good quality studies which provide support for the approach of Alcoholics Anonymous and their abstinence-based 'Twelve Step Facilitation Programme'. However, to be fair to AA, it should be emphasized that their perfectly reasonable insistence on anonymity and the associated difficulty of forming properly randomised control groups makes it difficult to evaluate. The AA has also created an unrivalled global infrastructure for tackling alcoholism.

FUTURE RESEARCH

1 Clarification of the health risks and possible benefits of light to moderate drinking, including heart disease and risks to the unborn child.
2 Studies to examine the role of learning processes, including classical and operant conditioning and social learning in the development of alcohol dependence and problem drinking.
3 Studies to assess the relative merits of abstinence versus controlled drinking as an objective for people with drinking problems. What types of client are best advised to aim respectively for abstinence and for moderation?
4 Investigations to establish what are the physiological and psychological mechanisms of dependence, tolerance and withdrawal symptoms.
5 Research into barriers to the adoption of policies which are known to be effective in reducing levels of alcohol problems, including taxation, restrictions on availability and advertising; and reasons for the persistence of policies known to be ineffective, including educational initiatives. Such research should be designed to take account of socio-economic and other cultural differences applicable in different countries and social groups.
6 Evaluation of the effectiveness of self-help, mutual aid and other interventions outside the formal treatment system, since the latter will never have the capacity to respond to the alcohol problems of all those who need help.

Summary

1. Most cultures both past and present have an ambivalent view of the use of alcohol, its benefits and undesirable effects. This ambivalence is often associated with the view that alcohol is harmless, possibly beneficial, in moderation, but harmful in excess.
2. There is a sharp conflict between addiction and disease models of alcoholism, particularly prevalent in North America, where lifelong abstinence is considered to be the only cure for the alcoholic, and psychological models, more common in Europe, where drinking in moderation is sometimes considered to be a viable objective.
3. Drinking has been shown to cause liver cirrhosis, pancreatitis, strokes, various cancers and, in the case of drinking during pregnancy, damage to the unborn child. Most of these physical health risks are confined to the heavy drinker. There is some evidence that light alcohol consumption may be protective against heart disease.
4. The greatest physical risk taken by the moderate drinker and by the occasional binge drinker is the risk of accidental injury or death, especially, but not exclusively, traffic accidents.
5. Heavy drinking has been shown to be associated with a substantial proportion of violent assaults and homicide, marital violence, marital breakdown and child abuse.
6. It is not clear to what extent drinking problems cause psychological disorders or are a consequence of pre-existing disorders. However, whichever is the case, drinking has the effect of exacerbating these disorders and making them more difficult to treat.
7. It has proved difficult to assess the relative contribution of hereditary and environmental factors to the development of different patterns of drinking; on balance, the evidence suggests that both factors make a substantial contribution but that environmental factors play the larger role.
8. The nature of physical and psychological dependence on alcohol is not well understood; at present, conditioning and learning models represent the most promising approach.
9. The most effective methods for preventing alcohol problems are measures that have the effect of reducing overall levels of consumption, including high taxation, advertising bans and restricted availability. However, in many countries the drinks industry acts as a powerful lobby against these measures and few politicians would risk unpopularity by introducing them.
10. Educational programmes have had little effect in reducing alcohol problems.
11. Brief interventions from general practitioners, including ‘opportunistic interventions’ given to individuals attending for other reasons, have been shown to be particularly effective in producing substantial reductions in levels of consumption.
12. For individuals seeking treatment for alcohol problems, motivational interviewing has been shown to be very effective. This approach contrasts sharply with traditional confrontational approaches.

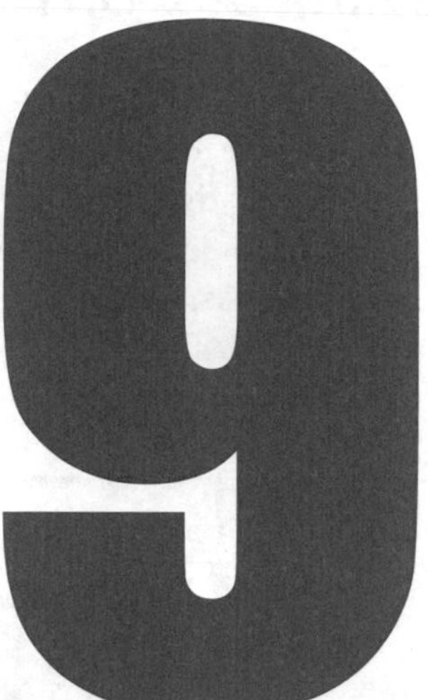

Tobacco and Smoking

This vice brings in one hundred million francs in taxes every year. I will certainly forbid it at once – as soon as you can name a virtue that brings in as much revenue.

Napoleon III, 1808–73

Outline

With the accumulation of evidence on the negative aspects of smoking, Western governments have promoted measures to reduce the prevalence. These measures have met with substantial success, in spite of attempts by the tobacco industry to deliberately misinform the public. Smoking prevalence is increasing throughout the developing world and many people continue to smoke in the industrialized world. This chapter documents the extent of smoking, its major health impacts, and factors that help to explain its continued popularity. Smoking is a complex practice involving a mixture of biopsychosocial processes. Three main theories, the biological, psychological and social, are outlined. The primary methods to assist smokers to quit are reviewed together with the results of evaluation studies. Methodological issues with placebos and vested interests of industry suggest caution in interpreting studies funded by the pharmaceutical industry.

BRIEF HISTORY OF TOBACCO AND SMOKING

In the first century BC the Mayans in Central America are alleged to have smoked tobacco in religious ceremonies. The Aztecs took the smoking custom from the Mayans who later settled in the Mississippi Valley and smoking was adopted by neighbouring tribes (see Figure 9.1). Amazonian Indians also used tobacco in their religious rituals. This group colonized the Bahamas, later discovered by Columbus in 1492.

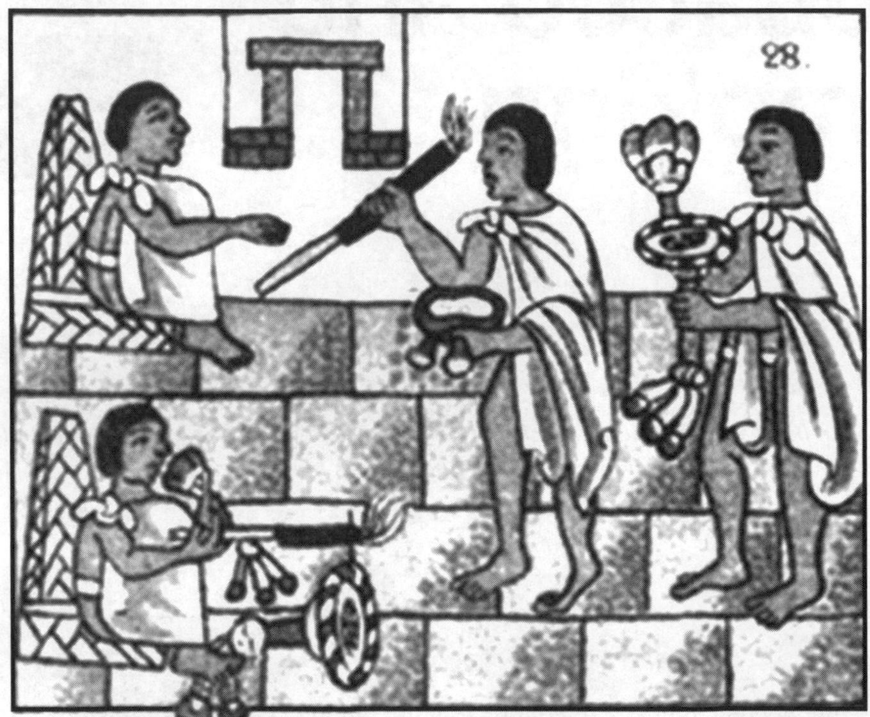

Figure 9.1 Aztec guests being presented with a tobacco tube and a sunflower
Source: The Florentine Codex

The English adventurer Sir Walter Raleigh is alleged to have introduced both potatoes and tobacco to England. Raleigh's public health legacy of tobacco and potato (in their fried form) would be hard to rival. Raleigh popularized tobacco at court, and apparently believed that it was a good cure for coughs and so he often smoked a pipe. Indeed, it is alleged that Raleigh's final request before his beheading by James I at the Tower of London in 1618 was a smoke of tobacco, a legacy to all subsequent prisoners facing execution.

Cigarette smoking was reintroduced to England by British soldiers returning from Wellington's Napoleonic campaigns in the Iberian Peninsula (1808–14). Following this, veterans returning from the Crimean War (1853–56) increased cigarette smoking in Britain. In addition to bringing many millions of deaths and injuries to service personnel, war has always been a great addicter to tobacco and, in the case of the Royal Navy, to rum.

The economics and politics of tobacco are complicated with many dilemmas and contradictions. Over the last 450 years tobacco has become a major contributor to the economy. Tobacco tax makes a significant contribution to the wealth of nations, exceeding the cost of treating smoking-related diseases in health systems. Tax revenue from tobacco products in the UK reached £10 billion in 2008/9. Cheaper cigarettes, purchased abroad or smuggled, result in substantial revenue loss to the Treasury of around £4–5 billion per year. In this, as in other domains, government policy involves a conflict of interests. Many farms on the European continent grow tobacco and the European Union (EU) subsidizes tobacco growers by paying EU farmers €3650 million each year. At the same time the EU has a policy of discouraging smoking by restricting tobacco advertising, and mandating health warnings on cigarette packets.

Table 9.1 Tobacco consumption in 2000 and 2010

TOBACCO: CONSUMPTION 000 tonnes	ACTUAL 2000	PROJECTED 2010
World	6769.1	7151.5
China	2627.5	2659.5
EU (15)	724.1	690.6
India	470.3	563.8
USSR (Former Area)	442.4	442.3
USA	434.4	433.8
Brazil	202.5	257.9
Japan	169.5	–
Indonesia	156.1	–
Turkey	133.6	–
Pakistan	90.0	–

Source: http://www.fao.org/english/newsroom/news/2003/26919-en.html

The Food and Agriculture Organization of the United Nations projected a global increase in tobacco consumption between 2000 and 2010 (see Table 9.1). China is the largest consumer, with the EU in second place, and India third.

PREVALENCE AND DISTRIBUTION

Although tobacco was popular during the nineteenth century, it was largely smoked using pipes and confined to men. The development of cigarettes towards the end of the nineteenth century was followed by a rapid increase in tobacco consumption. In the first half of the twentieth century, cigarette smoking became a hugely popular activity, especially among men in the western world. In the USA cigarette consumption doubled in the 1920s and again in the 1930s and peaked at about 67 per cent in the 1940s and 1950s. However, between 1965 and 2004, cigarette smoking among adults aged 18 and older declined by half from 42 per cent to 21 per cent and rates declined to 20 per cent in 2007. An estimated 43.4 million Americans currently smoke (American Cancer Society, 2009).

In Britain it was estimated that the prevalence among men reached almost 80 per cent during the 40s and 50s (Wald, Kiryluk, Darby, Doll, Pike & Peto, 1988). Since then, the prevalence has declined overall, with sex, social class, regional and other differences. The World Health Organization (2004) estimated that 47 per cent of men and 12 per cent of women smoked, including 42 per cent of men and 24 per cent of women in developed countries, and 48 per cent of men and 7 per cent of women in developing countries. Prevalence in developing countries is rising dramatically where there is extensive promotion of smoking by the tobacco industry.

Though fewer women than men are smokers, there have been dramatic increases in smoking among women and the gap in smoking rates between men and women is narrowing in most places. In Europe, there was a consistent decline in the prevalence of smoking among men from about 70–90 per cent to about 30–50 per cent between 1950 and 1990. However, among women the same period saw a rise in the prevalence of smoking followed by a slow decline reaching 20–40 per cent in 1990. The initial rise in prevalence was led by women from professional backgrounds, but they have also led the decline such that today smoking is more common among women from poorer backgrounds.

National variations in smoking behaviour have also been found across Europe. More than 40 per cent of men in Austria, Greece, Norway and Portugal smoked, while less than 25 per cent smoked in Belgium, Finland, Hungary and Sweden. In general the prevalence of smoking was lower among women and lowest (10 per cent) in Finland.

National surveys have also clearly established a growing link between smoking and various indicators of social deprivation. In Britain a national survey of health and lifestyles found that smoking is more prevalent among people on low incomes, the unemployed and those who are divorced or separated.

HEALTH EFFECTS OF SMOKING

The health effects of smoking have been studied for over 100 years. There is hardly a single organ in the body that is not deleteriously influenced by tobacco smoking. Today the only group still claiming that smoking is safe is the tobacco industry.

Effects on Active Smokers

The classic study by Doll and Hill (1952) linking smoking with cancer was followed by reports by the Royal College of Physicians in Britain (1962) and the Surgeon General in the United States (US Department of Health, Education and Welfare, 1964) demonstrating the harmful effects of smoking. The US Centers for Disease Control and Prevention (2005) give a useful guide to the health impacts of smoking. Cigarette smoking accounts for more than 440,000 deaths each year in the United States and 120,000 deaths in the UK, nearly 1 of every 5 deaths. More deaths are caused each year by tobacco than by all deaths from human immunodeficiency virus (HIV), illegal drug use, alcohol use, motor vehicle injuries, suicides and murders combined. The risk of dying from lung cancer is at least 22 times higher among men who smoke, and about 12 times higher among women who smoke compared with those who have never smoked.

Chemicals and radiation that are capable of triggering the development of cancer are called 'carcinogens.' **Carcinogens** initiate a series of genetic alterations ('mutations') which stimulate cells to proliferate uncontrollably. A delay of several decades occurs between exposure to carcinogens in tobacco smoke and the onset of cancer. People exposed to carcinogens from smoking cigarettes generally will not develop cancer for 20 to 30 years. In the USA there have been 29 Surgeon General's Reports on smoking and health during the period 1964–2006. Tobacco is the leading preventable cause of illness and death in the United States, resulting in an annual cost of more than $75 billion in direct medical costs. Nationally, smoking results in almost 6 million years of potential life lost each year. More than 6.4 million children living today will die prematurely because of their decision to smoke cigarettes.

The 2004 US Surgeon General's report on smoking and health revealed that smoking causes diseases in nearly every organ of the body. Published 40 years after the Surgeon General's first report on smoking – which had concluded that smoking was a definite cause of three serious diseases – the 2004 report found that cigarette smoking is conclusively linked to leukaemia, cataracts, pneumonia and cancers of the cervix, kidney, pancreas and stomach. On average, men who smoke cut their lives short by 13.2 years, and female smokers lose 14.5 years. Statistics indicate that more than 12 million Americans have died from smoking since the first Surgeon General's report in 1964, and another 25 million Americans alive today are likely to die of a smoking-related illness. The report concluded that quitting smoking has immediate and long-term benefits, reducing risks for diseases caused by smoking and improving health in general. Quitting smoking at age 65 or older reduces by nearly 50 per cent a person's risk of dying of a smoking-related disease.

Effects on Passive Smokers

For obvious reasons, tobacco smoke does most damage to the person who is actively inhaling. However, those consistently breathing **secondhand smoke** (SHS) also have a higher risk of cancer,

Case Study

INTERNATIONAL CASE STUDY Smoking deaths in India

In an epidemiological study, Jha et al. (2008) estimated that smoking accounts for 900,000 deaths a year in India. The authors predicted that one million people a year will die from tobacco smoking in India during the 2010s. The study warned that, without action, the death toll from smoking will climb still further. It predicts smoking could soon account for 20 per cent of all male deaths and 5 per cent of all female deaths in India between the ages of 30 and 69. The data showed a 6-year reduction in longevity for male smokers and a 8-year reduction for females (see Figure 9.2).

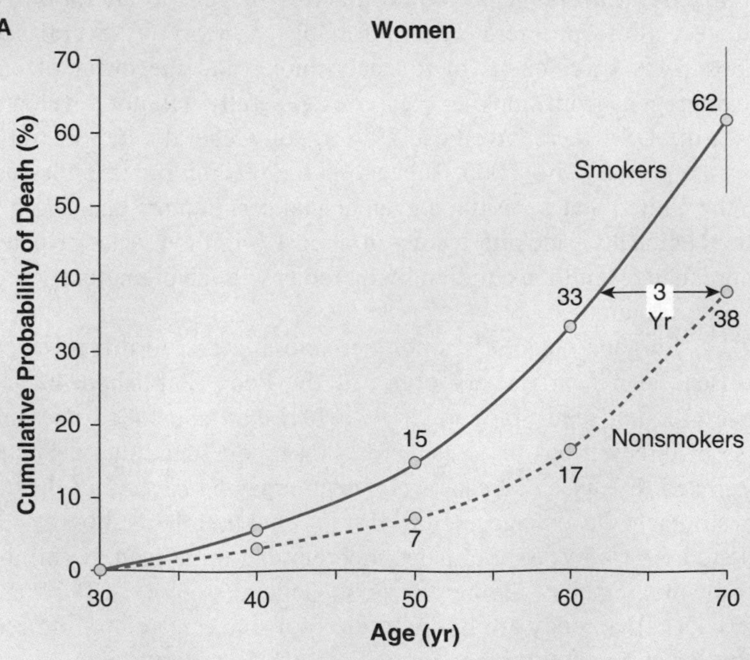

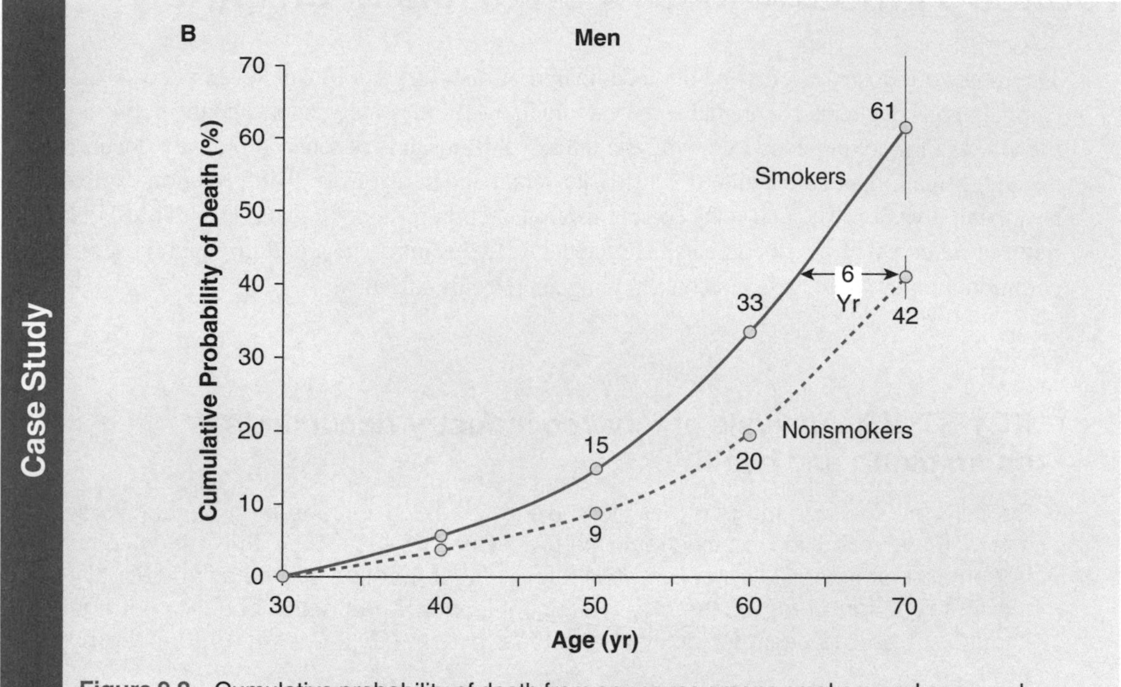

Figure 9.2 Cumulative probability of death from any cause among smokers and non-smokers between the ages of 30 and 69 years: women (Panel A, opposite) and men (Panel B)
Source: Jha et al. 2008.

heart disease, and respiratory disease, as well as sensory irritation. The Surgeon General estimated that exposure to SHS killed more than 3000 adult non-smokers from lung cancer each year, approximately 46,000 from coronary heart disease, and an estimated 430 newborns from sudden infant death syndrome. In addition, SHS causes other respiratory problems in non-smokers such as coughing, phlegm and reduced lung function. Passive smoking causes the premature death of thousands of non-smokers worldwide.

The Scientific Committee on Tobacco and Health (SCOTH, 1998) commissioned a review of the impact of secondary smoking on lung cancer. This review analysed 37 epidemiological studies of lung cancer in women who were life-long non-smokers living with smokers. The review found that the women had a statistically significant excess risk of lung cancer of 26 per cent. The analysis also showed that there was a dose response relationship between the risk of lung cancer and the number of cigarettes smoked by a person's partner, as well as the duration over which they had been exposed to their smoke. The report also concluded that parental smoking caused acute and chronic middle ear disease in children. Furthermore, it concluded that **sudden infant death syndrome** (SIDS), the main cause of post-neonatal death in the first year of life, is associated with exposure to environmental tobacco smoke. The association was judged to be one of cause and effect.

TOBACCO INDUSTRY CAMPAIGN OF DISINFORMATION

The tobacco industry has carried out a campaign of disinformation over several decades. This campaign has deliberately sought to create doubt in the minds of legislators and the public about the effects of smoking. However, with the release of thousands of tobacco industry documents through litigation and the action of whistleblowers, the details of the disinformation campaign have been revealed. The anti-tobacco organization, Action on Smoking and Health (ASH), carried out a survey of the documents, extracted 1200 relevant quotes, and grouped these under common themes (Source: Action on Smoking and Health, 2010).

KEY STUDY Analysis of tobacco industry documents on smoking and health

Publicly the tobacco industry has denied that smoking causes lung cancer – yet it has understood the carcinogenic nature of its product since the 1950s, e.g.: 'A demand for scientific proof is always a formula for inaction and delay and usually the first reaction of the guilty … in fact scientific proof has never been, is not and should not be the basis for political and legal action' (S. J. Green, 1980, cited by ASH, 2010).

- *Nicotine and addiction.* The industry routinely denied that tobacco is addictive yet it knew this since the 1960s. The idea of nicotine addiction destroyed the industry's stance that smoking is a matter of personal choice, e.g.: …the entire matter of addiction is the most potent weapon a prosecuting attorney can have in a lung cancer/cigarette case. We can't defend continued smoking as 'free choice' if the person was 'addicted'.' (The Tobacco Institute, 1980, cited by ASH, 2010).
- *Marketing to children.* The companies deny that they target the young. Yet company documents revealed the companies' pre-occupation with teenagers and younger children and methods to influence smoking behaviour in these age groups, e.g.: 'If the last ten years have taught us anything, it is that the industry is dominated by the companies who respond most to the needs of younger smokers' (Imperial Tobacco, Canada, cited by ASH, 2010).
- *Advertising.* The industry maintains that advertising is used only to fight for brand share, not to increase total consumption, while academic research shows otherwise, e.g.: 'I am always amused by the suggestion that advertising, a function that has been shown to increase consumption of virtually every other product, somehow miraculously fails to work for tobacco products' (Emerson Foote, former Chairman of McCann-Erickson, which handled US$20m of tobacco industry accounts, cited by ASH, 2010).

- *Cigarette design.* The industry promoted 'low-tar' cigarettes knowing that they were lacking any health benefits, or even made cigarettes more dangerous, e.g.: 'Are smokers entitled to expect that cigarettes shown as lower delivery in league tables will in fact deliver less to their lungs than cigarettes shown higher?' (BAT in 1977, cited by ASH, 2010).
- *Passive smoking.* The industry refused to accept the evidence of the harm caused by SHS, e.g.: 'All allegations that passive smoking is injurious to the health of non-smokers, in respect the social cost of smoking as well as unreasonable demands for no smoking areas in public places, should be countered strongly' (BAT in 1982, cited by ASH, 2010).
- '*Emerging markets'.* With reducing smoking levels in the West, the companies moved aggressively into developing countries and Eastern Europe, e.g.: 'They have to find a way to feed the monsters they've built. Just about the only way will be to increase sales to the developing world.' (Ex tobacco company employee, R. Morelli, cited by ASH, 2010).

Source: Action on Smoking and Health, 2010

Another study reached similar conclusions to those of ASH. SHS has been linked causally with sudden infant death syndrome (SIDS) in major reports such as the 2004 US Surgeon General report. Tong, England and Glantz (2005) discuss the tobacco industry's use of scientific consultants to attack the evidence that SHS causes disease, including lung cancer. Tobacco industry documents included 40 million pages of internal memos and reports made available in litigation settlements against the tobacco industry in the United States. From their analyses of these documents, Tong et al. concluded:

> *PM executives responded to corporate concerns about the possible adverse effects of SHS on maternal and child health by commissioning consultants to write review articles for publication in the medical literature. PM executives successfully encouraged one author to change his original conclusion that SHS is an independent risk factor for SIDS to state that the role of SHS is 'less well established'. (Tong et al., 2005: 356)*

Balbach, Smith and Malone (2006) argue that the Health Belief Model (see Chapter 6) helps the tobacco industry through its theoretical stance regarding individual choice, and 'information'. Balbach et al. analysed trial and deposition testimony of 14 high-level tobacco industry executives from six companies plus the Tobacco Institute to determine how they used the concepts of 'information' and 'choice' in relation to theoretical models of health behaviour change. They concluded that tobacco industry executives deployed the concept of 'information' to shift full moral responsibility for the harms caused by tobacco products to consumers. The industry executives characterized the tobacco industry as 'that of impartial supplier of value-free "information", without regard to its quality, accuracy and truthfulness … Over-reliance on individual and interpersonal rational choice models may have the effect of validating the industry's model of smoking and cessation behaviour, absolving it of responsibility and rendering invisible the "choices" the industry has made and continues to make in promoting the most deadly consumer product ever made' (Balbach et al., 2006). Discourses about smoking have a powerful influence on attributions of responsibility, whether the consumer or the provider is ultimately to blame. Our 'blame culture' can easily swing in either direction.

TOBACCO PROMOTION AND THE SOCIAL AND ECONOMIC CONTEXT OF SMOKING

The tobacco industry spends billions worldwide advertising and promoting tobacco products. Research shows that tobacco advertising encourages children to start smoking and reinforces the social acceptability of the habit among adults. The US Surgeon General (1989) stated that tobacco advertising increases consumption by:

- Encouraging children or young adults to experiment with tobacco and thereby slip into regular use;
- Encouraging smokers to increase consumption;
- Reducing smokers' motivation to quit;
- Encouraging former smokers to resume;
- Discouraging full and open discussion of the hazards of smoking as a result of media dependence on advertising revenues;
- Muting opposition to controls on tobacco as a result of the dependence of organizations receiving sponsorship from tobacco companies;
- Creating, through the ubiquity of advertising and sponsorship, an environment in which tobacco use is seen as familiar and acceptable and the warnings about its health impacts are undermined.

Hastings and MacFadyen (2000) analysed internal tobacco company documents and found that the companies worked with advertising agencies to target young people. The companies used advertising to increase overall consumption as well as brand share, in contrast to their public assertions that they only advertise to encourage existing smokers to switch brands.

Most econometric studies have found that increased expenditure on tobacco advertising increases demand for cigarettes, while banning advertising leads to a reduction in tobacco consumption. In 1991, a meta-analysis of 48 econometric studies found that tobacco advertising significantly increased tobacco sales. The UK Department of Health's Chief Economic Adviser found that there was a drop in tobacco consumption of between 4 and 16 per cent in countries that had implemented a tobacco-advertising ban (Smee, Parsenage, Anderson, & Duckworth, 1992). Given the huge numbers of people who die from smoking related diseases, it seems illogical that tobacco companies are allowed legally to advertise their harmful products. However, many issues are intertwined and the abolition of tobacco advertising has not been as simple and straightforward as it might first appear.

First, there is the argument that there is a lack of evidence to suggest that tobacco advertising significantly influences smoking behaviour. The 'magical potency' of tobacco advertising could be questioned since most advertisements are directed to target audiences who already use the product. Researchers claimed that econometric studies have found either no overall relationship between advertising and sales or a small, statistically significant positive relationship. However, this view can be contested and the results of such studies are equivocal as much depends on who supplies data for the studies: the tobacco industry or the public health authorities.

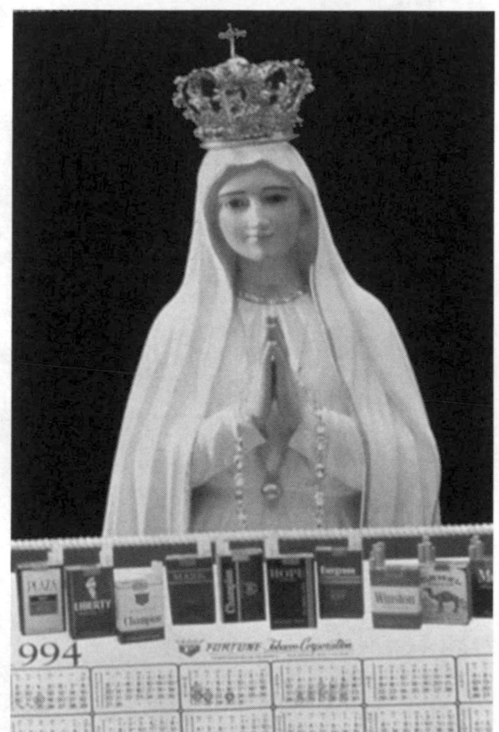

Figure 9.3 The Virgin Mary praying over leading brands – a calendar from the Fortune Tobacco Corporation, Philippines, 1994

The issue of banning tobacco advertising is further tangled when politics are included. The epitome of this can be seen within the European Union (EU) that, on the one hand, supports and finances the tobacco industry through the Common Agricultural Policy, and on the other, recognizes the health effects of tobacco in funding its 'Europe Against Cancer' campaign. However, in financial terms, the former greatly exceeds the latter. Despite this, attempts have been made to persuade tobacco growers to change their crops. Yet the fact remains that in 1994 the EU provided €41,165 million in tobacco subsidies and a mere €415 million to the 'Europe Against Cancer' campaign.

As we saw in Chapter 2, demographic changes are occurring with decreasing birth rates and increasing life expectancy. Smokers who die before the average life expectancy are helping to reduce expenditure on an already expensive elderly population. Between 4 and 5 per cent of government revenue comes from tobacco sales tax. By killing off smokers early, the tobacco industry is helping the economy. This fact may help to explain why policies to control tobacco over many years have been so ineffectual.

THEORIES OF SMOKING

The resistance shown by smokers to large-scale campaigns to discourage the practice has prompted a massive amount of research to help to explain the continuing popularity of smoking. It is agreed that smoking is an extremely complex practice involving a mixture of processes. The biopsychosocial model indicates three influences on health that are mirrored in theories of smoking: the biological, the psychological and the social theories of smoking (see Box 9.1). The theories are complementary and slightly overlapping, hence the term 'biopsychosocial' is an apt one in this context.

Box 9.1

The three main theoretical approaches to the understanding of smoking

Theory	Main elements of the theory
Biological	1 Tobacco contains nicotine, an addictive substance. 2 Nicotine activates brain circuits that regulate feelings of pleasure, the 'reward pathways' of the brain. 3 Nicotine increases the amounts of the neurotransmitter dopamine. 4 The acute effects of nicotine disappear in a few minutes, causing the smoker to repeat the dose of nicotine. 5 Smoking is an addiction that is repeatedly and immediately reinforced with each new intake of nicotine.
Psychological	1 Smoking is a learned habit, which becomes an automatic response to stimuli following repeated reinforcement – a conditioned response. 2 The pleasant associations of smoking generalize to a range of settings and situations. 3 The smoker learns to discriminate between those situations in which smoking is rewarded and those in which it is punished. 4 The smoker develops responses to a number of conditioned stimuli (internal and external 'triggers') that elicit smoking. 5 Smoking is an escape/avoidance response to certain aversive states. The smoker will light up a cigarette to escape or avoid an uncomfortable situation.

(Continued)

Theory	Main elements of the theory
Social	1 Initially, smoking is physically unpleasant but this is overruled because of social reinforcement from peers. 2 Smoking is a social activity in which the smoker identifies with others who smoke. There is a rebellious feeling associated with the activity. 3 The social identity of the smoker is changed once he/she forms the habit. 4 Smokers group together socially and share their experiences, which smokers finds pleasurable and empowering. The in-group feeling is heightened by social norms and health advice to quit. 5 The strong associations between social identity, in-group feelings, and a smoking sub-culture are difficult to change.

Biological Theory

Nicotine, the main active ingredient in tobacco smoke, is a substance that if taken in large quantities can be toxic. However, delivered in small amounts via cigarette smoke it has a range of psychophysiological effects including tranquillization, weight loss, decreased irritability, increased alertness and improved cognitive functioning. However, tolerance to the effect of nicotine develops such that there is less evidence of performance improvements among regular smokers (Jarvis, 2004). Over time the smoker develops a **physical dependence** on nicotine. In 1997 the smallest of the big five US tobacco companies (the Liggett Group) admitted that it had raised the nicotine content in cigarettes to increase their addictiveness. Nicotine is a naturally occurring colourless liquid that turns brown when burned and smells of tobacco when exposed to air. It has complex but predictable effects on the brain and body. Most cigarettes contain 10 milligrams (mg) or more of nicotine. The typical smoker takes in 1 to 2 mg nicotine per cigarette. Nicotine is absorbed through the skin and lining of the mouth and nose or by inhalation in the lungs. In cigarettes nicotine reaches peak levels in the bloodstream and brain rapidly, within 7–10 seconds of inhalation. Cigar and pipe smokers, on the other hand, typically do not inhale the smoke, so nicotine is absorbed more slowly through the mucosal membranes of their mouths. Nicotine from smokeless tobacco also is absorbed through the mucosal membranes.

Nicotine is addictive because it activates brain circuits that regulate feelings of pleasure, the 'reward pathways' of the brain. A key chemical involved is the neurotransmitter **dopamine** that nicotine increases. The acute effects of nicotine disappear in a few minutes, causing the smoker to repeat the dose of nicotine to maintain the drug's pleasurable effects and prevent withdrawal symptoms.

The cigarette is an efficient and highly engineered drug-delivery system. By inhaling, the smoker can get nicotine to the brain rapidly with each and every puff. A typical smoker will take 10 puffs on a cigarette over a period of 5 minutes that the cigarette is lit. Thus, a person who smokes 30 cigarettes daily gets 300 'hits' of nicotine every day. That is over 100,000 hits a year or one million every ten years! This is why cigarette smoking is so highly addictive. Smoking behaviour is rewarded and reinforced hundreds of thousands or millions of times over the smoker's lifetime. An enzyme called monoamineoxidase (MAO) shows a marked decrease during smoking. MAO is responsible for breaking down dopamine. An ingredient other than nicotine causes the change in MAO, since it is known that nicotine does not dramatically alter MAO levels. Smokers may be increasing central dopamine levels by reducing monoamine oxidase inhibitor activity, reinforcing smoking by keeping high satisfaction levels through repeated tobacco use.

There is evidence that tobacco is a highly addictive drug. More than 30 per cent of people who try tobacco for the first time develop a dependency on tobacco, while for other drugs, this percentage is generally lower. However, there are variations in the speed and strength of **addiction** to nicotine among smokers. One obvious way to explain individual differences in smoking is our genetic makeup. Genetic factors could play a role in several aspects of nicotine addiction, from the tendency to begin smoking, to the chances of quitting.

Twin studies produced evidence of a genetic link to smoking. Heath and Madden (1995) found that genetic factors increased the likelihood of becoming a regular smoker ('initiation') and of these smokers becoming long-term smokers ('persistence'). In a large follow-up survey of male twin pairs from the US Vietnam Era Twin Registry, True et al. (1997) found that genetic factors account for 50 per cent of the risk of smoking and environmental factors accounted for a further 30 per cent. In addition, genetic factors accounted for 70 per cent of the risk variance of becoming a regular smoker whereas environmental factors were not important.

With the decline in the overall prevalence a group of 'refractory' smokers has emerged who are more likely to have other problems such as depression, anxiety and bulimia (Pomerlau, 1979). In ancient times these patterns may have been biologically adaptive or neutral. However, in contemporary society, a more active fight or flight response is inappropriate. Smoking would be valuable to this population because it can produce small but reliable adjustments to levels of arousal. Evolutionary approaches to addictions tend to ignore the psychological and social influences that create the conditions for tobacco use (Marks, 1998). It is to these influences that we now turn.

Psychological Theory

Probably the most frequently used model of smoking is that based on learning theory. Basically, it argues that people become smokers because of the positive reinforcement they obtain from smoking. The mechanisms are similar to those described in Chapter 8 in reference to alcohol drinking. Initially, smoking is physically unpleasant (to a greater extent than is the case for alcohol) but this is overruled because of the social reinforcement from peers. The pleasant associations of smoking then generalize to a range of other settings. In addition, the smoker learns to discriminate between those situations in which smoking is rewarded and those in which it is punished. He or she also develops responses to **conditioned stimuli** (both internal and external) that elicit smoking. Smoking can be conceptualized as an escape/avoidance response to certain aversive states (Pomerlau, 1979). The smoker will light up a cigarette to escape or avoid an uncomfortable situation.

In 1966 Tomkins proposed his 'affect management model' of smoking that was subsequently revised and extended by Ikard, Green and Horn (1969) who conducted a survey of a national (US) probability sample. In a factor analysis of the responses they identified six smoking motivation factors: reduction of negative affect, habit, addiction, pleasure, stimulation and sensorimotor manipulation. Subsequent surveys produced similar factors. Women more than men report that they smoked for reduction of negative affect and pleasure.

In their study of smoking among young adults, Murray et al. (1988) added two additional reasons: boredom and nothing to do. In a survey they asked young adults to indicate which of these factors were important reasons for smoking in different situations. In all situations relaxation and control of negative affect were considered the most important reasons. At home boredom was also considered important, perhaps reflecting these young people's frustration with family life. At work addiction was considered important, perhaps reflecting the extent to which it disrupted their work routine, while socially habit was rated important.

According to Zuckerman (1979) individuals engage in **sensation seeking** so as to maintain a certain level of physiological arousal. More specifically, Zuckerman emphasized that sensation seeking was designed to maintain an optimal level of catecholaminergic activity. In a French sample, smokers score higher on a measure of sensation seeking, in particular on disinhibition, experience seeking and boredom susceptibility subscales. From a physiological perspective these sensation seekers have a low level of tonic arousal and seek exciting, novel or intense stimulation to raise the level of cortical arousal. This argument is similar to that of Eysenck, Tarrant and Woolf (1960) who found that smokers scored higher on measures of *extraversion.* This personality dimension is also supposed to reflect a lower level of cortical arousal that could be raised by engaging in risky activities such as smoking.

Besides sensation seeking and extraversion, a variety of personality characteristics have been found to be associated with smoking. In a sample of Scottish adults, Whiteman, Fowkes Deary and Lee (1997) found that smoking was associated with hostility. However, they accept that 'presence of an association does not help in determining if the relationship is causal'. Indeed, they hypothesize that deprivation of smoking that was required for the study may have increased hostility.

A variety of different types of studies have found that stress is associated with smoking. For example, among smokers, consumption is higher in experimental stressful laboratory situations. In surveys, people with higher self-reports of stress are more likely to be heavy smokers. In a study of nurses' smoking practices, Murray et al. (1983) found that those who reported the most stress were more likely to smoke. This relationship remained after controlling for the effect of family and friends' smoking practices. Finally, in a macro-social study, US states that have the highest levels of stress as measured by a range of social indicators also have the highest levels of smoking and of smoking related diseases.

Other researchers have looked for evidence of personality differences between people who smoke and non-smokers. Sensation seeking, neuroticism and psychoticism are all correlated with smoking (Marks, 1998). However the relationships are fairly weak and it can be concluded that anybody has the potential to become addicted to nicotine.

Social Theory

Smoking is a social activity. Even when the smoker smokes alone he or she still smokes in a society where cigarettes are widely available and promoted. A number of qualitative studies have considered the social meaning of smoking. Murray et al. (1988) conducted detailed interviews with a sample of young adults from the English Midlands. These suggested that smoking had different meanings in different settings. For example, at work going for a cigarette provided an opportunity to escape from the everyday routine. For these workers, to have a cigarette meant to have a break and conversely not to have a cigarette meant not to have a break. The cigarette was a marker, a means to regulating their work routine.

Outside work, smoking was perceived as a means of reaffirming social relationships. For those young people who went to the pub, the sharing of cigarettes was a means of initiating, maintaining and strengthening social bonds. Those who did not share cigarettes were frowned upon.

Graham's (1976) series of qualitative studies has provided a detailed understanding of the meaning of smoking to working-class women. In one of her studies, she asked a group of low-income mothers to complete a 24-hour diary detailing their everyday activities. Like the young workers in the study by Murray et al. (1988), smoking was used as a means of organizing these women's daily routine. Further, for these women smoking was not just a means of resting after completing certain household tasks but also a means of coping when there was a sort of breakdown in normal household routines. This was especially apparent when the demands of childcare became excessive. Graham describes smoking as 'not simply a way of structuring caring: it is also part of the way smokers re-impose structure when it breaks down' (1987: 54).

Graham (1987) argued that for these women smoking is an essential means of coping with everyday difficulties. It is also a link to an adult consumer society. Through smoking the women were reaffirming their adult identity. Similarly, in Bancroft, Wiltshire, Parry and Amos' (2003) Scottish study, both men and women reported integrating smoking into contrasting periods of their lives. They smoked as a means of coping with stress at work and often because of boredom at home.

Smoking is not only embedded in the immediate material circumstances in which the smoker lives, but also in the wider social and cultural context within which smoking is widely promoted. Admittedly, in most Western societies there are considerable restrictions on the sale and promotion of cigarettes. Despite these, tobacco manufacturers continue to find ways to promote their products, e.g. through the sponsorship of sporting and cultural activities. In the USA it is estimated that the tobacco companies spend approximately $6 billion per annum on advertising and promotion. As illustrated above, the tobacco industry is a powerful lobby group having considerable influence on government and policymaking.

SMOKING CESSATION

In the last 10 years smoking prevalence in adults has been driven down in many Western countries to around 15–30 per cent. Yet millions are still harmed by tobacco, and to an increasing extent in developing countries, deepening health inequalities. This has led to attempts to develop a more sophisticated understanding of the process of giving up smoking. There is more clarity today about the best ways to proceed in helping individual smokers.

The majority of smokers spend a considerable portion of their smoking career wishing they could quit. When they do finally quit, the vast majority do so on their own, without professional help, and they quit using 'cold turkey', i.e. by abrupt withdrawal. The American Cancer Society (2003) reports that 91.4 per cent of former smokers quit 'cold turkey' or by slowly decreasing the amount smoked. Doran, Valenti, Robinson, Britt and Mattick (2006) surveyed adult patients attending Australian GPs in 2002 and 2003. Over a quarter of patients were former smokers and one in five were current smokers. Doran et al. reported that 92 per cent of former and 80 per cent of current smokers used only one method in their last quit attempt, 'cold turkey' being the most common method used by both former (88 per cent) and current (62 per cent) smokers.

For those who seek help, guidelines such as those of the US Surgeon General (2008) can be followed. For smokers who are willing to quit, the 5 As are a useful framework:

- **A**sk about tobacco use. Identify and document tobacco use status for every patient at every visit.
- **A**dvise to quit. In a clear, strong and personalized manner urge every tobacco user to quit.
- **A**ssess willingness to make a quit attempt. Is the tobacco user willing to make a quit attempt at this time?
- **A**ssist in quit attempt. For the patient willing to make a quit attempt, offer medication and provide or refer for counselling or additional treatment to help the patient quit. For patients unwilling to quit at the time, provide interventions designed to increase future quit attempts.
- **A**rrange follow-up. For the patient willing to make a quit attempt, arrange for follow-up contacts, beginning within the first week after the quit date. For patients unwilling to make a quit attempt at the time, address tobacco dependence and willingness to quit at next clinic visit.

For smokers unwilling to quit, it is recommended to implement the 5 Rs: explain the **r**elevance, **r**isks, **r**ewards, **r**un over the roadblocks, and **r**epeat at every available opportunity. In the next section we review the three main approaches to smoking cessation which are available singly or in combination: pharmacological, psychological and social.

Pharmacological Approach to Cessation

It is well established that **cessation** of smoking by regular smokers leads to a variety of symptoms such as irritability, difficulty concentrating, anxiety, restlessness, increased hunger, depressed mood and a craving for tobacco. Important evidence that these withdrawal symptoms are due to the loss of nicotine is the finding that it is relieved by administration of nicotine but not of a **placebo**.

This evidence has led to the development of a variety of pharmacologic products aimed at aiding smoking cessation. There are three distinct kinds.

1 **Nicotine replacement therapy** (NRT) reduces symptoms of nicotine withdrawal, thereby increasing the likelihood of smoking cessation. NRT is designed to deliver nicotine directly rather than through cigarette smoke. Five forms of NRT have been found to be effective: nicotine gum, nicotine transdermal patch, nasal spray, inhaler and lozenge. Evidence from clinical trials has been interpreted by advocates as demonstrating that these NRT techniques are effective (e.g. Stolerman and Jarvis, 1995). NRT company websites, and also 'independent' sites that are viewed as authoritative such as the US Surgeon General's, among others, proclaim that the nicotine patch, available over-the-counter, will 'double your chances of quitting'. The NHS Smokefree website

claims that: 'If you also use medicines such as patches or gum to manage your cravings, you are up to four times more likely to successfully go smokefree!' (National Health Service, 2010). It appears that the latter claim is exaggerated as no reputable review has shown a four-fold increase in abstinence rates. The best abstinence rate reported by the Surgeon General (2008) reported with 8 sessions of counselling and behaviour therapy plus medication had an odds ratio of 1.7 and an estimated abstinence rate of 32.5 per cent. The typical placebo abstinence rate is around 11.5 per cent, and so even this high rate of 32.5 per cent is less than a three-fold increase compared to placebo.

There are methodological problems with randomized controlled trials which compared NRT to placebos. The use of placebos in trials of nicotine replacement products treatments has been contested on the grounds that the smokers in the placebo condition can detect that they are not receiving any nicotine (Mooney, White, & Hatsukami, 2004; Polito, 2008). These critics suggest that the trials are based on a false premise, namely that researchers were able to hide the onset of nicotine withdrawal symptoms from placebo control groups. Mooney and colleagues found that studies of nicotine replacement therapies are generally not blind in that participants correctly guess assignment at rates significantly above chance. Dar, Stronguin and Etter (2005) found that control group members were 3.3 times more likely to correctly guess that they had received placebo than to incorrectly guess that they had received nicotine (54.5 per cent v. 16.4 per cent). If the trials are not double blind, the results are compromised and the findings give a misleading picture of treatment effectiveness.

2 **Bupropion** (Zyban) is a weak dopamine and nor-epinephrine re-uptake inhibitor. Initially employed as an antidepressant, bupropion was found to be effective as a smoking treatment. One of the primary symptoms of smoking cessation has been depressive symptoms and it is known that central dopamine levels are reduced by lowered monoamine oxidase inhibitor activity which occurs on quitting. The mechanism of action of bupropion, therefore, may be to maintain central levels of dopamine during cessation. Bupropion reduces the severity of nicotine cravings and withdrawal symptoms. The treatment normally lasts for seven to twelve weeks, with the patient halting the use of tobacco about ten days into the course. The efficacy of bupropion is similar to that of nicotine replacement therapy. Bupropion approximately doubles the chance of quitting smoking successfully after three months. Wu, Wilson, Dimoulas and Mills' (2006) meta-analysis found that after one year of treatment, the odds of maintaining quitting were 1.5 times higher in the bupropion group than in a placebo group. However, the combination of bupropion and nicotine does not to appear to increase the cessation rate.

3 A third pharmacotherapy is **Varenicline** (Chantix) which is a nicotinic acetylcholine receptor partial agonist. Agonists at this receptor may stimulate the release of dopamine to reduce craving and withdrawal while simultaneously acting as a partial

antagonist by blocking the binding and consequent reinforcing effects of smoked nicotine. In a direct comparison of buproprion with varenicline, Jorenby et al. (2006) found varenicline had superior efficacy: after one year, the rate of continuous abstinence was 10 per cent for placebo, 15 per cent for bupropion, and 23 per cent for varenicline.

Critics claim that research carried out by the pharmaceutical industry should be treated with suspicion as the investigators have received industry funding as consultants, a hidden bias which can affect their ability to remain independent. Lexchin, Bero, Djulbegovic and Clark (2003) carried out a systematic review of the effect of pharmaceutical industry sponsorship on research outcome and quality. They found that pharmaceutically sponsored studies were less likely to be published in peer-reviewed journals. Also, studies sponsored by pharmaceutical companies were more likely to have outcomes favouring the sponsor than were studies with other sponsors (odds ratio 4.05; 95 per cent confidence interval 2.98 – 5.51). They found a systematic bias favouring products made by the company funding the research.

KEY STUDY The National Health Service (NHS) in England's Smoking Cessation Service.

This service is based on pharmacotherapy in combination with counselling support. An ASH report claims that the average cost per life year gained for every smoker successfully treated by these services is less than £1000, below the NICE guidelines of £20,000 per QALY (quality-adjusted life year). However, the investment in NHS stop smoking services is relatively low. A comparison with treatment costs for illicit drug users shows that £585 million is committed for 350,000 problem drug users compared to £56 million for 9 million users of tobacco. This is £6.20 for each smoker, compared to £1670 per illegal drug user (Action on Smoking & Health, 2008).

Disappointingly, the claims for high efficacy and cost-effectiveness of NRT have not been substantiated in real-world effectiveness studies (e.g. Pierce & Gilpin, 2002; Ferguson, Bauld, Chesterman & Judge, 2005; Doran et al., 2006). Pierce and Gilpin (2002) stated: 'Since becoming available over the counter, NRT appears no longer effective in increasing long-term successful cessation' (p. 1260). Efficacy studies, using randomized controlled trials, do not transfer well to real-world effectiveness. Bauld, Bell, McCullough, Richardson and Greaves (2009) reviewed 20 studies of the effectiveness of intensive NHS treatments for smoking cessation published between 1990 and 2007. Quit rates showed a dramatic decrease between 4-weeks and one year. A quit rate of 53 per cent at four weeks fell to only 15 per cent at 1 year. Younger smokers, females, pregnant smokers and more deprived smokers had lower quit rates than other groups.

The NHS evaluation data prove that NRT produces *poorer* outcomes than non-pharmacological methods (Health and Social Care Information Centre, Lifestyles Statistics, 2008). In 2007/08, 680,000 people set a quit date and 88 per cent of these had received pharmacotherapy at a cost of £61M. Of these, 49 per cent successfully quit for four weeks compared to 55 per cent of people who had received no pharmacotherapy. Smokers who used NRT had a lower quit rate than those who did not use NRT. On that basis, the NRT system needs to be replaced by a more effective system.

Another issue concerning NRT is lack of safety. In 2005 the MHRA relaxed the restrictions on NRT use allowing the combined use of patches and gum, and permission for its use by pregnant and young smokers, smokers with cardiovascular disease and smokers who want to reduce their smoking. However, a critical review concluded that NRT use by pregnant women and children would pose a significant risk to neurological development in infants and children (Ginzel et al., 2007). That NRT is used so widely in health-care systems in spite of the poor outcomes and lack of safety is a win for the pharmaceutical industry, but a questionable return for taxpayers and smokers.

Learning Points: (1) Adoption of a therapeutic strategy for smoking should look beyond a purely medical model. (2) A psychosocial model would yield a radically different approach. (3) Efficacy and cost-effectiveness will be higher when treatment strategies address the causes, not the symptoms.

Psychological Approach To Cessation

Quitting smoking or, if that is impossible, reducing cigarette consumption, are both viable targets for a smoking cessation programme. In order to achieve these aims, it is necessary for an intervention to help smokers to control both their physical and their **psychological dependency** on smoking. The US Surgeon General's (2008) guidelines on 'Treating Tobacco Use and Dependence' recommended the use of individual, group and telephone counselling. The report concluded that two components of counselling are especially effective, practical counselling concerning problem solving and skills training, and social support. The results of the meta-analysis are shown in Table 9.2. While counselling and medication are effective alone, a combination of counselling and medication is the most effective. The report found a strong association between the number of sessions of counselling when combined with medication, and smoking abstinence. The best abstinence rate was obtained with more than 8 sessions of counselling and behaviour therapy plus medication giving an odds ratio of 1.7 and an abstinence rate of 32.5 per cent.

The Guidelines give specific recommendations about particular behavioural and social elements to include in smoking treatments (see Table 9.2). There has been increasing

Table 9.2 Meta-analysis of the effectiveness of and estimated abstinence rates for various types of counselling and behavioural therapies (n = 64 studies)

Type of counselling and behavioural therapy	Number of arms	Estimated odds ratio (95 per cent CI)	Estimated abstinence rate (95 per cent CI)
No counselling/ behavioural therapy	35	1.0	11.2
Relaxation/breathing	31	1.0 (0.7, 1.3)	10.8 (7.9, 13.8)
Contingency contracting	22	1.0 (0.7, 1.4)	11.2 (7.8, 14.6)
Weight/diet	19	1.0 (0.8, 1.3)	11.2 (8.5, 14.0)
Cigarette fading	25	1.1 (0.8, 1.5)	11.8 (8.4, 15.3)
Negative affect	8	1.2 (0.8, 1.9)	13.6 (8.7, 18.5)
Intra-treatment social support	50	1.3 (1.1, 1.6)	14.4 (12.3, 16.5)
Extra-treatment social support	19	1.5 (1.1, 2.1)	16.2 (11.8, 20.6)
Other aversive smoking	19	1.7 (1.04, 2.8)	17.7 (11.2, 24.9)
Rapid smoking	19	2.0 (1.1, 3.5)	19.9 (11.2, 29.0)

Source: Surgeon General, 2008

interest in the use of cognitive behavioural therapy (CBT) for the control of smoking and other health-related behaviours. These therapies can be delivered as a brief intervention in one or more sessions to groups of smokers who are at the action stage. One example of a treatment programme which integrates a variety of effective behavioural techniques is the QUIT FOR LIFE (QFL) Programme (Sulzberger & Marks, 1977). This multi-modal programme includes all of the methods listed in Table 9.3 (Marks, 1993, 2005). QFL encourages a steady reduction of cigarette consumption over seven to 10 days followed by complete abstinence. The QFL programme is delivered in several alternative ways: as a group therapy of 10 sessions, as a self-help programme following a single, one-hour group therapy session, or on the Internet.

A preliminary observational study suggested that the therapy could be particularly effective when delivered to groups of self-referring smokers (Marks, 1992). Randomized controlled trials showed that the QFL programme is capable of delivering relatively high quit rates among lower SES smokers with only one intensive session (Marks & Sykes, 2000; Sykes & Marks, 2001). These results suggest that this CBT intervention has the potential to reduce smoking among lower SES smokers at relatively low cost.

Table 9.3 Elements of problem-solving and skills training recommended in the Surgeon General's (2008) Guidelines

Practical counselling (problem solving/ skills training) treatment component	Examples
Recognize danger situations – Identify events, internal states, or activities that increase the risk of smoking or **relapse**.	Negative affect and stress. Being around other tobacco users. Drinking alcohol. Experiencing urges. Smoking cues and availability of cigarettes
Develop coping skills – Identify and practise coping or problem-solving skills. Typically, these skills are intended to cope with danger situations.	Learning to anticipate and avoid temptation and trigger situations. Learning cognitive strategies that will reduce negative moods. Accomplishing lifestyle changes that reduce stress, improve quality of life, and reduce exposure to smoking cues. Learning cognitive and behavioural activities to cope with smoking urges (e.g., distracting attention; changing routines).
Provide basic information – provide basic information about smoking and successful quitting.	The fact that any smoking (even a single puff) increases the likelihood of a full relapse. Withdrawal symptoms typically peak within 1–2 weeks after quitting but may persist for months. These symptoms include negative mood, urges to smoke and difficulty concentrating. The addictive nature of smoking.

The most popular method of smoking cessation remains 'cold turkey' (abrupt cessation). The Australian study by Doran et al. (2006) reported success rates among 2207 former smokers and 928 current smokers as follows: cold turkey 77.2 per cent; nicotine patch 35.9 per cent; nicotine gum 35.9 per cent; nicotine inhaler 35.3 per cent; and bupropion 22.8 per cent. According to these data, NRT and bupropion *reduced* the odds of quitting when considered across the whole population of quitters. Health-care professionals tend to see only those smokers who have the most difficulty quitting by themselves. It is therefore likely that, as the smoking population shrinks over time, those who seek help become harder to treat.

Social Approach To Cessation

Smoking is deeply embedded in everyday social activities. Today, smoking has become almost taboo, and smokers are seen as 'outsiders'. Cessation attempts must take these aspects into consideration, including the increasing social gradient in smoking prevalence.

Smoking is becoming confined to people who live in poor circumstances. As Graham (1987) demonstrated, smoking serves an immediate reward function such that attempts to discourage smoking will be resisted.

Stewart et al. (1996) conducted a qualitative study of the role of smoking in the lives of such women and their perception of smoking cessation efforts. In reading the interviews with these women Stewart et al. felt that 'due to the pressing nature of the participants' life circumstances, many were caught in a daily struggle for survival. Consequently, the long-term benefits of quitting had little relevance for them' (p. 45). Smoking was a means of coping with the 'stress, chaos and crises in their lives'. In addition, the women felt that they did not have the self-esteem and confidence to quit smoking.

As regards attempts to quit, the women mentioned lack of social support from their partners, immediate family and friends. They felt that if there were peer support groups it would

Box 9.2

Internet sites supporting quitters

WhyQuit's Freedom from Nicotine: designed for 'cold turkey' quitters only without use of any product, pill or procedure. This leading site has an archive of more than 100,000 member posts on 19 subject message boards. The forum claims a six month nicotine cessation rate of 35 to 39 per cent self-reported continuous nicotine cessation for new members posting to the group at least once. However this claim has not been independently verified. http://whyquit.com/

KillTheCan.org: advocates abrupt nicotine cessation for smokeless tobacco quitters but provides support for all methods including NRTs. The site claims that: 'Its 7 founders chewed for over 100 years collectively and now represent over 10 collective years of cessation.' http://www.killthecan.org/

Nicotine-Anonymous.org: a non-profit 12-Step programme for those using quitting products or abrupt nicotine cessation quitters. http://nicotine-anonymous.org/meetings_internet_meetings.php

Quit Smokeless.org: for Smokeless tobacco quitters only. http://www.quitsmokeless.org/index.php

QUIT FOR LIFE Programme: provides a psychological therapy for smokers based on gradual withdrawal. http://www.staff.city.ac.uk/quitforlife/contents.html

be easier to quit. In concluding, Stewart et al. emphasized the disempowering character of the immediate social circumstances of some women's lives. Smoking cessation efforts need to provide not only social support but also attempt to enhance the women's sense of control and mastery through changing their social conditions. Smoking cessation may thus form a part of a more general community intervention to promote empowerment and health advocacy (see Chapters 6 and 14).

Many group treatment programmes use the 'buddy system' in which smokers are paired up to provide mutual support. A variety of organizations also offer group support for quitters. These are organized at a local level by health-care providers and charities. The NHS Stop Smoking Services offer free local group sessions which start a week or two before the official quit date. The group then meets weekly for four weeks to give advice and motivation. Some people prefer to talk one-to-one with a professional advisor, but many find the group support helpful. Many support systems are provided by hospitals and clinics. For example, in South Bend, Indiana, USA, the Memorial Health System's Lung Center offers a quit smoking programme called 'Freedom From Smoking Program'. Smoking cessation classes are offered to people using a behaviour change approach.

The Internet also provides social networking through specialized forum sites which aim to support quitters using diverse methods. A few non-commercial sites are listed in Box 9.2. However excellent the social support, the quitter must finally make a decision to quit as an individual.

ADOLESCENTS, SPECIAL POPULATIONS, MOBILE PHONES AND THE INTERNET

In this section we review a few meta-analyses on smoking cessation efforts with adolescents, special populations and new technology. First, we summarize a review of studies of adolescent smoking cessation. Garrison, Christakis, Ebel, Wiehe and Rivara (2003) reviewed controlled trials for adolescent smoking cessation up to June 2002. Only six of 281 studies met the selection criteria, three school-based studies, a study in pregnant adolescent girls, a hospital-based study, and a trial of laser acupuncture. None had follow-up times greater than 5 months. The authors concluded that 'there is very limited evidence demonstrating efficacy of smoking-cessation interventions in adolescents, and no evidence on the long-term effectiveness of such interventions. Smoking-cessation interventions that have proven most effective in adults, such as nicotine replacement and antidepressant use, have not been studied in adolescents in a controlled manner' (p. 363). In spite of this lack of research, and the possible risks involved, administration of NRT to adolescent smokers in now being actively encouraged by zealots of this form of treatment, including, we are sorry to say, a few health psychologists.

Turning now to adults and hospitalized populations, Ranney, Melvin, Lux, McClain and Lohr (2006) systematically reviewed smoking cessation intervention strategies for adults and adults in special populations. Ranney et al. reviewed systematic reviews, randomized, controlled trials, and observational studies of strategies for effective smoking cessation treatment in adults and special populations published from 1 January 1980 to 10 June 2005. Ranney et al.'s review included studies evaluating the efficacy of cessation strategies, such as self-help, counselling, single pharmaceutical agents, combined pharmacotherapies, and pharmacotherapies combined with psychological counselling. Research findings were consistent with previous reviews in showing that self-help strategies alone are ineffective, but counselling and pharmacotherapy used either alone or in combination can improve rates of success with quit attempts. There were few studies focused on ways to reach or treat special populations. Three studies with hospitalized patients were consistent with a previous review in showing little evidence that clinical diagnosis affected quit rates.

Recent reviews have reviewed the use of electronic media in smoking cessation, specifically mobile phones and the Internet. Whittaker, Borland, Bullen, Lin, McRobbie and Rodgers (2009) reviewed trials of mobile phones used as a medium for smoking cessation. Participants were smokers of any age who wanted to quit. Studies included any intervention aimed at mobile phone users, based around delivery via mobile phone with follow-up of at least six months. Four trials were included: a text message programme in New Zealand; a text message programme in the UK; and an Internet and mobile phone programme involving two different groups in Norway. In a meta-analysis the text message programme trials showed a significant increase in short-term self-reported quitting rate ratio (RR 2.18, 95 per cent CI 1.80 to 2.65). This review found text message mobile phone programmes to be effective in the short-term (six weeks), and a combined Internet–mobile phone programme to be effective up to 12 months. More evidence is needed to determine if programmes delivered over mobile phones can help people to stop smoking.

Shahab and McEwen (2009) reviewed the efficacy and acceptability of online, interactive interventions for smoking cessation and identified moderators and mediators of treatment effects in the literature from 1990–2008. Shahab and McEwan found 11 relevant randomized controlled trials of variable quality. Web-based, tailored, interactive smoking cessation interventions were found to be effective compared with untailored booklet or e-mail interventions (rate ratio (RR) 1.8; 95 per cent confidence interval (CI) 1.4 – 2.3) increasing 6-month abstinence by 17 per cent (95 per cent CI 12–21 per cent). Pooled results suggest that only interventions aimed at smokers motivated to quit were effective (RR 1.3, 95 per cent CI 1.0–1.7). Fully automated interventions increased smoking cessation rates (RR 1.4, 95 per cent CI 1.0–2.0), but evidence was less clear-cut for non-automated interventions. The web-based interventions were considered acceptable and user satisfaction was generally high. The authors concluded that interactive, web-based interventions for smoking cessation can be an effective aid in smoking cessation.

FUTURE RESEARCH

1. There is still limited understanding of cigarette smoking among young people. In particular, there is a need for increased understanding of the social, ethnic and gender variations in smoking among young people.
2. Although there has been a plethora of prevention programmes, there is a need for greater understanding of the variations in their effectiveness.
3. More research on the influence of tobacco advertising on the uptake of smoking in young people is necessary in those countries where advertising is permitted. This evidence will be significant in eventually gaining a worldwide advertising ban.
4. Randomized controlled trials with sound methodological controls of both psychological therapy and nicotine replacement therapy are necessary to determine their relative efficacy and cost effectiveness.
5. More research funding on smoking prevention and cessation is necessary from bodies independent of the tobacco industry.

Summary

1. About 25 per cent of adults in most Western societies smoke, while prevalence rates in the developing world are higher than this and increasing. The prevalence of smoking varies according to sex, social class and ethnicity.
2. Biological, psychological and social factors contribute to the smoking epidemic.
3. Effective tobacco control requires a multi-level approach including economic, political, social and psychological interventions.
4. Most smokers report difficulty in quitting the habit. However, significant progress has been made in our understanding of smoking cessation.
5. Efficacy and cost-effectiveness are higher when treatment strategies address the causes, not the symptoms.
6. Smokers wishing to quit are helped using the 5 As: Ask about tobacco use; Advise to quit; Assess willingness to make a quit attempt; Assist in quit attempt; Arrange follow-up.
7. Smokers unwilling to quit are helped using the 5 Rs: explain the Relevance; Risks; Rewards; run over the Roadblocks; and Repeat at every available opportunity.
8. Doubts have been raised about the methodology and funding of clinical trials of pharmaceutical products used in smoking cessation. Studies sponsored by pharmaceutical companies are more likely to have outcomes favouring the sponsor's products.

(Continued)

(Continued)

9. Evaluation studies using real world observation produce outcomes that are significantly less favourable to pharmaceutical products such as NRT than randomized trials.
10. A psychosocial model focuses on the experience of smoking, its motivation, and its emotional and social associations.
11. Brief psychological therapies for smoking cessation based on cognitive behavioural therapy are showing considerable promise.
12. The most effective strategy for smoking cessation to date uses elements from each of the biological, psychological and social approaches, a combination of medication, cognitive behavioural therapy and social support.

10

Physical Activity and Exercise

By equating certain types of behaviour with virtue and others with vice, the secular moralists … threaten to undermine the critical task of educating the public in general … to the very real dangers lurking behind everyday behavioural choices.

Leichter, 1997: 360–1

Outline

Recent years have seen an increased official concern at the apparent widespread decline in the participation of people in all types of physical activity. This chapter reviews the evidence for this and for its potential impact on health. It also considers the social and psychological factors associated with participation. It then considers the varying meanings of different forms of physical activity and the strategies that have been used to promote greater participation.

EXTENT OF PHYSICAL ACTIVITY

Physical Activity Definitions

The term '**physical activity**' is used to describe a wide range of activities that involve energy expenditure by the human body. It has been defined as 'any force exerted by skeletal muscles that result in energy expenditure above resting level' (Caspersen, Powell & Christenson, 1985: 126). This definition moves beyond the popular concern with sports and exercise to be more inclusive of a wide range of activities including walking, dancing, DIY, gardening and housework. With such an inclusive definition it is difficult to measure and 'difficult to understand, because it changes from day to day, hour to hour, and is influenced by both the seasons and weather' (Flannery Pearce, 2009: 879). Despite these challenges a wide range of governmental reports have drawn attention to the supposed decline of participation in physical activity and the consequences for public health. A range of public campaigns designed to promote greater participation in physical activity has followed this. The evidence from this wide range of research is considered in this chapter.

Modern Lifestyle

We discussed in Chapter 7 the evidence that human beings traditionally required considerable energy expenditure for survive. In ancient times the hunter–gatherer needed to expend substantial energy on a regular basis so as to ensure access to food and shelter. This need to expend substantial energy remained well into this century and continues in much of the developing world. However, the rapid increase in technology in industrialized societies over the past generation has led to a much more sedentary lifestyle. This decline in physical activity is a consequence of the reduced need for energy expenditure in all spheres of human life, including work, transportation and home maintenance. Technological developments in entertainment have reduced the role of physical activity in leisure time (King, 1994).

Evidence from a variety of social surveys has confirmed the more **sedentary** lifestyle of modern society. A recent UK survey indicated that 60 per cent of men and 72 per cent of women do not exercise to recommended levels (Information Centre for Health and Social Care, 2009; see Figure 10.1). A similar scenario exists in Australia where 70 per cent of individuals who are 15 years or over are classified as sedentary or having low exercise levels (Australian Bureau of Statistics, 2006).

According to the UK Time Use Survey 2000 among those who are most active the most common activities are walking, gardening, DIY and 'ball games'. However, there is evidence that even walking is becoming less common. For example, according to the National Travel Survey the total miles walked per annum fell by 26 per cent between 1975 and 2001 and the amount travelled by bicycle fell by 26 per cent during the same period. It was estimated that this meant approximately 66 fewer miles walked per annum per person in that

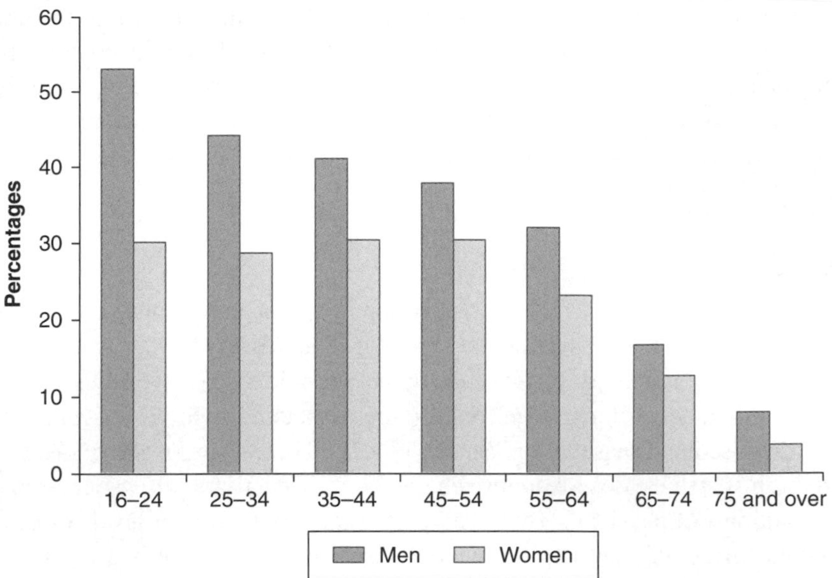

Figure 10.1 Percentage of adults who meet the physical activity recommendations: by sex and age, 2003, England

Source: Office for National Statistics, 2010

period. Fortunately, there is some lesser evidence that people are taking up more leisure-time physical activity such as walks over two miles, swimming, keep fit and yoga.

Variation in Participation

Most studies confirm that the extent of participation in physical activity is linked not only to age and sex but also to socio-economic and education background. The Health Survey for England (Prescott-Clarke and Primatesta, 1998) found that men from manual social classes are more active but this was due to greater occupational activity. In general, adults from manual social classes participated less in sporting and leisure-related exercise activities.

One problem with many of the estimates of participation of physical activity is that they often focus on leisure time activity, especially organized sports. Attempts to measure the extent of physical activity in work and at home are more limited. The study by Cochrane et al. (2009) used the *International Physical Ability Questionnaire* (http://www.ipaq.ki.se/downloads.htm) which requires participants to complete a daily record for seven days activity in four domains: work related, active transport, gardening and domestic, and leisure. It is then possible to obtain a measure of energy in each of these domains. In the survey of a sample of residents of an English Midlands city they found that work accounted for 43.9 per cent of reports of physical activity compared to 32.2 per cent for garden and domestic activity, and 12 per cent for both active transport (walking and cycling) and leisure. However, the median level of physical activity at work was zero for both men and women and also zero for leisure activity for women. This would suggest that the majority of people have very sedentary working styles and most women participate little in leisure-time physical activity.

Physical Activity and Health

The reason for governmental interest in this apparent decline in physical activity is the increasing evidence of a negative impact on health. The World Health Organization identified physical activity as a major cause of death and chronic disease worldwide. Rates of the following chronic diseases have been found to be associated with higher rates of physical activity: cardiovascular disease, colon cancer, type 2 diabetes, stroke and breast cancer. The WHO also highlighted the dose-response character of this activity–disease relationship with the greater amounts of physical activity being associated with greater levels of health.

A particular impact of inactivity has been the increase in levels of obesity in the population. Since increased levels of obesity is due to an imbalance between energy intake and energy expenditure it is not surprising that evidence of a decrease in physical activity has been followed by evidence of an increase in rates of obesity. Between 1980 and 2002 the rates of obesity in England increased threefold.

In England it has been estimated that approximately one quarter of the adult population can now be classed as clinically obese. Again this is associated with age and social class. About two thirds of women and three quarters of men aged 55–74 years are classed as overweight or obese. Rates of obesity are higher among those from manual social classes. It was estimated that 23 per cent of men and 29 per cent of women from unskilled manual social classes were classed as obese compared with 16 per cent of men and women from professional social classes.

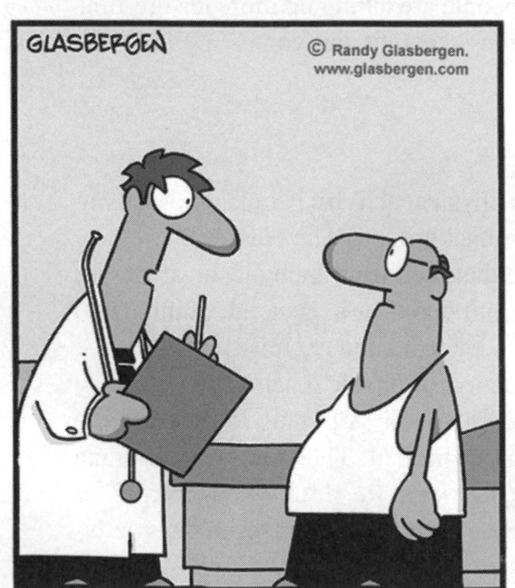

"What fits your busy schedule better, exercising one hour a day or being dead 24 hours a day?"

This has led to a series of governmental reports recommending increased participation in physical activity. In England the Department of Health (2004) issued a report highlighting the preventive benefits of physical activity but also the therapeutic benefits for those with particular chronic conditions such as cardiovascular disease, cancer and diabetes. Often these reports adopt a victim-blaming stance to those who participate little in physical activity and ignore the broad social context.

CONTEXT OF PHYSICAL ACTIVITY

Environmental Context

Environmental psychologists emphasize the importance of considering the 'behavioural setting' or the physical and social context within which the behaviour occurs (Stokols, 1996). This includes the **built environment**, the buildings in which we live and work, and the communities in which we reside. Modern buildings are not designed with increasing physical activity in mind. The architects have created environments which foster inactivity, and hence obesification (see Chapter 7). For example, stairways are often more difficult to access than either escalators or elevators. Communities often have poor play facilities. This is especially the case in low-income neighbourhoods. The most common means of transport is cars so that cycling and walking are discouraged or dangerous (Sallis, Bauman & Pratt,1998).

A study of participation levels among residents of an English Midlands city helped clarify the relative importance of the physical environment. Cochrane et al. (2009) obtained environmental data from various official sources including data on access to shops, traffic density, crime statistics, etc. and combined this data with information from a community survey of participation in physical activity and attitudes toward physical activity. Statistical analysis of this complicated dataset identified a number of environmental predictors of physical activity including ease of access to shops and to work suggesting that, the more accessible those places, the more likely people are to walk to them. Other factors of importance identified included moderate levels of road traffic and lower rates of road traffic accidents suggesting that such environments are more conducive to walking. However, although these environmental factors were important, they were of lesser importance than beliefs and intentions about participation in physical activity as measured in the community survey.

An Australian study by Salmon and Hall (2003) produced similar findings. They found that personal barriers such as lack of time, other priorities, work and family commitments predicted extent of involvement in physical activities more than environmental barriers such as weather, cost and safety. It is worth noting that these immediate personal barriers are a reflection of broader social demands. Another Australian study by Giles-Corti and Donovan (2002) also found that individual and social environmental factors were more important than physical environmental factors in predicting exercise participation. They found that the most important predictors of participation in recreational physical activity were perceived behavioural control, behavioural intention, habit and exercising peer. The most important environmental predictor was accessibility to recreational facilities.

In the United States, Wilson, Ainsworth and Bowles (2007) conducted a telephone survey of physical activity among residents of South Carolina. They found that those residents who reported that they lived in a pleasant neighbourhood, that were trusting of their neighbours and who had sidewalks in their neighbourhood were less likely to report being physically inactive. Finally, a study in Chicago found that residents of suburbs and those who had high levels of fear about their neighbourhoods were less likely to walk (Ross, 2000). While these studies demonstrate the importance of environmental factors, it is important to consider the distribution of activity-friendly neighbourhoods and the greater exposure to various environmental threats for people from working class communities.

Cultural Context

Physical activities are conducted within a wider cultural context that promotes different ideals about physicality. For example, the muscular physique is presented as the ideal male form in Western societies. As Luschen, Cockerham and Kunz (1996) noted, the emergence of bodybuilding exercises aimed at building muscular strength and fitness 'reflects a bodily culture that is in line with American values of masculine prowess' (p. 201). He continues: 'activities like American football, weightlifting, and boxing set a premium on brute physical force and place much less emphasis on endurance and relaxation' (p. 202). Ability to attain this physical shape is promised to those who participate in various fitness gyms. However, access to these somewhat elite facilities is often restricted to those with money. In addition, aggressive sporting activities are also promoted among the middle class as a training ground for developing an aggressive business attitude, not to mention the making of useful social contacts. This begins at an early age as is illustrated in studies of school sporting activities (Wright, MacDonald & Groom, 2003).

An important aspect of culture is religion. Different religions have different concepts of the body (see Chapter 4). For example, certain forms of Christianity have traditionally held a negative view of excessive concern about the body. It has been suggested that this is a reason for the poorer performance of athletes from more Catholic countries in sporting events (Curtis and White, 1992). Conversely, in more Protestant or secular societies concern with body shape and performance is promoted. Indeed, Turner (1984) has argued that contemporary concern for the body could be described as the new Protestant ethic.

An understanding of the variations in the extent of participation in physical activities requires attention to the socio-cultural context within which they have meaning and which promote or discourage involvement in such pursuits.

PSYCHOLOGICAL MODELS

Various **social cognition** models of health behaviour have been used to explain variations in the extent of participation in physical activity among adults. The three that have attracted most research interest are the Theories of Reasoned Action and Planned Behaviour, the Social Cognitive Model, and the Transtheoretical Model. We provide further details of these models in Chapter 6. In addition, recently there has been increasing interest in the role of body image in explaining exercise participation.

Theories of Reasoned Action and Planned Behaviour

The Theory of Reasoned Action (TRA) was developed by Ajzen and Fishbein (1980). This model proposes that behaviour, such as physical activity and exercise, is predicted by intention to engage in such behaviour, which in turn is predicted by the individual's attitude towards exercise and the perceived social norm. The attitudinal component is a function of the perceived consequences of participating and a personal evaluation of those consequences while the perceived norm is a function of the perceived expectations to participate and the motivation to comply with those expectations.

The Theory of Planned Behaviour (TPB) developed by Ajzen (1985) introduced *perceived behavioural control* into the basic TRA model and suggested that, besides the attitudinal and social norm components, whether someone intended to behave in a certain way depended upon the extent to which they believed they had control over a particular behaviour (see Figure 6.7).

There have been several meta-analytic studies that have used the TPB to explain involvement in physical activity. In a review of more than 30 studies Hausenblas, Carron and Mack (1997) found that there were significant mean correlations between exercise intention and attitude (0.52), subjective norm (0.27) and perceived behavioural control (0.43). A subsequent review by Hagger, Chatzisarantis and Biddle (2002) also found significant but lower correlations. However, a large proportion of the variance in studies of physical activity remains unexplained.

Hamilton and White (2010) explored salient behavioural, normative, and control beliefs among mothers and fathers of young children drawing on the TPB belief framework. Interview data were analysed using thematic content analysis. Hamilton and White identified a range of advantages (e.g., improves parenting practices), disadvantages (e.g., interferes with commitments), barriers (e.g., time), and facilitators (e.g., social support) to performing physical activity and also normative pressures.

Extensions of the TPB have investigated the role of a range of other psychological factors such as moral norms, affect, self-efficacy and past behaviour (Conner & Armitage, 1998). An example of the use of an extended TPB model is the study by Abraham and Sheeran (2004). This found that **anticipated regret** explained an additional proportion of the variance besides the core TPB variables in explaining exercise intentions.

Social Cognitive Theory

Bandura's (1986, 2001) social cognitive theory has been used extensively to explain participation in physical activity. In particular, Bandura's argument that **self-efficacy** is the common cognitive mechanism that mediates behavioural responses has been applied. It is argued that whether a person persists in a particular behaviour in different circumstances depends upon his/her perception of individual mastery over the behaviour. This sense of self-efficacy develops through personal experiences of success, but also from verbal support from others and the perceived level of physiological arousal. This theory is bidirectional such that not only can self-efficacy contribute to increased behavioural effort, but also success in the behaviour can contribute to increased self-efficacy.

In physical activity and exercise research it has been found that self-efficacy predicts greater involvement (e.g. McAuley & Jacobson, 1991). A number of variants of self-efficacy have been found to predict involvement. These include *barrier self-efficacy* or the confidence in ones' ability to overcome barriers to regular exercise attendance (Brawley, Martin & Gyurcsik, 1998), *scheduling self-efficacy* (DuCharme & Brawley, 1995) and *exercise self-efficacy* (Poag-DuCharme & Brawley, 1993). Some studies have found a negative relationship such that lower levels of self-efficacy statistically predicted more physical activity. Rimal (2001) in a longitudinal study found evidence of this and suggested that those with lower self-efficacy improved their self-efficacy over time which in turn led to greater exercise behaviour. Together these findings would confirm the interactive nature of self-efficacy beliefs and physical activity.

A related factor to self-efficacy is **self-determination**. According to Deci and Ryan's (1985) self-determination theory people will engage in many activities simply because of pure enjoyment or *intrinsic motivation*. A study in Wales (Ingledew, Markland & Medley, 1998) found that participants in the early stages of exercising attributed participation more to extrinsic motives (e.g. appearance/weight management) whereas in the later stages they referred to intrinsic motives such as enjoyment. It was concluded that intrinsic motives are important for progression to and maintenance of the exercise.

Bandura distinguishes between three forms of agency or efficacy: personal, collective and proxy. *Proxy efficacy* is the belief in the role of others in aiding achievement of desired outcomes. Although at first this might seem to be the converse of self-efficacy, evidence suggests that it can be an important compliment. The proxy is seen by the others as someone who will provide assistance and help them achieve their goals. A study of participants in a fitness class found that fitness instructor efficacy as well as self-efficacy beliefs were predictive of class attendance for class initiates (Bray, Gyurcsik, Culos-Reed, Dawson & Martin, 2001). However, Bandura (1997) does caution that an over-reliance on the proxy may reduce the cultivation of personal competencies. In a study to test this possible negative effect Shields and Brawley (2007) conducted a questionnaire study of participants in an exercise class. They found an interactive effect such that those participants who preferred proxy assistance expressed lower self-regulatory and task self-efficacy when faced with a class without a proxy. They conclude that to promote sustainability of exercise behaviour change proxy-agents (exercise instructors) should balance between providing assistance to participants and encouraging greater self-regulation by them.

Transtheoretical Model

The Transtheoretical Model (TTM) was originally developed by Prochaska and DiClemente (1983) to explain why anti-smoking messages were more successful for some people than for others. According to the TTM, people adopting a new behaviour move through a series of stages of change within which they utilize different processes to support the changes. These stages are described in Chapter 6. Movement across the stages is dependent on *decisional balance* and *perceived self-efficacy*. *Decisional balance* is a cognitive assessment of the relative merits of the pros and cons of the exercise behaviour while *self-efficacy* is the belief in one's ability to perform the exercise.

This model has been applied to physical activity by many researchers to describe the so-called five stages of exercise behaviour change (Marcus, Banspach, Lefebvre, Rossi, Carleton & Abrams, 1992). These stages are:

1 *Precontemplation:* Sedentary, no intention of becoming active within six months
2 *Contemplation:* Still sedentary but accepts the value of the need for physical activity
3 *Preparation:* Person is intending to become more active in the very near future
4 *Action:* Person is physically active but only in the last six months
5 *Maintenance*: Person has been active for more than six months

In addition to these five stages an integral part of the TTM are the processes of change which explain movement from one stage to the next. Marcus et al. (1992) found that the five experiential change processes were more important in predicting progress in the early stages of exercise behaviour change while the five behavioural processes were more important in the later stages (see Box 10.1).

Box 10.1

Five experiential exercise change processes

Cognitive	
Consciousness raising	Gathering information about benefits of exercise
Dramatic relief	Feelings about inactivity and its consequences
Environmental re-evaluation	Consideration of consequences of inactivity on others
Self re-evaluation	Reconsidering consequences of physical activity for self
Social liberation	Awareness of social norms
Behavioural	
Counter conditioning	Substituting alternatives to sedentary behaviours
Helping relationships	Support of others while becoming physically active
Reinforcement management	Rewards for physical activity
Self-liberation	Commitment to physical activity
Stimulus control	Avoiding environmental stimuli associated with physical inactivity

Source: Marcus et al., 1992

A Scottish study also found support for the role of these processes in explaining exercise behaviour change (Lowther, Mutrie & Scott, 2007). Over 300 urban residents who had volunteered to participate in an exercise programme were assessed by questionnaire prior to the programme and at various intervals after the programme. They found that self-liberation was the most important change process at every stage movement but other processes were more important at particular stage movements. Stimulus control was more important when progressing from contemplation to preparation while social liberation and helping relationships were more important progressing from action to maintenance. The authors recommended that future exercise interventions should be matched to the particular stage of change of the participants and should target the specific influential change processes.

Moving across the stages is dependent upon **decisional balance**. In a study that compared the reasons for and against participation in exercise given by a group of non-exercisers and regular exercisers Cropley, Ayers and Nokes (2003) found that the pre-contemplators provided relatively more *con* reasons while the maintainers provided relatively more *pro* reasons. It was concluded that one reason why people do not exercise is that they cannot think of reasons to do so.

Evidence of the importance of self-efficacy was provided by Marcus et al. (1992) who found that those who were regularly participating in physical activity (action or maintenance stages) scored higher on this measure. They concluded that this suggests that those who are at the early stages (pre-contemplation and contemplation) have little confidence in their ability to exercise.

Although the TTM continues to attract research interest it has also attracted ongoing criticism. Sutton (2000) argues that the TTM is not really a theoretical model at all but merely a description of 'pseudo stages' which are really arbitrary steps on a continuum of motivation. Armitage (2009) is sympathetic to this critique and suggests an alternative two stage motivational-volitional model. However, he also argues that the focus of the critique on the stages of change has diverted attention away from the more interesting processes of change.

Self-Concept or Body Image

Recent versions of the social cognition models have suggested introducing a variety of additional psychological variables. Hagger, Chatzisarantis, Culverhouse and Biddle (2003) suggested introducing *perceived competence* (similar to self-efficacy) and **self-concept**. There is evidence that there is a positive relationship between physical self-concept and participation in physical activity. It is supposed that a person who feels positively about himself or herself in one domain (physical) is more likely to perform well in that domain. Marsh (1990) has argued that this relationship is reciprocal such that prior self-concept affects subsequent physical activity and vice versa. Marsh, Papaioannou and Theodorakis (2006) confirmed this reciprocal relationship and found that physical self-concept had an independent effect in prediction of exercise intention beyond perceived control.

Another term for physical self-concept is **body image**, which has been defined by Grogan (2006) as 'a person's perceptions, feelings and thoughts about his or her body'. There has been extensive research exploring the relationship between exercise participation and body image. In an extensive review of over 100 studies, Hausenblas and Fallon (2006) concluded that exercise participation was associated with a more positively perceived body image. In addition, this relationship was apparent not only in correlational studies but also in intervention studies such that those who participated in physical exercise programmes reported an enhanced body image following the programme. This led Hausenblas and Fallon (2006) to conclude that exercise programmes may be an effective intervention for people with poor body image. However, they also caution that there may be a negative effect with some sub-groups. For example, Slater and Tiggemann (2006) found that women who exercise a lot have higher levels of body dissatisfaction and a great drive for thinness. This follows the general critique of modern representations of women equating beauty with slimness. Not surprisingly, it has been found that women and girls who weigh more are more dissatisfied with their body (Healey, 2006) although this relationship depends upon various social and cultural factors.

There is less research on male body image. Most studies have investigated the dimensions of adiposity and muscularity. As expected, males have reported a greater desire than females to become more muscular (Grogan & Richards, 2002). Adolescents who engage in sporting activities have reported a more positive body image (Ferron, Narring, Cauderay & Michaud, 1999). However, it would seem that there is less investment in body image for males (Hargreaves & Tiggemann, 2006) than for females although this would be influenced by various social and cultural factors. Tiggemann, Martins and Churchett (2008) investigated aspects of men's body images beyond simply adiposity and muscularity: head hair, body hair, height and penis size, in addition to body weight and muscularity. Online questionnaires were completed by 200 heterosexual men. Men were dissatisfied with all six aspects of their bodies, but particularly concerned about their body weight, penis size and height. Men's weight, muscularity, height and penis size, but not head or body hair, were related to overall self-esteem about appearance. This study suggests that men's body image is less unidimensional than is often assumed.

Campbell and Hausenblas (2009) conducted a meta-analysis of the effects of exercise interventions on body image and also participant, intervention and design features associated with larger effects. They identified 57 interventions with pre- and post-data for the exercise and control groups and found a small random effect indicating that exercise interventions had improved body image compared to control conditions.

Although there is increasing research on the role of body image in explaining extent of physical activity there is a need to be aware that body image is not simply an intrapsychic phenomenon. Rather it is one that develops in interaction with others and within a specific socio-cultural context. As Gleeson and Frith (2006) emphasize 'it is more useful to consider *body imaging* as a process, an activity, rather than a product' (p. 88). This re-orientation away from a static definition of body image emphasizes the need for more sophisticated qualitative work to explore the connection between body imaging and physical activity.

Comments

Social cognition models (SCMs), such as those described above, have focused on identifying the psychological determinants of physical activity. These models continue to attract substantial research interest. As we saw in Chapter 6, they have also attracted criticism for their methodological and theoretical shortcomings. There remain fundamental concerns that the models are too mechanistic in conceptualization. Stainton-Rogers (1991) provided a coherent critique of these models describing them as portraying: 'thinking as a passive, mindless activity rather than an active striving after meaning, and portray people as thinking-machines rather than as aware and insightful, open to being beguiled by convincing tales and rhetoric, and inventive story-tellers' (p. 55).

More than this they locate the thinking in the head of the individual rather than as something that unfolds in interaction with others leading to an individualistic focus in health promotion. A social interactionist views the individual as part of a group and of a society. His or her behaviour, thoughts and beliefs can be considered as unfolding in interaction with the groups and society as a means of adapting to changing circumstances. Their decision to become involved in physical activity is the result of an ongoing engagement with their immediate social world. Further criticisms of SCMs can be found in Chapter 6. There is a need for more qualitative research work to grasp the various meanings of physical activity.

MEANINGS OF PHYSICAL ACTIVITY AMONG ADULTS

An understanding of the extent of participation in physical activity requires an understanding of the different meanings of physical activity. This depends upon the character of everyday social experience.

Social Class

People from diverse social background perceive physical activity differently. Calnan and Williams (1991) conducted detailed interviews with a sample of middle-aged men and women from the southeast of England. The participants were from different social backgrounds. They found clear social class differences in perceptions of exercise. Those from working-class backgrounds perceived exercise in relation to everyday tasks, activities and duties at home and at work. They adopted a functional definition of health and fitness. For them their ability to 'exercise' their everyday tasks both confirmed and reaffirmed their health. For example, one farm-worker said: 'I get enough exercise when I am working on the farm shoveling corn all day, you get enough exercise. In the garden out there, I take the dog for a walk, yet I get enough exercise' (p. 518). They tended to be satisfied with their physical health that they could enhance during their everyday activities.

Middle-class people tended to perceive exercise as not being part of their everyday activities. They preferred to define it with reference to recreational or leisure activities that they sometimes felt they could not engage in because of lack of time. Fitness for these individuals was defined in terms of athleticism not in ability to perform everyday tasks. This group also made more reference to the health-promoting effects of exercise in terms of 'well-being' and relief from routine daily obligations. In discussing these class differences in perceptions of exercise Calnan and Williams (1991) referred to the work of Bourdieu (1984) who suggested that whereas working-class people express an instrumental relation to their bodily practices, middle-class people engage in health practices which are 'entirely opposed to (such) total, practically oriented movements' (p. 214).

In a large-scale survey of young people's physical activity in Norway, Oygard and Anderssen (1998) also considered the importance of the meaning of exercise and the physical body. In discussing the relationship between social class and exercise they also refer to the work of Bourdieu (1984) who suggested that this relationship derives from social class differences in attitude toward the body. In Western society the legitimized body emphasizes both inner and outer characteristics. While the former is concerned with the healthy body, the latter refers to the fit and slim body. The middle and upper classes are more able to produce this legitimized body since it requires investment in time and money. Working-class people with less time free from necessity have a more instrumental view of their body and view concern with exercise and fitness as pretentious. Conversely, middle-class people with more leisure time and resources to expend promote a cult of health and a concern with physical appearance.

Gender

Men and women perceive physical activity differently dependent upon their social and cultural background. In their survey Oygard and Anderssen found that level of education was positively associated with extent of participation in physical activity among females but not among males. In reviewing this finding, they refer to the suggestion that concern with the body is more common among those belonging to the cultural elite who are more anxious about their appearance and their 'body for others' (Bourdieu, 1984: 213). Oygard and Anderssen concluded: 'For females in higher social positions, it may be of importance to show others who they are by developing healthy and "delicate" bodies, i.e. they are more concerned with the inner and outer body than females in lower social positions' (1998: 65). However, they also added more prosaically that the lesser involvement of less educated females in physical activity may be due to them having limited access to leisure facilities. They found little relationship between education and physical activity among males and suggest that this may reflect the greater promotion of male sporting activities and the greater integration of physical activity into male culture.

Age

It is well established that participation in physical activity declines steadily with age. This may reflect a variety of factors including limited socialization into physical activity among that generation to perceived social exclusion. A study in New Zealand found that older people who participated in sporting activities reported that they were often confronted by a discouraging stance from younger people (Markula, Grant & Denison, 2001). This negative social value regarding seniors and sports would seem to be internalized such that many elderly people report limited participation for fear that they might incur an injury (O'Brien Cousins, 2000).

Hardy and Grogan (2009) investigated older adults' influences and motivations to engage in physical activity in 48 52–87-year-old participants. Preventing disability through exercise was a key factor in determining physical activity participation. Other influences included enjoyment of exercise, having support from others as motivators to exercise and a perception of limited appreciation for older people's needs.

Ethnicity

People from ethnic minorities participate less in various physical activities. This is due both to the social and environmental constraints and differences in the perceived nature of physical activity. Henderson and Ainsworth (2003) conducted interviews with African–American and African–Indian women about their perception of physical activity. These women emphasized not only the physiological but also the spiritual benefits of physical activity. As one woman said: 'I love being outside. Mostly I love taking walks. I love the quietness with that' (p. 319). Despite this positive view of physical activity these women identified various obstacles to participation. This included perceived lack of time, although they also wondered about the legitimacy of this perceived obstacle. As one woman said: 'I talk about lack of time, et cetera, but you know, time is the sort of thing you can make available when you want' (p. 315). Other perceived constraints included job demands, tiredness, illness, family needs and safety issues. These constraints are not peculiar to women from ethnic minorities. Other studies (e.g. Verhoef, Love & Rose, 2003) have identified similar constraints as being common among other groups of women.

EXERCISE AMONG CHILDREN

In the UK it has been estimated that among 2–15 year olds, four out of 10 boys and six out of 10 girls are not participating sufficiently in physical activity (Prescott-Clarke & Primatesta, 1999). As with adults the extent of participation varies substantially. In a study in Norway, Oygard and Anderssen (1998) found that teenage girls with higher levels of education were more physically active whereas among boys there was less evidence of a relationship with level of education. This is discussed further in the section below on school physical education.

It would seem that physical activity levels established in childhood are maintained across the lifespan. Friedman et al. (2008) extracted data from the American Terman life-cycle study that began in 1922 and collected data on participants at regular intervals in subsequent decades. Statistical analysis of this longitudinal dataset found that children who were physically active were also likely to report greater participation in physical activity in adulthood and in later life. This was especially the case for males although it was suggested that this might have been due to the 'restrictions on the physical activity of females during the 20th century' (p. 1100). This longitudinal linkage of physical activity levels has added to government concern at the evidence of a decline in involvement of children in physical activity and exercise.

Meaning of Physical Activity For Young People

An increasing number of qualitative studies have begun to clarify the changing experiences of physical activity among young people. Kunesh, Hasbrook and Lewthwaite (1992) conducted a detailed investigation of the school play activities of a sample of 11- to 12-year-old girls in central USA. In interviews the girls reported that they found physically active games at home and at school enjoyable. However, in the school playground the girls preferred to stand in a group and talk while the boys participated in various games. When the girls did participate in games they were often criticized by the boys for their supposed inferior skill performance. To avoid this negative treatment the girls excluded themselves. The girls reported that when playing at school they felt nervous and embarrassed. These findings would suggest that while at an early age boys and girls both enjoy physical activities by the time they reach puberty the girls feel that they are being excluded.

As they enter adolescence the gender difference in participation in physical activities becomes more pronounced. From a series of interviews with young people from southeast London, Coakley and White (1992) identified five factors that help explain young people's decisions about participation in sporting activities. These are detailed in Box 10.2.

Box 10.2

Young people's decisions about sport participation

- Consideration of the future, especially the transition to adulthood
- Desire to display and extend personal competence and autonomy
- Constraints related to money, parents and opposite-sex friends
- Support and encouragement from parents, relatives, and/or peers
- Past experiences in school sports and physical education

Source: Coakley & White, 1992; Reproduced with permission

This study emphasized that perceived identity was a central concern in the extent and character of sports preferred. Young people actively sought out or rejected involvement in certain physical activities dependent upon a variety of factors including previous experiences and ongoing changing circumstances. As Coakley and White (1992) state: 'young people become involved in sport through a series of shifting, back-and-forth decisions made within the structural, ideological, and cultural context of their social worlds' (p. 21).

Qualitative studies have investigated gender and social class factors that encourage different forms of participation of children in various forms of physical activity. In a study of the images in teenage girls' magazines Cockburn (2001) found two polarized female images: one actively involved in romantic activities; the aberrant female involved in physical activity. Teenage girls who she interviewed resented these stereotypical images and felt that it did not accord with the everyday conflicts they experienced. However, they also voiced concern at the increasing social restraints on their involvement in sporting activities. For example, one girl said: '… when I was at primary school I just used to go out there and I'd do anything … I wouldn't care what other people thought, I'd just go out and enjoy it … now it's more, 'Oh my god can I do this?' And you know, like everybody's looking at you … I hate it …'

Together, these studies confirm the importance of the various meanings associated with physical activity among children and young people.

PROMOTING PHYSICAL ACTIVITY

With the growing evidence on the health benefits of physical activity and exercise, governments and health authorities have become keen to promote greater participation. For example, in Britain, the Department of Health requires all health authorities to contribute to local programmes designed to promote greater physical activity (Department of Health, 2001). These have included population, community, school and clinic based interventions.

Population-Based Strategies

Population-based strategies are designed to promote more widespread participation in physical activity in society. The strategies range from ones with an environmental focus, such as the introduction of cycle lanes in cities and reducing traffic speed, to mass media campaigns. A number of studies have illustrated the variable impact of these interventions. An evaluation of an intervention designed to promote physical activity (Sallis, King, Sirard & Albright, 2007) found that it had a greater impact among women in the area that reported no unattended dogs and low crime in their neighbourhood and among men who reported often seeing people being active in their neighbourhood.

However, these environmental supports for physical activity are not equally distributed in society. In a review of the literature Taylor, Carlos Poston, Jones and Kraft (2006) identified the strong inverse relationship between what they termed physical-activity friendly environments and low-income and ethnic minority groups. To promote an activity friendly environment requires an 'environmental justice' approach which aims to redress these social inequalities in exposure to environmental hazards.

In public buildings a number of physical strategies have been employed to promote greater physical activity. It has been found that simply displaying posters near stairwells promotes greater usage (e.g. Andersen, Franckowiak, Snyder, Bartlett & Fontaine, 1998). A variant of this is the positioning of health promotion messages on the actual stair rises. A study of a shopping centre in England found that such an initiative more than doubled stair usage (Kerr, Eves & Carroll, 2001). While these measures are important they cannot ignore the many other occupational hazards in the workplace that are again unfairly distributed. An example of a participatory approach to challenging occupational and environmental hazards is given below.

Case Study

INTERNATIONAL CASE STUDY Promoting environmental justice through 'Theatre of the Oppressed'

Environmental justice is concerned with challenging the environmental hazards in any communities which act to increase exposure to noxious pollutants and reduce opportunities for healthy activities. An example of an environmental justice campaign is that developed by John Sullivan and his colleagues in various low income communities in Texas. The campaigns were participatory and informed by Augusto Boal's Theatre of the Oppressed.

This approach uses drama as a means of expressing the community's dissatisfaction with current environmental arrangements and demanding improved living and working conditions. During the drama, or Forum, the participants are encouraged to reflect upon the current arrangements and to identify strategies for change.

The Forum is not expected to be a passive affair but rather the spectator is transformed into a 'spect–actor'. 'There is no place for passivity at a Forum; Theatre of the Oppressed primes spectators to apply their powers to deconstruct what they see and "prepare for action"' (Sullivan et al.: 171).

Source: Sullivan, Petronella, Brooks, Murillo, Primeau & Ward, 2008

The third population-based strategy places an emphasis on mass media campaigns. A survey of European countries found that residents of those countries who perceived that public policy was promoting physical activity were more likely to report participating in such activity (Von Lengerke et al., 2004). However, these moves to promote exercise through healthy public policy must be distinguished from the further promotion of the ideology of individualistic self-control (Murray et al., 2003). While middle class adults may be attracted to this message, many people from working class and more deprived background may treat it with deserved cynicism (Crossley, 2003). Healthy public policy needs to connect with the material circumstances of people's everyday lives if it is to achieve an echo (Murray and Campbell, 2003). Otherwise, it invites the same 'victim-blaming' (Crawford, 1980) criticism as traditional health education.

Community-Based Strategies

Interventions that have attempted to increase participation in communities have often been based upon various social cognition models, especially the TTM. Marcus et al. (1992) designed an exercise intervention for volunteers recruited from a community. The character of the intervention was matched to the initial stage of change of the volunteers. On follow-up there was evidence of a significant increase in involvement in exercise commensurate with the initial stage. In a subsequent randomized controlled trial, Marcus, Eaton, Rossi and Harlow (1994) found further supportive evidence. At three months follow-up the subjects in the stage-matched group showed stage progression (i.e. greater interest or involvement in exercise) while those in the standard group showed stage stability or regression.

Clarke and Eves (1997) found partial support for the value of the TTM to explain the willingness of a sample of sedentary adults to participate in an exercise programme prescribed by their family doctor. They classified the participants into the pre-contemplation, contemplation and preparation stages reflecting the fact that at this stage they had not begun the programme. The cons of participation in the exercise programme decreased across the stages as predicted although there was little change in the pros. The barriers to participation identified were lack of support, lack of facilities, dislike of exercise and lack of time. The importance of dislike of exercise declined across the stages while the importance of lack of facilities increased. The finding that lack of time was used as frequently by those in the pre-contemplation as those in the preparation stage was interpreted as evidence that it is more a justification for lack of participation rather than a convincing reason.

Other studies have expanded the basic TTM to consider the importance of *outcome expectancies* (Williams, Anderson & Winett, 2005). For example, Dunton and Vaughan (2008) investigated the role of anticipated positive and negative emotions. This study was a three-month follow-up of a sample of healthy, community dwelling adults who agreed to participate in an exercise programme. It found that anticipated emotions interacted with stage of behaviour change in predicting activity adoption and maintenance. At baseline, they found that anticipated positive emotions of success were lowest in those classed in the precontemplation stage while anticipated negative emotions of failure were highest in those classed in the maintenance stage. Further, anticipated positive emotions of success predicted physical activity adoption and maintenance.

Finally, a large number of studies have considered the role of body image in evaluating the impact of exercise interventions. A review of 41 such studies by Hausenblas and Fallon (2006) concluded that exercisers had a more positive body image and that participants had a more positive body image post intervention.

School Physical Education

There is a long history of physical education (PE) in schools. This tradition, especially in British schools, has been based upon a nineteenth century model of teaching children to perform a range of very masculinistic and militaristic physical exercises (Paechter, 2003). Not surprisingly, girls are rather reluctant to participate actively in many of these exercises. In their study of teenage girls Cockburn and Clarke (2002) noted that 'Many of these traditional and stereotypical rituals in PE contradict the notion of acceptable/desirable "appearance" within the teenage feminine culture and cause conflict for girls' (p. 654). Indeed, this conflict with the dominant image of femininity can lead to a clash between what Cockburn and Clarke describe as two polarized identities. 'A girl can identify herself as a masculinized "doer" of PE (a "tomboy"), or a feminized ("girlie") "non-doer" of sport and physical activity. It is highly unlikely that girls can achieve both physically active *and* (heterosexually) desirable, so they are obliged to choose *between* these images' (p. 661). Further, in her study Paechter (2003) found that some girls demonstrate their femininity through deliberate resistance to PE.

Boys who are poor at school sporting activities also often attract ridicule from their more athletic peers. This is especially the case in those schools that emphasize the more physical sports. These games in which the boys are expected to demonstrate their strength have many similarities with military exploits (Paechter, 2003).

In a study of PE in Australian schools Wright et al. (2003) showed how its character was clearly related to social class. Boys, especially those from affluent backgrounds, participated in organized team sports from an early age. For these boys, participation in sports was a very important part of the school ethos and identity. This led Wright et al. (2003) to describe the social practices around sport as 'powerful disciplinary technologies (Foucault, 1980) whereby particular kinds of citizens, forms of masculinity and ways of interacting with physical activity are shaped' (p. 25). In this setting the young people are being trained to strongly identify with their school team and to act in a particularly aggressive way towards others. Sport thus becomes part of the training for a form of officer class.

An alternative to this technology of disciplining young people through physical activity is one that offers emancipatory potential. This approach is one informed by Freire's pedagogy and that aims to enhance the children's experience of themselves as physical beings in the world (see Lloyd, 2008). It is an approach infused with happiness and laughter in the present as well as a questioning and curiosity about the future. This approach is designed to experiment with forms of physical activity and explore new ways through which the students can enhance their bodies.

Clinic-Based Physical Activity Programmes

Exercise interventions are often targeted at certain sub-groups of the population including people who are overweight, elderly people or those who suffer from particular health problems. The evaluations of these programmes have often been quantitative in design and have identified a limited number of social cognition variables that predict adherence to the programmes. In a review of the impact of exercise programmes for coronary heart disease Woodgate and Brawley (2008) identified the importance of personal efficacy. They distinguished between task self-efficacy and self-regulatory-efficacy.

A common problem with exercise programmes is that while many people sign up for such programmes it has been estimated that 50 per cent or more drop out after a short period of participation (Dishman, 1986). Box 10.3 provides a summary of four behavioural strategies identified by Robinson and Rogers (1994) as being associated with increased adherence. However, this is a very schematic outline and there is a need for further research into the dynamic nature of the exercise behaviour change process.

Box 10.3

Behavioural strategies to improve adherence to exercise programmes

Stimulus control: providing cues that remind people of the programme.

Consequent control: providing rewards and punishments for participation.

Cognitive behaviour modification: increasing people's belief that they have control over the design and conduct of the programme.

Behavioural treatment packages: combining behavioural and cognitive strategies.

Source: Robinson & Rogers, 1994; Reproduced with permission

Most of the interventions targeted at enhancing physical activity have used quantitative assessments. This restricts the opportunity to clarify what the participants actually feel about the various interventions. Several recent evaluations that have used qualitative methods have emphasized the importance of perceived enjoyment. A study by Daley, Copeland, Wright and Wales (2008) included a qualitative study within the larger randomized controlled trial of an exercise intervention for obese adolescents. This revealed that the participants expressed a variety of feelings including feeling more energetic and pleased about potential weight loss. The research emphasized the importance of positive feelings and enjoyment in the programme as being central to its success. The researchers concluded that 'it is unlikely that young people who are obese will commit to a regular active lifestyle unless they have opportunities to experience positive feelings from engagement' (p. 816).

Another qualitative study (Graham, Kremer & Wheeler, 2008) explored the experiences of people with chronic illness and disability who participated in a physical exercise programme. Analysis of the interviews identified three polarized themes, which are summarized in Box 10.4. In reviewing these themes it is apparent that the intervention is effective not just through improving physical ability but also on more social and psychological processes. In particular, the value of the activity intervention in enhancing mood, social connections and identity.

Box 10.4

Reactions to participating in an exercise programme for people with disability

1 ***Passive distress vs. active mood management:*** whereas disability can contribute to a passive inactive lifestyle, participation can enhance mood and reduce patterns of rumination. For example: 'My energy wasn't great. I would get into the house and just sit down and say, 'I can't be bothered'. I was doing nothing at all. I was just going home, watching TV all day. I don't do that now because I think of the exercises ... I imagine myself within the group and I do a few [exercises] at home. I'm sort of motivated now.

2 ***Identity erosion vs. identity renewal:*** whereas disability and chronic illness can lead to feelings of identity loss, participation in physical activity contributed to a new identity of physical competence. For example: 'From being an outgoing, physical sort of person you were bedridden. That was mind-blowing. Terrible. Shattered. Suddenly this residual bit of fitness I had all my life was going out the window.' The exercise programme stopped that slide into inactivity.

3 ***Detachment vs. connection:*** while disability can lead to detachment from the familiar valued aspects of everyday life such as friends and familiar bodily functioning the intervention provided new connections. For example: 'Since getting so unwell I have lost contact with a lot of people I would have met when I was out and about. Now I don't have those kinds of contacts because I'm inside most of the time. I meet people here [day centre]. It's a bit like being exiled or being cast out – you'd think I'd leprosy sometimes! *[laughs]* Maybe I'll get a bell to warn people off.'

Source: Graham et al., 2008; Reproduced with permission

Further, these strategies are largely focused at the individual level. They ignore the social context and the social meaning of exercise and physical activity. Social approaches attempt to widen the traditional individual change approach to include: 'changes in social networks and structures, organizational norms, regulatory policies, and the physical environment as a means of enhancing long-term maintenance of the target behavior' (King, 1994: 1406).

ALTERNATIVE FORMS OF PHYSICAL ACTIVITY

There is increasing challenge to the dominance of the functional approaches to promoting physical activity with its attendant emphasis on physical health. Alternative strategies consider such issues as the more social, emotional and aesthetic aspects of physical activity. Three such alternative forms are dance, walking groups and lifestyle sports.

Dance

There has been a recent growth of interest in the health benefits of dance. It is considered a very non-intrusive means of promoting participation in physical activity. However, participation in dance is more than just a means of enhancing physical health. Fensham and Gardner (2005) argue that within dance 'the body is not simply an object upon or through which discipline or utility must be imposed, but [...] through which values, meanings and pleasures are enacted and created' (p. 15). Dancing can be considered a means of developing cultural capital (Bourdieu, 1986). This form of capital allows one to withdraw from the economic necessities of life and distance oneself from 'practical urgencies'.

Dance is attractive to men and women from different social backgrounds. For example, Baker (2002) notes that especially for younger people dance is an important way of playing being sexual in which 'they try a more sexual presence on for size' (p. 18). Among older people it is a very enjoyable means of developing social interaction (Paulson, 2005). The intrinsic joy of dancing with others gives this physical activity a meaning beyond simply that of exercise for exercise sake.

Walking Groups

KEY STUDY The 'Healing Balm' effect. Using a walking group to feel better

Research suggests that the setting in which activity occurs is a major influence on the therapeutic effects of the activity on well-being and enjoyment. This study took place in a mental health day service in a rural town in the UK with 14 participant collaborators, all members of a walking group who went together to the countryside. The study combined methods from grounded theory and ethnography, exploring members' experience of a mental health day service walking group. Participant observation, interviews and a group discussion were analysed using a grounded theory approach. Priest created a model of 'the Healing Balm Effect', which brought together seven categories concerning the healing properties of the experience. The categories are: Closer to What is More Natural; Feeling Safe; Being Part; Striving; Getting Away; Being Me; and Finding Meaning. The model is illustrated below.

Source: Priest, 2007

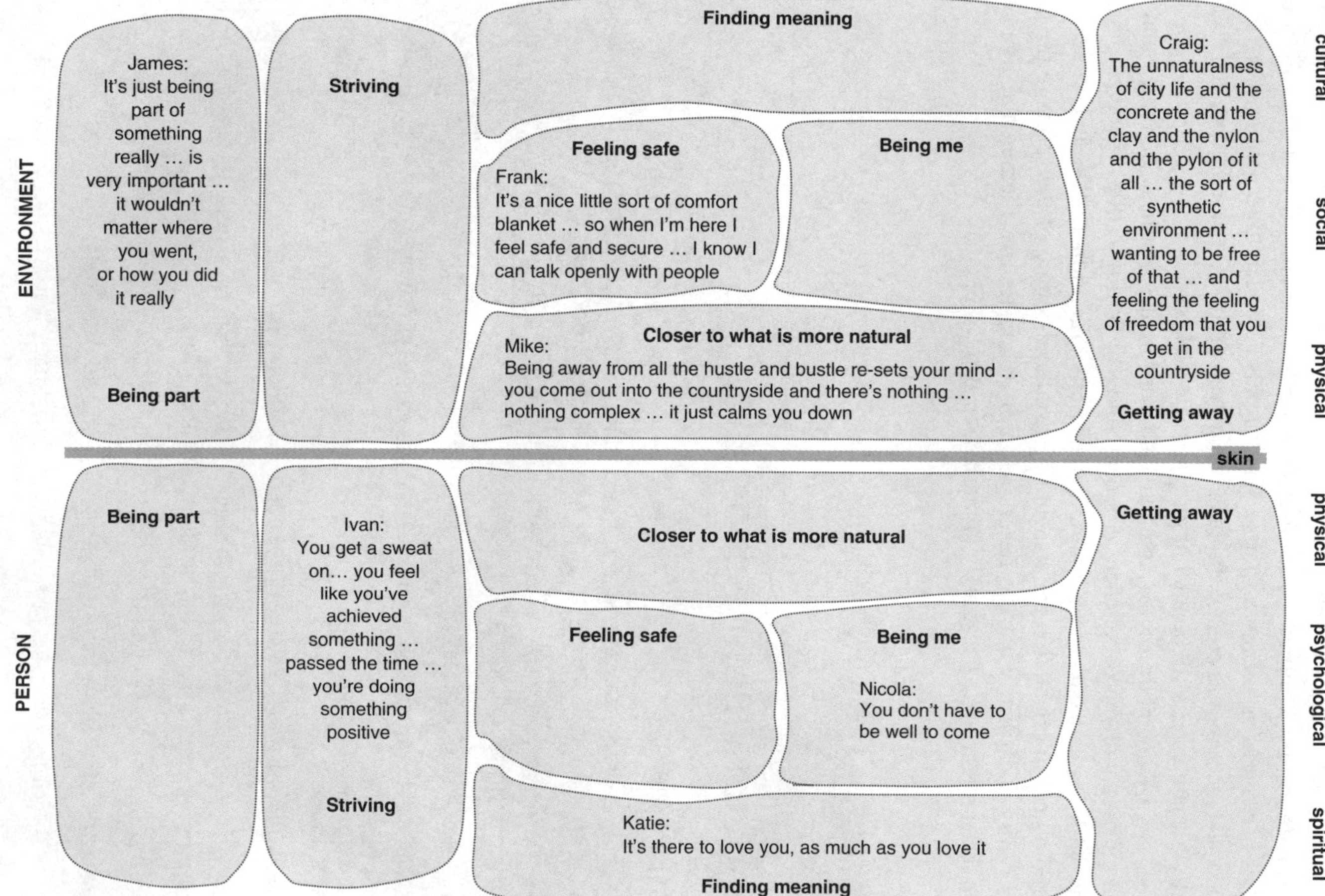

Source: Priest, 2007; Figure reproduced with permission

Lifestyle Sports

Over the past 10–20 years a counter-establishment form of sporting activity has grown in popularity. A report by Tomlinson, Ravenscroft, Wheaton and Gilchrist (2005) collectively termed these activities as 'lifestyle sports'. They are also frequently termed *extreme sports* and include such activities as bungee jumping, white water rafting, rock-climbing and surfing. These activities are especially popular among young people.

There is a growing body of research on who participates in these activities and the perceived character of the experience. A recent study by Willig (2008) involved detailed interviews with a small sample of eight extreme sports practitioners. The interviews were phenomenological in orientation and sought to grasp the meaning of the sports to the practitioners. Willig identified what she described as four constitutive themes and five other themes in these interviews. These are summarized in Box 10.5.

Box 10.5

Meanings of extreme sports

Constitutive themes

Context: the environmental or social context within which the sport has a particular enhanced meaning, e.g. solitude and the experience of mountain climbing.

Challenge: the opportunity to push oneself to the limits both physically and mentally, e.g. overcoming the fear of jumping from a great height.

Suffering: the possibility of pain, injury or death.

Other people: other people being aware that they were practising these sports; being different from others.

Additional theme

Mastery and skill: the need for specialized knowledge and skill.

Contrasts: the presence of two apparently contradictory qualities, e.g. the beauty/calmness of the landscape and the challenge of the sport.

Being in the present: the focus on the immediate to the exclusion of other thoughts.

Compulsion: the strongly felt need to engage in these activities.

Pleasure: the heightened feelings of pleasure and excitement.

Source: Willig, 2008

Unlike populist characterizations of these activities as reckless or sensation seeking it was apparent from these interviews that the participants carefully considered them. Willig suggested that participation in these activities enabled the participants to attain a particular state of being comparable to what Csikszentmihalyi (1997) has termed 'flow'. This is the experience of a sort of unity of the self, world and activity in which the more mundane, everyday worries and concerns become less important. As such, it could be argued that participation in these sports is a reaction to broader cultural demands on young people in our consumer society, which provides limited opportunity for such experiences. However, the individualistic nature of such activities can pose potential threats. For example, Willig cautions that while participation in these activities may be therapeutic they may also lead to dependency.

FUTURE RESEARCH

1 Public participation in physical activity is continuing to decline, including children and young people. There is a need to develop a more sophisticated understanding of this using a variety of methods of investigation.
2 There is still a need to explore the specific impact of exercise interventions on the health of different population groups to demonstrate that increased activity actually improves health.
3 Physical activity has different meanings for different sub-groups of the population. Research is needed to develop our understanding of these different meanings.
4 There is scope for further research on the social embeddedness of exercise.
5 Participatory action research offers an opportunity to increase our understanding of different perceptions of physical activity programmes.

Summary

1 Interest in exercise has waxed and waned over the years. The past generation has witnessed increasing interest in the health benefits of exercise.
2 Results of several comprehensive surveys indicate that moderate degrees of physical activity have both physical and psychological benefits.
3 There is some evidence to suggest that excessive exercise can have negative health effects.
4 A large proportion of the populations of western societies are sedentary.
5 The degree of participation declines during adolescence, especially among girls.
6 In adulthood, participation is lesser among females, those from poorer social positions and those from ethnic minorities.

7. Various psychological factors have been found to be associated with participation in both childhood and adulthood.
8. The meaning of exercise is linked to the varying social contexts.
9. Exercise participation programmes can be either population based or aimed at high-risk groups. The main problem with both forms of programme is the generally low adherence.
10. Alternative methods of activity such as dance, group walking and lifestyle sports are capable of evoking joy, excitement and pleasure which means that the activity is more likely to be repeated.

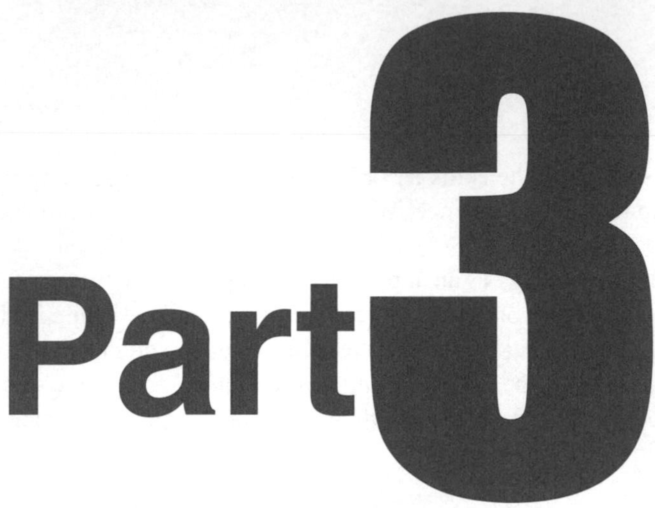

Part 3

Health Promotion and Disease Prevention

In Part 3 we review health promotion and disease prevention. In Chapter 11 we begin with an introduction to communication theory and examine some questions that need to be considered for effective communication. Emerging areas of research on health communication are then discussed. We explore the general approaches to the study of health care professional–patient communication, social marketing, message framing and e-health. We also consider the impact and limitations of information dissemination as an approach to health promotion.

Chapter 12 discusses theoretical approaches to the study of stress and coping, and research on stress as a cause of physical illness. It begins with an account of stimulus, response and interactional perspectives, and includes a critical analysis of them. Consideration is given to the effects of stress on the immune system and to ways in which people react to trauma. A discussion of methodological problems confronting research on stress and illness is followed by an examination of evidence linking stress to cardiovascular disease, cancer and infectious diseases.

Chapter 13 considers two main forms of disease prevention available within modern healthcare systems: screening and immunization. These prevention programmes are premised on the basis of controlling risk. Screening programmes are designed to identify those individuals who, because of certain personal characteristics, are considered as being at risk of developing a certain disease. Immunization programmes are designed to inoculate people who are at risk of developing a certain disease because of their exposure to environmental pathogens. Various social and psychological processes are involved in explaining these processes of risk management.

Chapter 14 provides a general discussion of health literacy and its relevance to health promotion. We begin with a discussion of why information dissemination is not enough in health promotion and where health literacy fits into the picture. We present some of its key definitions and the scales developed to measure it. We also discuss the skills associated with health literacy and its implications to health processes, outcomes and experience. We finally discuss possible ways to promote health literacy and equal access for all.

Chapter 15 reviews community health psychology as an approach based upon promoting strategies for social change at the local level that can contribute to health and well-being. While such approaches offer much potential for reducing health inequalities they can potentially distract attention from the broader structural causes of ill-health. The chapter summarizes the character of this approach and considers some examples of it applied to health inequalities, social engagament, safety and sexual health.

11 Information and Communication[1]

The problem with communication ... is the illusion that it has been accomplished.

George Bernard Shaw

Outline

In this chapter, we begin with an introduction to communication theory and examine some questions that need to be considered for effective communication. Emerging areas of research on health communication are then discussed. We explore the general approaches to the study of health care professional–patient communication, social marketing, message framing and e-health. We also consider the impact and limitations of information dissemination as an approach to health promotion.

[1]An earlier version of the section on health care professional–patient communication was prepared by Carla Willig for the first and second editions of this textbook.

WHAT IS HEALTH COMMUNICATION?

Health communication refers to all interpersonal, organizational or mass communication that concerns health. Normally, such communication is intended to improve the health status of individuals or populations. Health communication can:

- Occur in various *contexts* (e.g. health-care professional–patient relations, community-based health promotion, public health communication)
- Be applied in a variety of *settings* (e.g. clinics, schools, homes, workplaces, churches, clubs, online communities)
- Use a variety of *channels* (e.g. face-to-face communication, pamphlets, posters, television, radio, Internet)
- Deliver a variety of *messages* (e.g. healthy eating, smoking cessation, safe sex, physical activity); and
- Be used for a variety of *reasons* (e.g. risk assessment, communication of diagnosis and treatment, disease prevention, service awareness, advocacy)

Health communication is important for both providers and consumers of health information. For the providers, effective health communication is vital in ensuring that the intended message reaches and influences its target audience. For the consumers, effective health communication can enable them to access information that can help them, for example, make sense of their health condition or make them become aware of health risks and relevant health services. Communication feedbacks between providers and consumers are also useful to generate information that can be used in the design, implementation, monitoring and evaluation of health interventions.

COMMUNICATION THEORY

To understand health communication, let us first discuss what communication means. Communication is the exchange of information from one entity to another. For communication to occur, you will need a *sender*, a *receiver*, a *message* and a *medium* for transmitting the message. Writing and reading this book, for example, is a form of communication. As authors, we send a message to you, our reader, using printed text on paper as the medium for transmitting this message. To describe how messages are transmitted in the communication process, Shannon and Weaver (1949) proposed one of the best-known models of communication as illustrated in Figure 11.1 below.

As shown here, Shannon and Weaver's (1949) model of communication has five main components:

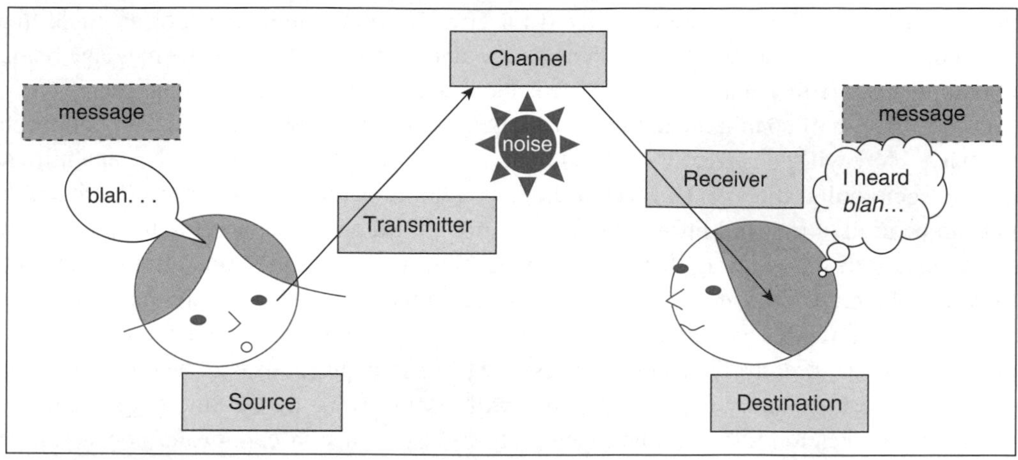

Figure 11.1 Shannon and Weaver's Model of Communication

1 Source – where the message is coming from
2 Transmitter – something that 'encodes' the message into signals
3 Channel – where encoded signals are transmitted
4 Receiver – something that 'decodes' the signal back into the message
5 Destination – where the message goes

As an example, say you have an idea that you want to communicate to a friend. In this case, you are considered the *source* of the message (i.e. your mind to be more specific). To communicate this, the message needs to be 'encoded'. You therefore use words to encode the message and then transmit it using your mouth as the *transmitter*. Your message is then converted into sound waves that travel through a *channel*, which in this case, is air. Your friend's ear then *receives* the sound waves and the brain decodes it and translates the sound waves so the message reaches its *destination* (your friend) in a recognizable format.

A sixth component in Shannon and Weaver's model is *noise*. This is any interference between the sender and the destination. In Figure 11.1, noise could be translated literally as *physical noise* (e.g. loud music in the background). However, noise can also be *cognitive* (e.g. the sender is using words that the receiver finds difficult to understand), *psychological* (e.g. the receiver hesitates to listen), or *socio-cultural* (e.g. the socio-cultural context influences the way the message is interpreted).

The simplicity of Shannon and Weaver's communication model can be considered both a strength and a weakness. Originally developed as part of a technical report for a telephone company, this model has evolved over time and is one of the most influential models of communication. In health communication, Shannon and Weaver's model provides insights into the factors that need to be considered for effective communication. For example, for recipients, it is important to consider the *message* and its *source*. What is the message being communicated? How reliable and accurate is the source? For senders, it is important to consider the *purpose* of communication and the target *destination* – who are you trying to reach and why? How will you effectively reach them considering their backgrounds, capabilities, and the socio-cultural context in which they operate? Considering the variety of *channels* that can be used to transmit information, which one would be best to achieve the purpose of communication? Considering that *noises* can interfere with message transmission, how can distortions be minimized and clarity in understanding maximized? What are the factors that compete for the recipients' attention and what strategies can be used to ensure the communication aims are effectively achieved? These are just some questions health communication research could look into. In this chapter, we will discuss some of the emerging strands of health communication research that touch on these issues: health-care professional–patient communication; social marketing; message framing; and E-health.

HEALTH-CARE PROFESSIONAL–PATIENT COMMUNICATION

Good communication between health-care professionals (HCP) and patients is essential to health promotion, disease prevention and treatment. For example, good communication can enable patients to relay information about their physical and/or mental state that can allow early identification of symptoms, diagnosis and treatment of their condition. Through good communication, HCPs and patients can discuss shared understandings of the condition and consider treatment options or adjustments in lifestyle as necessary. Good communication can also enable HCPs to provide useful health-related information to the patient to prevent disease and promote health. Thus, good communication can serve as the foundation of an effective HCP–patient partnership.

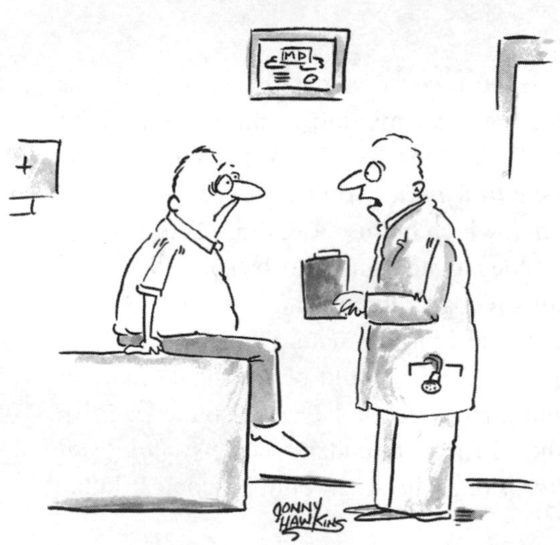

"Unfortunately, we won't know what's wrong with you untill we do an autopsy."

Reproduced with permission from www.cartoonstock.com

Despite its importance, HCP–patient communication may not always be effective. For example, there could be gaps between what the HCP conveys and what the patient understands. The HCP may provide information or treatment directives but not confirm whether these were clearly understood by the patient.

There could also be gaps between messages patients would like to express and what the practitioner receives. For example, patients might not feel comfortable expressing major worries and expectations during the consultation process. HCPs might also be unable to detect subtle non-verbal cues from the patient, or perhaps due to time constraints, it may be possible that HCPs and patients are not able to discuss personal, family or social circumstances that could be relevant to the patient's condition. There could also be inadequacies in communication concerning the diagnosis and treatment options, as well as lack of reassurance from the HCP which can increase patients' anxieties. Patient dissatisfaction, inaccurate diagnosis or understanding of the patient's condition, non-compliance or non-adherence to treatment, poor understanding and recall of information, and poor patient health outcomes are some of the dire consequences poor HCP–patient communication can bring (Ong, de Haes, Hoos & Lammes, 1995).

There are three general approaches to the study of HCP–patient communication: the 'deviant patient' perspective; the 'authoritarian doctor' perspective; and the 'interactive dyad' perspective.

The 'Deviant Patient' Perspective

Early studies focused on patient characteristics in their attempt to account for failures in doctor–patient communication. For example, Balint's (1964) psychoanalytic approach assumed that in their presentations to the doctor, patients were routinely masking the 'real' problem and that it was the doctor's task to uncover it. However, the search for patient characteristics responsible for non-adherence to treatment regimens met with little success. Instead, it was found that there was a link between **patient satisfaction** and **compliance** or **adherence** (i.e. satisfied patients were more likely to co-operate with their doctor's advice). This, together with wider social developments of the late 1960s that challenged traditional concepts of 'authority', led to a shift of focus onto the role of the doctor.

The 'Authoritarian Doctor' Perspective

In this approach researchers looked at the ways in which doctors use their authority in order to control the doctor–patient interaction. Much emphasis was placed upon the inbuilt asymmetry in the doctor–patient interaction. In a classic study, Byrne and Long (1976) identified different doctors' styles of communicating with patients. They analysed audiotape interactions from 71 GPs and approximately 2500 patients and identified four diagnostic styles and seven prescriptive styles used by the doctors. These styles constitute a continuum from 'patient-centred' to 'doctor-centred' styles. A **patient-centred style** makes use of the patient's knowledge and experience through techniques such as silence, listening and reflection, whereas a **doctor-centred style** makes use of the doctor's knowledge and skill, for example, through asking questions. Byrne and Long observed that doctors adopted a habitual style that they tended to use with most patients.

The major criticism of doctors' traditional communication style was that it was characterized by working to rigid agendas, little listening to patients' accounts and little open discussion of treatment options. A more patient-centred approach was thus called for. Table 11.1 summarizes the six interactive components of the patient-centred approach.

Table 11.1 The patient-centred approach to doctor–patient communication (Brown et al., 2003)

Component	Description
Exploring both the disease and illness experience	• Differential diagnosis (history, physical, lab) • Dimensions of illness (ideas, feelings, expectations and effects)
Understanding the whole experience	• The person (life history and personal development) • The proximal context (family, employment, social support) • The distal context (culture, community, ecosystem)
Finding common ground regarding management	• Problems and priorities • Goals of treatment and/or management • Roles of patient and doctor
Incorporating prevention and health promotion	• Health enhancement • Risk avoidance • Risk reduction • Early detection of disease • Complication reduction
Enhancing the patient–doctor relationship	• Characteristics of the therapeutic relationship (compassion) • Sharing power • Healing • Self-awareness • Transference and counter-transference
Being realistic	• Time and timing • Team building and teamwork • Wise stewardship of resources

It was suggested that patient-centred styles increase patient adherence as well as satisfaction (Brown, Stewart, Weston & Freeman, 2003). One corollary of this approach was the attempt to provide medical students with effective training in doctor–patient communication (e.g. Maguire, Fairbairn & Fletcher, 1989). However, success has been limited. Previous studies have also not found as strong and positive a relationship between patient-centredness and satisfaction (Winefield, Murrell, Clifford & Farmer, 1996). Kreps (1996) advocated a consumer orientation to health care and health promotion in order to address the imbalance of power between providers and consumers. (Kreps, 2001, provides further discussion of issues relevant to health communication – see Reading 18 in Marks, 2002a.)

The 'Interactive Dyad' Perspective

In the 1990s the focus on HCP–patient communication shifted again. Researchers began looking at the communicative event to which both doctor and patient contribute. Thus, both HCP and patient are seen to be shaping the conversation as they make use of culturally available discursive resources. Both HCP and patient use language in order to achieve interpersonal objectives, such as disclaiming or attributing responsibility for the patient's ill health or projecting a 'brave face' to avoid categorization as a hypochondriac. A focus on the communicative event as a joint achievement can shed light on the reasons for communication failure. For example, serious misunderstandings can arise when the doctor takes at face value patient statements that are in fact designed to communicate relational or self-presentational meanings, such as responding 'Fine, thank you' when being asked 'How are you?' (e.g. Coupland, Robinson & Coupland, 1994).

The importance of non-verbal communication in the form of eye contact, facial expression, gestures and other forms of communication has also been highlighted (Bensing, 1991). A focus on the *communicative event*, as opposed to the individual characteristics of HCPs and/or patients, also allows the role of culture specificity in HCP–patient interactions to be explored.

SOCIAL MARKETING

Social marketing (SM) is the application of consumer-oriented marketing techniques in the design, implementation and evaluation of programmes aimed to influence behaviour change for public benefit. Social marketing draws on concepts from *behavioural theory*, *persuasion psychology*, and *marketing science* and incorporates the 'four Ps' of marketing (i.e. Place, Price, Product and Promotion) (Evans, 2006). The key concepts to social marketing are as follows (Department of Health, 2008):

- Consumer orientation. The consumer is at the core of this approach. It uses consumer research to gain insight into their knowledge, attitudes and beliefs, and the social context in which they live and work so it can be used to inform the design and implementation of the intervention.
- Existing behaviour and behavioural goals. This approach bases its behaviour change strategies on existing behaviours and the factors that influence it. Clear behavioural goals to change existing behaviours are developed which are divided into actionable and measurable steps, which are phased over time.
- **'Intervention mix'** or 'marketing mix'. This approach uses a range of interventions or methods to achieve its goals.

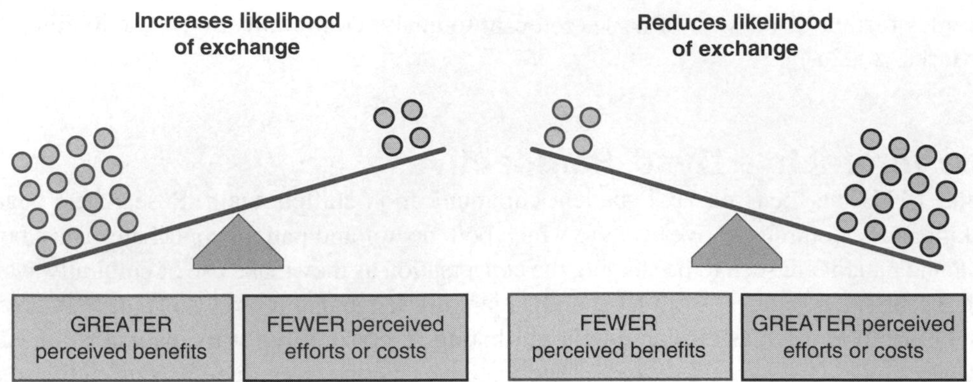

Figure 11.2 Exchange in social marketing
Source: Department of Health, 2008: 9; Reproduced with permission

- **Audience segmentation.** This approach classifies its audience into segments so that the intervention can be tailored according to the specific needs of each segment.
- **Exchange.** This approach takes into consideration what people must give up or pay to receive the benefits of behaviour change. To increase the likelihood of behaviour change, the intervention is designed in such a way that it maximizes perceived benefits while minimizing the perceived costs (see Figure 11.2).
- **Competition.** This approach takes into consideration all other factors that compete for people's attention and willingness to adopt the behaviour being promoted.

Social marketing has been widely used to inform the development, implementation and evaluation of health promotion campaigns. In a systematic review of 54 social marketing interventions, there was evidence to suggest that interventions adopting social marketing principles could be effective in improving diet, increasing exercise, and tackling the misuse of substances like alcohol, tobacco and illicit drugs. It was also suggested to be effective with a range of target groups, in different settings, and can influence policy and professional practice as well as individuals (Stead, Gordon, Angus & McDermott, 2007). For example, as part of a comprehensive programme of tobacco control and smoking cessation intervention in Nottingham, a local team of National Health Service staff developed, implemented and evaluated a social marketing campaign which aimed to reduce smoking in adults living in its most deprived areas (see De Gruchy & Coppel, 2008). Insights into the smoking behaviour of the target groups were developed through geo-demographic profiling, literature review, and qualitative research in semi-structured sessions and street interviews. A marketing agency developed the intervention mix, which included billboards, bus and tram banners, posters and beer mats. Box 11.1 provides a detailed description of this social marketing project.

Box 11.1

'Listening to Reason': A Social Marketing Stop-Smoking Campaign in Nottingham

Context: Nottingham City NHS Primary Care Trust (PCT) established a multidisciplinary team to co-ordinate a social marketing campaign to get adults to stop smoking, targeting the over-40-year-old population living in the most deprived areas of the city.

Consumer research: Information from the geo-demographic classification system (Mosaic) was supplemented with local information to profile the target group. A marketing research company was also sub-contracted to gain insight into the incentives and barriers to stopping smoking, what could be offered in exchange, and the competing personal behaviours and external factors which would limit interventions to smoking cessation. A qualitative research was also undertaken which suggested that there are three distinct groups of smokers: those who would give up now, those who would give up sometime, and those who would never give up.

Developing the campaign: Using the information from the consumer research, the team considered what the *'exchange'* would be in this context (i.e. what was the benefit of giving up smoking compared to the cost). Participants for instance, expressed having the health and energy to spend time with children and grandchildren as a benefit for quitting smoking.

"I missed seeing my kids grow up because I worked shifts. Now I have to make sure I'm fit enough to keep up with all my grandchildren." Cyril, 60, Aspley

listen to reason... stop!
for more great reasons to stop smoking call
0115 934 9526
www.listentoreason.org.uk
SMOKEFREE
ONE

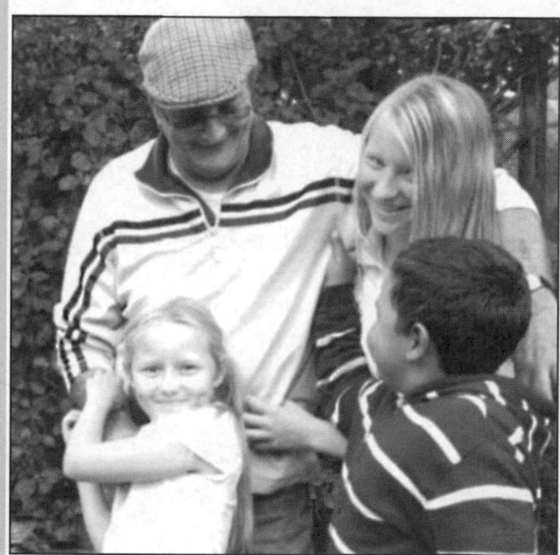

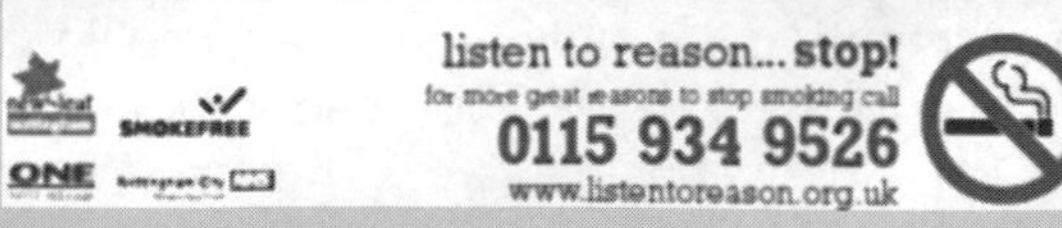

Figure 11.3 Sample poster for the 'Listen to Reason' Campaign
(Reproduced with permission)

(Continued)

(Continued)

Other benefits included financial savings and being fitter and therefore able to do more leisure activities. Both internal and external *'competition'* was also considered. Based on the Mosaic profiling information, it was found that the target groups were more likely than the general population to feel negatively about the then impending legislation on smoke-free public places. Thus the team delayed the launch of the local campaign to have some distance from the implementation of this legislation on 1 July 2007. Another issue was the use of the NHS brand (i.e. while the team was aware that the target groups tended to resist health professionals telling them to stop smoking, it was thought the NHS brand was an important way of indicating that there was free support available). The campaign was also explicitly linked to the stop-smoking service to promote the fact that support was readily available.

A *'media mix'* was developed by a marketing agency which used the by-line 'listen to reason' which revolved around the idea of knowing the arguments for stopping smoking and considering the testimony of local people about why they had given up smoking and the benefits they had experienced (i.e. 'My reason is. . .'). The strategies used considered accessibility to the target audience and cost. These included:

- *A3 posters* using the testimonies of nine local volunteers identified through the stop-smoking service
- *Banners* for trams, buses and billboards carrying the same visual images of the volunteers on the posters with shortened testimonies
- *Beer mats* for pubs in target areas
- *A campaign website* (www.listentoreason.com) to support the campaign and provide free access to campaign materials and additional information about smoking

The materials were pre-tested through a stakeholder event, which involved approximately 50 people, including local people, service users, stop-smoking advisors, PCT staff and others.

Implementing the campaign: The campaign was launched in mid-August 2007. Local people whose images appeared in the campaign were asked to participate in the launch. Good local media coverage was received. The team also undertook distribution of the posters through front-line NHS staff, to aid their engagement and improve distribution to appropriate venues. The beer mats were distributed by the marketing agency directly to 75 pubs in the target areas. The website was accessed by over 350 people during the eight weeks of the campaign.

Source: De Gruchy & Coppel, 2008

MESSAGE FRAMING

It has been suggested that the way messages are framed could influence people's motivation to undertake the health behaviour being promoted in health campaign materials (Rothman & Salovey, 1997). The idea that shifting how information is framed influences individual's behavioural decisions was influenced by Tversky and Kahneman's (1981) **prospect theory**. According to this theory, people consider their 'prospects' (i.e. potential gains and losses) when making a decision. It was suggested that people's preferences are sensitive to how information is framed and that people will act to avoid risks when considering the potential gains, but will be willing to take risks when considering the potential losses. Researchers in health **message framing** pursued this theory and investigated whether gain- or loss-framed messages can be tailored to specific target behaviour to maximize its effectiveness. **Gain-framed appeals** are information about a health behaviour that emphasizes the benefits of taking action; whereas **loss-framed appeals** are information about a health behaviour that emphasizes the costs of failing to take action. Table 11.2 lists some examples of message-framed health information used by health communication researchers.

Table 11.2 Examples of message-framed health information

Health-related behaviour	Gain-framed	Loss-framed
Breast self examination (Meyerowitz & Chaiken, 1987)	By doing BSE now, you can learn what your normal, healthy breasts feel like, so that you will be better prepared to notice any small, abnormal changes that might occur as you get older. Research shows that women who do BSE have an increased chance of finding a tumor in the early, more treatable stage of the disease. You can gain several potential health benefits by spending only 5 minutes each month doing BSE. Take advantage of this opportunity.	By not doing BSE now, you will not learn what your normal, healthy breasts feel like, so that you will be ill prepared to notice any small, abnormal changes that might occur as you get older. Research shows that women who do not do BSE have a decreased chance of finding a tumor in the early, more treatable stage of the disease. You can lose several potential health benefits by failing to spend only 5 minutes each month doing BSE. Do not fail to take advantage of this opportunity.
HIV testing (Apanovitch, McCarthy & Salovey, 2003)	There are many benefits, or good things, you may experience if you get tested for HIV. If you decide to get HIV tested, you may feel the peace of mind that comes with knowing about your health. There are many problems, or bad things,	There are many benefits, or good things, you may not experience if you do not get tested for HIV. If you decide not to get HIV tested, you will not feel the peace of mind that comes with knowing about your health. There are many problems,

(Continued)

Table 11.2 (Continued)

Health-related behaviour	Gain-framed	Loss-framed
	you may not experience if you get tested for HIV. If you decide to get HIV tested, you may feel less anxious because you would not wonder if you are ill.	or bad things, you may experience if you do not get tested for HIV. If you decide not to get HIV tested, you may feel more anxious because you may wonder if you are ill.
Dental flossing (Mann, Sherman & Updegraff, 2004)	Flossing your teeth daily removes particles of food in the mouth, avoiding bacteria, which promotes great breath.	If you do not floss your teeth daily, particles of food remain in the mouth, collecting bacteria, which causes bad breath.

Source: Rothman, Bartels, Wlachin & Salovey, 2006: S204; Reproduced with permission

Detweiler, Bedell Salovey, Pronin and Rothman (1999) compared the effectiveness of 4 differently framed messages (2 highlighting gains, 2 highlighting losses) to persuade 217 beach-goers to obtain and use sunscreen. Attitudes and intentions were measured before and immediately following the delivery of the framed information. After completing the questionnaire, participants were given a coupon redeemable for a small bottle of sunscreen later that same day. It was found that people who read either of the 2 gain-framed brochures, compared with those who read either of the 2 loss-framed brochures, were significantly more likely to: 1) request sunscreen; 2) intend to repeatedly apply sunscreen while at the beach; and 3) intend to use sunscreen with a sun protection factor of 15 or higher. Similarly, Rivers, Salovey, Pizarro, Pizarro and Schneider (2005) investigated the influence of message framing on pap test utilization among women attending a community health clinic. In a randomized experiment, 441 women watched either a loss- or gain-framed video emphasizing the prevention or detection functions of the pap test to examine whether loss- and gain-framed messages differentially influence health behaviours depending on the risk involved in performing the behaviour. Findings showed that gain-framed messages emphasizing the benefits of preventing cervical cancer were most persuasive in motivating women to obtain a pap test rather than loss-framed messages emphasizing the costs of not detecting cervical cancer early. In general, it is now widely recognized that:

- *Gain-framed* messages are expected to be more effective when targeting behaviours that *prevent* the onset of disease; whereas
- *Loss-framed* messages are expected to be more effective when targeting behaviours that *detect* the presence of a disease.

While the application of message framing research has focused exclusively on efforts to promote specific health behaviours, it is acknowledged that practitioners frequently face the challenge of encouraging people to perform a series of behaviours and sustain such actions (Rothman et al., 2006). Thus, it was suggested that future research and theory on message framing are needed that will help inform efforts to promote both the initiation and the maintenance of health practices. Furthermore, a huge majority research on message framing is quantitative in nature, which examines changes in attitude and behaviour change using self-completed questionnaires. Qualitative approaches however could provide valuable insights into how message framing can influence people's subjective experiences. As an example, try to examine the posters presented in Figure 11.4 developed by the NHS to promote breastfeeding. Following a discourse analytic approach, examine the messages being communicated here. Examine the words and images used. What are its connotations? How is the message framed? What do you think it achieves by framing it in this way? Do you think it will be effective? How do you think it will affect its target audience? How will it make them think, feel and behave?

If you would like to share your thoughts on these questions and view other readers' comments, then feel free to visit this textbook's companion website at www.sagepub.co.uk/marks3.

E-HEALTH

The convergence of multi-media (e.g. radio, television, print, audio, computers, telephone, etc.) and the emergence of the Internet have created a vast opportunity to extend the reach of health communication. **E-health** is a general term used to refer to the application of information and communication technology to health or health care. Three broad examples of e-health research will be presented in the next section: Health information on the Internet; Online support groups; and Patient-provider email contact.

Health Information on the Internet

With the fast-paced growth and influence of the World Wide Web, individuals are now able to disseminate and access information right at their fingertips. In 2003, the Health Information National Trends Survey (HINTS) in the US showed that out of the 6369 individuals aged 18 years or older who participated in this study, 63 per cent reported ever going online, of which 63.7 per cent have looked for health information for themselves or others at least once in the previous 12 months (Hesse et al., 2005). In a literature review carried out by McMullan (2006), it was found that the majority of health-related Internet searches by patients are made to seek information for specific medical conditions and are usually carried out *before the clinical encounter* to inform how to manage their own health care independently and/or to decide whether they needed professional help. The Internet searches are also carried out *after the clinical encounter* for reassurance or due

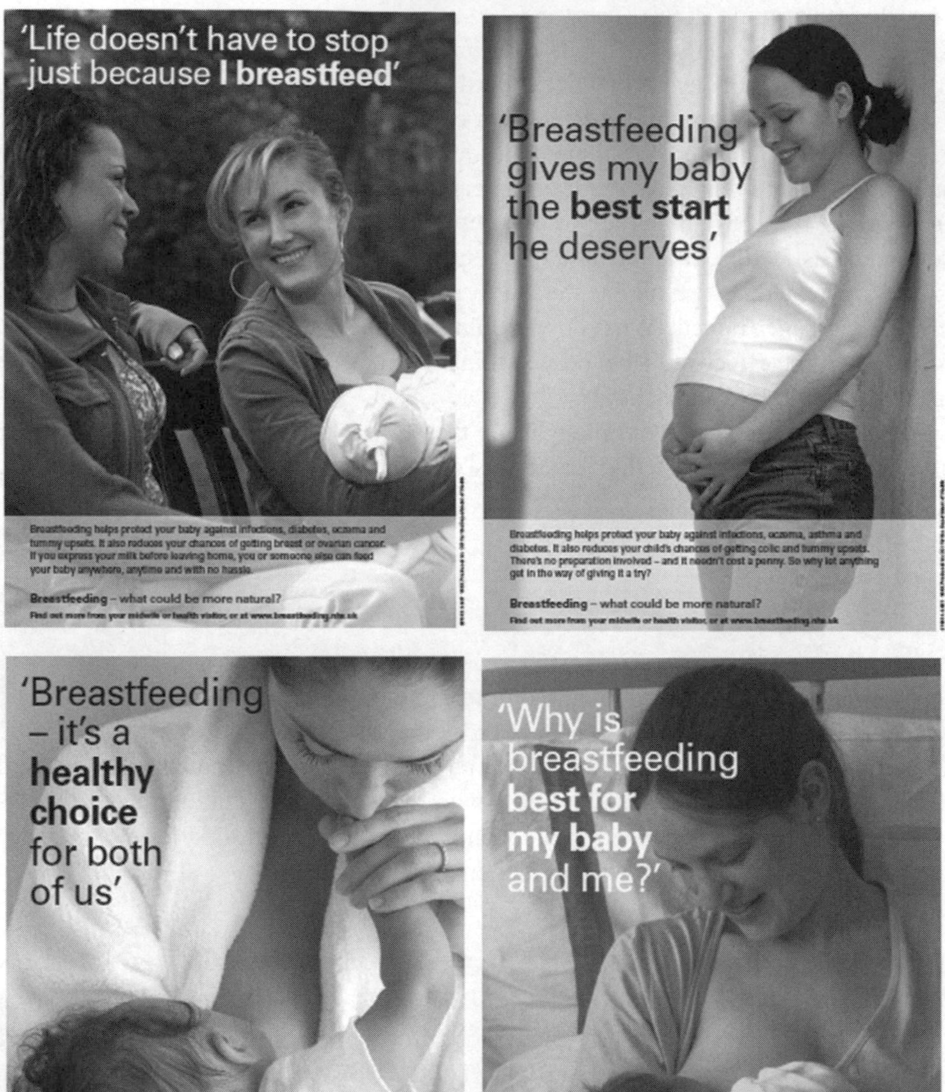

Figure 11.4 NHS breastfeeding campaign posters

Source: www.breastfeeding.nhs.uk; Reproduced with permission

to dissatisfaction with the information provided by the health professional. This shows a shift in the role of the patient from the *passive recipient* of information to *active consumers* and it was suggested that health professionals are responding to the more 'Internet informed' patient in various ways. HCPs may, for example, *feel threatened* and respond defensively by asserting their 'expert opinion'; they may also *collaborate* with patients in obtaining and analysing the information brought by the patient; and they may *guide* patients to reliable health information websites (McMullan, 2006).

Although health information is available online, health professionals are still generally seen as main sources of reliable information by patients. For example, in a qualitative research exploring the impact of information seeking behaviour of patients on the Internet on consultations with health professionals, it was found that patients still acknowledge the primary role of health professionals in delivering health and medical information, and that Internet searches *complement rather than oppose* medical expertise (Kivits, 2006). Increased accessibility of health information on the Internet can thus have its empowering and disempowering consequences on individual patients, HCPs and society in general as summarized in Table 11.3 below.

I'VE ALREADY GOT A DIAGNOSIS FROM HOMEDOC.COM.. BUT I THOUGHT I'D SEE YOU FOR A SECOND OPINION!
FRAN

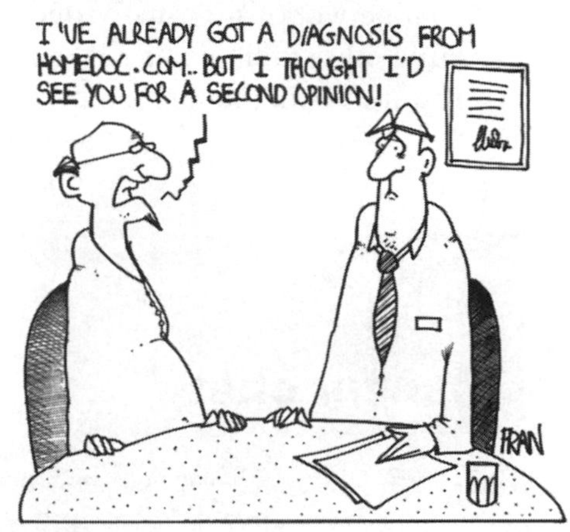

Source: www.cartoonstock.com

Table 11.3 Empowering and disempowering aspects of health on the Internet (Korp, 2006)

Empowering	Disempowering
Enabling of advanced information and knowledge retrieval	A shift towards the expert control and evaluation of sources of health information
Anonymity and convenience in accessing information	Widens the gap between 'information rich' and 'information poor' users, thus reproducing existing social divisions
Creation of social contacts and support independent of time and space	The increase in 'lexicalization' and 'healthism' results in increased anxiety and poorer health
Challenging the expert–lay actor relationship	

In practice, health professionals need to acknowledge that patients generally want to be informed regarding their health concerns and that this information, whether it is reliable or not, may be available, searched and accessed by patients online. **Patient informatics** can thus be a useful addition to the education and training of HCPs (McMullan, 2006).

Online Support Groups

Online networks and discussion boards are also becoming common sources of health information and social support for people affected by health-related conditions. These social networks are usually open for people who would like to talk, share information or find other individuals who share similar experiences as themselves. This could be as a result of being diagnosed or living with chronic illness, taking care of someone with

Box 11.2

Cancer chat

Cancer Chat is a free online forum run by Cancer Research UK where people affected by cancer can talk together, share their experiences, and find information and support. Discussion topics on this website include risk and prevention, symptoms, testing and diagnosis, clinical trials and research, treatment, living with cancer, moving forward, and dying with cancer. Visitors can also post additional discussion topics on the discussion board. There are also links on how to contact the information nurse if more support is required.

Specialist nurses support a team of moderators who regulate this website to ensure that Cancer Chat is a secure and welcoming environment. Accuracy of information posted on the forum is checked regularly and a number of 'house rules' are observed. Users are discouraged from using offensive language which includes swear words and material that could be considered obscene, abusive, vulgar, hateful, threatening or defamatory. Discrimination on the grounds of race, sex, age, religion, ethnic origin or any other basis are also discouraged and threatening other users or threats of physical violence are unacceptable on this website. Visitors are also encouraged to respect other users' views and opinions and are encouraged to 'be safe' in terms of sharing personal details on the forum.

Sources: Cancer Research UK, 2010; http://www.cancerchat.org.uk

a medical condition, or just simply being interested in health issues and sharing views with others online. Some of these sites have chat rooms, discussion boards, e-mail listings, information sheets and links to other useful websites for further information regarding the health condition, relevant treatments and services (see Box 11.2 for an example).

A systematic review was carried out to investigate the effects on health and social outcomes of computer based peer-to-peer communities and electronic self-support groups (Eysenbach, Powell, Englesakis, Rizo & Stern, 2004). Forty-five publications describing 38 distinct studies met the inclusion criteria in this review: 20 were randomized trials, 3 meta-analyses, 3 non-randomized controlled trials, 1 cohort study, and 11 before and after studies. Only six of these evaluated 'pure' peer-to-peer communities, and one had a factorial design with a 'peer to peer only' arm, whereas 31 studies evaluated complex interventions, which often included psycho-educational programmes or one-to-one communication with health-care professionals. The outcomes measured most often were depression and social support measures. Most studies did not show an effect and there was no evidence to support concerns over virtual communities harming people. It was concluded that there was no robust evidence to support consumer led peer-to-peer communities, partly because most of these evaluations were done in conjunction with more complex interventions or involvement with health professionals.

Gender differences in online health-related support groups have also been investigated. Mo, Malik and Coulson (2009) carried out a systematic review and found that gender differences in communication styles among online health support groups exist. For example, in a study comparing messages posted to a breast and a prostate cancer board, it was found that for the breast cancer group, most messages posted online contained support (45.5 per cent), followed by medical/treatment issues (28.9 per cent); whereas for the prostate cancer group, medical/treatment issues were the most prevalent (43.2 per cent), followed by support (36.1 per cent) (Blank & Adams-Blodnieks, 2007). These findings were supported by previous research carried out by Klemm, Hurst, Dearholt and Trone (1999) comparing messages posted to prostate, breast, and mixed cancer support groups using content analysis. It was found that while *information giving/seeking* was ranked the first in the prostate cancer group (36.4 per cent), *sharing of personal experience* was most evident in the breast cancer group (27.9 per cent). Similarly, in a study comparing ovarian and prostate cancer support groups using phenomenological thematic analysis, Sullivan (2003) found that members in the ovarian cancer group appeared to post messages that provided *positive communication and emotional support*. On the other hand, members in the prostate cancer group tended to *share medical information* predominantly with regards to treatment-related issues. In contrast however, Gooden and Winefield (2007) compared the messages posted to a prostate and breast cancer support group using grounded theory and a quasi-quantitative approach but did not find any significant differences in the number of informational or emotional support messages posted to the two groups. In terms of the language used in messages, one study has shown that members in the prostate cancer group tended to engage in more discussion about sexual dysfunction, cite more medical findings, and use lengthier jokes or humorous exchanges compared to members in the breast cancer group. They were also more likely to imply their emotions, and use 'battle-like' terminology when offering encouragement (e.g. Gooden & Winefield, 2007).

Research has shown empowering benefits for participants of online health-related groups. For example, Van Uden-Kraan, Drossaert, Taal, Shaw, Seydel and van de Laar (2008) investigated the empowering processes and outcomes of participation in online support groups for patients with breast cancer, arthritis, or fibromyalgia and interviewed 32 participants of these online support groups. This analysis suggested that members felt empowered by participating in these groups and felt that it helped them to facilitate information exchange, encounter emotional support, find recognition, share experiences, help others, and be amused. In turn, participants felt that they were better informed, felt more confident in the relationship with their physician, their treatment, and their social environment, improved acceptance of the disease, increased optimism and control, and enhanced self-esteem and social well-being. Furthermore, it also fostered collective action among its members. Although disempowering processes were also mentioned in this study (e.g. being unsure about the quality of the information, being confronted with negative sides of the disease, or being confronted with complainers) these were far less mentioned in comparison to its positive consequences.

Apart from online support groups that help people to cope with chronic illnesses, there are also websites that encourage unhealthy behaviours. For example, in an interpretative phenomenological analysis examining the meaning of participation in pro-anorexia sites and its relationship with disordered eating (Mulveen & Hepworth, 2006), it was found that some participants of these websites routinely report their attempts of losing weight and pass on their 'tips and techniques' to other members. Members of the 'pro-anorexia community' also appear to distinguish between *anorexia as a mental illness* versus *anorexia as a lifestyle choice* (also referred to as 'ana'). Describing anorexia as a personal choice is often backed up with challenges to the medical and health authorities and compares it with earlier psychiatric discourses that defined homosexuality as a mental illness. Social support is also often offered in these websites where its members feel that they have the freedom to speak openly about their eating disorders while at the same time have a safe space to express these thoughts. These findings suggest that participation in these sites was multi-purpose and provided coping function in relation to weight loss. It was concluded that the contribution of pro-anorexia websites to increased levels of eating disorders is not inevitable.

Patient-Provider E-mail Contact

In many developed societies, electronic mail is considered a common and convenient medium of communication. The use of e-mail in health communication has the potential to revolutionize the design, delivery and evaluation of health care and promotion. It was suggested that correspondence between HCPs and patients through e-mail can be seen as an opportunity to *increase accessibility to expert advise, increase speed, convenience and access to medical care* (Neill, Mainous, Clark & Hagen, 1994). E-mail communication also has the potential to *reduce missed appointments* by sending reminders to patients through e-mail, *facilitate clinical management* by improving HCP–patient contact, and *improve concordance and follow-up* by enabling patients to report and feedback to health professionals by e-mail (Car & Sheikh, 2004a). Listed in Table 11.4 are some of the potential advantages and disadvantages of delivering health care by e-mail.

In a review of 71 articles on the impact of electronic communication on the HCP–patient relationship, it was found that patients are generally satisfied with the use of secure physician messaging systems and find such services to be convenient, time-saving and useful. Physicians also do not report adverse effects from their use – however legal concerns with electronic messaging were raised (Wallwiener, Wallwiener, Kansy, Seeger & Rajab, 2009). Furthermore there have been concerns on the quality of consultations, confidentiality, liability and the challenge of recovering fees. Car and Sheikh (2004b) argued that while early e-mail use in health care has grown, there was no adequate supporting infrastructure to address security issues. Ensuring privacy, confidentiality and security of information are considered vital for e-mail consultations, and various user friendly safeguards are now becoming available. Thus e-mail consultations would require education and awareness for both patients and doctors on how to use them safely and effectively. In 2002, the American Medical Association published some guidelines on patient–health professional electronic communication as shown in Box 11.3.

BEYOND HEALTH INFORMATION AND COMMUNICATION

Dissemination of health messages through various means of communication has been widely used in health promotion and health care. But the question is – *does health communication actually make a positive impact on health-related behaviours and outcomes*? In a 10-year retrospective review carried out by Noar (2006), it was suggested that targeted, well-executed health mass media campaigns can have small-to-moderate effects on health knowledge, beliefs, attitudes and behaviours, which can translate into major public health impact given the wide reach of mass media. This is supported by a review of existing meta-analyses and other literature on the impact of health communication campaigns on health behaviour (Snyder, 2007), which found that campaigns that 1) pay attention to the specific behavioural goals of the intervention; 2) target specific populations; 3) consider

Table 11.4 Advantages and disadvantages of HCP–patient e-mail communication (adapted from Car & Sheikh, 2004a)

Factors	Advantages	Disadvantages
Face-to-face consultation	May reduce the need for face-to-face consultations which may be convenient for both patients and practitioners	Makes practitioners unable to examine patients and detect non-verbal cues which may increase the risk of diagnostic or communication errors
Information sharing	For patients: may allow them to discuss content of messages with family or friends to improve understanding For practitioners: may consult with colleagues and other professionals to provide a more considered response	Potential threats to patient privacy including unauthorized interception of unencrypted e-mails, receipt or retrieval of e-mails by unauthorized people
Speed	May be more efficient in terms of responses to routine messages	Potentially slow responses to messages that might require emergency actions
Volume and length	Can enable practitioners to offer routine transactions and patient education information to several people simultaneously; users can also send virtually any kind of electronic file as an attachment	Users may be overwhelmed by the volume and length of e-mails
Social inequalities	Increased access to care (e.g. for those with physical disabilities or those living in a remote area)	Widening social disparities by allowing preferential access to wealthier people and young middle class adults

communication activities and channels, message content and presentation; and 4) include techniques for feedback and evaluation; are able to affect health-related behaviour change. However, it is also worth noting that strategies that aim to inform, educate and modify patients' health-related behaviours to promote health must recognize the role of **health literacy** (see Chapter 14) and the wider determinants of health when designing, implementing and evaluating such interventions. The use of alternative and creative approaches to promote health messages and the value of community-based interventions are also worth considering (see Chapter 15).

Box 11.3

Guidelines for patient–health professional electronic communication

Timing and speed of response

- Establish turnaround time for messages
- Exercise caution when using e-mail for urgent matters
- Remind patients about the importance of alternative forms of communication for emergencies

Message efficiency

- Establish types of transactions (e.g. prescription refill, appointment scheduling) permitted over e-mail. Instruct patients to put the category of transaction in the subject line of the message for filtering: prescription, appointment, medical advice, billing question. Request that patients put their name and patient identification number in the body of the message
- Explain to patients that their messages should be concise
- Configure automatic reply to acknowledge receipt of messages; send a new message to inform patient of completion of request; request patients to use auto-reply feature to acknowledge reading clinicians message
- When e-mail messages become too lengthy or the correspondence is prolonged, notify patients to come in to discuss or call them

Record keeping

- Whenever possible and appropriate, physicians should retain electronic and/or paper copies of e-mail communications with patients
- Develop archival and retrieval mechanisms

Privacy

- Inform patient about privacy issues
- Patients should know who besides addressee processes messages during addressee's usual business hours and during addressee's vacation or illness
- Maintain a mailing list of patients, but do not send group mailings where recipients are visible to each other. Use blind copy feature in software

(Continued)

(Continued)

- Append a standard block of text to the end of e-mail messages to patients, which contains the physician's full name, contact information, and reminders about security
- Consider sensitivity of subject matter (HIV, mental health) in e-mail transactions

Etiquette

- Avoid anger, sarcasm, harsh criticism and libelous references to third parties in messages
- Remind patients when they do not adhere to the guidelines
- For patients who repeatedly do not adhere to the guidelines, it is acceptable to terminate the e-mail relationship

Source: American Medical Association, 2002

FUTURE RESEARCH

1 Longitudinal studies on the impact of social marketing strategies on quality of life.
2 Qualitative studies exploring message framing and subjective experiences.
3 Cost-effectiveness evaluation on the use of e-mail communication on health care delivery.

Summary

1 Health communication refers to all interpersonal, organizational or mass communication that concerns health.
2 Health communication can occur in various contexts, be applied in a variety of settings, use a variety of channels, deliver a variety of messages, and be used for a variety of reasons.
3 Shannon and Weaver's model of communication considers five key components to communication: 1) source; 2) transmitter; 3) channel; 4) receiver; and 5) destination. A sixth component, noise, is also considered in the model.
4 Good communication between health-care professionals (HCP) and patients is essential to health promotion, disease prevention and treatment and can serve as the foundation of an effective HCP–patient partnership.

5 There are three general approaches to the study of HCP–patient communication: 1) the 'deviant patient' perspective; 2) the 'authoritarian doctor' perspective; and 3) the 'interactive dyad' perspective.
6 Social marketing is the application of consumer-oriented marketing techniques in the design, implementation and evaluation of programmes aimed to influence behaviour change for public benefit.
7 The key characteristics of social marketing include: consumer orientation; understanding existing behaviour and setting behavioural goals; intervention or marketing mix; audience segmentation; exchange; and competition.
8 Social marketing has been widely used to inform the development, implementation and evaluation of health promotion campaigns.
9 The way messages are framed could influence people's motivation to undertake the health behaviour. Gain-framed messages are expected to be more effective when targeting behaviours that prevent the onset of disease; whereas loss-framed messages are expected to be more effective when targeting behaviours that detect the presence of a disease.
10 E-health is a general term used to refer to the application of information and communication technology to health or health care. The wider accessibility of health information on the Internet, the existence of online support groups and the use of electronic communication are revolutionizing the way health care and promotion are being designed, delivered and evaluated.

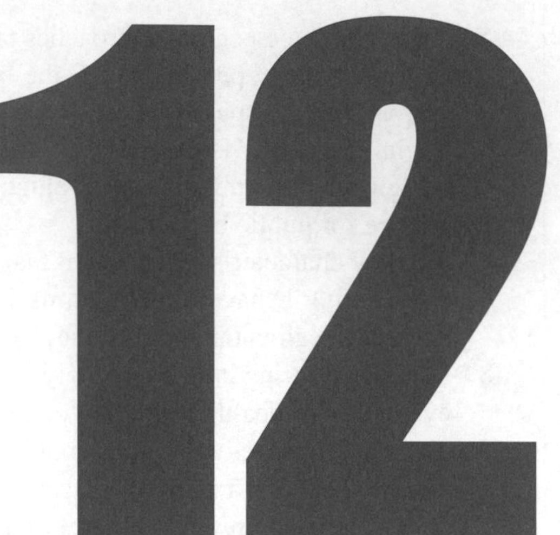

Stress and Coping

Though the faculties of the mind are improved by exercise, yet they must not be put to a stress beyond their strength.

John Locke, *Of the Conducting of the Understanding*, 1706

Outline

This chapter discusses theoretical approaches to the study of stress and coping, and research on stress as a cause of physical illness. It begins with an account of stimulus, response and interactional perspectives, and includes a critical analysis of them. Consideration is given to the effects of stress on the immune system and to ways in which people react to trauma. A discussion of methodological problems confronting research on stress and illness is followed by an examination of evidence linking stress to cardiovascular disease, cancer and infectious diseases.

WHAT IS STRESS?

It is widely believed that stress has become a major feature of modern living, as a result of changes in the type of work that we do, the increased pace of life, and many features of the contemporary urban environment. Life today may be less obviously stressful than the life of our hunter–gatherer ancestors, but it seems that modern humans have created an environment that is far from optimal for mental and physical health. Stress is thought to be a principal cause of psychological distress and physical illness and millions of working days every year are believed to be lost as a consequence of this. The ability to cope successfully with stress (see Figure 12.1) is frequently held to be the key to human happiness.

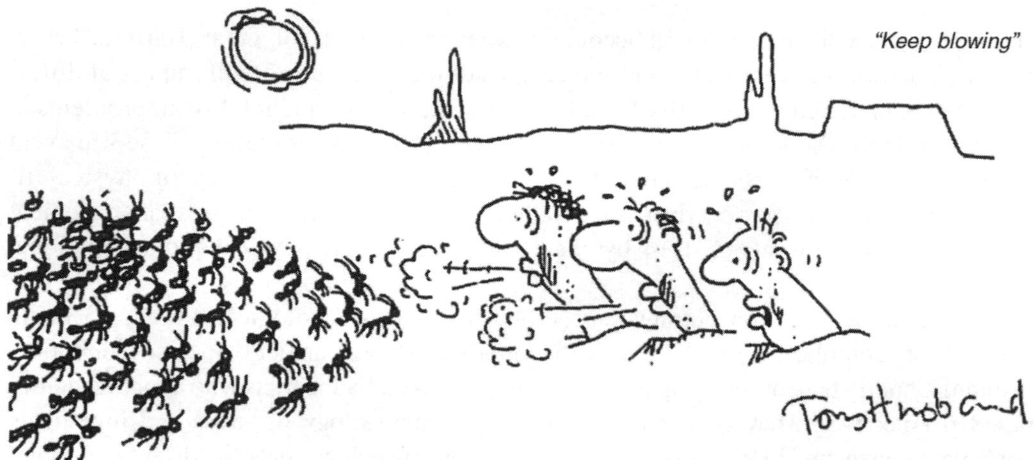

Figure 12.1 Coping with stress
Source: *Private Eye*, 4 October 1996: 22; Reproduced with permission

But what exactly do we mean by the term 'stress', and how convincing is the evidence in support of these popular beliefs? If you ask people what they mean by stress you will find that their answers fall into one of three categories, each of which finds its echo in the academic literature. These three categories are summarized in Table 12.1.

The first answer is that stress is 'when you are under a lot of pressure', or 'when things are getting on top of you'. This is essentially the position taken by researchers who adopt stimulus-based perspectives. These derive, to some extent, from the engineering approach to the elasticity of materials, where *stress* refers to a load applied to an object or structure, setting up a force, known as *strain*, that can result in damage once the *elastic limit* is exceeded. Applied to human beings, it is assumed that individuals have a

Table 12.1 Alternative approaches to stress

Theoretical perspective	Popular conception	Major theories and techniques	Approaches to stress management
Stimulus-based	'When things are getting on top of you'	Life event and 'daily hassles' scales	Making jobs and environments less stressful
Response-based	'When you feel stressed-out'	General adaptation syndrome, psychoneuroimmunology	Biofeedback, relaxation exercises, yoga and meditation
Interactional	'When you think that you cannot cope'	Interactional theories, coping scales	Cognitive-behaviour modification, stress inoculation training

certain tolerance to stress but will become ill when the stress is too great (Bartlett, 1998). Stimulus theorists have tried to devise measures of the relative stressful impact of different life events, ranging in severity from bereavement, divorce and job loss to problems in personal relationships, environmental disturbances and work pressures. These life event measures have in turn been used to investigate the role of stress as a cause of physical illness. Stimulus-based perspectives are associated with approaches to stress management that seek to reduce levels of stress by changing aspects of the physical and occupational environments.

The second answer concentrates on the physical and psychological feeling of 'being stressed' or 'completely stressed out' with symptoms such as anxiety, poor concentration, insomnia, bodily tension and fatigue. This position is taken by theorists who adopt response-based perspectives. They concentrate on the psychophysiology of stress and investigate possible mechanisms linking stress to physical illnesses such as coronary disease and viral infections, by way of the cardiovascular and immune systems respectively. Response-based perspectives have also provided the impetus for the introduction of stress management programmes that focus on controlling the psychophysiology of stress using techniques such as relaxation and breathing exercises, yoga, meditation, aerobics and other forms of physical exercise.

The third answer is that stress is 'when you think you can't cope' or 'when you have too much strain put on you and you do not have the ability to deal with it'. This is the position developed in interactional perspectives by theorists who argue that stress occurs when there is an imbalance between the perceived demands placed on the individual and the ability to meet those demands, often described as *coping resources*. These theories are attractive because they overcome a problem inherent in stimulus and response perspectives; individuals differ as to what events or demands they find stressful and in the way that they respond to them. Interactional perspectives have led to the study of coping and to the development of techniques aimed at helping individuals to overcome stress by increasing the effectiveness of their coping strategies. These are taught in **stress management workshops** and **stress innoculation training**.

The above three approaches are not mutually exclusive and it is possible to contemplate the emergence of a very broad 'general theory of stress' that incorporates elements of all of them. However the classification is useful because it enables us to focus on the rather different styles of research that have emanated from each and to discuss the major criticisms that have been directed at them.

STIMULUS-BASED PERSPECTIVES AND LIFE EVENT SCALES

Holmes and Rahe (1967) conducted influential research into the types of life events that people rate as being most stressful. They began by choosing 43 probably stressful life events, and then asked 400 US adults to rate the relative amount of readjustment that they judged would be required by each of the 43 events. The 10 highest rated of these are listed in Box 12.1. They then used their results to construct a **Social Readjustment Rating Scale (SRRS)** that assigns points values to different kinds of stress and that is still being used in research on stress and physical illness.

Box 12.1

Stressful life events and daily Hassles Scales

Listed below in order of severity are the 10 life events rated as highly stressful by a sample of the US adult population studied by Holmes and Rahe (1967), and the 10 daily hassles endorsed most frequently by a New Zealand student population studied by Chamberlain and Zika (1990) using a scale derived from Kanner, Coyne, Schaefer and Lazarus (1981).

Life events

1. Death of spouse
2. Divorce
3. Marital separation
4. Jail term
5. Death of close family member
6. Personal injury or illness
7. Marriage
8. Fired at work
9. Marital reconciliation
10. Retirement

Daily hassles

1. Not enough time
2. Too many things to do
3. Troubling thoughts about future
4. Too many interruptions
5. Misplacing or losing things
6. Health of a family member
7. Social obligations
8. Concerns about standards
9. Concerns about getting ahead
10. Too many responsibilities

Some researchers felt dissatisfied with the SRRS because many of the events listed in it occur relatively rarely in anyone's life. There was a need for a scale that reflected to a greater degree the day-to-day variation experienced by people in the levels of the stress to which they are exposed. This led Kanner et al. (1981), using similar techniques to those of Holmes and Rahe, to devise two further scales, a **Hassles Scale** consisting of everyday events that cause annoyance or frustration, and an **Uplifts Scale** consisting of events that make them feel good. Of the two, the Hassles Scale has been the more widely used for research that parallels that using the SRRS. Box 12.1 lists, as an example, the findings of Chamberlain and Zika (1990), using an adaptation of the Kanner et al. scale, of the 10 most frequently endorsed hassles by a sample of 161 students in New Zealand.

The SRRS, the Hassles Scale and research using them have been the subject of extensive criticism since their original publication (e.g. Schroeder & Costa, 1984). These criticisms focus on the choice of items for inclusion in the scale, items that often seem highly arbitrary, vague, ambiguous, insensitive to individual differences and sometimes likely to assess the individual's level of neuroticism rather than experienced life event stress.

The arbitrariness of items included in the scales is probably inevitable. It is trivially easy to think of stressful life events and hassles that have not found their way into the existing scales, but a complete listing of all such events would be endless. The vagueness and ambiguity of some items is another serious problem. Items such as *change in recreation* or *change in responsibilities at work*, taken from the SRRS, and most items on the Hassles Scale can be criticized in this way. Items such as bereavement may also create problems because bereavement may have very different stressful impacts on different people as a function of length and quality of relationship, whether or not the death was unexpected, and so on.

Much of the research linking physical illness to stressful life events has consisted of retrospective studies in which participants are asked about events occurring prior to the onset of physical illness. These studies have been criticized because people who have recently been ill may very well be predisposed to recollect and report recent stressful events to a greater extent than control group individuals who have remained well. Any such tendency will lead to an overestimation of the association between stress and illness. The inclusion of vague and ambiguous items in the scales is clearly likely to maximize the differential reporting of stressful events.

The question as to whether the scales may be partially measuring neuroticism arises because they include a lot of items such as *too many things to do* or *troubling thoughts about the future* that could equally find a place in scales designed to measure anxiety or depression. This leads to a problem in interpreting the results even of prospective studies that investigate the association between scores on Life Events and Hassles Scales and subsequently occurring physical illness over a period of time. In principle this can establish whether stress really does predict the development of illness. Most prospective studies have relied on self-reports of illness; but it is highly probable that neurotic individuals will not only give high scores on Life Events and Hassles Scales but also be more likely to interpret minor symptoms as indicative of physical illness in comparison with individuals low on neuroticism. Here an empirical association between stress and illness may occur as a result of a reporting bias rather than a genuine causal link. A better approach is to rely on biologically verified assessments of illness.

Recent researchers investigating stress–illness links have shown a trend away from the use of standardized checklists in favour of the structured interview techniques developed by Brown and Harris. Their **Life Events and Difficulties Schedule (LEDS)** is used to assess, classify and rate the severity of each stressful event, making allowance for individual circumstances. Originally developed to study the social origins of depression in women, the LEDS has since been used to study links between life event stress and physical illness (Harris, 2007).

RESPONSE-BASED PERSPECTIVES AND THE PHYSIOLOGY OF STRESS

Since any catalogue of potentially stressful events is endless and individuals differ greatly as to what they find stressful, an alternative is to seek to identify a characteristic stress response that occurs whatever the nature of the stress. This could theoretically include physiological, psychological and behavioural consequences of stress, although in practice researchers have tended to concentrate on physiological effects, especially those that may be associated with the development of physical illness.

Research on the physiology of stress originated in the work of Walter Cannon in the first half of the twentieth century. Cannon's theories revolve around the concept of *homeostasis*, whereby the physiological mechanisms of the body are considered as feedback systems functioning as far as possible to maintain a steady state. Homeostatic balance is disrupted not only by basic bodily needs, as in the case of hunger and thirst, but by any environmental stimulus that disrupts the body's state of equilibrium (e.g. excessive heat or cold, bacterial and virus infections, emotion provoking stimuli), thereby causing a reaction that has the function of re-establishing the inner balance. Anything that disrupts equilibrium may be regarded as stressful (Cannon, 1932).

Under Cannon's influence, Hans Selye began a programme of animal experimentation into the physiological effects of noxious stimuli and other types of stress from the early 1930s until shortly before his death in 1982 (Selye, 1976). He argued for the existence of a generalized response, known as the **General Adaptation Syndrome (GAS)**, that occurs whenever the body defends itself against noxious stimuli. The GAS occurs primarily in the pituitary-adrenocortical system and consists of three stages, an *alarm reaction* in which the body's defences are mobilized, a *resistance stage* in which the body adapts to the cause of stress, and an *exhaustion stage* when the body's capacity to resist finally breaks down. Selye particularly drew attention to the abnormal physiology of the animal during the resistance stage that, if protracted, could lead to what he called the *diseases of adaptation*. These include ulcers, cardiovascular disease and asthma.

Although Selye's views have been very influential in the history of stress research, they are no longer widely accepted following extensive criticism by Mason (1971, 1975). Mason argued that the body's reaction to different types of stress is not uniform at all. Those common physiological reactions that are found are caused by the emotional reaction of the animal to the stressful event rather than to a direct physiological effect. In many studies of the effects of stress, laboratory animals have been exposed to some highly unpleasant conditions (to put it more bluntly, they have been tortured) and it seems likely that the researchers have been, and perhaps still are, effectively studying the physiology of fear. It is not easy to find an ethical justification for this type of animal experimentation and such studies will not be considered any further.

The tradition of psychosomatic medicine, described in more detail in Chapter 17, spans a similar historical period as the work of Cannon and Selye but focuses much more on the human response to stress. Franz Alexander and his associates drew a distinction between the temporary and biologically adaptive changes in the physiology of the animal facing an emergency necessitating flight or fight and the protracted and maladaptive physiological changes taking place in the anxious or stressed human being. Of particular significance are the physiological changes that are activated by the sympathetic branch of the autonomic nervous system.

The proponents of psychosomatic medicine emphasized the effects of stress and anxiety on the cardiovascular, gastro-enteritic and respiratory systems. Some of their theories have an attractive plausibility, but their broad theoretical sweep and the range of physiological mechanisms proposed was never matched by an appropriate level of careful empirical research. Health psychologists have made some progress in investigating the relationship between stress and cardiovascular disease, but other areas considered by the schools of psychosomatic medicine remain, from a research point of view, largely virgin territory. At present the two most active areas of investigation into responses to stress are, firstly, the study of the effects of stress on the immune system, usually referred to as **psychoneuroimmunology (PNI)** and, secondly, the study of the long-term effects of extreme or traumatic stress, usually referred to as **post-traumatic stress disorder (PTSD)**. We will now consider these two areas of research.

PSYCHONEUROIMMUNOLOGY (PNI)

The AIDS epidemic was one reason for an increased interest in psychological influences on the immune system, but there are also other considerations. The immune system is implicated not only in the body's defences against all infectious diseases but also in cancer and in autoimmune diseases such as rheumatoid arthritis. If psychological factors can be shown to have a significant role as causes of upregulation and downregulation of the immune system, then it is possible that psychological interventions could play an important role in the treatment of a very wide range of diseases.

Reviews of modern research findings in PNI have been provided by Bachen, Cohen and Marsland (2007), Segerstrom and Miller (2004), Biondi (2001) and Evans, Hucklebridge and Clow (2000). At a theoretical level, Maier and Watkins (1998) attempt to synthesize current knowledge from an evolutionary perspective to account for psychological and behavioural effects of physical illness as well as the effects of stress on the immune system. These authors all emphasize that the immune system is complicated as it involves a range of different types of cell with distinct functions. A brief synopsis of these is given in Box 12.2.

Box 12.2

Cells of the human immune system

The main cells of the immune system are *leucocytes*, usually known as white blood cells. The three most important types of leucocytes are *granulocytic cells, monocytes/ macrophages* and *lymphocytes*. These in turn divide into the following categories:

- *Granulocytic leucocytes*: the main types are *neutrophils*, which are *phagocytes* (eating cells) that engulf and destroy bacteria, *eosinophils* that similarly engulf antigen-antibody complexes and *basophils*, which have effects that promote the migration of other immune cells to the region.
- *Monocytes/macrophages*: these cells have a number of functions including 'recognition' of certain carbohydrates on the surfaces of micro-organisms.
- *Lymphocytes*: these cells have the function of attacking specific targets. They can be subdivided into *B cells*, *NK cells* and *T cells*. B cells produce antibodies that proliferate rapidly, thereby controlling infection. NK (natural killer) cells destroy virus infected and tumour cells. T cells further subdivide into *T helper cells*, which enhance immune responses by stimulating the replication of immune system cells and antibodies, *cytotoxic T cells*, which destroy virus, parasite and tumour infected cells, and *T suppressor cells*, that inhibit immune responses.

It can be seen that the human immune system is not simple. Much as one might like to do so, it is not possible to talk in a general sense of heightened or reduced immunity, because the immune system is volatile with changes constantly taking place in one or more of its parts. At any particular time one measure may indicate heightened immunity while another may indicate reduced immunity. An important example is the distinction between *cell-mediated immunity* and *humoral immunity*. In recent years there has been considerable interest in the relationship between psychological stress and increases in levels of the hormone cortisol that has the effect of inhibiting cell-mediated immunity while enhancing humoral immunity (Evans et al., 2000; Dickerson & Kemeny, 2004). This provides some support for the much earlier conjecture of the psychosomatic schools (see Chapter 17) that asthma and other allergic conditions can have psychological origins. High levels of **cortisol** are associated with these conditions (Evans et al., 2000). Further support for this conjecture comes from the research of Sandberg et al. (2000) that demonstrated that acute and chronic stress is associated with subsequent asthma attacks in children who suffer from the condition.

A major difficulty when interpreting PNI research is that the preponderance of different kinds of immune cells varies considerably among healthy individuals and in the same healthy individual from day to day. O'Leary (1990) was one of the first to point out that the demonstration of statistically significant effects of stress on one or more parameters of the immune system does not necessarily entail that these changes have clinical significance as regards disease outcomes. Changes that have been shown to occur are invariably within the normal range of variation to be found in healthy individuals. There has been little progress on this important issue as is evident from the fact that 17 years later Bachen et al. (2007) make exactly the same point.

Research on stress and immunity can be broadly divided into studies of the short-term effects of *acute stress* and of the longer term effects of *chronic stress.* Types of acute stress that have been studied include sleep deprivation, space flight, taking examinations, exposure to the objects of phobias such as snakes, violent exercise, loud noises, electric shocks and attempting to solve difficult or impossible problems. Types of chronic or long-term stress that have been studied include bereavement, unemployment, marital conflict, separation and divorce, and caring for relatives suffering from Alzheimer's disease. No study has investigated the effects of any one kind of stress on all aspects of immune function and it is therefore necessary to piece together findings from different studies in order to obtain a general picture.

It has been a fairly consistent finding that chronic stress is associated with some degree of down regulation of immune systems with changes found particularly in the number of NK cells, the total number of T cells and the proportion of T helper cells to T suppressor cells. Findings for the effects of acute stress have been more variable, with some indications of upregulation, some of downregulation, and some null findings (Evans et al., 2000; Segerstrom & Miller, 2004; Bachen et al., 2007). Segerstrom and Miller also note that subjective reports of stress are not usually associated with immune changes.

While most research in this field is concerned with establishing the effects of stress on the immune system, there have also been a number of studies investigating the effects of psychological interventions, including stress management, on immune measures. If successful these interventions could have considerable potential benefit in reducing susceptibility to disease and improving recovery rates. Miller and Cohen (2001) reviewed 85 studies with rather disappointing conclusions. Positive findings were mainly for interventions using hypnosis and conditioning while stress management and relaxation techniques rarely produced substantial effects. However they warn against jumping to the conclusion that the immune system cannot be much influenced by psychological interventions, pointing out a range of research problems that need to be overcome before firm conclusions can be drawn.

There is general agreement that a number of methodological difficulties need to be overcome before we can safely conclude that stress has direct effects on the immune system with disease consequences. Firstly, it is important to distinguish between direct effects of stress and other physiological pathways that may be activated by stressful experiences such as sleep deprivation and space flight. Secondly, it is necessary to rule out indirect effects that may be obtained when stress provokes health hazardous behaviour, such as smoking and alcohol consumption, that may in turn have effects on the immune system. Thirdly, where significant effects of stress on immune function have been adequately demonstrated, it is also necessary to show that these effects have clinical significance as regards disease outcomes. We shall return to this last point later in this chapter when we examine research on the relationship between stress and biologically verified disease.

POST-TRAUMATIC STRESS DISORDER (PTSD)

Can a characteristic response to stress be found in individuals who have been subjected to extreme levels of stress, such as soldiers in battles, victims of rape and other violent crimes and survivors of disasters such as earthquakes, floods and nuclear accidents? The term 'PTSD' was introduced by researchers studying psychological symptoms reported by soldiers returning to the USA from the Vietnam War. It was subsequently extended to studies of other types of traumatic stress. It was first accepted as a diagnostic label by the American Psychiatric Association in 1980. The symptoms that are most often used to characterize PTSD are insomnia, nightmares, flashbacks, problems of memory and concentration, acting or feeling as if the event is recurring and a greatly increased sensitivity to new stressful events (Posluszny, Spencer & Baum, 2007). A variety of physiological changes have also been found in persons suffering from PTSD.

As in the other areas of enquiry that focus on stress reactions, our understanding of PTSD is complicated by the existence of large individual differences. Not everyone exposed to traumatic stress develops the symptoms of PTSD. Prevalence rates among individuals exposed to extreme stress vary widely according to the nature of the stress, most commonly from 10 per cent to 30 per cent. There are also large individual differences in the types of symptoms encountered and their severity. Some recent attempts have been made to review the voluminous literature on PTSD to establish whether differences in emotional reactions occurring at the time of and immediately after traumatic stress can predict the subsequent development of PTSD, although so far with little agreement (Harvey & Bryant, 2002; Ozer, Best, Lipsey & Weiss, 2003). Neither is it clear whether reactions to different kinds of traumatic stress are basically the same or whether they depend on the particular type of stress involved.

The psychophysiological differences found between PTSD sufferers and others are real enough, but it has not been established whether they have occurred purely as a result of exposure to traumatic stress, or are at least partly determined by pre-existing characteristics of the individuals who develop PTSD. It is quite often found that these individuals have a history of psychological problems, including childhood trauma, abnormal adolescent development, depression and anxiety disorders (Posluszny et al., 2007). This in turn raises the question, in any particular case, as to whether the traumatic stress is the primary cause of subsequent psychological reactions or the 'straw that breaks the camel's back'.

While there has been at least one recent attempt to develop a theoretical model of PTSD (Brewin, Dalgleish & Joseph, 1996), others question its usefulness as a clinical diagnosis. A trenchant critique is given by the Canadian anthropologist Allan Young (1995) who combines an historical analysis of the concept with an ethnographic study conducted in a psychiatric unit specializing in the treatment of PTSD. He argues that PTSD is not, as its proponents would have us believe, a psychiatric condition that has been vividly described throughout human history, but a cultural phenomenon of the modern era. He traces it to the work of Freud and others in the late nineteenth century, work that has contributed to the **medicalization** of certain types of human unhappiness. While not disputing the extent of the suffering that is caused by traumatic experiences, he does challenge the usefulness of the diagnosis of PTSD as a step towards helping people to deal with their suffering.

Summerfield (2001) takes some of these criticisms further. He points out that the diagnosis of PTSD now has an important legal advantage for people seeking financial compensation for distress suffered while performing functions that might be thought to be part of their job, such as ambulance personnel attending road accidents and police officers on duty at disasters. He comments:

> *There is a veritable trauma industry comprising experts, lawyers, claimants and other interested parties. It is a kind of social movement trading on the authority of medical pronouncements. An encounter between a sympathetic psychiatrist and a claimant is primed to produce a report of post-traumatic stress disorder if that is what the lawyer says the rules require and what has, in effect, been commissioned. In the United Kingdom awards for psychological damage based on the diagnosis can be several times higher than, say, the £30,000 to £40,000 limit that the Criminal Injuries Compensation Authority applies for the traumatic loss of a leg. (Summerfield, 2001: 95)*

Mezey and Robbins (2001) challenge Summerfield's view. While agreeing that the diagnosis of PTSD has been used indiscriminately in civil litigation, they argue that PTSD involves a level of distress that transcends ordinary human misery and unhappiness and that the diagnosis has the positive function of taking away blame from the sufferer who experiences guilt, shame and failure, so that the symptoms can be experienced as a normal response to an abnormal event rather than a pathological condition. They also argue that the psychophysiological characteristics of PTSD can be clearly distinguished from those associated with other psychiatric diagnoses.

INTERACTIONAL PERSPECTIVES AND COPING SCALES

It is apparent from the above discussion that a key problem for both stimulus and response based perspectives on stress is individual differences. Different people find different things stressful, and react to the same potentially stressful events and circumstances in different ways. A number of theorists have sought to overcome this problem by conceptualizing stress as a relationship between the individual and the environment and developing *interactional models*. The most influential of these was put forward by Lazarus and developed by Lazarus and Folkman (1984). In this model psychological stress is defined as 'a particular relationship between the person and the environment that is appraised by the person as taxing or exceeding his or her resources and endangering his or her well-being' (p.10). A distinction is made between *primary appraisal* whereby an event may be perceived as benign and non-threatening, potentially harmful, threatening to one's self-esteem, or challenging, and *secondary appraisal* in which an assessment is made of one's ability to cope with the threat or challenge. Stress occurs whenever there is a mismatch between perceived threat and perceived ability to cope.

These ideas have been developed at considerable length in a number of books and articles, but they do raise the question as to whether they amount to much more than just another way of saying that stress is when you think you cannot cope. Although this may seem a modest enough assertion, it can in fact be criticized for its implication that stress results only from a purely subjective mismatch between demands and coping resources. One can ask, what about the person who thinks that they can cope when objectively the demands of the situation exceed their actual ability to cope? Are such optimists not stressed? This problem is partially solved by Trumbull and Appley (1986) who extended the model of Lazarus and Folkman by proposing that stress can occur whenever either the real or the perceived demands exceed either the real or the perceived capacity to cope. It might be felt that Trumbull and Appley's definition is so broad and all-encompassing that it amounts to no more than a statement of the obvious. A critical question might be, what is the relative importance of mismatches between real demands and coping resources and those between perceived demands and coping resources in determining whether an individual suffers the effects of stress?

In some ways it is probably better to think of interactional models of stress as *frameworks* for thinking about the subject rather than as specific and testable theories or models. Another way of representing an interactional framework is the flowchart model of Cox (1978) shown in Figure 12.2. One of the useful features of this flowchart is that it incorporates feedback between responses, demands and appraisal. For example, behavioural responses, depending on whether they are appropriate or inappropriate, may result in a reduction or an increase

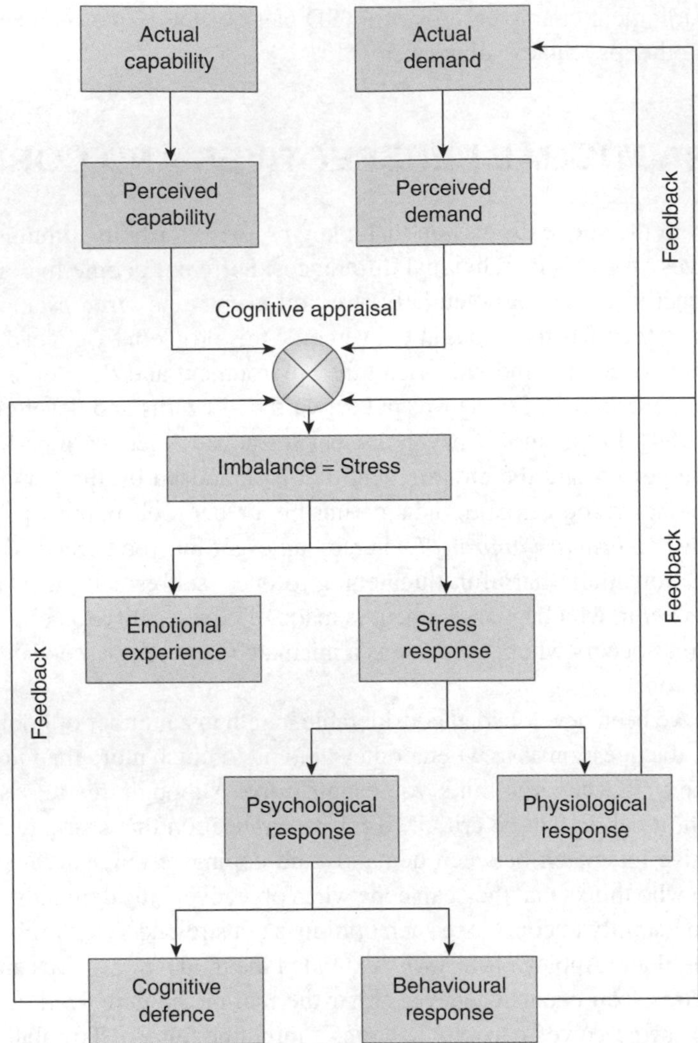

Figure 12.2 Flowchart for an interactional model of stress (Cox, 1978: 19; reproduced with permission)

in actual demand; psychological defence mechanisms may become activated leading to changes in the cognitive appraisal of mismatches between perceived demand and perceived capability, and so on.

One consequence of the emergence of interactional models of stress has been the development of checklists designed to assess the individual's predominant coping strategies. An example is the COPE questionnaire devised by Carver, Scheier and Weintraub (1989) that consists of 15 sub-scales each made up of a number of items for which the individual indicates agreement or disagreement on a four-point scale. The 15 sub-scales with an example of a checklist statement from each are shown in Box 12.3.

Box 12.3

Assessing coping strategies: the COPE scale

In the COPE scale, you are asked how you respond when confronting difficult or stressful events in your life. To each item you use the following rating system:

1 I usually don't do this at all.
2 I usually do this a little bit.
3 I usually do this a medium amount.
4 I usually do this a lot.

The 15 COPE sub-scales with an example of a checklist from each (the complete version contained four items per sub-scale) are:

1 **Active coping:** I take additional action to get rid of the problem.
2 **Planning:** I try to come up with a strategy about what to do.
3 **Suppression of competing activities**: I put aside other activities in order to concentrate on this.
4 **Restraint coping**: I force myself to wait until the right time to do something.
5 **Seeking social support for emotional reasons**: I ask people who have had similar experience what they did.
6 **Seeking social support for instrumental reasons**: I talk to someone about how I feel.
7 **Positive reinterpretation and growth**: I look for something good in what is happening.
8 **Acceptance**: I learn to live with it.
9 **Turning to religion**: I seek God's help.
10 **Focus on and venting of emotions**: I get upset and let my emotions out.
11 **Denial**: I refuse to believe that it has happened.
12 **Behavioural disengagement:** I give up the attempt to get what I want.
13 **Mental disengagement:** I turn to work or other substitute activities to take my mind off things.
14 **Alcohol-drug disengagement**: I drink alcohol, or take drugs, in order to think about it less.
15 **Humour**: I make fun of the situation.

Source: Carver et al., 1989

Problems and issues for coping research were discussed by Folkman and Moskowitz (2004). Coping scales have been criticized for adopting a 'blunderbuss' approach to the complex mechanisms involved in coping with different types of stress, and failing to take account of the fact that individuals may vary greatly in the way they cope with different stressful situations (Somerfield, 1997; Aldwin & Park, 2004). They may also be criticized for relying too much on introspective judgements unsupported by other types of evidence. If it is a feature of the psychology of stress that people tend to behave irrationally when exposed to high levels of stress, then the reports of individuals about their personal ways of coping may be particularly inaccurate. For example, *denial,* the refusal to acknowledge the existence of a real danger, may be observed when an individual ignores or denies the significance of symptoms of life-threatening disease, but it is unlikely to be a fully conscious process. How is such an individual likely to respond to the denial items on the COPE questionnaire when asked, for example, how often when confronted with stressful life events, he or she 'refuses to believe that it has happened'? Surely the whole point about denial is that it only works as a defence if the person does not realize she/her is doing it.

ARE STRESS THEORIES NECESSARY?

The stress theories that we have been considering were, for the most part, fully developed by the mid-1980s. Since that time there has been a sharp decline in interest in the development of general theories in favour of a piecemeal approach to research, mostly concerning possible links between specific types of stress and susceptibility to physical illness. Many critics have argued that the development of general theories of stress is not a viable scientific objective. For example, while it seems worthwhile to study the effects respectively of bereavement, living in noisy environments and of poor role definition at the workplace, it is not necessarily the case that such studies would yield results that have enough in common to be incorporated into a broad general theory. Critics have pointed out that stress is an umbrella term that has been applied to so many quite different phenomena as to become virtually meaningless from a scientific point of view (for example, Pollock, 1988; Brown, 1996). In an effort to encompass such diverse phenomena the concept has become so vague and ambiguous that it lacks any practical value. But if the stress concept is such a nebulous one, why has it come to play such a significant role in popular discourse and media presentations? Pollock, Brown and others have attempted to answer this question by analysing stress as a social construct. To illustrate these fairly complex modes of analysis, here are two illustrations of the way in which this approach can be revealing.

First, stress is often used as a device for legitimating behaviour that might otherwise be seen as the result of anxiety, neurosis or personal inadequacy. For example, to phone up your workplace to say that you will not be coming in today, or to excuse yourself for not sitting an examination on the grounds that you are too worried, not sleeping well, too tired, or simply feel inadequate would not be considered acceptable. To give as the reason that you are suffering from stress, preferably supported by a letter from a doctor or counsellor, could be considered perfectly reasonable. In spite of the differences between stimulus, response and interactional models of stress, what they all have in common is that they draw attention to current events in one's life or one's immediate environment as provoking a reaction, rather than focusing exclusively on the individual. But it may very well be that an inability to cope with the demands of everyday life may be more appropriately seen as indicative of a long-standing psychological problem such as anxiety or depression.

Second, stress often has the function of explaining the otherwise inexplicable, whether this be psychological or physical symptoms or actual illness. Suppose that someone has a consultation with the doctor after suffering a heart attack. The doctor is expected to provide an explanation as to why the heart attack occurred. Does the patient smoke, avoid exercise, drink a lot of alcohol, eat too much fatty food, have high blood pressure or a family history of heart disease? If the answer to all these questions is 'no', the next question is likely to be, 'have you been experiencing a lot of stress lately?', a question to which most people are likely to reply 'yes', especially if they are urgently seeking an explanation for an otherwise inexplicable complaint. But is the explanation a valid one or merely a convenient pseudo-explanation? Clearly the role of stress in the aetiology of physical illness needs to be investigated just as carefully as any other proposed causal agent.

For a more detailed review of arguments against stress theories and analysis of the concept as a social construct, the reader is referred to the useful summaries that have been provided by Bartlett (1998) and Jones and Bright (2001). For the rest of this chapter we focus on the evidence for associations between stress and physical illness.

DOES STRESS MAKE US MORE SUSCEPTIBLE TO PHYSICAL ILLNESS?

This topic has generated a great deal of research and it is easy to see why. If stress can be shown to be an important influence on our susceptibility to disease, then the possibility exists that interventions designed to reduce stress, or to help individuals to cope better with unavoidable stress, may lower the incidence of disease and assist the recovery of those who are already ill. The belief that stress is a major cause of physical illness is not convincingly supported by existing research findings, but neither is the opposite belief that stress plays only an insignificant role. The problem is that it is extremely difficult to carry out well-controlled research in this area and most of what has been done is open to a range of possible interpretations. We have already noted two shortcomings that apply to the majority of studies. First, retrospective studies may have a substantial response bias because people are more likely to recall experiencing stress in periods preceding illness than at other times. Second, all studies that rely on self-reports of illness may have a response bias because people who consider themselves to be suffering from stress are more likely than non-stressed individuals to interpret minor ailments as symptoms of illness.

The better designed studies that investigate the association between exposure to stress and subsequent and biologically verified illness may still present problems of interpretation. For example, it has been shown that people who are experiencing stress are more likely than others to indulge in health hazardous behaviour such as heavy smoking, a high fat diet and lack of exercise (Ng & Jeffery, 2003). Thus it could be that stress acts only indirectly as a cause of illness insofar as it influences health behaviour, rather than through direct physiological pathways.

The methodological problems that we have discussed so far are all likely to lead to inflated estimates of the strength of the association between stress and illness. Further issues have been raised that point in the opposite direction, to the possibility that current research may produce underestimates. These issues derive partly from work on the relationship between personality and illness considered in Chapter 17. One argument is that some individuals possess personal characteristics that make them resistant to the effects of stress. Among the personal characteristics that have been suggested as having this function are *internal locus of control, self-efficacy, hardiness and sense of coherence*. If stress only causes illness in people with vulnerable personalities, then it may be misleading to calculate the size of the effect of stress on illness by using general population samples that include many who are relatively insensitive to these effects. A further issue is the potential mediating effect of *social support* on the relationship between stress and illness. There is extensive evidence that people with strong networks of social support live longer and enjoy better health than relatively isolated individuals (Cohen, 2004). In seeking to explain this relationship, Cohen argues that social support has a *buffering effect* against the effects of stress, so that stress is only likely to cause illness among individuals with relatively low levels of support.

If the above considerations are valid, then stress is only likely to have a strong effect on susceptibility to illness among individuals who score low on internal locus of control, self-efficacy, hardiness and sense of coherence, and who have a low level of perceived social support. Therefore, studies of stress–illness links that are based on representative population samples may greatly underestimate the potential effects of stress because they include many individuals for whom the effect is likely to be small. Would-be researchers, who consider these issues alongside our previous observations on factors that may lead to overestimates, could be excused if they were to throw up their hands in despair. As a research topic it is not an easy one and certainly no study published to date has succeeded in overcoming all or even most of the potential problems. Nevertheless, recent and relatively well-designed studies have thrown up a number of interesting findings, particularly in the areas of coronary heart disease (CHD), cancer and infectious diseases, and to these we now turn.

Coronary Heart Disease (CHD)

Studies of the relationship between stress and subsequent CHD have produced a mixture of positive and negative findings. In a 12-year follow-up study of 6935 healthy men, Rosengren, Tibblin and Wilhelmsen (1991) found that those who had initially reported substantial stress were more likely to experience coronary artery disease subsequently, after controlling for the effects of smoking, alcohol consumption and lack of physical exercise. Similarly, in a more recent but relatively small scale 3-year follow up of 335 healthy men, Kamarck, Muldoon, Shiffman and Sutton-Tyrrell (2007) found that initial ratings of high demand and low levels of control in daily life were associated with the subsequent development of objectively measured cardiovascular symptoms. In contrast, in a six-year follow-up of 12,866 men who were at high risk, Hollis, Connett, Stevens and Greenlick (1990) found no relationship between stress and subsequent mortality. Macleod, Davey Smith, Heslop, Metcalfe, Carroll and Hart (2002) describe a 21-year follow-up study of 2623 Scottish men in which self-reported stress was strongly associated with subsequent angina but not with objective measures of CHD, including mortality. However, the diagnosis of angina is usually based on self-reported chest pain and Macleod et al. conclude that the stress–angina relationship probably results from a tendency of participants reporting higher stress to also report more symptoms.

There has also been extensive research into the possible relationship between occupational stress and CHD (Byrne & Espnes, 2008). Studies of workers in European countries, with follow-up periods ranging from 5 to 10 years, all found an association between assessments of job strain and subsequent risk of CHD (e.g. Kivimäki, Leino-Arjas, Luukkonen, Riihimäki, Vahtera & Kirjonen, 2002, and Kuper & Marmot, 2003), but Reed, LaCroix, Karasek, Miller & MacLean (1989) found no association in an 18-year follow-up of 8006 Hawaiian men of Japanese ancestry and Eaker, Sullivan, Kelly-Hayes, Agostino and Benjamin (2004) found no association in a 10-year follow-up of 1711 men and 1328 women in the USA.

In view of the conflicting nature of the findings to date, it is not possible to draw any definite conclusions as to whether stress increases susceptibility to CHD. It is to be hoped that future studies will clarify the picture. It is apparent that such studies should rely on objective measures of heart disease, rather than the diagnosis of angina, and attention will need to be given to possible differences between results for self reported stress and life event measures, for gender, socio-cultural and national differences, and for different kinds of stress.

Cancer

Studies that have considered the subsequent occurrence of all forms of cancer following periods of stress have generally failed to find evidence of an association. The few positive findings have come from small and poorly designed studies, whereas large prospective studies have produced negative findings. There is, for example, no indication of a higher cancer rate among the bereaved (Fox, 1988; Jones, Goldblatt & Leon,1984), and Keehn (1980) found no increased rate of cancer among former prisoners of war, men who had suffered extreme forms of mental and physical hardship. Joffress, Reed and Nomura (1985) found no relationship between stressful life events and subsequent cancer in a study of Japanese men living in Hawaii. With regard to the prognosis for individuals already suffering from cancer, the most impressive study involved over 14,000 women in Norway and found no increased risk of recurrence or death for those who had lost a spouse or had been divorced (Kvikstad, Vatten & Tretli, 1995) or who had lost a child (Kvikstad & Vatten, 1996). Reviewing the evidence from 26 studies on coping styles and survival and recurrence in people with cancer, Petticrew, Bell and Hunter (2002) conclude that there are few indications of significant associations.

Over the last 20 years particular attention has been given to the possible relationship between stress and breast cancer. This is understandable because breast cancer is the most common cause of premature death in women and epidemiological studies have so far failed to establish its causes. McGee (1999) notes that speculation about stress as a cause of breast cancer may be found in medical opinion at least as far back as 1893. He gives examples of relatively recent poorly designed studies that sometimes produce dramatic positive findings, while large prospective studies have not found an association. Duijts, Zeegers and Borne (2003) confirmed this conclusion in a detailed meta-analysis, with the single exception that there was a significant, albeit modest, association with death of spouse. In a further quite surprising finding, Nielsen, Zhang, Kristensen, Netterstrøm, Schnohr and Grønbæk (2005) found evidence that stress may actually reduce the likelihood of women developing breast cancer (see Box 12.4).

Box 12.4

International data on stress and breast cancer: Recent Danish evidence

Nielsen et al. (2005) followed up 6689 initially healthy women over 18 years after obtaining self-reported stress measures in 1981–3, when the women were participants in the Copenhagen City heart study. During follow-up 251 women were diagnosed with breast cancer. Surprisingly, the women with high stress levels were significantly less likely to be subsequently diagnosed with breast cancer than those with low stress levels. For each increase in stress level on a 6 point scale an 8 per cent lower risk of primary breast cancer was found. However the authors caution that lower breast cancer risk may be counterbalanced by possible effects of stress in increasing risks of other diseases.

In addition to research into the relationship between stress and the subsequent diagnosis of breast cancer, there has also been a good deal of interest in studies of the relationship between stressful life events and survival and recurrence for women who have already been diagnosed and treated. Some dramatic findings of a poorer prognosis for patients who experience stressful events after diagnosis were given considerable publicity although other researchers were reporting negative findings (see Petticrew, Fraser & Regan, 1999). All of these studies had serious methodological flaws that have been largely overcome in a major prospective study by Graham, Ramirez, Love, Richards, and Burgess (2002). They carried out a five-year follow-up of 170 women who had received surgery for breast cancer and found no evidence of a positive relationship between stressful events and increased risk of relapse; in fact they found a significant *decrease* in recurrence for women who had experienced one or more severely stressful events since diagnosis, a finding of the possible beneficial effects of stress that parallels that of Nielsen et al. (2005) described in Box 12.4.

It is unfortunate that occasional positive findings concerning stress and cancer are given a great deal of publicity while the many negative findings are ignored. Studies with negative findings may also not be submitted or accepted for publication. The assumption that stress is a cause of cancer plays a major role in justifying complementary therapies of uncertain efficacy. But, as McGee (1999) points out:

> *Recriminations over real or imagined life stress may be counterproductive for individuals with cancer and their families. They should be reassured that the available scientific evidence does not support any direct role for stressful life events leading to a diagnosis of cancer. (McGee, 1999: 1016)*

Infectious Diseases

If stress causes changes in the immune system, then this could lead to altered susceptibility to infectious diseases. We have already seen that there is extensive evidence that stress does have statistically significant effects on a variety of measures of immune functioning, but that these effects are generally well within the range of normal variation for healthy people. This leaves the question open as to whether they are sufficiently large to lead to altered susceptibility to disease. The obvious way to find out is to examine the evidence for a direct relationship between stress and the incidence of infectious disease. Over the last 20 years Sheldon Cohen and his associates have been conducting a thorough and detailed analysis of this issue.

Cohen and Williamson (1991) dismiss evidence drawn from retrospective studies and all studies that rely on self-reported illness for reasons that we have already explained. Much of the research in this area is concerned with minor viral infections, such as the common cold, and these are likely to be particularly susceptible to reporting bias. For example, a mild sore throat and headache may be self-diagnosed as a viral infection by the more hypochondriacal individual while others will attribute the same symptoms to staying up too late at a party or pollution from traffic fumes. It is easy to see how correlations may occur between such self-reported illness and perceived levels of stress, even if there is no true causal relationship between stress and susceptibility to viral infections.

A further problem pointed out by Cohen and Williamson is that stress may be associated with greater exposure to viruses, perhaps because stressed individuals seek the company of others to a greater extent than non-stressed individuals. An illustration of this methodological problem is given in Box 12.5. An ingenious way of avoiding the difficulty comes from **viral challenge studies** in which volunteers are deliberately exposed to viruses, usually cold viruses, and then followed up to determine whether those reporting high levels of stress prior to exposure are more likely than others to catch the virus, biologically verified by the researchers.

Box 12.5

Stress and exposure to viral infections: A research problem

A popular source of volunteers for researchers studying stress and illness has been medical students taking examinations, no doubt because they are the most readily available and cooperative participants to be found at institutions where medical research is conducted. However, as a method for studying the effect of stress on susceptibility to viral infections, the method is deeply flawed. Can you see why?

While it is true that taking examinations is very stressful for medical students, it is also the case that sitting in an examination hall with a large number of other students for several hours is likely to provide a high level of exposure to whatever minor viruses happen to be around at the time. Note also that, prior to taking examinations, for several days or more, students are likely to spend a lot of time alone in their own rooms preparing for the examinations, and relatively little time socializing with other students. They are unlikely to be exposed to viruses. After the examinations the reverse is the case. Students spend very little time on their own and a great deal of time socializing, once again at the mercy of whatever viruses are around. Researchers are likely to find that the students develop the symptoms of viral infections consistent with exposure at or shortly after the high stress period of taking examinations but only rarely consistent with exposure in the period prior to the examinations. They might draw the unwarranted conclusion that students have a heightened level of immunity in the stressful period prior to the examinations and a much reduced level afterwards.

Since 1986 Cohen and his associates have been conducting viral challenge studies on stress and the common cold, and Cohen and Miller (2001) summarize their findings. The first major study was conducted in the UK, where 394 participants were exposed to one of five different cold viruses. It was found that stress levels predicted increased likelihood of catching a cold, that this was equally true for all five viruses, and that the higher the level of reported stress, the greater the susceptibility. They also found that this relationship remained the same after controlling for the effects of smoking, drinking, diet, exercise and sleep quality. In a second major study, this time conducted in the USA, 276 participants were exposed to one or other of two types of cold virus, after completing the LEDS semi-structured interview, described earlier in this chapter. The main purpose of the study was to ascertain what types of stress were associated with increased susceptibility to the cold viruses. It was found that, the longer the duration of stress, the greater the probability of catching a cold, and that interpersonal problems with family and friends and work problems were the main culprits. Short term acute stress did not appear to increase susceptibility.

A question discussed frequently in recent years is whether stress is a factor in the onset or development of HIV/AIDS. Not everyone exposed to the HIV virus becomes infected and the rate at which the disease progresses varies from person to person. Since much of this variability is currently unexplained it is not surprising that there has been considerable interest in the possibility that stress is a factor. Unfortunately the topic is an extremely difficult one to investigate. It is rarely possible to know when an individual was initially exposed to the HIV virus with any degree of precision and subsequent diagnosis and disease progression is associated with much stress, lifestyle changes and the occurrence of other infections, so that it is not easy to disentangle the variables.

Following a detailed review of studies conducted from 1990 to 2007 Leserman (2008) finds consistent evidence that the occurrence of stressful life events is associated with a range of indicators of disease progression, including mortality. However, it is unclear whether this is the result of direct effects of stress on the immune system or changes in stress-related behaviour; Gore-Felton and Koopman (2008) note that the demands of coping with the side effects of medication and related illnesses may influence behaviour such as adherence to medication, substance use, sexual risk taking, and lack of exercise, all of which may cause more rapid disease progression.

FUTURE RESEARCH

1 Studies focusing on the psychological and physiological effects of different types of stress (e.g. bereavement, excessive work load, physical assault). Such research need not proceed on the assumption that very general psychophysiological models of stress are being tested.
2 Prospective stress–disease studies that combine measures of a wide variety of physiological characteristics (e.g. of the immune system) with biologically verified assessments of disease status.

3 Research into the effects of stress on the gastro-enteritic and respiratory systems in addition to its effects on the cardiovascular and immune systems.
4 Assessment of the effectiveness of therapeutic interventions designed to alleviate the psychological and physiological effects of stress for those already suffering from stress-related diseases.
5 Clarification of the relationship between stress, physiological reactions, health behaviours, social support and stress-immunizing personality characteristics using large-scale population-based studies.

Summary

1 Stress is sometimes conceptualized as environmental stimuli or life events that impinge on the individual, sometimes as a particular type of response or reaction to stressful events, and sometimes as a mismatch between demands placed on the individual and the perceived ability to cope with these demands.
2 Various methods have been proposed for assessing life events stress. The main problem is that individuals differ greatly as to what they find stressful. For this reason structured interviews are to be preferred to standardized questionnaires.
3 Investigations into physiological reactions to stress have identified many different types of reaction. Physiological reactions vary considerably from individual to individual and according to the nature of the stressor.
4 Significant effects of stress on the immune system have been demonstrated although it is not yet clear whether these effects are large enough to alter susceptibility to disease.
5 A variety of physiological and psychological effects associated with exposure to traumatic stress have been shown to exist, although it is arguable whether they can be used to establish post-traumatic stress disorder as a psychiatric condition.
6 Interactional models of stress are intrinsically attractive because they take account of individual differences in reactions to stress and methods of coping. They have the disadvantage that they depend very much on the reliability of subjective assessments and, for this reason, may not be scientifically testable.
7 Empirical studies of the relationship between stress and disease have frequently been unsatisfactory because they are retrospective and rely on self-reported stress and illness. They also frequently fail to distinguish between physiological effects of stress and influences on health behaviour.
8 Theoretical models of the relationship between stress and disease are difficult to test because they involve complex interactions between stress, social support and personality variables.
9 There is conflicting evidence as to whether stress does or does not contribute to risk of coronary heart disease.
10 There is no convincing evidence for a significant role of stress in the aetiology and prognosis for cancer.

11 Viral challenge studies have established that stress does increase susceptibility to some infectious diseases, especially colds and flu. It has not yet been established whether this association is the direct result of effects on the immune system or indirectly caused by changes in health behaviour.

12 There is evidence that occurrence of stressful life events is associated with HIV disease progression but it is unclear whether this is the result of direct effects of stress on the immune system or changes in stress-related behaviour.

13 Screening and Immunization

We are living in a world that is beyond controllability.

Ulrich Beck

Outline

This chapter considers two main forms of disease prevention available within modern health-care systems: screening and immunization. These prevention programmes are premised on the basis of controlling risk. Screening programmes are designed to identify those individuals who because of certain personal characteristics are considered as being at risk of developing a certain disease. Immunization programmes are designed to inoculate people who are at risk of developing a certain disease because of their exposure to environmental pathogens. Various social and psychological processes are involved in explaining these processes of risk management.

RISK AND RISK CONTROL

According to various sociologists we live in a 'risk society' (Beck, 1992) by which is meant that people feel that they are under threat from an increasing range of hazards. The role of the state in this later modern era is promoted as being to identify and bring under control these many hazards. Joffe (1999) argues that while risk in general is defined in the language of science, behind it is a 'more moralistic endeavour, one that routes dangers back to those responsible for them' (p.4).

The control of risk is a central theme in contemporary health care. Once again, the dominant language of science conceals a more moralistic message about personal responsibility. Preventive health care has been predicated upon epidemiological research that has estimated the statistical importance of various so-called risk factors. According to these statistical models individuals or groups who are exposed to certain pathogens, either internally or externally, or behave in a certain manner are at higher risk of developing a particular health problem. The task of preventive health programmes then becomes a task of identifying individual risks for particular health problems and bringing these risks under control. A central challenge is the extent to which people are willing to participate in these programmes.

Health psychology has contributed to attempts to explore this issue by investigating various cognitive and societal processes that can help clarify risk control actions. Research on preventive health services such as screening and immunization has been dominated by the cognitive approach that focuses on the information-processing model of the single individual in contrast to a more socio-cultural approach that considers the interaction between the individual and the socio-cultural context. Both of these approaches are considered below.

SCREENING

One of the main forms of health risk management is the early detection of disease through **screening**. This is the procedure whereby those sections of the population that are considered statistically more at risk of developing a particular disease are examined to see whether they have any early indications of that disease. The rationale behind this strategy is that the earlier the disease is identified and treated, the less likely it is to develop into its full-blown form. Within public health circles there has been sustained debate as regards the value of this strategy. A variety of criteria have been identified for deciding to implement screening (Wilson & Jungner, 1968). These include the character of the evidence on its effectiveness, benefits, harms and costs.

In Western countries there have been several attempts to introduce mass screening for a limited number of conditions that satisfy all or most of these criteria. However, despite the supposed benefits of these programmes there has been a variety of problems in their implementation. It was generally assumed by their proponents that the major problem would be the introduction of the programmes. However, the challenge has been not a technical one of implementing the programme but rather a human one concerned with the reluctance of at least a proportion of the targeted population to make use of these programmes and the unexpected negative side effects of participation. In addition, there continues to be debate about the effectiveness of particular forms of screening.

Screening for Cancer

Over the past decade there has been a concerted effort in most industrialized societies to introduce screening programmes for breast cancer. The reason for this was that it is a common health problem and there was evidence that those detected and treated at an early stage had better survival prospects. It is currently the most prevalent or the second most prevalent form of female cancer in Western society. It is estimated that one in nine women will develop breast cancer at some point in their lives. In England there were about 38,000 new cases diagnosed in 2007 and about 10,000 died from the disease (Office for National Statistics, 2009).

Partly in response to the epidemiological and medical evidence about the widespread prevalence of the disease and the association between stage of identification and success of treatment, there has been a demand not only from health authorities but also from women's organizations for the introduction of breast cancer screening programmes. Initially, the method favoured was breast self-examination (BSE) but due to debate about the accuracy of this procedure the many health authorities now favour **mammography** coupled (sometimes) with clinical breast examination by a health professional. In most countries mammography programmes have been targeted at all women aged 50 to 69 years, although some countries will also attempt to cover younger and older women.

Despite widespread support for breast cancer screening there is concern that some of the evidence on the effectiveness of particular approaches is not as definite as originally suggested. In a recent review of the evidence, Kearney and Murray (2009) highlighted the limitations of previous evaluative research. For example, evidence suggesting that BSE was of limited benefit in reducing mortality has been drawn from trials of BSE education, not of BSE practice. Instead it has been discouraged on the grounds that BSE would also lead to heightened anxiety among women and unnecessary visits to the family doctor. However, there is little evidence for the latter. Rather, there is evidence that the majority of breast cancers tumours are discovered by the women themselves. There is a need for further research on breast self-examination.

Conversely although mammography is widely promoted by health authorities, evaluations of its effectiveness have not been conclusive. The Cochrane Collaboration review estimated that the breast cancer mortality reduction due to mammography was 15 per cent rather than the 29 per cent previously reported (Gøtzsche & Nielsen, 2009). They concluded that while on a societal level mammography may be beneficial 'the chances that a woman will benefit from attending screening is very small, and considerably smaller than the risk that she will experience harm.' The authors refer to a range of harmful consequences of mammography that have often been ignored in evaluations including heightened levels of distress among the women, harmful effects of radiation, and overdiagnosis (cases that would never become clinically detectable or pose a threat to health without screening) leading to surgery and other forms of treatment. A recent commentary noted that 'it seems likely that little of the decline in breast cancer mortality since 1990 is due to mammography screening, and nearly all to improved therapy of breast cancer' (Miller, 2008: 485). The continued promotion of mammography over BSE or CBE indicates the power of the interests of medical technology.

Cervical cancer is a much less prevalent condition. In 2006, almost 3000 new cases of cervical cancer were diagnosed in the UK, making it the twelfth most common cancer in women and accounting for around 2 per cent of all female cancers (ONS, 2009). Incidence rate for cervical cancer is highest for those aged 30–40 reaching around 17 per 100,000 women. In 2007, there were 941 deaths from cervical cancer in the UK. It has been established that the human papillomavirus (HPV) is the main risk factor and a necessary cause of cervical cancer. This virus is spread particularly through sexual activity.

There is evidence that the precancerous stage of the disease can be detected at an early stage using a simple cervical smear test (pap test). Most Western countries have introduced campaigns to encourage women to attend regular smear tests, usually at least once every three to five years. Another prevention strategy has been the introduction of the HPV vaccination. In many countries a HPV immunization programme has been introduced into schools for teenage girls.

Evidence from several countries suggests that a large proportion of women do not avail themselves of cancer screening programmes. Approximately 2.2 million women aged 50–70 were invited for breast cancer screening in 2007–08 in England. Of these, 73 per cent were screened. The cervical smear test has been around for a longer period but it also has encountered a reluctance of a substantial proportion of targeted women to participate. In England the proportion of eligible women attending cervical smear tests increased from approximately 40 per cent in 1989 to 82 per cent in 1995 but fell to 78.6 per cent in 2007–08 (ONS, 2009). Several studies in the United States (e.g. Mickey, Durski, Worden and Danigelis, 1995) have shown that use of cancer screening programmes is lower among women from low socio-economic status (SES) backgrounds and, to a lesser extent, among those from ethnic minorities.

More recently there have been attempts to introduce screening for other forms of cancer. There has been particular interest in developing screening for colorectal cancer, which is the second major cause of cancer in Western society and affects both men and women. Early indications are that in various trials of different forms of screening for colorectal cancer the uptake has been lower among people from lower SES backgrounds (Wardle, McCaffery, Nadel & Atkin, 2004).

Health Beliefs and Cancer Screening

The dominant approach used by health psychologists to explain participation in screening programmes has been underpinned by various social cognition models especially the *Health*

Belief Model (HBM) and the *Theory of Reasoned Action* (TRA). (For further details, please see Chapter 6.) These models argue that it is possible to identify a certain typical belief pattern that will predict use of health services such as screening.

In the case of breast cancer screening, most of the studies have considered participation in mammography programmes and fewer have considered breast self-examination. The most frequently cited predictors of participation in both are perceived susceptibility and perceived barriers. A meta-analysis of a large number of US studies (McCaul, Dyche Branstetter, Schroeder & Glasgow, 1996) found a strong relationship between family history (actual risk) and mammography utilization but also a moderate relationship between perceived vulnerability (perceived risk) and use of mammography. In a UK study, Sutton, Bickler, Aldridge and Saidi (1994) also found a relationship between perceived risk and attendance. Stein et al. (1992) found that perceived susceptibility to breast cancer was the best predictor of future intention to participate in mammography. However, they add that 'it is questionable … whether heightened feelings of susceptibility alone will sufficiently motivate women to obtain mammograms in the absence of a physician's recommendation' (p. 458).

Various barriers to attendance for mammography, both physical and psychological, have been reported. Rimer et al. (1989) found in their survey of women in the USA that those who did not attend for mammography had a stronger belief that screening was not necessary in the absence of symptoms, a preference not to think about it and a worry about the effect of radiation. Murray and McMillan (1993b) found that perceived barriers were the most important predictor of attendance for a smear test. The barriers they considered included dislike of the health service, fear of the examination, and fear of the result. Moore, Barling and Hood (1998) found that the main barriers to both breast and testicular self-examination were embarrassment, perceived unpleasantness and difficulty, reliability concerns and concerns about the findings.

McCaul et al. (1996) found that women who worry about breast cancer are more likely to engage in various self-protective actions such as breast self-examination and attendance for mammography. Sutton et al. (1994) found a non-linear relationship with the highest attendance among women who were 'a bit worried', while those at the two extremes of worry were less likely to attend. They concluded that health promotion campaigns must balance advice to women on perceived risk with the negative impact of excessive worry. Other barriers reported include belief that a mammogram is appropriate only when there are symptoms, concern about radiation exposure, cost and access-related factors (Slenker and Grant, 1989).

With respect to benefits, several studies have indicated that the most frequently given reason for non-participation in cancer screening is that the women do not feel it necessary – they were healthy so they did not feel it was necessary to use it. It was thought that it was only necessary to have mammograms when one was sick. Potvin et al. (1995) found that perceiving one's health as good was inversely associated with recent mammography. Harlan, Bernstein and Kessler (1991) found that the most frequently given reason for not having a cervical smear was not believing it necessary.

Although the HBM has been widely used in studies designed to predict attendance for breast cancer screening the results have not always been consistent. Hyman et al. (1994) found that women who never scheduled a mammogram were more likely to perceive both fewer benefits of and barriers to mammography. They did not find any relationship between perceived susceptibility and mammography usage. They suggested that possibly other variables such as knowledge was a more important overriding factor. Many women are either unaware of the availability of the services or do not understand the character of the investigation. For example, Gregory and McKie (1991) found that many women did not understand that the early stages of *cervical carcinoma* are not accompanied by any symptoms. Similarly, Harlan et al. (1991) found that the main reason for non-participation in cervical screening was that women did not think it necessary because they did not have any symptoms.

A criticism of many of these studies of breast cancer screening is that they used a cross-sectional design. One study that used a longitudinal design (Norman & Brain, 2005) found that previous experience of breast self-examination was the best predictor of the practice. Of the HBM factors considered the best predictors were perceived emotion barriers (e.g. 'Finding breast cancer is emotionally distressing') and perceived self-efficacy barriers (e.g. 'I am confident that I can examine my own breasts regularly'). This would suggest that the barriers dimension should be considered in more detail. In addition, this study found that those women who scored low on perceived self-efficacy barriers and high on breast cancer worries and perceived severity of cancer were more likely to conduct breast self-examination excessively. It was suggested that these women may carry out more frequent but less thorough breast self-examination.

In a survey of a large sample of Scottish residents invited to participate in colorectal cancer screening, Wardle et al. (2004) found that interest in participating in screening was predicted by perceived higher risk, worry and benefits, and lower perceived barriers, fears and fatalism. They also found that those from lower SES backgrounds perceived the benefits of screening less and the barriers to it as more. Although their study was not formally based on the HBM, it does agree with other studies of cancer screening.

The *theory of reasoned action (TRA)* has met with some success in predicting cancer screening behaviour. In a large survey of women in Seattle, Montano and Taplin (1991) found that attitude and subjective norm both predicted participation in mammography as did affect, which was a measure of the emotions associated with having a mammogram. They also found that facilitating conditions (a measure of logistics that is somewhat similar to the barriers factor in the HBM) and habit (a measure of previous use of mammography) also independently predicted usage.

Several researchers have used the *Transtheoretical Model (TTM) of change* (Prochaska and DiClemente, 1983) to explore the extent of participation in screening programmes. Rakowski et al. (1992) found that women who were classified as precontemplators (i.e. those who never had a mammogram and did not plan to have one) scored higher on a measure of negative beliefs including the beliefs that mammograms lead to unnecessary surgery and that they are only advisable if you have some breast symptoms. Skinner et al. (1997) found that action/maintainers were less likely to agree with the various psychological and physical barriers to screening.

There is a tendency in these health belief studies to adopt a **deficit model** to explain non-participation in screening. Those who do not use the service tend to be characterized as lacking in knowledge and concern about their health. This is especially the case when there are attempts to explain the lower utilization by people from low SES and from ethnic minorities. An alternative perspective is to view this non-attendance within its socio-cultural context and as a form of resistance to what is perceived as an unnecessary interference in their lives or even of something that could increase the likelihood of cancer.

Meaning of Cancer and Cancer Screening

Despite the advances in the treatment of cancer, or indeed partly due to the character of these advances, cancer remains the most feared disease in Western society. Murray and McMillan (1993a) conducted a survey of a random sample of adults resident in Northern Ireland. They found that cancer was the most feared disease especially among women. The reason for this fear was because cancer was perceived as incurable and as leading to a painful death. Slenker and Spreitzer (1989) conducted a survey of a random sample of adults in Ohio. They found that not only was cancer the most feared disease but approximately half the respondents felt there was little you could do about the disease.

Several qualitative studies have explored women's fear of cancer and their reluctance to use the various screening services. Blaxter (1983) conducted interviews with women from Glasgow about their views on health and illness. She found that the women were reluctant to talk about cancer. Blaxter suggested that this lack of reference to cancer was a coping strategy used by the women to protect themselves from cancer: 'to talk about it was to invoke it, to speak briefly or in a lowered voice was to leave it sleeping'. Participation in screening would threaten this form of psychological defence.

Murray and McMillan (1988) conducted interviews with a sample of working-class women from Northern Ireland. Again they found evidence of a fear of cancer and a reluctance to interfere. One woman explained why she had not had a smear test taken:

> *I think you have the fear, you see, of it. But they say they can get it in time … but sure how do they know they've got it in time. They don't know until they start opening you up and if they open you up, it would spread. So I would say, leave well enough alone.* (Murray and McMillan, 1988: 42)

A similar finding was reported by Gregg and Curry (1994). They conducted detailed interviews with a sample of African–American low income women on their beliefs about cancer. Not surprisingly, they had a very negative image of the disease. They not only believed that cancer was deadly but they felt that if the cancer could be detected by mammography then it was already beyond cure. An example of this attitude is the case of the 62-year-old woman who had received a negative result from her pap test. Her reaction was a refusal to obtain a follow-up test:

> *My last pap didn't come back good and they want me to go over to Grady, but I didn't go because I'm afraid they're going to tell me that I've got cancer. I've just had so much experience with cancer, and I know that if they operate on me its going to get worse. So I'm just going to prolong it as much as I can … We all got to die anyway … Its too late now.* (Gregg and Curry, 1994: 524)

Balshem (1991) linked these negative beliefs about cancer with the life experiences of the women. She conducted an ethnographic study of a working-class community in Philadelphia that seemed very resistant to a health promotion campaign aimed at encouraging healthier lifestyles including attendance for breast cancer screening. When she interviewed these women, Balshem found that the health promotion message was counter to their experience. They believed that fate determined who got cancer and who survived. To look for cancer was to tempt fate; it was 'looking for trouble'. To quote Balshem: 'Challenging fate is a risky business. Cancer inspires not challenge but taboo.' Thus the women preferred not to think about cancer.

Other qualitative work would suggest that some women would prefer to conduct self-examination rather than attend a medical centre for investigation. For example, Tessaro et al. (1994) interviewed a sample of older African–American women and found that they did not think it necessary to use the health service since after self-examination they had found no lumps. Other women felt that they accepted lumps and bumps as part of life and were more concerned about other people's health rather than their own. One woman had this to say:

> *I think the black woman don't realize herself she has a tendency to leave herself alone and worry about other people. So she doesn't have a chance to examine her body and see what is really wrong with it because she is so used to bumps and knocks and hurts until she ignores it.* (Tessaro et al., 1994: 291)

Another important issue to consider is the sexual connotations of both breast and cervical cancer. Breasts are at the centre of a woman's sexual identity. Women fear breast cancer partly because of the threat to this identity (Murray and McMillan, 1988). Also, the evidence that a sexually transmitted virus may contribute to cervical cancer has been widely discussed. This has contributed to some women's reluctance to have a smear test. McKie (1993, 1995) considered the views of a sample of English working-class women. She found that in the minds of some of the women the test was associated with sexual promiscuity, a label that if they did not want to have. By avoiding the test they sought to avoid the label.

Kearney (2006) conducted a series of focus groups with women about their perceptions of cancer and cancer screening. This study was organized using feminist action research with the two groups of women meeting regularly to discuss the issues over several weeks. Over the course of this study the women became more critical of the medical establishment. One woman described the promotion of mammography as the preferred method for breast cancer screening as an example of 'boys with toys' and as reflecting the masculine preference for technology within health care in general. Another woman described as 'chilling' her growing awareness of the role of medical technology.

The women in these studies were often from lower socio-economic backgrounds or from ethnic minorities who tend to have a higher rate of cancer but a lower uptake of mammography. Rather than acquiescing with scientific medical advice these women protected themselves from the threat of cancer either by refusing to discuss it, by associating it with other people, or by characterizing cancer screening as a potential cause of the disease itself. This accords with Joffe's (1999) argument that 'people are motivated to represent the risks which they face in a way that protects them, and the groups with which they identify, from threat. They make meaning of the threat in line with self-protective motivations rather than with rational dictums' (p. 10).

Experience of Cancer Screening

Most of the research on cancer screening has concentrated on describing those factors associated with initial attendance for mammography. However, according to current guidelines women are expected to attend not once but on a regular basis. Fewer studies have examined this process of re-attendance although the evidence does suggest that rate of attendance for follow-up is lower than for initial examination (Sutton et al., 1994). One important factor in re-attendance is the woman's reaction to the initial test. Evidence suggests that this is not always positive.

Women will often find mammography screening painful. Keefe, Hauck, Egert, Rimer, Kornguth (1994) reviewed several studies on the experience of pain during mammography and found that the percentage of women reporting pain varied widely across studies with a range of 1–62 per cent. Admittedly, four of the eight studies reviewed by Keefe et al. (1994) found that at least one-third of the women reported some degree of pain during mammography. Lightfoot et al. (1994) reported that 40 per cent out of a sample of 315 women undergoing screening mammography agreed that it hurt. Admittedly, it would seem that many will accept the pain and discomfort since it is short-term and has perceived long-term benefits. However, some are less accepting and indeed feel that the pain may actually increase their risk of cancer. For example, one woman commented in Eardley and Elkind's (1990) study: 'The straight answer is – if I don't have cancer now, I'll have it after this [the pressure of the machine].' Such a viewpoint may act as a disincentive for repeat mammography.

There is also evidence that cervical screening can be uncomfortable for some women. Schwartz et al. (1989) found in her survey of women in the East End of London that 54 per cent rated having a smear test as painful or uncomfortable and 46 per cent found it embarrassing. Again, such experiences would not be expected to encourage re-attendance.

In her study in the East Midlands of England Armstrong (2007) contrasted the official discourse on cervical screening with that of the women. Whereas the former presented the smear test as a simple, painless and non-intrusive procedure the women characterized it as invasive and very uncomfortable. Armstrong, using Foucauldian discourse analysis, referred to three resources on which the women drew to challenge the official discourse. The first of these was their emotional experiences through which the women could explain their particular feelings. For example, one woman said:

> *It's just something that I just hate, I think it's, you know I don't know what it is and I know to the nurse it's nothing but I think it's just, perhaps because I'm such a private person* (p. 77).

In this case the woman is emphasizing her particular 'private' nature that led to her feeling particularly uncomfortable about the test. A second resource was the actual physical experiences in that the women drew attention to their particular physical experiences. For example, one woman said:

> *...every time uncomfortable and painful, they're just horrible ... apparently, erm, I've got a funny shape so when the instrument is put in it goes in to open your cervix up it doesn't always go properly because of the shape* (p. 79).

The third resource was the changing body that was an extension to the physical experiences. In talking about the smear test these women were not trying to find a way to avoid attending for the test but rather challenging the official medical discourse of smear test as routine.

Psychological Consequences of Cancer Screening

In the initial haste to establish screening programmes, the psychological costs in terms of increased anxiety were overlooked. Wardle and Pope (1992) classified research on the psychological impact into five groups:

1 *Impact of screening publicity*: there is limited evidence of increased public anxiety about cancer as a result of publicity campaigns for screening. Some studies (e.g. Eardley and Elkind, 1990) found that women were alarmed when they received an invitation to attend. Gram and Slenker (1992) found a lower level of anxiety about breast cancer among those who did not attend a mammography screening programme in Norway.

2 *Psychological costs of participation*: participation in screening programmes is not always positive (Eardley and Elkind, 1990). The psychological effects may be disguised because of a selection effect such that the more anxious women avoid screening. Bowling (1990) has suggested that the middle-class women who tend to attend are more comfortable with the whole medical/scientific approach, whereas women from other social groups and cultures may be much more uncomfortable.

3 *Psychological costs of diagnosis of cancer*: not surprisingly the evidence suggests that a diagnosis of cancer is met by alarm and despair. Allebeck et al. (1989) found an increased rate of suicide among women positively screened in Scandinavia. Also, a Swedish study found that the increased rate of cardiovascular mortality following cancer screening offset the cancer mortality reduction (Andersson et al., 1988)
4 *Psychological response to diagnosis of abnormality*: although the screening test does not definitively identify cancer, evidence would suggest that any indication of abnormality is usually interpreted by the woman as such. Lidbrink et al. (1995) found that women who had been recalled because of inconclusive findings on mammograms had heightened levels of anxiety. Until the possibility of cancer is ruled out these women will experience distress similar to being diagnosed with cancer. Indeed Lerman et al. (1991) found that this distress often continued after cancer had been ruled out. The extensive nature of this distress led Schmidt (1990) to conclude that the life years of mood impairment outweighed the benefits of cancer screening in terms of additional life years.
5 *Psychological costs of false positive diagnosis*: a large proportion of women with an initial positive diagnosis from the mammogram will later be declared negative on further examination. These are known as false positive cases. Not surprisingly, women will be extremely alarmed at being informed that there may be something wrong. In a three-month follow-up of women who participated in mammography, Lerman et al. (1991) found that 47 per cent of those who had suspicious readings reported that they had substantial anxiety about the procedure. This anxiety can last for a considerable period. In Norway, Gram et al. (1990) found that 29 per cent of women with a false positive diagnosis reported anxiety about breast cancer compared to 13 per cent of those with negative results. The false positive result is followed by further anxiety provoking investigation that will include clinical examination and possibly surgery. In a 10-year follow-up, Elmore, Barton, Moceri, Polk, Arena and Fletcher (1998) found that one-third of the women who obtained some positive results were required to undergo additional investigations, including *biopsies,* even though it turned out that they did not have breast cancer.

Several studies have suggested that this anxiety remains even after the women have been cleared. Lerman and Rimer (1993) found that distress and anxiety continued after further examination had excluded cancer. Admittedly, not all women continue to experience anxiety. Although most cancer agencies will attempt to reduce anxiety by speeding up the process between evidence of a positive finding on the mammogram and subsequent surgical clearance, this is not always possible. An analysis of the tests conducted on a sample of women eventually declared false positive in Sweden found that they sometimes took up to two years (Lidbrink et al., 1996).

Health Service Organization for Cancer Screening

Several studies have found that the most important factor in explaining variation in participation is the extent to which the woman's doctor recommends participation (Fulton et al.,

1991). Further, Lurie et al. (1993) found that women are more likely to undergo screening with pap smears or mammograms if they see female rather than male physicians. There is evidence to suggest that some physicians are reluctant to advise mammography for a variety of reasons including scepticism about its effectiveness in general or for certain groups of women and fear of the effect of radiation. Smith and Herbert (1993) found that family physicians did not recommend mammography because they did not think the patients would participate, because the test was not available, because they were concerned about the radiation risk and because of the cost. Physicians are especially less likely to refer older women for screening (Costanza, 1994). Further, Frazier, Jiles and Mayberry (1996) found that black women were more likely to report that their physician had not recommended participation.

A further reason for the hesitancy among some physicians in the USA as to recommending screening is fear of litigation. It has been suggested that in the USA many physicians may be reluctant to talk about screening with their patients because of the public controversy about screening guidelines (Leitch, 1995). This could lead to anxiety among some physicians, bearing in mind that delayed diagnosis of breast cancer is one of the most common causes of malpractice complaint. In the USA women who have developed cervical or uterine cancer after smear tests have won legal cases because of inappropriate treatment. In commenting on these cases Austin and McLendon (1997) state that 'this trend is having a chilling effect on those professionals in the field of cytotechnology and cytopathology and potentially threatens the availability of this procedure for many of our patients' (p. 754).

More countries and regions are now establishing dedicated cancer screening programmes with postal invitations to women to attend on a regular basis. Despite these moves a proportion of women are still reluctant to participate in these programmes. Richards et al. (2001) report a randomised controlled trial of the effectiveness of different intervention in family practices designed to increase the uptake of breast cancer screening. They found a significant increase in uptake among women who had been sent a letter from their GP and those women whose patient notes had been flagged. However, they note that the letter was the more cost effective of the interventions.

GENETIC SCREENING

The recent rapid advances in genetic research now hold out the prospect of genetic screening for different diseases. This can take various forms (see Lerman, 1997). *Carrier* testing investigates people who are likely to be carriers of the genes for such diseases as *cystic fibrosis* or *Tay-Sachs disease.* This form of testing is usually conducted in the context of reproductive decision making. *Presymptomatic* testing allows the identification of a disease before the symptoms actually develop. This form of testing is used to determine the person's risk of developing such late-onset diseases as Huntington's disease. *Susceptibility* testing is designed to test for a person's susceptibility to develop a disease, although whether or not that disease develops depends upon a variety of environmental and nutritional factors partly outside the person's control.

Although the general principles underlying genetic screening are similar to those of other forms of screening there are certain unique features. Lerman (1997) described several distinguishing features that need to be taken into consideration when investigating the psychological aspects (see Table 13.1). These factors need to be accounted for in exploring the development of these services.

Table 13.1 Features of genetic screening (Lerman, 1997: 4)

Type of information	Genetic information is probabilistic and uncertain. In some cases you can say with certainty that a person will develop a disease (e.g. Huntington's disease). In other cases it is unclear whether the person will develop the disease at all (e.g. cancer).
Medical value	Control over disease onset is limited for certain diseases (e.g. cancer) and nonexistent for others (e.g. Huntington's disease).
Timescale	The timescale is variable in that the results of genetic testing concern events that may occur far in the future.
Impact of results	The results not only affect the individual but the family since genetic susceptibility is transmitted within families.

A common feature in use of genetic testing is its perceived benefit. An extension of cancer screening programmes has been genetic testing for cancer. This is still not a very common procedure but has attracted substantial interest among certain population sub-groups. In a study in New Zealand, Cameron and Reeve (2006) found that worry about cancer was associated with interest in obtaining such a test although perceived risk was not. It was suggested that this may be due to perceived risk leading to more cautious appraisals of the benefits of genetic testing.

The importance of the patients' assessment of the benefit of the test was shown in a qualitative study of patients, patient group representatives and health professionals involved in clinical genetic services (McAllister, Payne, Macleod, Nicholls, Donnai and Davies, 2008). This study found that a common integrating theme in the patients' accounts was perceived empowerment. By this was meant that participating in the genetic testing enhanced the patients' feelings of control over their disease. As one patient group representative said:

> *Information is power, [you're] powerless if you don't have information and that's one of the problems that we've come across. Families feel isolated, they have anxiety because they have no information therefore they have no power … I mean power to make the right decisions.*

Psychological Consequences of Genetic Screening

Unlike cancer screening, genetic testing is often initiated by individuals when they suspect that because of family history they may be carriers. Thus they would be expected to be in a heightened state of anxiety. Several studies have found a reduction in such anxiety following testing (e.g., Tibben et al., 1993). However, in some cases there was evidence of subsequent psychological distress. Lawson, Wiggins, Green, Adam, Bloch and Hayden (1996) found that of 95 individuals receiving the results of a test for Huntington's disease, two made plans for suicide and seven had clinical depression. Interestingly, there was no difference between those tested positive and those tested negative. Tibben et al. (1993) found that carriers tended to minimize the impact of the test results on their futures.

There is evidence that the positive effect of screening is only short term. At six-month follow-up Tibben et al. (1993) found that one-quarter of the carriers exhibited signs of psychopathology. They continued to follow the group for three years (Tibben et al., 1997) and found that for the first six months there was a rise in avoidant thoughts and a decrease in intrusive feelings. This was followed by a reversal of this pattern. It was suggested that this was evidence of a coping strategy whereby the carriers 'dose themselves' with tolerable levels of intrusive thoughts as they begin to process and accept the test results.

Genetic screening can also have a dramatic impact on the family of the carrier. Hans and Koeppen (1989) found that partners often reacted with disbelief and denial. However, this turned to resentment and hostility as they became aware of the threat of transmission to their children. The partners can play an important role in helping the carrier cope with the diagnosis (Tibben et al., 1993).

The evidence of the psychological impact of genetic screening has been followed by calls for greater provision of psychological support services (Marteau, 1990). It is suggested that such services be made available both prior to testing such that the testees are fully aware of the issues and also afterwards so that they and their families can begin to come to terms with the findings.

Some Ethical Issues

The prospect of widespread genetic screening has provoked sustained debate about the ethical issues. Harper (1992) voiced concern that the needs of individuals and families are being made subservient to broader eugenic goals. Stone and Stewart (1996) have claimed that the voice of the public is rarely heard in this debate. They argue that the advocates of genetic screening often falsely claim that their programmes are based on the public's right to know. Yet there is little evidence that the public wants to know. Stone and Stewart also raised a variety of other questions about genetic screening such as the ability of lay people to interpret genetic information, the competence of health personnel in explaining aspects of genetic screening and the use made of genetic information. Future programme development needs to consider these and other ethical issues.

In a review of the social impact and ethical implications of genetic testing, Davison, Macintyre and Davey Smith (1994) identified three areas of popular perception that have implications for predictive testing for Huntington's disease:

1 Both positive and negative results can lead to personal and family anguish. While the former is expected there is also evidence that those who are cleared suffer from survivor guilt and a feeling they do not belong to their family.
2 Some families who inherit the gene have developed ways of deciding who in the family will be sufferers. This lay procedure is undermined by medical investigation.
3 Knowing about possible futures may decrease the quality of a person's life. They note that this finding 'is not easily accommodated within the essentially rationalist or utilitarian philosophy underlying the idea of screening' (p. 354).

One particular aspect of remaining ignorant is that it allows the maintenance of hope. Many lay people are happy to tolerate uncertainty because of the hope that they will survive.

The premise of much genetic testing is that people understand the basic principles of inheritance. However, there is evidence that this is not always the case. In a qualitative interview study of members of families at risk of familial adenomatous polyposis (FAP), which geneticists consider almost 100 per cent genetic, Michie et al. (1996) found that many referred to what they considered to be the vital role of the environment. Many of the family members also minimized the threat posed by the disease. While advising these people that they are at risk may be formally correct, it has immense implications for the future quality of their lives.

IMMUNIZATION

Immunization or vaccination is the procedure whereby those individuals who are most susceptible to contracting certain communicable diseases are administered a vaccine. This procedure is aimed at both immediate protection of individuals and also immunity across the whole community where the uptake rate is high. Over the years various vaccines have been developed for specific diseases.

In the mid to late nineteenth century several countries began to introduce vaccines to prevent specific diseases. In the UK laws were passed making smallpox vaccination of children compulsory. However, this was not always met with approval and in some countries led to the development of anti-vaccination societies (Blume, 2006). This was perhaps not surprising in view of the organization of public health practice at that time but gradually this opposition declined and a range of vaccines have been introduced over the past century. According to current public health agencies immunization is now one of the most successful examples of the primary prevention of disease. However, as McKeown (1979) emphasized, the specific impact of vaccination programmes should not be confused with the health benefits of improvements in living and working conditions.

Despite the apparent success of mass immunization programmes, a large proportion of individuals in Western societies are not immunized against certain diseases. Indeed, this has given rise to what has been described as a new anti-vaccination movement (Blume, 2006). An understanding of this participation of people in mass vaccination programmes requires an understanding of both individuals' perceptions and of the broader social context.

Psychological Models of Immunization

There is a large body of research using different social cognition models to predict uptake of vaccination. A common feature of these models is risk perception. In a meta-analysis of 48 such studies, Brewer, Chapman, Gibbons, Gerrard, McCaul and Weinstein (2007) distinguished between three dimensions of risk that were termed perceived likelihood, perceived susceptibility and perceived severity. These dimensions are detailed further in Table 13.2. A fourth dimension – perceived risk if you do not take the health-protection action – was also noted. However, since this dimension was seldom reported in research it was not included it in the meta-analysis.

Table 13.2 Dimensions of risk

Dimension	Description	Example
Perceived likelihood	Probability that one will be harmed by the hazard	If I don't get immunized, there is a high chance I'll get the flu
Perceived susceptibility	Constitutional vulnerability to a hazard	I get sick more easily than others my age
Perceived severity	Extent of harm that hazard would cause	The flu can kill you.

Source: Brewer et al., 2007

The results of the meta-analysis showed:

1 those perceiving a higher likelihood of getting an illness were more likely to be vaccinated;
2 those who perceived themselves to be more susceptible to a particular illness were more likely to be vaccinated;
3 those who perceived the severity of the particular illness to be higher were more likely to be vaccinated.

It could be argued that these relationships were simply *post-hoc* rationalizations for receiving the vaccinations, i.e. after being vaccinated the individuals justified their actions by emphasizing their perceived risk. However, the effect sizes for the prospective studies were larger than for the cross-sectional studies suggesting that this was not the case.

It was also noted that the effect sizes were larger for influenza vaccination than for other forms of vaccination. This may have been due to a variety of factors including:

1 the non-flu studies included a wide range of vaccines, each with particular perceived characteristics;
2 flu vaccination is more familiar and contributes to a clearer perceived risk;
3 the non-flu vaccine (e.g. hepatitis) requires multiple vaccinations that may attenuate the risk perception.

A final result of this meta-analysis was that the effect sizes were smaller for medical personnel. Brewer et al. suggest that this may be due to the fact that perceived risk to the medical personnel themselves may be a lesser motivator than reducing the risk to their patients. In addition, it may be the case that medical personnel are required by their employers to be vaccinated. Some evidence on the importance of health professional identity was provided by a study conducted by Falomir-Pichastor, Toscani and Despointes (2008) conducted in Switzerland. This study conducted a survey of nurses' intention to receive the flu vaccination. They found that the more the nurses identified with their profession the more likely they were to perceive vaccination as a professional duty and the more likely they were to have been vaccinated.

Recently there have been attempts to expand the various social cognition models of health behaviour to include various emotional components. In the case of immunization, this has included such emotions as worry and regret. In a study of university employees Chapman and Coups (2006) found that anticipated regret and worry were stronger predictors of vaccination than perceived risk. This would confirm that humans are less concerned about statistical estimates of risk and more with how they feel about the likelihood of something happening.

Socio-cultural Context of Immunization

As with our earlier discussion of screening, there is a need to locate the cognitive view of the risk associated with immunization within a broader understanding of the meaning of immunization and infectious diseases and the particular socio-cultural context.

The widespread introduction of immunization programmes over the past two centuries is a major example of the power of medical science. However, this power has not been accepted unquestionably. Blume (2006) has reviewed the growth of anti-vaccination movements over the past two centuries. When compulsory vaccination was introduced in the mid-nineteenth century it was opposed by a wide range of groups of people including the middle class who were concerned with threats to individual liberty but especially the organized working class that opposed the growing power of the state in the disciplining of the body. In the 1970s the public concern about the safety of the pertussis vaccine led to a substantial fall in its uptake. More recently, moves to introduce a range of new vaccines have been met with varying degrees of support.

The swine flu vaccine was introduced into many countries in 2009. Although in some countries it was enthusiastically received in others this was not the case. For example, in North America there were active campaigns for mass vaccination against swine flu whereas in the UK after some initial debate support for it declined as evidence for the severity of the epidemic declined. This is probably a reflection of the greater medicalization of American society.

Dew (1999) in his review of changing media representations of measles argues that the dominant approach of the media has been an acceptance of the medical viewpoint. However, in this age of risk (Beck, 1992) the media can become a forum for challenging the accepted medical approach. A review of British newspapers during the 1990s found a substantial increase in reportage of vaccine-related topics (Cookson, 2002). Of particular note was the finding that an increasing proportion of these articles dealt specifically with concerns about the safety of vaccines. In addition, there are an increasing number of websites devoted to critical views of vaccination. This would suggest that the debates about the value of immunization that were current in the nineteenth century are again growing. It is within this context of confusion that individuals attempt to develop an approach that is personally and socially responsible.

Health Care Providers and Immunization

Besides the media health professionals also have a very important role to play in creating a climate of support or opposition to immunization. Several projects have illustrated the variable view of medical practitioners. While public health officials may enthusiastically promote immunization other health professionals may be less supportive. For example, there is evidence that family doctors have played a role in spreading fear about particular vaccines. A report in Britain (Peckham, Bedford, Senturia & Ades, 1989) concluded that the main obstacle to parents having their child immunized was misconceptions concerning contraindications by the family doctor.

New and Senior (1991) in their interview study of mothers in North West England found that 53 out of 71 mothers who had not had their children fully immunized claimed that either their child was contra-indicated to pertussis vaccine or their doctor had advised them against it. Further, many of the mothers said they had received conflicting advice from different health professionals that led to confusion and loss of confidence in such advice. Indeed, some mothers said it was the actual attempt by the health professionals to convince them of the minimal risk which deterred them. As one mother said: 'Until they find a safe vaccine, one in 300,000 is still too large; I wouldn't play Russian roulette with my child.'

In addition to the family doctor, ancillary health staff can contribute to parents' anxiety about immunization. For example, Reddy (1989) conducted a survey of parents in a town in South East England. He found that a frequent reason given for non-vaccination was that their child was ill at the appointed time. However, Reddy found that when he telephoned the parents most of those children who were supposedly ill only had a minor cold. When questioned the parents said they were concerned about the dangers of vaccinating a sick child and that this concern had been shared by the health centre receptionist leading the parent to defer the appointment.

Immunization Among Children

Much of the debate and research on immunization has focused on children and their parents. The reason for this is that from a very early age it is expected that children receive immunization against a range of diseases such as whooping cough, polio and measles. Despite substantial health-care expenditure immunization uptake among children is not comprehensive. For example, more than two thirds of Primary Care Trusts (PCTs) in England (221 of 294) reported less than 85 per cent coverage for MMR during 2003–2004. Indeed, the coverage fell below 70 per cent in 19 PCTs (Henderson et al., 2008). As with adults, rates of immunization have been found to be lower among children from more disadvantaged communities and from certain minority ethnic communities.

New and Senior (1991) conducted detailed interviews with over 250 mothers from North West England. They found that mothers with lower educational qualifications, mothers living alone, mothers with large families and having a sick child were the best predictors of non-immunization. A study in the north of England (Reading et al., 1994) found that even after the establishment of an immunization programme, the relationship between immunization uptake and social deprivation remained. In this study the immunization of four birth cohorts between 1981 and 1990 was examined. Although there was an overall increase in uptake, the rates remained lowest in the children from the most deprived areas.

Several studies have identified a variety of reasons expressed by parents for not having their children immunized. These have been summarized by Meszaros, Asch, Baron, Hershey, Kunreuther, and Schwartz-Buzaglo (1996) under five categories which, similar to the meta-analysis of Brewer et al. (2007), focused on perceptions of risk and risk management (see Table 13.3).

In their study, Meszaros et al. (1996) attempted to assess the relative importance of each of these explanations in a questionnaire survey of readers of *Mothering*, a popular magazine read by mothers in the USA. They found that the most important predictors of parents having their child immunized were the perceived dangers of the vaccine, doubts about medical claims that vaccines are effective, omission bias, belief that physicians overestimate the dangerousness of the disease, perceived ability to protect their child and perceived assessment of the likelihood of their child contracting the disease.

Table 13.3 Parental reasons for non-immunization

Risk/benefit ratio	Perception that the risks of contracting the disease outweigh the benefits of being immunized.
Individual risk	Belief that the societal statistics that public health planners use do not apply to their child. Further, the parents believe that they can protect the child from exposure.
Ambiguity aversion	Aversity to options with ambiguous outcomes such that parents will prefer a straightforward Yes/No assessment of the likelihood of their child contracting a disease. When there is disagreement about potential risk they will err on the side of caution. Further, some parents may already be sceptical of medical information.
Omission bias	Preference for acts of omission over acts of commission.
'Free riding'	Assumption that since most of their children's peers have been vaccinated they are protected.

Source: Meszaros et al., 1996: 698

This fear of the adverse effect of immunization may be particularly high in certain communities. In a study in England (Loewenthal and Bradley, 1996) it was found that the uptake of childhood immunization was particularly low among Orthodox Jews. It was suggested by mothers interviewed that the main reason for their low uptake was their fear of a negative reaction, logistical difficulties and unsympathetic treatment by health staff. According to the health professionals, the mothers' fears were exaggerated because they lived in a close-knit community that perpetuated tales of bad reactions. A more recent study of a similar community by Henderson et al. (2008) emphasized the importance of the closed nature of the community within which rumours about the harm done by immunization were combined with a general concern about the negative influence of the outside world on the Jewish community. Table 13.4 summarizes the main findings of the study.

Table 13.4 Childhood immunization in an Orthodox Jewish community

Social network	Advice circulated through local networks
Media	Stories from mass media coupled with negative feelings about outside world
Safety	Separation of community from outside influence led to feelings of safety
Danger	Immunization was perceived a 'putting the disease in the child'

Source: Henderson et al., 2008

Besides these factors, an additional factor is the perceived relative risk. In a qualitative investigation of the views of a sample of inner-city parents in Baltimore, Keane et al. (1993) found that although some parents accepted that they or their children might be vulnerable to infectious diseases, other threats such as drugs, street violence and 'the wrong crowd' were considered more severe. Further, vaccines were viewed as only partly successful.

The continued occurrence of chickenpox was frequently cited as evidence of vaccine failure.

A frequent explanation given by mothers in several studies is the natural/unnatural distinction. New and Senior (1991) found that whereas vaccination was perceived by some mothers as unnatural, by implication whooping cough was natural and therefore acceptable. Admittedly, some other women had weighed up the benefits and risks of immunization and decided in favour of immunization. It would be expected that these were the women who were more accepting of the medical viewpoint.

This natural/unnatural distinction was also alluded to in a large German study by Weitkunat et al. (1998). They found that the most significant predictors of measles immunization were parental natural health orientation, advice of pediatrician, birth order position, dangerousness of measles, marital status, reliability of vaccination and smoking. They suggested that natural health orientation and advice of pediatricians may be interactive since individuals with a natural health orientation may select like-minded physicians. In a more detailed analysis of what they described as the subjective relevance of measles they found that those who assessed the likelihood of contracting measles as high and the latency as low were more likely to have their children immunized.

Parental concern about the possible risks of vaccination is also expressed in homeopathic beliefs. In a survey of parents of children in South West England (Simpson et al., 1995) it was found that the commonest reasons given for non-immunization of their children were homeopathy and religious beliefs. With regard to homeopathy, one parent said:

> *I believe that the body's defences are best strengthened by optimum nutrition and good hygiene and by allowing the body to experience normal illnesses without suppression during the normal course of events. To enhance this process I consult our family homeopath for acute and chronic assistance as necessary. I am actually thoroughly opposed to current practices in vaccination programmes; the onslaught of several vaccinations at once on a tiny body for the sake of convenience and getting them done, I find very disturbing. I am sure high prices are paid for this in terms of autoimmune diseases and weakened immune systems.* (Simpson et al., 1995: 227)

Taken together these findings would suggest that while parents may be hesitant about having their child immunized because of their anxiety about the potential risk, this image is compounded by media speculation and by the contradictory advice they sometimes receive from health professionals.

A final point needs to be made about a more recent form of childhood immunization. The recent introduction of HPV immunization for 11–12-year-old-girls has attracted substantial media and increasing research interest. A survey of parents of adolescent girls resident in North Carolina (Reiter, Brewer, Gottlieb, McRee & Smith, 2009) found that the various dimensions of the Health Belief Model were predictors of vaccine uptake by their daughters. Parents who reported their daughter had been vaccinated were more likely to perceive the HPV vaccine as effective, perceived fewer barriers and harms and were also likely to be confident their insurance covered the cost. Although there has been media discussion about the sexual connotations of HPV immunization they did not find that anticipated regret about greater sexual activity by their daughter was an independent predictor of HPV uptake although another study did find some evidence of such a relationship (Ziarnowski, Brewer & Weber, 2009). This is a new form of immunization and the role of socio-cultural factors is of obvious importance.

The role of industry in promoting the uptake of HPV, despite limited evidence on its effectiveness, also draws attention to the importance of the socio-cultural context. A large amount of money has been used by industry to promote this vaccine and further medicalize the lives of people (Porta et al., 2008). While psychology can identify the immediate factors that promote its uptake it needs also to consider these contextual factors.

CONCLUSIONS ABOUT DISEASE PREVENTION

The development of screening and immunization programmes designed to prevent the onset of specific diseases is premised upon a scientific model of risk with less attention given to the social and psychological features. While psychological research has tended to focus on the role of individual perceptions of risk, these need to be studied within the broader socio-cultural context.

FUTURE RESEARCH

1. Modern health care is pervaded by notions of risk control. There is a need to critique the relative contribution of various prevention programmes.
2. Perceptions of risk have often been studied in isolation without reference to their changing meaning. There is a need for research to connect risk perceptions to their socio-cultural context.
3. There are substantial social and ethnic variations in participation in screening and immunization programmes. Research needs to explain the varying meanings of these programmes to particular population sub-groups.
4. The media plays an important role in shaping lay people's understanding of vaccination. There is a need for research to consider the influence of different forms of media.
5. Genetic research has rapidly produced a host of social, psychological and ethical issues. There is a need for an expanded programme of research to investigate both professional and public perceptions of genetic screening and the impact on different populations.

Summary

1. Many countries have implemented screening programmes for different forms of cancer. Participation in these programmes varies substantially.
2. Psychological factors associated with use of these programmes connect with the socio-cultural context.
3. The health professional, especially the family doctor, is central to explaining participation in these programmes.
4. The so-called genetic revolution has many implications for screening.
5. Both the general public and people who are at risk of certain diseases have a variety of concerns about genetic screening.
6. A wide range of immunization programmes have been developed for adults and children.
7. A central feature in the uptake of immunization is perceived risk but this needs to be considered within its socio-cultural context.
8. The health professional plays a central role in deciding whether parents have their children immunized.
9. Parents have a range of fears and anxieties about childhood immunization.

14 Health Literacy

Literacy arouses hopes, not only in society as a whole but also in the individual who is striving for fulfilment, happiness and personal benefit by learning how to read and write. Literacy ... means far more than learning how to read and write ... The aim is to transmit ... knowledge and promote social participation.

UNESCO Institute for Education, Hamburg

Outline

This chapter provides a general discussion of health literacy and its relevance to health promotion. We begin with a discussion of why information dissemination is not enough in health promotion and where health literacy fits into the picture. We present some of its key definitions and the scales developed to measure it. We also discuss the skills associated with health literacy and its implications to health processes, outcomes and experience. We finally discuss possible ways to promote health literacy and equal access for all.

INTRODUCTION

One way to influence health-related behaviour is through health communication, as discussed in Chapter 11. Dissemination of health information through communication has been one of the most prominent approaches to health promotion over the past decades. This has been influenced by the changing pattern in the causes of mortality and morbidity in many developed countries. As deaths caused by infectious diseases began to decline with improvements in living and working conditions and developments in health care and treatment, the health communication message also began to shift towards personal responsibility over health where individuals were being encouraged to adopt healthier lifestyles to prevent illness and disability. The proliferation of epidemiological research linking *health conditions* (e.g. cancer and cardiovascular disease) with *lifestyle factors* (e.g. smoking, diet and lack of physical activity) helped develop the argument that individuals have the responsibility to take control over their own health by making responsible lifestyle choices (see Matarazzo, 1982). Therefore, to promote health, individuals should be provided with sufficient information that will encourage them to make 'healthy' choices and to modify certain behaviours that are considered 'hazardous'. In the end, it is assumed to be the individual's responsibility to make 'rational' choices and to look after their own health based on the information provided.

This approach to health promotion acknowledges the relevance of human agency, autonomy and personal choice in determining one's health status and treats individuals as active processors of data rather than passive responders to environmental stimuli. This frame of thought lies at the very heart of **social cognition models** (SCMs) designed by psychologists who argue that knowledge, perceived social norms, beliefs, attitudes and self-efficacy are associated with behavioural intentions and behaviour itself (see Chapter 6). Examples include the Health Belief Model (Rosenstock, 1966), the Theory of Reasoned Action (Fishbein & Ajzen, 1975), its revised version, the Theory of Planned Behaviour (Ajzen, 1985), the Protection Motivation Theory (Rogers, 1975), the Information-Motivation-Behavioral Skills Model (Fisher & Fisher, 1992), Self-Regulation Theory (Leventhal et al., 1980), Social Cognitive Theory (Bandura, 1986) and the Transtheoretical Model (DiClemente & Prochaska, 1982). As health psychology theories in the form of SCMs gained prominence in the design of health information and education programmes, researchers in the health communication field were also making developments as **social marketing** approaches paved their way to influence health information dissemination (see Chapter 11). Despite these efforts, interventions that have relied primarily on health information dissemination have often failed to achieve sustainable behaviour change and have made little impact in helping to narrow the gap in social and economic inequalities in health (Nutbeam, 2000).

WHY INFORMATION DISSEMINATION IS NOT ENOUGH

Health promotion is more than just giving people information about health. As psychologists, we understand that influencing human behaviour is more complicated than that. Just imagine this scenario as an example: you are on your way to grab something to eat when somebody from the street hands you a flyer. You took it, looked at it and got the impression that it's about obesity and how to prevent it. As a keen reader of health-related materials, let's pretend that you decided to read it and that you understood what was written there. What will you do with the information you read? Will you follow the recommendations on the flyer? If so, do you think you will be able to do it? Will you know how to do it and will you be able to do it considering your personal and social circumstances? Will you have the confidence, skills and resources to do it? If so, will you be able to maintain it? If you need to know more about it, do you know where to find it? If so, will you have access to the information you need?

While disseminating health information through communication may seem a straight-forward way to influence health-related behaviours, as shown in this series of questions, information processing, attitude formation and its relationship with behaviour intention, implementation and maintenance is not a simple process. The point is: just because individuals are given information about health doesn't mean that they will simply adopt the information given, understand it, or even read it in the first place!

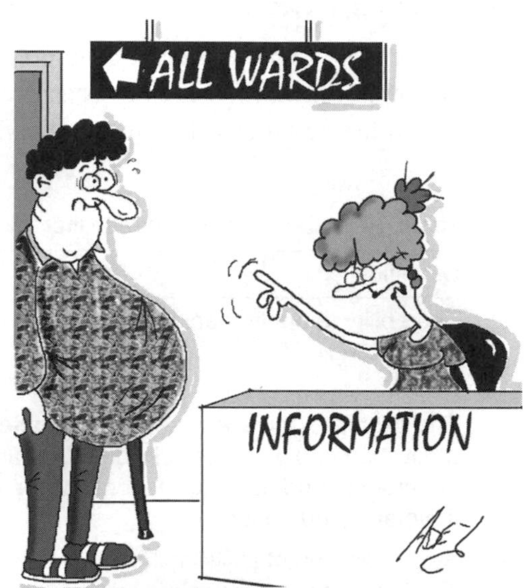

"Cardiac day patients? Up the corridor, left at x-ray, right at critical care, straight up the stairs to the fourth floor, fork left at pathology, bear right at neurology and it's dead opposite the mortuary."

Information dissemination is not enough as far as health promotion is concerned because it is based on the assumption that knowledge alone is sufficient to influence health-related behaviours and health outcomes. It assumes that individuals have equal access to information and that the information disseminated is at a level understood by its intended recipients. It also assumes that knowledge can lead to attitude change, which as assumed by SCMs, can lead to behavioural intentions, which then can lead to behaviour change itself. But the problem is that these assumptions are still unsupported. Despite efforts to improve SCMs, there is still little evidence to confirm these causal links and more than half of the variance in health behaviour remains unexplained by these models (Mielewczyk & Willig, 2007). When it comes to using information dissemination as an approach to influence behaviour change to improve health, it is worth considering whether: 1) *the information* reaches and is understood by its intended recipients; 2) *the recipients* have the necessary skills to adopt the information; and 3) *the environmental and structural conditions* are supportive of the behaviours advocated. This is where the concept of **health literacy** comes in.

WHAT IS HEALTH LITERACY?

Definition

There is no single universal definition of health literacy. As shown in Table 14.1 below, the concept of health literacy has been evolving over the past two decades. Early definitions of health literacy focused on the application of *cognitive skills* such as reading and numeracy

Table 14.1 Definitions of health literacy

Definition	Source
The ability to apply reading and numeracy skills in a health-care setting	USA National Adult Literacy Survey (Kirsch, Jungleblut, Jenkins and Kolstad, 1993)
The cognitive and social skills which determine the motivation and ability of individuals to gain access to, understand and use information in ways which promote and maintain good health	WHO health promotion glossary (Nutbeam, 1998)
A constellation of skills, including the ability to perform basic reading and numeracy skills required to function in a health-care environment	Ad Hoc Committee on Health Literacy (1999)
The degree to which individuals have the capacity to obtain, process and understand basic health information and services needed to make appropriate health decisions	Cited in the Institute of Medicine (2004) and the US Department of Health and Human Services (2000) from Selden et al. (2000)
The ability to make sound health decisions in the context of everyday life – at home, in the community, at the workplace, in the health-care system, the marketplace and the political arena. It is a critical empowerment strategy to increase people's control over their health, their ability to seek out information and their ability to take responsibility	Kickbusch, Wait and Maag (2005)
The ability of individuals to access and use health information to make appropriate health decisions and maintain basic health	Murray, Rudd, Kirsch, Yamamoto and Grenier (2007)
The ability to access, understand, evaluate and communicate information as a way to promote, maintain and improve health in a variety of settings across the life course	Rootman and Gordon-El-Bihbety (2008)

skills to *understand* and *use* information to *function* in the health-care setting. Later definitions expanded the concept to include *social skills* and applying these skills to include one's ability to *access* information to *promote* and *maintain* health. More recent definitions incorporated ideas from health promotion and empowerment to include *evaluation* and *communication* skills that can enable individuals to *improve* their health by making *informed decisions, increasing control* and *taking responsibility* for health in *various contexts*.

Levels and Domains of Health Literacy

The evolution of the concept of health literacy is reflective of the three levels of health literacy proposed by Nutbeam (2000):

- Level 1 (**functional health literacy**) – refers to the basic reading and writing skills that can help individuals to function effectively in the health-care context. Activities associated with this level involve communication of factual information on health risks and health services utilization. It is directed towards improving knowledge and usually involves the use of leaflets and other available media to disseminate information.
- Level 2 (**interactive health literacy**) – refers to the development of personal skills in a supportive environment to improve personal capacity to enable individuals to act independently based on knowledge. It focuses specifically on improving motivation and self-confidence to act on the advice received. Examples of activities in this level include tailored health communication, community self-help and social support groups.
- Level 3 (**critical health literacy**) – refers to the ability to critically evaluate and use information to actively participate in health promotion. Activities associated with this level involve cognitive and social skills development, as well as capacity building to enable individuals and communities to act on the social and environmental determinants of health.

Zarcadoolas, Pleasant and Greer (2005) similarly proposed a multidimensional framework for understanding health literacy which organized the concept into four central domains (p.197):

- Domain 1 (**fundamental literacy**) – refers to reading, writing, speaking and numeracy skills
- Domain 2 (**scientific literacy**) – refers to competence with fundamental scientific concepts, comprehension of technological complexity, scientific uncertainty, and an understanding that rapid change in the accepted science is possible
- Domain 3 (**civic literacy**) – refers to skills that enable people to become aware of public issues and to become involved in the decision-making process
- Domain 4 (**cultural literacy**) – refers to the ability to recognize and use collective beliefs, customs, worldview and social identity in order to interpret and act on health information.

Measuring Health Literacy

Various standardized psychometric scales have been developed over the years to measure health literacy. As shown in Table 14.2 , early assessment tools on health literacy formed part of general literacy tests that measure word recognition, reading comprehension and numeracy. As health literacy research gained momentum, assessment tools became more specific to health-care contexts. In the US, two of the most commonly used tools to assess health literacy levels of patients in clinical practice are the Rapid Estimate of Adult Literacy in Medicine (REALM, Davis et al., 1993) and the Test of Functional Health Literacy in Adults (TOFHLA, Parker, Baker, Williams, Gazmararian & Nurss, 1995). Box 14.1 and 14.2 show sample extracts from these tests.

Table 14.2 Health literacy scales

Tool	Description
The Instrument for the Diagnosis of Reading (IDL)	A bilingual (English–Spanish) tool. Participants are asked to read a text at different grade levels and are later tested by being asked a series of multiple-choice questions of varying difficulty about the material (Blanchard, Garcia & Carter, 1989)
The Slosson Oral Reading Test-Revised (SORT-R)	Often used in educational settings but also appropriate in medical contexts. Participants are asked to pronounce a word from a list of 20 words representing each grade level from kindergarten to high school. Words are counted as incorrect if 1) they are mispronounced or omitted; 2) the individual takes longer than 5 seconds to pronounce the word, or; 3) more than one pronunciation is given (Slosson, 1990)
Wide Range Achievement Test (WRAT)	A nationally standardized achievement test consisting of three sub-tests: 1) *reading* which involves word recognition, naming letters and pronunciation of printed words; 2) *spelling* which involves copying marks resembling letters, writing one's name, and printing words; and 3) *arithmetic* which involves counting, reading number symbols, and oral and written computation (Jastak & Wilkinson, 1993)
Rapid Estimate of Adult Literacy in Medicine (REALM)	A word recognition test using a laminated sheet containing 22 common medical words or layman's terms for body parts and illnesses. The words are written in large font and arranged in order of difficulty. Patients are asked to pronounce each word aloud (Davis et al., 1993)
Test of Functional Health Literacy in Adults (TOFHLA)	This tool assesses both reading comprehension and numeracy skills. To assess *reading skills*, participants are asked to complete missing sections of selected passages about an upper gastrointestinal series, a Medicaid application, and a procedure informed consent form. To test *numeracy skills*, participants are asked about directions on prescription labels, blood glucose values, and appointment slips. Although it is comprehensive, administering this test can be time consuming thus a shortened version was later developed (Parker et al., 1995; Baker, Williams, Parker, Gazmaraian & Nurss, 1999)

Table 14.2 (Continued)

Tool	Description
The Medical Terminology Achievement Reading Test (MART)	This was modelled after the WRAT but was later developed to measure health literacy in a way that is less threatening to patients. A variety of medically related words are printed in small font and pasted on a prescription bottle. The bottles are covered with a glossy finish. To make this test less intimidating to participants, examiners explain that the small print and the glare from the glossy bottle may make words difficult to read (Hanson-Divers, 1997)
The Peabody Individual Achievement Test-Revised (PIAT-R)	This tool assesses both recognition and comprehension. The *recognition* sub-test has varying levels of difficulty from preschool through high school. The *comprehension* sub-test contains 66 items and is given only if the participant completes a majority of the preschool items on the recognition test. In this section, participants are asked to read a sentence silently and then choose, from among four pictures, the one that best represents its meaning. The sentences become progressively more difficult, and the test is stopped when five of seven consecutive items are answered incorrectly (Markwardt, 1997)
Literacy Assessment for Diabetes (LAD)	The LAD is a diabetes-specific literacy test. It is a word recognition test with a word list ordered by difficulty. It measures a patient's ability to pronounce terms that they would encounter during clinic visits and in reading menu and self-care instructions. The majority of the terms are on a 4th-grade reading level, with the remaining words ranging from the 6th- through 16th-grade levels (Nath, Sylvester, Yasek & Gunel, 2001)
Newest vital sign (NVS)	This uses a nutrition label from an ice cream container where patients are asked 6 questions about how they would interpret and act on the information contained on the label (Weiss et al., 2005)
E-health literacy scale	A tool measuring combined knowledge, comfort and perceived skills at finding, evaluating and applying electronic health information to health problems (Norman & Skinner, 2006)
Single Item Literacy Screener (SILS)	A single item instrument designed to identify patients who need help with reading health-related information. The question asked here is *'How often do you need to have someone help you when you read instructions, pamphlets, or other written material from your doctor or pharmacy?'* Possible responses range from 1 (never) to 5 (always). The authors identified the cut-off point as '2' to capture potential patients needing assistance (Morris, MacLean, Chew, Littenberg, 2006)
Nutritional Literacy Scale (NLS)	It is designed to evaluate patients' understanding of current nutrition labels. The test includes actual nutritional labels that the patients refer to. The first 12 questions are open-ended, and the last 12 require the patient to decide between two response options. It can be administered without a time limit (Diamond, 2007)

Sources: Andrus and Roth, 2002; Gray and Coughlan, 2009

Box 14.1

Sample prompts for the Test of Functional Health Literacy in Adults (TOFHLA)

Prompt 1: The label will need to be printed and pasted on an actual prescription bottle which will be handed over to the participant and be asked the following questions:

- If you take your first tablet at 7:00am, when should you take the next one?
- And the next one after that?
- What about the last one for the day, when should you take that one?

GARFIELD IM 16 Apr 93
FF941858 Dr. Lubin, Michael

PENICILLIN VK
250MG 40/0
Take one tablet by mouth four times a day 02 (4 of 40)

Prompt 10: The label will be printed in a laminated card and handed over to the participant who will be asked this question:

Let's say that after deductions, your monthly income and other resources are $1,129. And let's say you have 3 children. Would you have to pay for your care at that clinic?Cipteluderi

You can get care at no cost if after deductions your monthly income and other resources are less than:

$581 for a family of one
$786 for a family of two
$991 for a family of three
$1,196 for a family of four
$1,401 for a family of five
$1,606 for a family of six

Source: Adapted from Parker et al. (1995) cited in Institute of Medicine (2004)

Although these scales have been useful in clinical practice and in research, the skills being assessed by these measures are limited. As will be discussed in the next section, health literacy is more than just reading, comprehension and numeracy; but involves a set of skills needed for people to gain control over the factors that influence health.

HEALTH LITERACY SKILLS

The World Health Organization (1986) defines **health promotion** as 'the process of enabling people to increase control over, and to improve, their health (p.1).' It is recognized that this process requires

BOX 14.2

Rapid Estimate of Adult Literacy in Medicine (REALM)

Patient Name/ Subject # ____________ Date of Birth ____________ Reading Level ____________
Date ________ Clinic _____ Examiner ____________ Grade Completed ____________

List 1	List 2	List 3
Fat	Fatigue	Allergic
Flu	Pelvic	Menstrual
Pill	Jaundice	Testicle
Dose	Infection	Colitis
Eye	Exercise	Emergency
Stress	Behaviour	Medication
Smear	Prescription	Occupation
…	…	…

SCORE
List 1 ____________
List 2 ____________
List 3 ____________
Raw Score ____________

the *strengthening of skills and capabilities* of individuals, communities and social groups by building *healthy public policy*, *creating supportive environments*, *strengthening community actions*, *developing personal skills*, and *reorienting health services* (Nutbeam, 1998). Thus, as shown in Table 14.3, health promotion goes beyond disseminating information and necessitates the development of numerous skills, including the ability to read, listen, comprehend and evaluate information to make informed choices; to implement the choices made; and to enable mobilization of action to improve social conditions to prevent disease and improve health.

HEALTH LITERACY, HEALTH OUTCOMES AND EXPERIENCE

The association between health literacy and health outcomes is clearly established. In a systematic review of the literature, DeWalt, Berkman, Sheridan, Lohr and Pignone (2004) showed

Table 14.3 Skills and tasks relevant to health promotion

Skills	Examples of tasks relevant to health promotion
Reading and comprehension	• Understanding written health information materials • Making sense of doctor's prescription, food labels, health risk precautions • Understanding policies on patient's rights
Listening and comprehension	• Understanding spoken medical advice • Making sense of significant others' health concerns • Listening to specific health issues relevant to the community
Speaking	• Reporting health status to health professional • Asking for clarifications regarding health condition or treatment • Communicating health information with others • Providing patient perspectives on how to improve health care
Writing	• Keeping personal records of medication intake • Communicating with health professional by e-mail • Writing a petition to improve equal access to health care for all
Numeracy	• Timing and applying appropriate dosage for prescribed medications • Budgeting personal finances to accommodate 'healthy living' • Interpreting relevance of statistical information concerning a public health issue
Analytical	• Making sense of medical test results • Evaluating credibility and accuracy of health information • Assessing implications of public issues on health
Decision-making	• Providing informed consent for treatment procedures • Working as partners with relevant professionals in the design, implementation and evaluation of health programmes • Voting on organizational or government policies affecting health
Navigation	• Locating health facilities • Navigating oneself through the health-care system
Negotiation	• Scheduling doctor's appointments • Negotiating treatment options • Negotiating ways to improve personal and public health
Awareness	• Being aware of physical symptoms and personal health status • Recognizing social barriers and opportunities to promote health • Recognizing collective understanding and shared social beliefs to improve environmental and structural conditions affecting health
Advocacy	• Obtaining information and resources needed to promote health • Mobilization of action to address public health issues

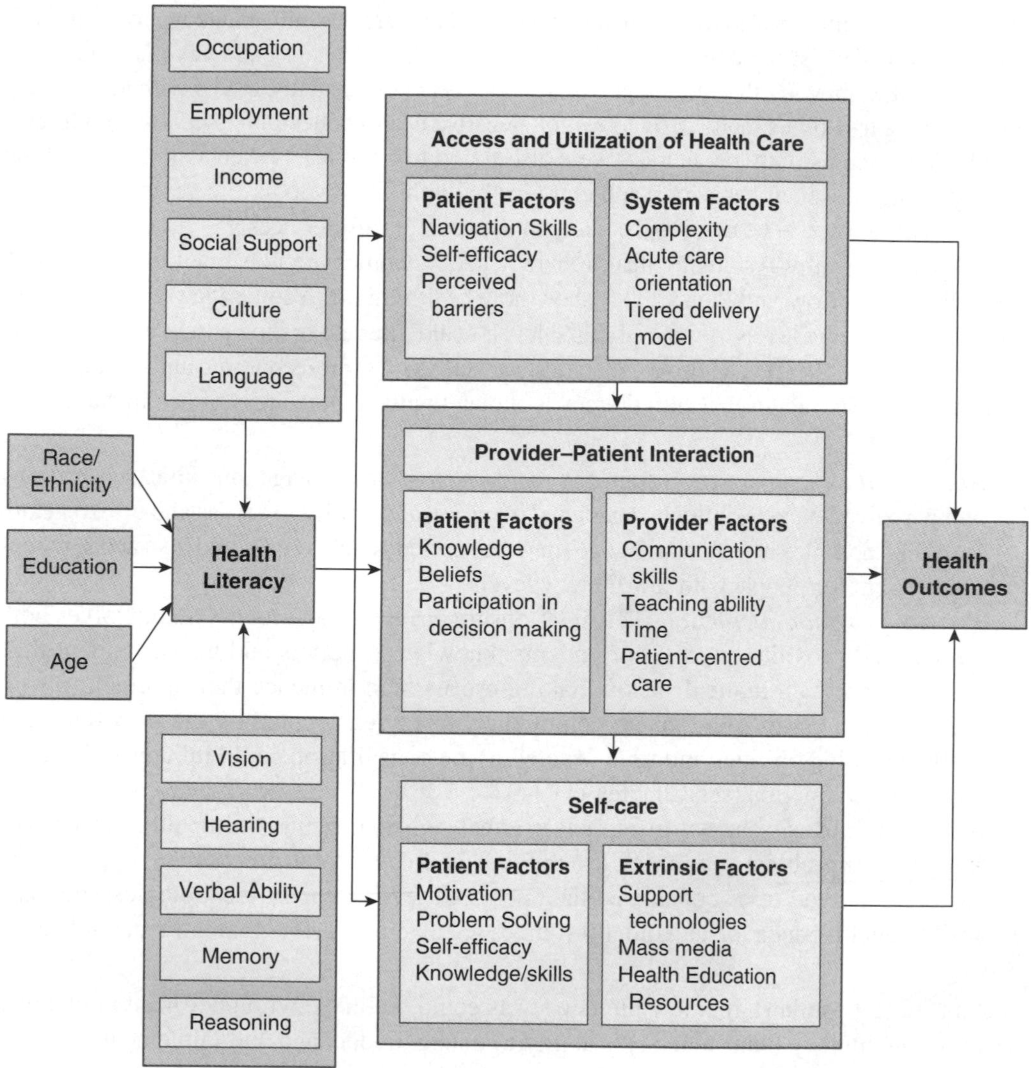

Figure 14.1 Causal pathways between limited health literacy and health outcomes
Source: Paasche-Orlow & Wolf, 2007: S21; Reproduced with permission

that patients with low literacy tend to have poorer health outcomes, including knowledge, intermediate disease markers, measures of morbidity, general health status, and use of health resources. Patients with low literacy were also found to be 1.5 to 3 times more likely to experience a given poor outcome. In a follow-up systematic review on health literacy and child health outcomes, DeWalt and Hink (2009) also found that children with low literacy had worse health behaviours and outcomes than those with higher literacy levels. Parents with low literacy levels also had less health knowledge and had behaviours that were less advantageous for their children's health. This is supported by Sanders, Federico, Klass, Abrams and Dreyer's (2009) systematic review showing that after adjusting for socio-economic status, adults with low literacy levels are 1.2 to 4 times more likely to exhibit negative health behaviours that affect children's health. Adolescents with low literacy were also found to be at least twice as likely to exhibit aggressive or antisocial behaviour, and chronically ill children who have caregivers with low literacy were shown to be twice more likely to use more health services.

The possible pathways linking health literacy and outcomes are illustrated in Figure 14.2. Here, Paasche-Orlow and Wolf (2007) show how health literacy can be viewed at both individual and systemic levels. At an individual level, health literacy is shown to be influenced by the person's sensory and cognitive capacities, as well as by socio-economic and demographic factors. At a systemic level, health literacy is shown to affect three areas of health care:

1 *Access and utilization*: It is recognized that factors such as navigation skills, self-efficacy and perceived barriers influence patients' intention and ability to access and utilize health care. The complexity, orientation and how the service is delivered could also act as potential barriers for people with low literacy levels.
2 *Patient–provider interaction*: This relationship is a two-way process that involves both patient and provider factors. For patients, knowledge, beliefs and how confident they feel to participate in the decision-making process can influence their interaction with the provider. On the other hand, communication styles adopted by the provider, their skills, teaching abilities and time devoted to the consultation could influence the quality of the interaction (see Chapter 11).
3 *Self-care*: Intrinsic and extrinsic factors affect self-management of health. Motivation, knowledge, problem-solving skills, the will and capacity to implement self-care are factors that need to be considered on a personal level. Support technologies, the mass media, health education and other resources are external factors that influence self-care.

It has been postulated that low literacy levels could be linked with poor health outcomes because low literacy limits a person's ability to obtain, understand and implement information for health care (Pignone & DeWalt, 2006). Although the relationship between literacy and adherence is still unclear (Powers & Bosworth, 2006), it is not surprising how low literacy can cause difficulties because of the patient's decreased ability to identify medications (Kripalani, Henderson, Chiu, Robertson, Kolm & Jacobson, 2006) or interpret prescription warning labels (David et al., 2006). Despite this, patients with low literacy levels may be reluctant to seek assistance when experiencing difficulties due to the stigma and shame attached with low literacy as expressed by patients in Figure 14.2 (Baker & Pitkin, 1996). It is important for health-care providers to be able to provide adequate support for people with low levels of health literacy when communicating health information. Being able to identify those who might need more support, without causing shame or intimidation to the patient,

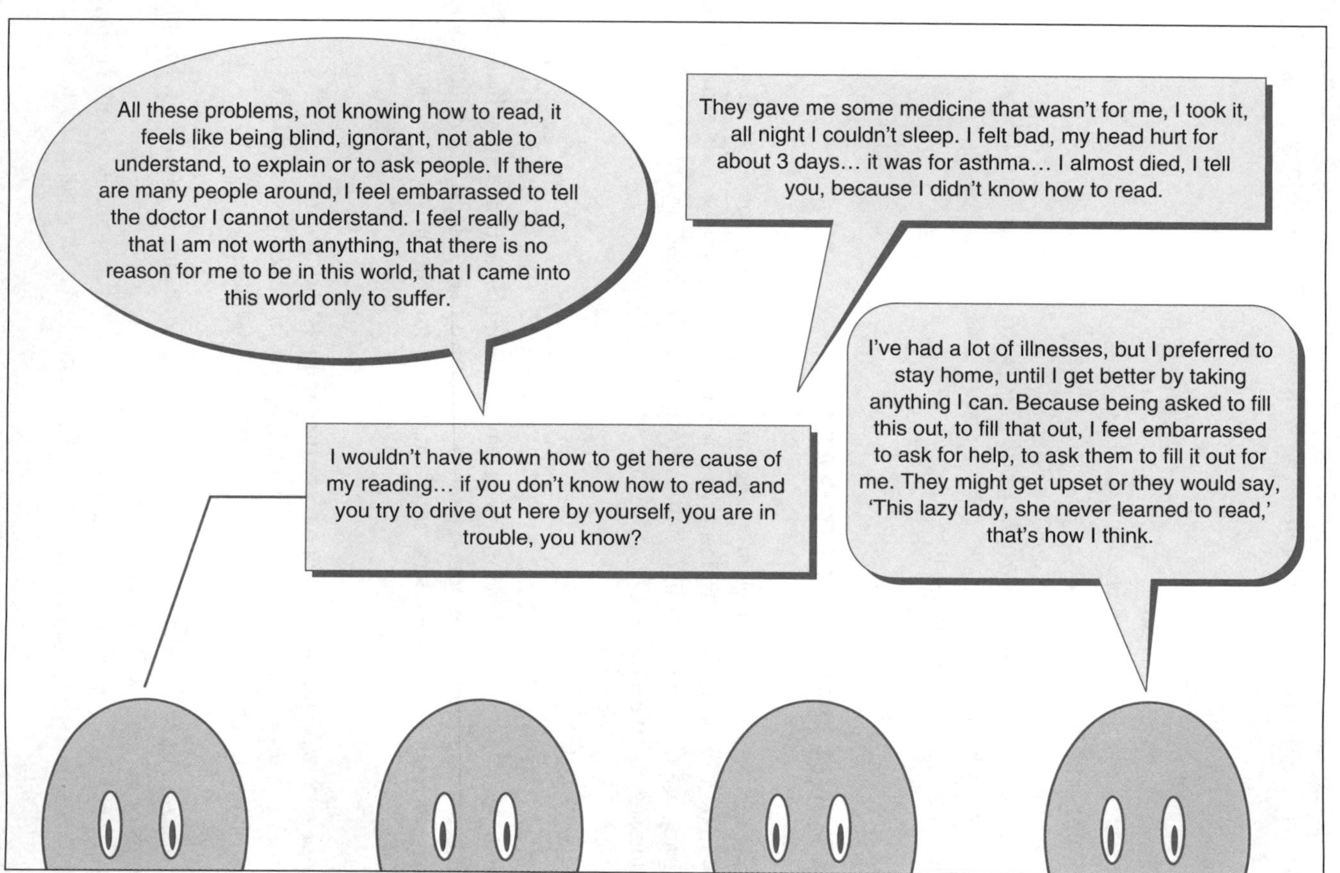

Figure 14.2 What patients with low literacy levels have to say interview extracts from Baker & Pitkin (1996: 330–2)

is a good step forward. The following are some behaviours suggestive of inadequate health literacy skills (Baker et al., 1996, cited in Safeer & Keenan, 2005: 646):

- Asking staff for help
- Bringing along someone who can read
- Inability to keep appointments
- Making excuses (*'I forgot my glasses'*)
- Non-compliance with medication
- Poor adherence to recommended interventions
- Postponing decision making (*'May I take the instructions home?'* or *'I'll read through this when I get home'*)
- Watching others (mimicking behaviour)

PROMOTING HEALTH LITERACY

As discussed earlier, when it comes to using information dissemination as an approach to health promotion, it is worth considering the following factors especially when levels of health literacy are taken into account: 1) the information; 2) the recipients; and 3) the environment and structural conditions.

Consider the Information: Improve Communication

In the health-care setting, it is important for health professionals to be aware of health literacy levels when communicating information to ensure effective interactions. Below are some recommended strategies to improve interactions and support for patients with low health literacy (Weiss, 2007: 29):

- *Slow down.* Speak slowly and spend some time talking with patients.
- *Use plain, non-medical language.* Use easy to understand language and avoid medical jargon. Table 14.4 lists some suggested plain language alternatives to medical terms.
- *Show or draw pictures.* Visuals can help enhance understanding and recall. Simple line drawings or cartoons will suffice.
- *Limit the amount of information provided – and repeat it.* Information is easier to understand and to remember when given in small doses. Repeating and highlighting key tasks can help enhance recall.
- *Use the 'teach back' technique.* Confirm that the information was understood by asking patients to repeat or demonstrate what they have been told.

Table 14.4 Plain language alternatives to medical terms

Medical term	Translation to plain language
Analgesic	Pain killer
Anti-inflammatory	Less swelling and irritation
Benign	Not cancer
Carcinoma	Cancer
Cardiac problem	Heart problem
Cellulitis	Skin infection
Contraception	Birth control
Enlarge	Get bigger
Heart failure	Heart isn't pumping well
Hypertension	High blood pressure
Infertility	Can't get pregnant
Lateral	Outside
Lipids	Fats in the blood
Menopause	Stopping periods
Menses	Period
Monitor	Keep track of, keep an eye on
Oral	By mouth
Osteoporosis	Soft, breakable bones
Referral	Send you to another doctor
Terminal	Going to die
Toxic	Poisonous

Source: Weiss, 2007: 31

- *Create a shame-free environment: Encourage questions*. Promote an attitude of helpfulness in the practice. Make patients feel comfortable about asking questions. The Ask-Me-3 programme can be a useful guide for patients and practitioners (see Key Study).

When it comes to written information, the following points can be considered when designing materials:

- ***Know your audience***. Consider their backgrounds, age, culture, interests, skills and literacy levels and develop the material appropriately.
- ***Keep focused***. Bear in mind what the material aims to achieve. Highlighting the information you want to communicate would be helpful to keep your readers focused. Too much information on the material can be confusing or can be off-putting to read.
- ***Consider the material's readability***. Is the material reader-friendly? Factors affecting this include the words used, the complexity of the sentences, the lay-out, font size, the use of

diagrams or tables, writing style and tone. There are **readability tests** that can be used to assess readability. An example is the *Flesch-Kincaid readability test* which weighs word lengths and sentence lengths in a text to provide a statistical measure of how easy or difficult it is to read. Although readability tests are useful, it would be more meaningful to also pilot materials with recipients to assess its readability rather than relying merely on numerical figures.

Consider the Recipient: Build Capacity

As discussed earlier, health promotion requires the development of various skills necessary to enable individuals and communities to take control over the determinants of health. Thus, **capacity building**, literacy skills development and health promotion are intertwined processes which are also linked with activities related with **empowerment** and **community development** (see Chapter 15). If skills are the tools individuals need to function in society, then developing people's skills can help enhance experiences and opportunities of individuals and the community in general. Capacity building through skills development has been strategically used for health promotion purposes, as shown in the case study on *Skilled for Health* in Box 14.3.

KEY STUDY The Ask-Me-3 Programme

The Ask-Me-3 programme is a patient education programme advocated by the US National Patient Safety Foundation designed to promote communication between patients and health-care providers. In this programme, patients are encouraged to ask health service providers (e.g. doctors, nurses, pharmacists, etc) these three questions:

What is my problem?
What do I need to do?
Why is it important for me to do this?

Miller et al. (2008) carried out a modified, separate-sample, pretest–posttest study to evaluate this programme. One-hundred and six community-dwelling, well-elderly participants were recruited from senior centres in Polk County between March 2006 and February 2007. Information on demographic characteristics, regularity of health care and medication use, health literacy level and multidimensional health locus of control were collected. Participants were randomly allocated to one of the three groups – pretest–posttest, pretest only; and posttest only – during each of the 12 'Ask-Me-3' educational sessions. The evaluation showed that the Ask-Me-3 programme increased the proportion of participants planning to or actively bringing a list of current medications when visiting the pharmacist ($p \leq 0.025$). It was concluded that this programme is a practical tool that can reinforce the principles of clear health communication. However, it was recommended that the programme needs to be evaluated in diverse pharmacy and health care settings with patients at high risk from poor health communication.

Source: http://www.npsf.org/askme3/

Box 14.3

Skilled for Health

Skilled for Health (SfH) is a UK-based initiative which aims to develop literacy, language and numeracy skills in a health improvement setting. It aims to address both the low-level skills and health inequalities prevalent within hard to reach communities by helping adult learners to gain a better understanding of their health and how to better utilize health services through the combination of basic skills development and health education. SfH is a partnership between the Department of Health (DH), the Department for Innovation, Universities and Skills (DIUS) and the learning and health charity ContinYou. The programme had two phases:

- Phase 1 focused on developing the SfH resources and was set in eight community-based projects using a variety of settings and user groups.
- Phase 2 expanded the learning from Phase 1 and applied the resources within different sectors and groups, including army families, prisons, museums, libraries and archives, the Nottingham City Council, Royal Mail, and Gateshead Health NHS Foundation Trust. Eleven community sites around the country also took part.

In April 2009, the final evaluation report for SfH was published and showed that the intervention managed to target and recruit individuals who do not usually participate in public health or adult learning programmes, thus showing the programme's effectiveness to reach marginalized groups. The motivation to learn basic skills was shown to be the key factor in engaging the participants. For participants whose first language was not English, learning the language had been a significant incentive for participation. The evaluation also reported increases in health knowledge, particularly in the areas of healthy eating, physical activity, smoking, alcohol consumption and looking after their mental health. Participants also reported that SfH positively affected their health choices. For example, about 85 per cent of learners who completed an SfH course reported that they were eating more healthily. The skills and knowledge participants developed were also passed on to their families. Retention and progression rates were also high.

Source: www.continyou.org.uk

Another way to build capacity through skills development is by engaging community members in **participatory action research** (see Chapters 5 and 15). Actively involving community members in the PAR process can help develop skills and raise critical consciousness at the same time. Thus the process helps develop all three levels of literacy (i.e. functional, interactive and critical) proposed by Nutbeam (2000). A case study using PAR to enhance skills and expand health literacy through the use of videos is shown below.

Consider the Environment: Simplify Health Care and Promote Healthy Communities

It has been acknowledged that health-care systems currently rely on complex processes that can be tedious even to those with high levels of health literacy (DeWalt, 2007).

Case Study

INTERNATIONAL CASE STUDY Expanding health literacy: Indigenous youth creating videos

This study is a participatory action research project with a group of Canadian indigenous youth and their teachers which aimed to generate knowledge about the community's health concerns through the creation of videos. Developed over a span of six years, the project used video making as a tool for artistic expression, as well as for the discovery of self and others. The project used a youth participation model and is based on a theoretical approach that integrates indigenous health and health literacy. The specific objectives of the project were (p.182):

1 To facilitate indigenous student investigation of topics that they perceive to be of importance for the promotion of healthy living and injury prevention;
2 To develop strategies for injury prevention and health promotion for indigenous young people that are based upon health concerns identified by the youth themselves;
3 To develop leadership skills and research expertise among indigenous young people through participation in conducting research about health and wellness; and
4 To develop an understanding of ways in which participatory action research can be used to develop school and community-based initiatives for indigenous health promotion.

In the course of producing the videos, participants also developed critical consciousness about community, culture, confidence and control thus expanding the notion of health literacy to include cultural conceptions of health and wellness. In the process, this action research improved health literacy not only by raising awareness on health and wellness but also by enhancing personal and community capabilities to enable the promotion of health.

Source: Stewart, Riecken, Scott, Tanaka & Riecken, 2008

There is a need to simplify these systems to enable both patients and practitioners to operate effectively within this environment. Paasche-Orlow, Schillinger, Greene and Wagner (2006) suggested the following recommendations to address the organization of health care:

- *Adopt a patient-centred system.* It is advisable to tailor health-care messages and interventions to suit the needs of patients. Actively involving patients in goal-setting and decision-making can help improve the effectiveness of health promotion and health-care services.
- *Simplify and explain procedures clearly.* Current procedures need to be simplified and explained clearly to enable both patients and practitioners to effectively navigate themselves through the system. Minimizing bureaucratic procedures and using plain and simple language to explain how the system operates will be beneficial to all regardless of health literacy level.
- *Develop structures that incentivize programmes that meet quality standards for vulnerable populations.* Developing structures that reward investments in technologies and interventions that support patient education, engagement and self-management, especially those most in need will be helpful in addressing social inequalities in health.

In addition to improvements in the health-care system, there is also a need to consider the wider social and environmental conditions that influence health-related behaviours of individuals and community members. Considering that health literacy is about having the capability and skills to implement informed choices to promote health, it is important that the environment is supportive of the decisions made by individuals that encourage healthy living.

ADVOCATING LITERACY FOR ALL

According to the Education for All Monitoring Report (EFA, 2008), there are an estimated 776 million adults who lack basic literacy skills; about two-thirds of whom are women. It is perhaps a misconception that poor literacy is a problem that exists only in developing countries. On the contrary, even the most economically advanced societies also suffer from this problem. In the Organization for Economic Cooperation and Development's (OECD) final report on the *International Adult Literacy Survey*, it was reported that 14 out of the 20 countries surveyed had at least 15 per cent of its adult population with very poor literacy skills. In fact, even in the country with the highest score on the test (Sweden), 8 per cent of its adult population still encountered severe literacy deficits (OECD, 2000).

It has been recognized that unequal access to literacy often coexists and interacts with other social vulnerabilities (Paasche-Orlow et al., 2006). In the US for example, those who are at risk of low literacy levels include indigenous communities, immigrants, racial and ethnic groups, those older than 65 years with limited schooling, low-income communities, acutely ill individuals and those who consistently encounter stressful hospital settings (Marks, 2009). On a global scale, such inequalities exist between developed and developing countries. In 2006, for example, pre-primary gross enrolment ratios averaged at 79 per cent in developed countries, whereas in developing countries it was 36 per cent. In sub-Saharan Africa, the level was as low as 14 per cent. These global disparities are mirrored in inequalities within countries where some children from the wealthiest 20 per cent of households are five times more likely to attend pre-school programmes than those from the poorest 20 per cent (EFA, 2008).

Literacy for All has been one of the main campaigns advocated by the international community. It was envisioned that for the United Nations Literacy Decade (2003–2012) significant progress will be made towards the EFA Dakar goals where *useable literacy, numeracy and other basic competencies* will be attained, *dynamic literate environments* will be encouraged, and *quality of life* will be improved as an impact of developing literacy (see Box 14.4).

Although some progress has been achieved since the development of the Dakar Goals in 2000, there are still challenges that pervade the accomplishment of these goals. These include (EFA, 2008):

- *Lack of political will* (e.g. low prioritization; inadequate policies and financial resources for literacy)
- *Lack of strategy and planning* (e.g. insufficient planning, coordination, organizational frameworks and partnerships)
- *Poor quality* (e.g. low quality of literacy provision)
- *Lack of community-based information* (e.g. poor understanding of context; insufficient data on literacy levels and needs; poor monitoring and evaluation; lack of examples of good practice)

It is therefore important to advocate more strongly for political commitment and financial resources to support activities towards equal access to literacy. Increased and improved effectiveness of international aid for basic education could be added to the global agenda to address this issue. In addition, as recognized by the EFA (2008), it is also important to understand the interconnectedness of *upstream functions* (e.g. planning, management, research and capacity development) and *downstream applications* (e.g. facilitators' training, material preparation, instructional methods, and regular

Box 14.4

The Dakar Goals

In April 2000 over a thousand delegates from 164 nations gathered in Dakar, Senegal as part of the international community's commitment to promote Education for All. Here are the Six Goals agreed from this convention:

1 Expand and improve comprehensive early childhood care and education, especially for the most vulnerable and disadvantaged children;
2 Ensure that by 2015 all children, particularly girls, children in difficult circumstances and those belonging to ethnic minorities, have access to and complete free and compulsory primary education of good quality;
3 Ensure that the learning needs of all young people and adults are met through equitable access to appropriate learning and life skills programmes;
4 Achieve a 50 per cent improvement in levels of adult literacy by 2015, especially for women, and equitable access to basic and continuing education for all adults;
5 Eliminate gender disparities in primary and secondary education by 2005, and achieve gender equality in education by 2015, with a focus on ensuring girls' full and equal access to and achievement in basic education of good quality;
6 Improve all aspects of the quality of education and ensure excellence of all so that recognized and measurable learning outcomes are achieved by all, especially in literacy, numeracy and essential life skills.

Source: UNESCO, 2000

monitoring and evaluation) in putting policy into practice. Structural and political conditions need to be supportive of promoting literacy for all to ensure that the promises made in Dakar are met to help break down social and economic inequalities in both literacy and health.

FUTURE RESEARCH

1 Current health literacy scales need to expand beyond measurement of reading skills, numeracy and comprehension.
2 More research on the application of health literacy in other contexts (e.g. workplace, schools, advocacy, etc.).

3 Development of community-based, capacity building and creative approaches to promote health literacy.
4 More rigorous evaluations and evidence of good practice on health literacy.

Summary

1 Using health information dissemination as an approach to health promotion is inadequate because influencing behaviour change requires more than just the transmission of knowledge.
2 In promoting health, it is important to consider whether the information communicated is understandable, that the recipients have the skills to implement choices, and that the environment is supportive of the choices made.
3 Health literacy considers the application of cognitive and psychosocial skills to access, understand and apply information to maintain and promote health in various contexts.
4 There are three general levels of health literacy: a) functional; b) interactive; and c) critical. Its domains include fundamental literacy, scientific literacy, civic literacy and cultural literacy.
5 Various standardized psychometric scales have been developed to measure health literacy.
6 There are a number of skills related with health literacy that are relevant to health promotion. These include communication skills, reading, writing, numeracy, analytical skills, decision-making, navigation, negotiation, awareness and advocacy.
7 Low literacy has been associated with poor health outcomes, including knowledge, intermediate disease markers, measures of morbidity, general health status and use of health resources.
8 Health literacy is influenced by the person's sensory and cognitive capacities, as well as by socio-economic and demographic factors. Health literacy also affects access and utilization to health care, the patient–provider interaction, and self-care.
9 Patients with low literacy may be reluctant to seek assistance due to the stigma and shame attached with it.
10 Health professionals need to be aware of health literacy levels when communicating information to ensure effective interactions with patients.
11 Improving communication between health-care professionals and patients can help address problems associated with poor health literacy.
12 Capacity building through literacy skills development is an approach that can be used to empower individuals and communities to promote health.

13 There is a need to simplify health-care systems to take into account varied levels of health literacy.
14 Progress towards equal access to literacy requires political will and commitment to help break down inequalities in both literacy and health.

15

Community Approaches Within Health Psychology

Imagination lights the fuse of possibility

Emily Dickinson

Outline

Community health psychology is an approach based upon promoting strategies for social change at the local level that can contribute to health and well-being. While such approaches offer much potential for reducing health inequalities they can potentially distract attention from the broader structural causes of ill-health. The chapter summarizes the character of this approach and considers some examples of it applied to health inequalities, social engagament, safety and sexual health.

Since its inception health psychology has developed different ways of understanding health and illness and different strategies for promoting health and well-being. Throughout this book we have emphasized the importance of broadening the focus of health psychology to consider the social and cultural context within which health and illness are located and to develop more social and collective strategies for promoting health. Recently there has been increasing interest in community-based approaches within health psychology. This chapter considers the background to this approach.

SOME HISTORY

Over the past decade there has been growing political interest in the concept **community**. The term itself has a long history. Williams (1971) (quoted in Carpenter, 2009a) noted that in the English language the term has been in use since at least the fourteenth century although its meaning has changed somewhat over the years. For example, in the eighteenth century it came to mean an alternative form of group living (e.g. New Lanark) apart from industrial society. It harked back to the supposed tranquil communal style of living that existed before the rise of the more conflictual and individualistic forms of living in the rising capitalist society. The cooperative movement grew out of this challenge to individual greed.

Box 15.1

New Lanark

New Lanark was an ideal vision of an industrial community that was developed by Robert Owen in the early nineteenth century. It was built on the River Clyde in Scotland and included a factory and housing for the workers and their families. Owen was a philanthropist and utopian socialist and he aimed to provide healthy working and living conditions. At its height the village had over 2500 residents. It remained in existence for over 150 years but when the mill closed the residents left and it is now a heritage site.

In the late twentieth century the term community was also used to describe various forms of oppositional culture and different ways of challenging the dominant styles of living of the nuclear family. One form was the growth of interest in communes as a way of building a more extended cooperative form of living.

In contemporary society we see once again increasing interest in community at both the popular and political levels of debate. At the popular level it is argued that modern consumer society has emptied all human relationships of affectionate bonds and replaced it with concern about taking advantage of your neighbour. At the political level it is argued by politicians that many of the ills of modern society are the result of the breakdown of community and there are various calls for the rebuilding of community. However, these calls for rebuilding community are fraught with conflicting political agendas to which health psychologists should be alert.

THE POLITICS OF COMMUNITY ACTION

Overlapping with this interest in community has been the growth of various forms of community or local social action which aims to challenge social oppression at a local level. However, the extent to which it actually is a challenge to wider political power depends upon its underlying assumptions. Community action draws upon different political heritages which are summarized by Carpenter (2009a):

1 The consumerist approach which is informed by contemporary neo-liberal ideology. This approach tends to underplay the importance of broader political forces, e.g. issues of power, de-industrialization, and adopts a very idealistic view of community change which can lead to community victim blaming.
2 The ordered community approach which harks back to some mythical past and is informed by neo-conservative and even fascist ideas. This approach tries to rearrange social relationships and behaviours without consideration of the wider social context.
3 The socially just community approach which emphasizes the importance of promoting social equality and celebrating diversity. This approach combines an awareness of and challenge to broader social injustices with local campaigns.

If we look at the evolution of community psychology we can see similar tensions.

COMMUNITY PSYCHOLOGY

In the 1960s increased social unrest in both developed and developing societies was reflected in new approaches within clinical psychology which had become focused on testing and individual psychotherapy. It was also closely tied with medicine and adopted the medical language of diagnosis and treatment. In North America this gave rise to a form of community psychology that was informed by the communitarian and humanitarian values of the liberal left while in South America – a more political community – social psychology developed that was informed by liberation theology and critical literacy. Both of these forms have influenced some evolving community approaches within health psychology.

After the initial radicalism of the 1960s the North American approach to community psychology became more accommodationist in its approach to society and also adopted the methods of mainstream psychology. Its concern was often around the evaluation of community-based social interventions rather than with attempts to challenge broader social injustices. There was a tendency for community psychology to become integrated into the practices of an unjust society rather than being part of the challenge to such injustices.

More recently there have been attempts to radicalize this tradition with a reaffirming of transformational values and attempts to connect with other critical movements within psychology in terms of both theories and methods. An example is the work of Prilletensky and Nelson (2004) who have deliberately affirmed a more political agenda in their work and have explicitly identified a series of social values for community psychology. These values were suggested as an approach that could inform a community health psychology (Murray, Nelson, Poland, Maticka-Tyndale & Ferris, 2004). These were defined as:

1 An awareness of the political dimensions of human problems and a concern to promote an empowerment approach that emphasizes self-determination, democratic participation and power-sharing;
2 A commitment to participation in broader social movements for social action and social justice;
3 An emotional commitment to social change through adopting a 'preferential option' for the poor and dispossessed;
4 A concern with promoting health and preventing disease and distress;
5 Respect for diversity.

While this affirmation of emancipatory values was an important correction to the accommodationist tendencies within mainstream community psychology there remains a need to work out how this translates into practice.

The South American approach to community psychology has traditionally been more explicitly political. Historically, it drew heavily on the critical pedagogy ideas of Paulo Freire (1910–1990), a Brazilian educator who argued that the campaign to increase literacy was a political struggle. He contrasted the traditional approach to literacy education with a more critical approach.

In the former approach the all knowledgeable educator pours his/her wisdom into the empty vessels who are the students. 'Education thus becomes an act of depositing, in which the students are the depositories and the teacher is the depositor' (Freire, 1970: 53). He described this as the 'banking' model of education.

In the more critical approach the educator engages with the student in an active dialogical manner to encourage them to consider the broader social and structural restraints on their lives and how they can begin to challenge these through collective action.

He used the term *conscientization* to describe this process of developing critical consciousness. 'Problem-posing education affirms men and women as beings in the process of *becoming* – as unfinished, uncompleted beings in and with a likewise unfinished reality' (p. 65).

Freire stressed that his work was 'rooted in concrete situations' working with poor peasants. He emphasized the collaborative nature of his work. He described the radical as someone who 'does not become the prisoner of a "circle of certainty" within which reality is also imprisoned ... This person does not consider himself or herself the proprietor of history or of all people, or the liberator of the oppressed; but he or she does commit himself or herself, within history, to fight at their side' (p. 21). These ideas were also developed further in the liberation psychology of Ignacio Martin-Baro (see Box 15.2).

Box 15.2

Liberation psychology

This approach draws its inspiration from the liberation theology developed by the worker–priest movement in different countries in Latin America during the 1950s and 1960s. This movement argued that it was the duty of Catholics to fight against social injustice and to adopt a ***preferential option for the poor.***

These ideas were given wider currency within psychology by Ignacio Martin-Baro (1942–1989) who was murdered by the Salvadoran army for his campaigning work in defence of the poor.

He developed a form of liberation psychology that set as its primary task the interests of the poor and oppressed. He criticized mainstream psychology for its scientistic mimicry and its lack of an adequate epistemology (including positivism, individualism and ahistoricism). This focus on individualism 'ends up reinforcing the existing structures, because it ignores the reality of social structures and reduces all structural problems to personal problems.'

Instead he argued that psychologists need to 'redesign our tools from the standpoint of the lives of our own people: from their sufferings, their aspirations, and their struggles' (Aron & Corne, 1994, p. 25). He proposed three elements in this new liberation psychology:

1. A new horizon: psychology must stop focusing on itself and being concerned about its scientific and social status but rather focus on the needs of the masses;
2. A new epistemology: psychology needs to consider what psychosocial processes look like from the perspective of the dominated;
3. A new praxis: psychology needs to consider itself as 'an activity of transforming reality that will let us know not only about what is but also about what is not, by which we may try to orient ourselves toward what ought to be' (Aron & Corne, 1994, p. 29).

Eliot Mishler states in the preface to the collection of his writings that they 'challenge us to align ourselves, as he did in El Salvador, with those struggling for equality and justice in our own country' (Aron & Corne, 1994, p. xii).

Both of these sets of ideas have been extremely influential in the shaping of community social psychology in Latin America. However, the growth of neo-liberalism has contributed to moves to dull the critical edge of community social psychology. Freitas (1990) notes that in Brazil there has been increasing attention within community psychology on specific issues with limited connection with the broader political context. She argues that such an approach was a backward step since: 'Specific issues in the daily life of communities are not going to be resolved by psychologists without taking into account the larger, material processes that are critically intertwined with specific situations' (p. 322). Instead, she argued for a return to the original ideals of community psychology including a clear political commitment to the interests of the less favoured sections of society and to their mobilization against injustices. She also recognized the need to connect more explicitly with other critical strands within psychology – both theoretical and methodological.

These are important points to consider with the development of community health psychology. There is a continuous need for critique and reflection if this approach is not to be drawn into the service of conservative political interests that act to entrench social inequalities in health rather than challenge them.

More recently, important developments in South Africa and other countries have served to revitalize community psychology in terms of its socio-political project. This includes projects concerned with the health challenges faced by indigenous people and also the issues of colonialism and post-colonialism (Duncan, Bowman, Naidoo, Pillay & Roos, 2007). These developments have introduced important ideas such as those of Franz Fanon who developed a sophisticated understanding of the psychology of political oppression, in particular, the processes by which oppressed people internalize ideas of inferiority and worthlessness.

This short overview of the growth of community psychology highlights its potential as a transformative agent but also one that can be compromised by conflicting political ideals.

COMMUNITY HEALTH PSYCHOLOGY

Over the past decade there has emerged increasing interest in developing a community health psychology. This has been defined as 'the theory and method of working with communities to combat disease and to promote health' (Campbell & Murray, 2004: 187). As within community psychology there are different orientations. The more accommodationist approach focuses on processes within the community while the more critical approaches aim to connect intra-community processes with the broader socio-political context. A primary aim of critical community psychologists is:

> *to promote analysis and action that challenges the restrictions imposed by exploitative economic and political relationships and dominant systems of knowledge production, often aligning themselves with broad democratic movements to challenge the social inequalities which flourish under global capitalism. (Campbell & Murray, 2004: 190)*

This emergent approach has deliberately attempted to connect with other developments in critical social and health psychology and with developments in community psychology. In devising strategies for social and community change health psychologists must be aware of the various dimensions of communities and the processes involved in encouraging participation in community activities.

The activist orientation of community health psychology distinguishes it from other forms of community-based health interventions. McLeroy, Norton, Kegler, Burdine and Sumaya (2003) distinguish between four different forms of community-based health promotion. These are community as setting, community as target, community as agent and community as resource. Community as setting is largely defined in geographical terms. This is a very common definition and assumes outside experts who are targeting a clearly defined community. The community as target is somewhat similar but is particularly concerned with creating a healthy environment through largely systemic changes. The community as resource is concerned with outside experts identifying and promoting the community strengths. Finally, the community as agent emphasizes working with the community to identify needs and resources and to support them in the processes of change. This approach is the most similar to that of community health psychology.

Although many health professionals have adopted different forms of community-based practice there is still a tendency to maintain a focus on individual change rather than broader social change. Dalton, Orford, Parry and Laburn-Peart (2008) conducted interviews with a sample of health professionals who were working in an urban regeneration area. They found that the most popular definition of health was in terms of lifestyle. While they also referred to the importance of the environment and to 'life as a struggle', the professionals had 'no compelling and coherent model to link community, the family and the individual' (p. 77). Community health psychology has begun to develop such a framework based upon a theoretical understanding of community processes together with reports from actual fieldwork.

Dimensions of Community

Community is often considered only in terms of location such that those people who live in a particular defined location are considered as being members of a community. Indeed, in North America the term community is often used where the term village is used in Britain. However, as many empirical projects have shown, people who live in the same locality often have different interests and affiliations. Indeed, there can be conflicts between sub-groups within any locality that may change or persist over time.

A more social psychological approach to community takes into consideration issues of shared values and identity. The framework developed by Howarth (2001) provides a useful approach to understanding the processes at work within communities as well as communities as potential sources of change. Deriving her ideas from social representation theory, Howarth describes community in terms of four dimensions:

1 A source of social knowledge: communities share common histories, meanings and ideas.
2 As a basis for common identities: community provides its members with a sense of shared identity which distinguishes its members from another;
3 As a means of marginalization and social exclusion: dominant groups can represent particular communities as inferior or threatening and thereby exclude its members from sustained social interaction with members of other groups or communities;
4 As a resource for empowerment: conversely communities can take action as a collective to challenge negative social representations. Through this very process the members of the community can engage in a process of personal and social transformation.

This description of the work of communities not only provides an understanding of what keeps a community together but also how a community can take action to challenge oppressive restraints and to promote healthier lives.

Community Participation

Much of the concern of community health psychology focuses on the process of working with the community to promote social change. It is well established that many community residents are apprehensive about participating in community health actions. This can be for a variety of reasons. Stephens (2007b) identifies three primary approaches to understanding community participation:

1 A focus on the immediate practical problems and successes and how the problems can be overcome. For example Nelson et al. (2004) identified language and cost as major problems that could be directly addressed. This approach considers all forms of participation positive and does not critique the nature of participation.

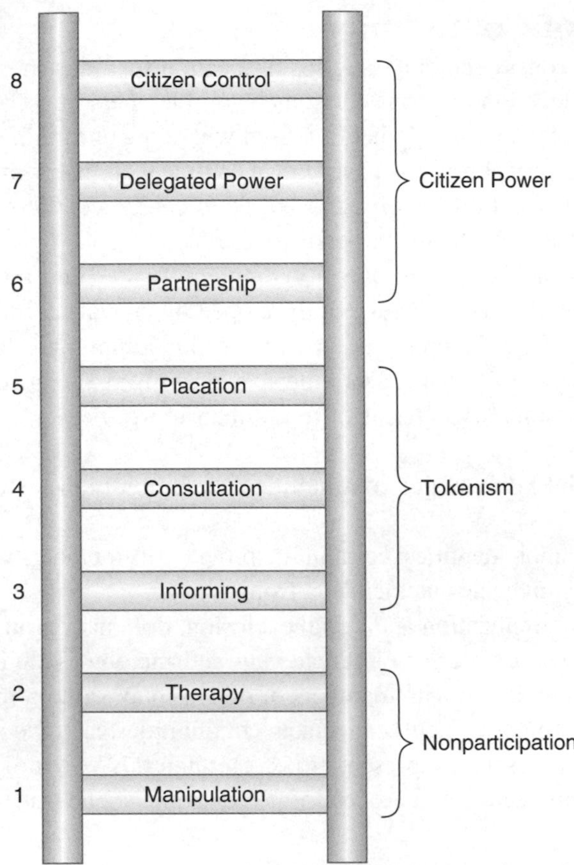

Figure 15.1 Arnstein's ladder of participation

2 A concern with different forms of and complexities of participation. A classic example is Arnstein's (1969) **ladder of participation** from token participation through to citizen power (see Figure 15.1). Although this approach is popular it lacks a clear understanding of the meaning of participation and why some people do not want to participate.

3 Then there is the more social psychological approach that draws upon the work of Campbell and Jovchelovitch (2000) and is similar to that of Howarth (2001) which we previously described. This approach starts with re-emphasizing the importance of social identity in participation. It is not simply the physical location but rather the extent to which the members identify with the community. This is a dialectical relationship in that the more they participate in community activities the more they identify with it and vice versa. In addition, there is the shared knowledge within the community. This knowledge can be both about contemporary processes or the history of the community. Finally, there is the issue of power. This can either facilitate or restrain active participation.

Power is central to discussion about community participation. As Campbell and Jovchelovitch (2000) state:

> *The power to act is always limited not only by material inequalities, but also by recognition others confer on what is done. Participation in conditions where material and symbolic obstacles prevent the possibility of real social change can be a hollow exercise. It legitimises the status quo rather than providing an opportunity for marginalised people to pursue their needs and interests (2000: 266).*

In participating in community action the residents of a community have the opportunity of challenging established power and also of growing in power themselves. The process of *empowerment* has been central to community action. It is a much debated concept particularly as regards the extent to which it is real or symbolic. Much research on empowerment is concentrated on feelings or sense of empowerment rather than actual change in power relationships.

As mentioned earlier it is essential that community health psychology adopts a reflexive stance so as to be aware of the broader socio-political forces that may coopt its activities for a more repressive aim. An overall criticism of concern with participation and empowerment is that it is part of a wider 'duties discourse' which uses appealing language of new social movements so that they become self-regulating while serving the goals of the state and other agencies (Stephens, 2007a). Thus while within community health psychology there is a notion that community empowerment is a progressive cause there is an ongoing need to connect with the broader socio-political context.

COMMUNITY HEALTH ACTIONS

As community health psychology has developed it has begun to work with different groups of people to take different forms of social action. A few examples are considered here.

Promoting Health Behaviour Change

The traditional focus of health psychology has been on promoting individual behaviour change. There have been various attempts to explore more community-based strategies. Previously we have discussed how there have been various government strategies designed to discourage unhealthy behaviours and to encourage more healthy behaviours. However, these strategies have adopted the traditional individualist focus. Community health psychology attempts to work with groups or communities to identify how they see the issue and to explore opportunities for change.

A sustained example of this approach is the work of Catherine Campbell in South Africa where she has been involved in several projects designed to reduce HIV infection. A central feature of her work has been the use of peer educators. These are people from the community who take a leading role in educating the residents about the risk of HIV infection. The ideal role adopted by the peer educators is to engage in participatory learning through, for example, games, drama and role-playing. Following the model of Friere the educator engages in a process of dialogue with the co-learners rather than imposing certain ideas. The participants are then active participants in the learning.

Despite considerable resources being expended in the development of such community interventions Campbell (2006) did not encounter sustained success. She identified a variety of reasons for this limited success both in the programme delivery and in the broader community context. The traditional didactic model of teaching in the schools meant that both the peer educators and the other students were unfamiliar with the participatory approach that underlay the programme. In addition, the strongly negative attitude of the community residents to HIV/AIDS discouraged the students from participating in the programme. Outside the school the students had limited opportunity to discuss these issues and the role models provided by adults were not supportive. Of particular importance, Campbell (2006) notes that

> *the young people's lives were blighted by macro-social environments characterised by poverty, lack of educational opportunities, unemployment, which undermined their confidence and their sense of personal agency to take control of their lives in general, or their sexual health in particular.*

This conclusion highlights the major impediments to promoting health behaviours in communities which are threatened by poverty. This highlights the importance of connecting community health interventions with attempts to promote economic empowerment of the residents.

In her subsequent work Campbell has been involved in programmes designed to promote AIDS-competent communities (Campbell, Nair & Maimane, 2007b). These are communities where a large proportion of the residents have HIV/AIDS. In these communities the aim is to reduce the stigma associated with the disease and to encourage support for sexual behaviour change and care of those with the disease. They have identified six factors that promote these sort of communities:

1 Building knowledge and basic skills
2 Creating social spaces for dialogue and critical thinking
3 Promoting a sense of local ownership of the problem and incentives for action
4 Emphasizing community strengths and resources
5 Mobilizing existing formal and informal networks
6 Building partnerships between marginalized communities and more powerful outside actors and agencies.

Although these factors were specifically developed in the context of building AIDS-competent communities they have broader relevance in other contexts.

Promoting Social Well-Being

The growth of interest in the connection between social interaction and health status has contributed to a more expansive definition of health including the extent and character of people's everyday social relationships. This research is informed by a variety of concepts, in particular social capital and collective efficacy. The concept social capital was popularized by the work of Putnam (2000). He argued that in modern society there has been a steady decline in social capital which he characterized as the character of civic participation, trust in others and reciprocity within a community. Other work by Bourdieu has characterized social capital in terms of resources that can be drawn upon. However, after initial enthusiasm about this concept confusion over its definition and its lack of connection with broader political processes have led researchers to consider other more specific concepts.

One such concept is the character of social interaction that people in any community enjoy. It has been established that in more disadvantaged neighbourhoods, older residents have more restricted social interaction. A study by Murray and Crummett (see Box 15.3) in one such neighbourhood found that the older residents were reluctant to access resources outside their immediate neighbourhood. They were however prepared to participate in locally organized social activities.

Box 15.3

Promoting social engagement through community arts

In a study in a British industrial city a group of older residents of a disadvantaged neighbourhood participated in a **community arts** project. This involved weekly meetings where they engaged in a variety of artistic activities including painting, writing and pottery. At the close of the project the participants organized an exhibition to which they invited other local residents and representatives of various local agencies. Reviewing the project the participants were extremely enthusiastic. A particular strength of this intervention was its collective nature. The enjoyment of art was a shared activity and as such strengthened social bonds between the participants.

Source: Murray & Crummett, 2010

Another concept is drawn from Beck's idea of the risk society and the extent to which this explains the extent of youth engagement or alienation from society. In a study conducted in Australia, Bradley, Deighton and Selby (2004) conducted a participatory action research project with rural youth. Theoretically they situated this project within Beck's concept of a risk society. According to this theory one of the consequences of modernization is the breakdown of established certainties which has a particular impact on young people who have no clear identity maps. This confusion can contribute to such problems as homelessness, suicide, unemployment, drug-use, crime and single parenthood. In this context Bradley et al. argue it is extremely important that young people have the opportunity of participating in community planning.

Their project involved three stages. In the first they organized a public conversation involving city councillors and various providers of services for young people. This led to little change in the provision of council support for young people. In the second stage young people themselves were invited to participate in a collaborative theatre group. This group used the theatrical techniques developed by Boal's theatre of the oppressed. In the third stage the young people had the opportunity of performing to a large audience. Later one member of the group had an opportunity of describing the project and the impact it had had on her and other participants. This led the council to reverse their earlier decision and fund a youth officer.

This project showed the deliberate attempt of the psychologists to not only work with their community of interest (young people) but also to involve them in a process of challenging the established authority (town council). Thus the project not only had an impact on the immediate participants but also on the wider audience. As Bradley et al. summarize the impact of the project:

> *The initial basis for commonality in the group appears to have been not the type of problems faced, but the fact that the members discovered they were not alone in having problems and the feeling they now had licence to express them. The licence empowered them to see their problems in a larger social and historical frame that led to the collective wish to change their community and to the idea of a public performance. (2004: 210)*

It was through the process of collective meaning making and action that the young people grew in confidence and were prepared to take further action to transform their situation. A further point stressed by Bradley et al. was the power of public display of the young people's experiences. The greater impact of this public display compared with previous scientific evidence provided some confirmation for Beck's argument on the declining power of expert knowledge.

Community Approaches to Combating Health Inequalities

A more critical community health psychology attempts at all times to connect local action with broader social change. For example, in their project Bradley and his colleagues deliberately attempted to challenge broader social assumptions of young people while in Campbell's studies she raised the issue of building linkages with outside powerful agencies. The extent to which community health psychologists make connections with the broader social context depends upon opportunity as well as orientation. Indeed, while community action projects can enthuse the participants they are often apprehensive about taking larger social action. The magnitude of the task is apparent in the various community projects that have sought to challenge social inequalities in health.

In previous chapters we have clearly outlined the substantial social inequalities in wealth and health that exist both within and between societies. As we have argued the traditional individualistic lifestyle approach to addressing these inequalities has met with limited success. There is an obvious need to address the material factors such as poverty and deprivation within which these unhealthy lifestyles are located. However, this does not negate the potential contribution of local community action to tackle local manifestations of this deprivation.

A detailed study of the impact of a community intervention to address the health inequalities in South Wales provides insight into these processes (Cropper et al., 2007). At the outset Williams (2007) argues that 'although poverty, inequality and other economic indicators of social development may remain the "base" condition underlying health inequalities, the "superstructure" is not irrelevant' (p. 9). He quotes Bourdieu (1986: 241) that 'the social world is accumulated history' that weighs heavily on people and undermines their capacity for change. This restricts the capacity of people in disadvantaged circumstances to initiate change but also opens up opportunities for community action.

In developing the participatory community health improvement programmes, Williams highlighted the importance of a socio-historical analysis of the community context. South Wales is an area that has recently experienced substantial deindustrialization. The impact of this has been tremendous on the local psyche. He says:

> *Whereas in the past solidarity provided the basis for union and political action, the decline over 30 years and more has created a situation in which the resources for hope and resistance are depleted. (2007: 12)*

Such resignation needs to be tackled at various levels. There is a need not just to tackle the structural inequalities but also from below to mobilize the communities to take action. Such action needs to be linked to the historical concerns of the community while at the same time opening up opportunities for change. The impact of one project may be small but it should be considered part of a larger programme to generate change. Cropper et al. concluded that their projects have shown 'that it is possible to establish a rallying point, or catalyst, for work towards a more social or communitarian model of health improvement' (2007: 211).

COMMUNITY LEVEL APPROACHES TO SEXUAL HEALTH

Community level approaches to sexual health mobilize skills and resources from communities who themselves can see that changes are necessary and who can develop strategies for making those changes. Communities may consist of ethnic groups, neighbourhood groups, or groups with particular social identities, e.g. men who have sex with men. These approaches are characterized as **'grass roots'** and **'bottom-up'** because the issues for change and change strategies are identified and applied by people themselves. The 'top-down' approach of theoretical models, government-led programmes and campaigns are rejected in favour of bottom-up approaches based on personal relationships and social networks. The concept that there needs to be adolescent participation in the promotion of their sexual and reproductive health is enjoying widespread popularity as part of a broader shift towards participatory (bottom-up) health promotion. Key policy statements by the World Health Organization (1986, 1997) endorse a participatory approach at the level of whole communities. The community approach is highly flexible and adapted from place to place according to the particular community issues and needs. In this section, we review three examples of community approaches to sexual health.

Adolescent Sexual Health in Peru

Ramella and de la Cruz (2000) describe an adolescent sexual health promotion project in Peru called 'SaRA' – 'Salud Reproductiva para Adolescentes'. SaRA was implemented in 15 communities located in deprived rural and urban/marginal areas in the Coastal Andean and Jungle regions of Peru. The project operates at a grass roots level in collaboration with existing community networks. SaRA's goal is to encourage positive changes in adolescent sexual health by working with relevant social actors and social networks. In each of the communities the project set up networks or 'Clubs'. The Clubs were created in open encounters jointly arranged by the SaRA team and local community networks. The Clubs organize a range of social activities designed to nurture the network of adolescents and to embed it within its community by seeking collaboration and exchange with other social agents. These activities are classified as informal, information or economic. However the three categories blend into each other when social activities take place. Adolescents decide for themselves the nature and content of events while the SaRA team facilitates assistance and collaboration from locally available services.

All Clubs were given access to video cameras, photographic cameras, tape recorders and paper and pencil. Some were given basic training in the use of audio-visual equipment and they have trained other adolescents in the group. The Clubs are thus encouraged to generate making use of these technologies in creating accounts of their activities, e.g. a football match, a visit to a health centre or a Salsa party, a fundraiser. The production of textual and audio-visual stories have a central role in SaRA. It is not only 'a fun thing to do' but acts as a catalyst for social activities. The stories open up opportunities for adolescents to talk about pressing issues felt by them and created a means of expression which can feedback into the adolescents' reflections and understanding of themselves. These stories contribute to SaRA's goal of promoting sexual health while helping adolescents to improve their communication skills and competence, which are a central aspect of sexual health. In all but four of these communities, the Clubs established themselves as key social players by becoming a social centre for local adolescents. A second output indicator was the increased use by adolescent Club members of locally available health services and products. A third output was a substantial decrease (90 per cent) in the level of unintended pregnancies among adolescent girls in SaRA.

Case Study

INTERNATIONAL CASE STUDY: HIV/AIDS stigma amelioration in South Africa

> *If you have AIDS you die twice because the first thing that kills you is being lonely when everyone discriminates against you, even your family members. The second one is the actual death.* (Young man, high school learner; quoted by Campbell et al., 2007a).

Campbell, Nair, Maimane and Nicholson (2007a) present a Stigma Amelioration Model (SMA) designed to reduce HIV/AIDS related stigma. They argue that **stigma** is a key driver of the epidemic 'through the role it plays in undermining the ability of individuals, families and societies to protect themselves from HIV and to provide assistance to those affected by AIDS' (p. 404). The authors present a multi-level model of the roots of AIDS stigma in two South African communities.

The SMA model highlights the complex interplay of psychological and social factors which generate stigma around AIDS. This project was carried out in two communities in KwaZulu-Natal, South Africa, Entabeni, a rural community near Eshowe, and Ekuthuleni, a peri-urban area near Durban, where around 40 per cent of pregnant women are HIV-positive. Entabeni and Ekuthuleni are typical Zulu-speaking communities in poverty and with high unemployment. When the study was carried out (2004) antiretroviral drugs were not available to the study communities. The society is patriarchal. HIV/AIDS-related community organizations invited the researchers to assist them in acquiring more understanding of the factors within the social environment that were facilitating or hindering their work.

Stigma is an obstacle to AIDS-care in these African communities:

> *Families hide the person away from the community once they discover they have AIDS. They take him away from the community and we end up not knowing what has happened to that person. They don't even allow him or her to go to the clinic or to seek out any help at all.* (Young woman, youth leader; Campbell, Nair, Maimane and Nicholson, 2007a).

Health workers reported that it was hard to persuade people to apply for AIDS grants when they kept their HIV status secret. Stigma might even deter people from asking for ARVT drugs once drug treatment took place.

(Continued)

Case Study

(Continued)

One hundred and twenty semi-structured interviews, and also focus groups, explored community responses to HIV/AIDS. The main drivers of stigma were observed to consist of six factors:

- fear
- lack of social spaces to engage in dialogue about HIV/AIDS
- the link between HIV/AIDS, sexual moralities and the control of women and young people
- the lack of adequate HIV/AIDS management services
- the way in which poverty shaped people's reactions to HIV/AIDS
- availability and relevance of AIDS-related information

Source: Campbell et al., 2007a

Campbell et al. (2007a) suggest four possible methods for the amelioration of the negative impacts of stigma in these regions:

1 generating debate and discussion about how stigma fuels the fear that facilitates the epidemic – with many people too frightened to seek out information about how to protect their sexual health through the creation of social contexts where people with AIDS are treated with care, love and respect.
2 discussion of stigma problems in group contexts, to help to empower people to identify their strengths, abilities and resources.
3 promoting community ownership of the HIV problem, to help bring about a sense of identification between community members and those who are suffering from HIV/AIDS.
4 encouraging participants to be creative about forging links with organizations that could help them to manage HIV/AIDS more effectively.

Campbell et al.'s Stigma Amelioration Model is an innovative example of using the community approach in a sexual health intervention. The SMA model has significant potential to promote sexual health internationally among vulnerable groups when the odds against this are fairly extreme. Stigma amelioration could also be applied to other stigmatized illness communities including those who suffer from obesity, drug addiction, obstructive pulmonary disease and mental ill health.

Confronting HIV/AIDS and Alcohol in Cambodia

Lubek and colleagues (2002) (Lee et al., 2010: Lubek et al. 2002) presents the Hybrid Capacity Building Model (HCBM) as another example of a community-level HIV intervention. The context is that of attempting to reduce, not the stigma of HIV/AIDS, but its actual transmission. The HCBM brings diverse stakeholders together, even when their interests initially appear conflicting, to help solve a shared problem. In rural Cambodia, where non-literacy rates are as high as 75 per cent, female workers face health and safety risks selling international beer brands in restaurants (e.g. Heineken, Three Horses, Budweiser, Stella Artois, Beck's and Tiger). These so-called 'beer girls' or 'beer promotion women' are underpaid by about 50 per cent, and are sometimes forced to trade sex for money. Twenty per cent are HIV-seropositive, quickly die, and are replaced by younger girls from the countryside. 'Beer girls' must wear the uniforms of the international beer brands that they sell in restaurants and beer gardens. The Siem Reap Citizens for Health, Educational and Social Issues (SiRCHESI, 2008) organization, which embodies the HCBM, has confronted the issues involved.

In 2002, 'beer girls' were set a sales quota of twenty four 33cl. cans/small bottles per night – each selling at US$1.50 on average totalling US$36 worth of beer daily or US$13,000 annually. In 2004–5, Heineken and Tiger Beer promotion women were put on fixed salaries of around US$55 per month. This amount is about half the income they need to support their families. One-third of the women support children as single mothers, and 90 per cent support rural families. About half become indirect sex workers, exchanging money for sex to supplement their income. 'Beer girls' consume unsafe quantities of alcohol when working, drinking over 1.2 litres of beer (about 5 standard drinks) nightly 27 days a month (Schuster et al., 2006). This reduces condom use, increasing risks for HIV/AIDS and STIs. Condom use following beer drinking is lowered. Averaged over the 7 years, 20 per cent of the female beer promotion women in Cambodia are seropositive for HIV/AIDS (Lubeck, 2005). It is estimated that there are approximately 200,000 people living with HIV/AIDS (PLWHAs) in Cambodia, with 10,000 in Siem Reap.

A clone of the life-prolonging antiretroviral therapy (ARVT) costs approximately US$360 per year. The annual wage of US$600–US$800 means that ARVT is not an option for HIV-positive 'beer girls'. Medicins Sans Frontieres and other NGOs provide free clone ARVT for a small number of Cambodians with HIV/AIDS. Death can follow three months to two years after diagnosis.

The spread of HIV/AIDS is accelerated by sexual tourism, poverty and lack of condom use – HIV seropositivity rates have averaged 32.7 per cent (1995–May 2005) for brothel-based (direct) sex-workers. Siem Reap is the largest tourist site in Cambodia and hosted 354,000 people in 2001, and over 1,000,000 in 2004. Many of the male tourists are 'sexual tourists'. In 2001, 23 brothels were registered in the 100 per cent condom use programme, employing 250 direct sex workers. An additional 350 indirect sex workers were 'beer promotion women', or worked as massage workers and karaoke singers (Lubeck, 2005). Infection patterns reflect a 'bridging' pattern involving sexual tourists, indirect and direct sex workers, local men their wives and newborns. Married women, men and young persons are increasingly at risk, with less than 10 per cent of the estimated 10,000 persons living with HIV/AIDS in Siem Reap in 2006 being given antiretrovirals. In 2006–8, SiRCHESI partnered with three Siem Reap hotels in a hotel apprenticeship programme. This removed

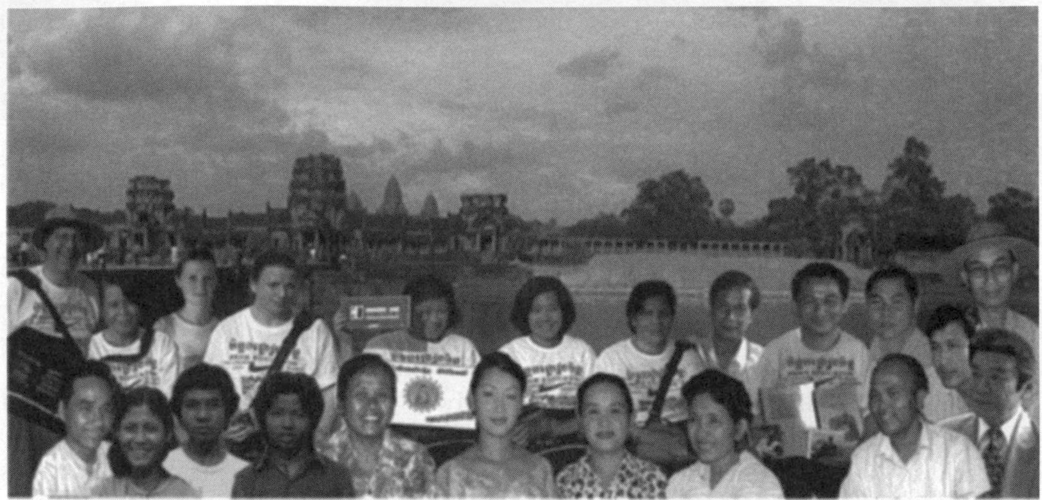

Figure 15.2 Health promotion by the local grass roots NGO, Siem Reap Citizens for Health, Educational and Social Issues shown at Angkor Wat. They offer HIV/AIDS prevention workshops to groups at risk

Source: http:// portal. psychology.uoguelph.ca/research/lubek/cambodia/index.html; Reproduced with permission

women from risky beer-selling jobs, sending them every morning to SiRCHESI's school to learn English, Khmer reading, health education, social and life skills, training them for safer careers inside the hotel industry. New advocacy, political and policy-formation skills and activism included trade union activities for beer sellers, meetings with government legislators, supplying data to ethical shareholders groups, and debating international beer executives in the press and scientific journals. Multiple actions are organized to tackle the issue at a number of different levels:

- workshops training women at risk for HIV/AIDS to be peer educators about health and alcohol overuse
- workshops to prevent the sexual exploitation and trafficking of children
- company sponsorship of HIV/prevention health education
- fair salaries to enable the women to adequately support their dependents
- monitoring voluntary HIV/AIDS testing (serology)
- free antiretroviral therapy (ARVT) for 'promotion girls' who are HIV positive
- breathalyzer testing in bars
- changes in community health behaviours and attitudes
- fund raising through the sale of fair-trade souvenirs

SiRCHESI uses a multi-sectoral Participatory Action Research (PAR) approach to confront the HIV/AIDS pandemic in Cambodia. The PAR approach emphasizes empowerment of local women and others increasingly at risk, as well as the development of a culturally and gender-sensitive health intervention /research programme, which eventually can be made self-sustaining. This approach succeeds best by facilitating collaboration between grass-root organizations and local and international corporate industries. All of these stakeholders need to take responsibility for the risk prevention of HIV. The HCBM provides a model for achieving this goal.

CRITIQUE OF COMMUNITY LEVEL THEORIES AND MODELS

- *Lack of evaluation.* The ability of an intervention to improve the health of individuals suffering from an illness needs to be evaluated if we are to place any confidence in its adoption in health care. Ideally, a similar, robust level of proof is required for all types of intervention. However, there is an uneven playing field because the same high level of proof available for individual-level interventions is not feasible for the vast majority of community-level interventions. Individual-level interventions of the top-down variety can be studied in randomized controlled trials and the data can be synthesized in meta-analysis. This is because the parameters can be systematically varied in the design of any trial and the conditions controlled accordingly. Bottom-up community interventions are by definition unique to each particular community and circumstance and the intervention(s) designed in light of the circumstances arising as the various stakeholders influence what actually happens. A community intervention often feels very messy, fluid and difficult to control, and certainly not amenable to a randomized controlled trial. In fact, it is almost impossible to run trials using matched controlled conditions in bottom-up interventions of the kind reviewed in this chapter. When any intervention is truly bottom-up, there is hardly ever going to be the opportunity to provide a controlled evaluation. However, evaluation using other types of design are not precluded, and should ideally be carried out, e.g. processes and outcomes should be monitored and compared at different time points. Unfortunately, for many community projects, evaluation ends up being a low priority, or tends to be overlooked.
- *Lack of detailed description.* Another problem with the community approach is community projects are often described in insufficient detail and clarity to enable people who were not directly involved to understand exactly what took place and how they could, if they wanted to, replicate the intervention at another time and place.
- *Empowerment – who empowers whom?* The idea of one group of people empowering others to do things that they otherwise could or would not do is a problematic concept. Who is to decide what exactly it is that the others should be encouraged to do? What right does the empowering group have to warrant this assumption? Who knows best what should be aimed for? Who are the power-brokers and how much control do they try to retain?

- *Victim blaming.* When community members are asked to participate in an intervention, their response can be quite variable. Participators can be perceived as an in-group or elite and those who do not participate as an out-group. Non-participation can then act as a vehicle for victim-blaming. The people in the in-group may well ask why others are not coming forward to join in and avail themselves of the organized events, which may be seen as a failure to help themselves.
- *Unexpected consequences.* Community change occurs as a consequence of a complex interplay of actors, circumstances and actions. The aims and objectives may well be noble and righteous, but the consequences are not always predictable or certain. The outcome could possibly be to the benefit of some and to the detriment of others. A kind of methodological hubris may cause unintended harm through externally led intervention techniques such as PAR (Estacio & Marks, in press).

ARTS AND COMMUNITY ACTION

A particularly popular means of mobilizing groups and communities is through a range of arts activities. **Community arts** is a descriptor for the range of activities in which participants are encouraged to explore new alternatives through different art forms. The success of the art is not in the classic sense of its aesthetic quality but rather to the extent that it contributes to some form of personal and social transformation. Meade and Shaw (2007) describe the subversive potential of community arts as being able to:

> *enter attentively into the experience of others, excavating and exploring causes of flaws and wounds in society, thinking critically about structures and relations of power and acting creatively and collectively to transform the world for the better. (2007: 414)*

As with other forms of community psychology, work in community arts can be compromised to serve the interests of the state more so than that of the community. Again, Meade and Shaw (2007) caution that the arts can provide 'a convenient means of political displacement, distracting attention from the real causes of social problems' (p. 416). In this sense we can contrast art as anaesthetic by which it dulls the power of the state with art as aesthetic which can enable people to see through the hidden veils of control and also assert a new agenda.

There are increasing examples of the power of arts to both communicate ideas and to promote community health action (see Murray & Gray, 2008). In the previous sections we have illustrated the work of theatre in mobilizing youth to assert their views. Another example was the role of the arts in increasing awareness of safety in the fishing industry (see Box 15.4)

Box 15.4

A community approach to promoting safety awareness

The fishing industry is one of the most dangerous occupations in the world. Attempts at reducing the rate of accidents have largely focused on a range of safety campaigns aimed at individual fish harvesters. However these have met with limited success. One study that attempted to adopt a more social and community approach was that reported by Murray & Tilley (2006).

In this study they worked with residents of small fishing villages in Canada to collaboratively raise awareness of the causes of accidents. The central theme of these initiatives was that it was not the responsibility of the fish harvester alone but of the whole community to become involved in safety action.

The project met with substantial success in terms of the interest it attracted and the number of residents who participated in the project. This was in contrast to the relatively small numbers who participated in government safety training programmes, again illustrating Beck's (1992) argument on the decline of expert power.

Source: Murray & Tilley, 2006

A series of projects have confirmed the powerful role of community drama in mobilizing communities for change. This interest in the use of drama parallels the so-called performance turn within social science that has been described by Denzin (2003). He described this as a means of moving beyond the representation of human experience through its transformation through performance. In this age of late capitalism with ongoing wars and increasing social inequality, social science needs to consciously connect with this approach to challenge the 'senseless, brutal violence that produces voiceless screams of terror and insanity' (p. 7). Different forms of performance should be considered central to community research practice.

An illustration of the power of drama is the work of Gray and Sinding (2002) with breast cancer patients, survivors, carers and health-care workers. Initially their project was aimed at using qualitative interviews to document in detail the experiences of people who had experienced cancer or who had been involved in some aspect of cancer care. With the help of professional dramatists it then moved on to the creation of a theatrical production that not only told the different stories to a wider audience but contributed to a wider process of consciousness raising about the experiences of people with cancer.

Photovoice

A particular art form that has attracted widespread adoption in community health action project is **Photovoice**. This is a process of collective photography and social action that was originally developed by Caroline Wang. In the original project women peasants in rural China collaborated with Wang and her colleagues in a project designed to draw attention to their poor living and working conditions (Wang, Burris & Xiang, 1996b). The project had the twofold effect of empowering the participants but also engaging them in a process of wider social action.

Wang (1999) has described the aims of Photovoice as threefold:

1 To enable people to record and reflect on both their own and their community's strengths and concerns through taking photographs;
2 To promote critical dialogue and review of the participants' lives through discussion around the photographs;
3 To deliberately connect with policy makers and decisions makers through public forums around exhibitions of the photographs.

Theoretically the approach has drawn inspiration from Freire's critical literacy and also from feminist theory and work on documentary photography. It emphasizes how within community health work the aim is to shift control over image-making from the professional to those with little power and influence. The participants both grow in confidence but can begin to exert influence to change social policy and to transform their lives.

With the rapid growth of the Internet and the availability of relatively cheap still and video cameras this approach has become extremely popular as a means of engaging communities. Unfortunately, it has also attracted negative connotations through the process of exposing people to ridicule and threats. This illustrates the conflicting use of technology to further both health and injury to both individuals and communities.

A related approach known as *digital storytelling* has also been used in community settings to involve people in recording and telling their stories about their communities. This is exciting new work that has as yet not involved health psychologists directly but could potentially be used in projects designed to promote social action. It is based upon the idea that not only can people become collectively involved in sharing their stories but that these can be video-recorded and used as part of a broader social action.

Community story-telling is an approach widely used in community work. The aim is to move from the individual story of threat and defeat to a shared story of threat and challenge. In the sharing of their stories the participants create a shared identity – a community. The work by Solinger, Fox and Irani (2008) provides a wide collection of examples of this process. Consider the work of Salas (2008) in which she worked with a group of immigrant women in New York state. Through the project the women shared their stories of personal threat and resistance which were subsequently performed. As a group the women then produced a book detailing their life experiences with stories and photographs. From this they moved to building a network of women throughout the state who shared their experiences and became involved in various campaigns to improve their living and working conditions.

All of these technological innovations have rapidly generated a whole range of Internet resources that can be accessed by community groups. The ready availability of these resources illustrates the opportunity for community health psychologists.

Comment

Community health psychology is an approach that is informed by an understanding of health and illness as being located within an unjust society with unequal distribution of resources and opportunities. It positions the health psychologist as a scholar–activist (Lykes, 2000) who engages collaboratively in community health action as part of a broader process of societal critique and action (Murray & Poland, 2008). While 'walking the walk' of social critique this approach also emphasises the importance of reflexivity in research and practice. This reflexivity promotes an awareness of one's social location and how this influences how we see the world, choose our theories and methods, and engage with others.

FUTURE RESEARCH

1. There is an ongoing need to clarify the processes that contribute to promoting community participation.
2. Different approaches to community engagement need to be explored.
3. The growth of the Internet opens up new types of community and of community participation.
4. Different art forms not only provide means of community participation but also of community research.

Summary

1. Community is a concept that has a long history and changing meaning.
2. The concept is used by people with different political interests.
3. Community psychology is an approach to encouraging involvement of people at a local level. It can have both radical and accommodationist approaches.
4. Community health psychology is concerned with promoting health through various forms of community action.
5. The arts are a popular means of involving people in community health action.
6. Community health psychology needs to consider the broader socio-political context within which it operates.

Part 4

Illness Experience and Health Care

In Part 4 we review illness experience and health care. In Chapter 16, we review lay representations of health and illness. The traditional biomedical approach to illness defines it in terms of physical symptoms and underlying physical pathology. However, to the lay person, illness is a much more complicated process. Psychologists have used a variety of theoretical perspectives to investigate popular representations of illness. This chapter contrasts research that has used a cognitive approach to the study of illness representations with those that have adopted phenomenological, discursive and social approaches. Whereas the former adopts a positivist perspective, the others adopt constructivist perspectives.

Chapter 17 examines the influence of individual differences in personality and other psychological characteristics on susceptibility to illness. It begins with a brief history of the contrasting approaches of practitioners of orthodox and wholistic medicine. It goes on to consider Freud's work on hysteria and contemporary approaches to medically unexplained symptoms such as chronic fatigue syndrome. After an account of some of the ways in which Freud's theories became applied to organic illness by the psychosomatic schools of psychoanalysis, there is an analysis of the problems involved in investigating and explaining links between personality and physical illness. The chapter concludes with an assessment of contemporary research on personality and illness with particular reference to coronary heart disease and cancer.

Chapter 18 reviews studies of adherence. Adherence and compliance are terms used to describe the extent to which patients adhere or comply with recommended treatment regimens. It is one of the most widely researched forms of health-related behaviour. The assumptions underlying the term compliance imply an authoritarian stance on the part of the physician or other health professional that is challenged by recent changes within health-care systems. This chapter considers the extent and character of treatment non-adherence and the issue of medical error. It also considers the patient-centred formulation of health care that focuses on shared decision-making and patient empowerment.

Chapter 19 discusses the nature of pain and the distinction between acute and chronic pain. The focus is chronic pain. We discuss the major theories, including direct line of transmission theories and multidimensional gate control theory, which acknowledges psychological influences. A range of psychosocial factors implicated in the mediation of the pain experience are considered. We summarize pain assessment methods. Finally, we explore the issue of pain management using psychological and other techniques.

Chapter 20 reviews three life-threatening and disabling diseases: cancer, coronary heart disease and HIV/AIDS. In each case we consider five issues: 'What is …?'; 'Interventions for …'; 'Living with …'; 'Adaptation to …'; and 'Caring for someone with …'. The contribution of psychosocial interventions for patients suffering from these conditions has been evaluated in systematic reviews. The evidence suggests that psychosocial interventions have not yet demonstrated their full potential. The quality of evaluation research with psychosocial interventions has generally been rather poor and the findings inconclusive. We suggest further research to strengthen psychological understanding of treatment and care for these conditions.

16

Lay Representations of Illness

As long as a particular disease is treated as an evil, invincible predator, not just a disease, most people with cancer will indeed be demoralized by learning what disease they have. The solution is hardly to stop telling cancer patients the truth, but to rectify the conception of the disease, to de-mythicize it.

Susan Sontag, 1978: 11

Outline

The traditional biomedical approach to illness defines it in terms of physical symptoms and underlying physical pathology. However, to the lay person, illness is a much more complicated process. Psychologists have used a variety of theoretical perspectives to investigate popular representations of illness. This chapter contrasts research that has used a cognitive approach to the study of illness representations with those that have adopted phenomenological, discursive and social approaches. Whereas the former adopts a positivist perspective the others adopt constructivist perspectives.

COGNITIVE APPROACHES

Illness Perceptions

The most developed cognitive model of illness was initially proposed by Howard Leventhal and his colleagues (Leventhal, Leventhal & Schaefer, 1989). This was derived from their work on the impact of fear communication. They found that, irrespective of the level of fear, the message conveyed was effective if it produced a plan of action. This led them to infer that the key factor was the way the threat was represented or understood. They developed a *dual processing model* to accommodate the representation of fear and of the threat (see Figure 16.1), an influential model that has undergone some elaboration by Leventhal (1999).

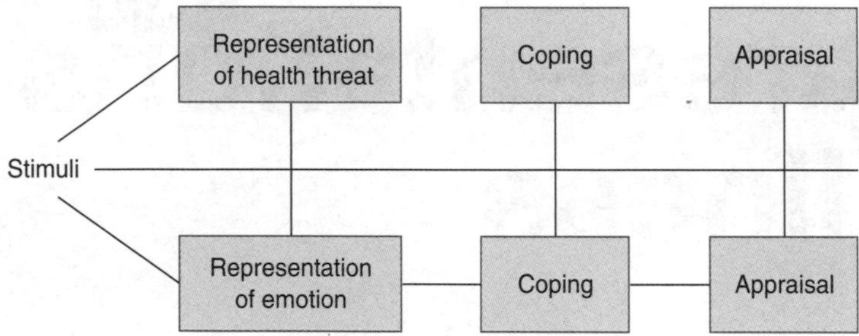

Figure 16.1 Self-regulatory model of illness behaviour
Source: Leventhal et al., 1989

Basically the model suggests that when faced with a threat the person forms a cognitive and emotional representation of that threat. They will cope with that threat depending upon the character of the threat representation. The consequences of these coping strategies will then be appraised and the representations and coping strategies revised accordingly. This model led the Leventhal group to explore how lay people represented specific threats such as illness. They conducted open-ended interviews with a sample of patients suffering from various diseases. From this information they proposed a *self-regulation model* of illness that suggested that lay people's thoughts on illness could be organized along four dimensions. Lau and Hartman (1983) suggested that since these dimensions were derived from a sample of patients with an acute, time-limited illness experience it was necessary to introduce a fifth dimension to cover those illnesses which were resistant to treatment (see Box 16.1). These five dimensions are often termed the **Common Sense** Model (CSM) of illness (see also Chapter 6).

Box 16.1

Dimensions of common sense illness perceptions

Identity: the signs, symptoms and the illness label.

Consequence: the perceived physical, social and economic consequences of the disease and the felt emotional consequences.

Causes: the perceived causes of the disease.

Time line: the perceived time frame for the development and duration of the illness threat.

Cure/Control: the extent to which the illness is responsive to treatment.

Sources: Leventhal et al., 1980; Lau & Hartman, 1983

A major impetus to research into this CSM was the development of the **Illness Perception Questionnaire** (IPQ) by Weinman, Petrie, Moss-Morris and Horne (1996) to measure the original five illness dimensions. This measure has been used extensively on a wide range of populations with varying degrees of success. It was originally used in a longitudinal study to investigate the relationship between illness representations and work behaviour after myocardial infarction (Petrie, Weinman, Sharpe & Buckley, 1996). This study found that attendance at a cardiac rehabilitation course was significantly predicted by a stronger belief during admission that the illness could be cured. Return to work was predicted by perception that the illness would last a short time and have less serious consequences. In conclusion, it was argued that these popular illness beliefs 'seem to be largely formed by information before becoming ill [and] are quite consistent over time'. A recent meta-analysis of 45 studies using this measure found some evidence that confirmed the five-fold structure of the CSM and also the relationship between the other components of the self-regulation model (Hagger & Orbell, 2003).

A revision of this questionnaire (Revised Illness Perception Questionnaire, IPQ-R) introduced a measure of *illness coherence* and of emotional representations of illness (Moss-Morris, Weinman, Petrie, Horne, Cameron & Buick, 2002). The former considers how the illness 'makes sense' as a whole to the patient. The emotional representations had been ignored in the previous model although they were explicit in the original formulation of the self-regulation model of illness. In addition, the IPQ-R divided the cure/control dimension into *personal control* and *treatment control*. This enabled researchers to distinguish between perceived control of the illness from perceived control of the treatment.

There continues to be research to explore the structure of this cognitive model of illness representations. It is generally agreed that this model should be applied lightly to different conditions to explore its relevance rather than assuming that it has universal validity. Recent researchers have attempted to expand the basic model. For example, in a study of patients undergoing surgery for coronary heart disease Hirani, Pugsley and Newman (2006) using the original IPQ confirmed what are considered the three core dimensions of the model which they labelled illness impact (consequences), duration (time-line), control (cure/control). They also identified a fourth dimension labelled self-image that they argued has been ignored in much research. They suggest that in the same way as the IPQ-R added an additional illness coherence component to the basic cognitive model future research should consider the overall impact of the disease on self-image.

A weakness in many of the studies that have used this framework is that they have been correlational. Thus although the CSM components have been found to be interrelated they do not provide firm evidence to support the self-regulation model. More recent studies have attempted to overcome this deficiency. An example is the work by Searle, Norman, Thompson and Vedhara (2007) in which they investigated the connection between illness representations (measured by the IPQ-R), illness cognitions and coping behaviours in a prospective study of patients with type-2 diabetes. They found that the illness representations were direct predictors of both coping cognitions and coping behaviours. This would suggest that intervention efforts to improve management of type-2 diabetes should focus on the patients' illness representations.

It is increasingly accepted among CSM researchers that illness representations are not simply the property of individual patients but reflect interpersonal and cultural experiences. For example, it has been found that the illness representations of patients and family are often similar (Weinman, Petrie, Sharpe & Walker, 2000) reflecting their shared experiences. Further, when they differ there is evidence to suggest that this has implications for the patients. An example of the consequences of conflicting perceptions is illustrated in the study of women's and men's perceptions of infertility by Benyamini, Leventhal and Leventhal (2009). They found different patterns in the relationship of illness perceptions between partners that were associated with different levels of distress. The highest distress was found among women who reported low levels of controllability whereas their partner reported high controllability. An awareness of these different perceptions could be used to provide psychological counselling for couples.

There have recently been attempts to use the CSM approach in investigations of lay representations of illness in developing countries. For example, Kart, Kinney, Subedi, Basnyat and Vadakkan (2007) conducted an interview survey of 3000 residents of Kathmandu, Nepal who had been diagnosed as having diabetes. They included two standardized assessment instruments: the revised version of the Illness Perception Questionnaire (IPQ-R) and the Summary of Diabetes Self-Care Activities (SDSCA) questionnaire. Both measures were translated into Nepali. Factor analysis of the responses to the IPQ-R revealed a similar structure to that in the original formulation of the measure (Moss-Morris et al., 2002). Only the 'Illness coherence' dimension was not identified. When the participants' ratings of the 18 causal categories in the IPQ-R were examined it revealed three causal clusters again similar to that found in other countries. Despite finding such similarities the authors were cautious in their conclusion. Their sample was educated and urban, in many ways unrepresentative of Nepal and more similar to people in developed countries. Also, they commented on the limitations of the quantitative assessment and concluded that there was a need for more qualitative research that could identify the particular cultural dimensions of Nepali illness representations.

Although the development of a standardized measure of lay representations of illness has contributed to a large body of research in this area it has also restricted its development. Fortunately, recently researchers using this framework have begun to explore other measures. For example, in a substantial study considering the differences between lay and professional representations of breathlessness, Insel, Meek and Leventhal (2005) administered a 'Perceived experience of breathlessness' scale to participants. This scale was not structured around the five dimensions of the CSM but rather inductively from concepts people with breathlessness used to describe the experience. A network analysis was conducted to explore the relationship between these concepts. This revealed a different network for the four groups of participants such that while for those with COPD the two central concepts were 'awareness of breathing' and 'worry about the next breath', the pulmonologists had a single central concept, 'breathlessness'. There were similarities in some of the nodes of the network with the dimensions of the CSM. This study illustrated new ways of investigating lay representations of illness but also connections between the various dimensions. Of particular note was the conclusion that there was need to integrate qualitative research with quantitative findings to develop a more sophisticated understanding of lay representations of illness.

Causes of Disease

Perceived cause is considered one of the central components in Leventhal's original model of lay illness representations. Psychological interest in how lay people explain the onset of disease derives from **attribution theory** (Heider, 1958). According to the basic tenets of attribution theory people attempt to provide a causal explanation for events in their world particularly if those events are unexpected and have personal relevance. Thus it is not surprising that people will generally seek a causal explanation for an illness, particularly one that is serious.

Swartzman and Lees (1996) considered the character of the causal explanations of various physical symptoms. Initial classification of the suggested causes revealed 14 categories. Multidimensional scaling analysis of the scores suggested three dimensions that they labelled: non-physical–physical, stable–unstable, and controllable–uncontrollable. The latter two labels are comparable to two of the original attributional dimensions while the first dimension is specific to explanations of illness. Physical causes included 'physical activity' and 'physical constitution' while non-physical causes included personality, mood and stress.

Murray and McMillan (1993a) asked a sample of over 700 adults to rate the relative importance of 24 potential causes of cancer. Factor analysis of their ratings revealed four factors that were labelled:

- Stress (which contained items referring to stress, worry, loneliness, unemployment).
- Environment (including such items as air pollution, work conditions, asbestos, nuclear radiation, a knock or hurt, X-rays and promiscuity).
- Health-related (such factors as childbirth, antibiotics, breast-feeding, virus or infection).
- Behaviour (fatty foods, smoking, drinking).

Although some of these factors could be redefined along the classic attributional dimensions, others (e.g. health-related) were more specific and would suggest that people combine general and specific casual explanations.

In the development of their revised illness perception questionnaire (IPQ-R) Moss-Morris et al. (2002) identified four causal dimensions: psychological **attributions**, risk factors, immunity, and accident or chance. They stressed that these four factors should not be considered universal or prescriptive but that they depend upon the illness, the culture and the population.

Comment

The common sense model of illness has attracted considerable research effort. The enthusiasm for this approach is partly explained by the development of a standardized assessment instrument. There is considerable theoretical and methodological debate about this approach. The first concerns the broad limitations of the cognitivist approach with its positivist epistemological assumptions and the information-processing model of thinking. The second concerns the neglect of social and cultural factors as well as the limitations of using a standardized instrument to assess a dynamic process. Some recent research shows an interest in exploring connections with more qualitative approaches.

PHENOMENOLOGICAL APPROACHES

A major criticism of the cognitive approach is that it adopts an information-processing approach and loses sight of the person who is actively trying to make sense of their world. One attempt to recover the person is the **phenomenological** approach. Here we will briefly consider, in particular, two forms of this approach – interpretative phenomenological analysis (IPA) and the **narrative** approach. These approaches share epistemological constructivist assumptions and a preference for qualitative methods of investigation. It is argued that since phenomenology is concerned with exploring the participant's perspective on the world rather than confirming that of the observer/researcher then the researcher should adopt an open-ended qualitative approach to research. The concern is with trying to understand the subjective experience of the patient in their own words.

Interpretative Phenomenological Analysis

The IPA approach has attracted considerable attention over the past decade. It was originally developed by Smith (1996) and since then has been applied extensively in health psychology. This approach argues that a human characteristic is a tendency towards self-reflection, an ongoing process in which humans try to make sense of their worlds. There is no presumed structure to this subjective experience and the challenge faced by the researcher is trying to describe the world from the perspective of the other. The primary source of information on the subjective world of the other is their verbal reports of their experiences.

Smith has provided detailed advice on how to obtain and analyse these verbal reports. In particular, he notes the importance of the researchers being explicit about their own interpretative framework. He has described this approach as being a double hermeneutic in that the researcher is trying to make sense of the patient's sense making. It is for this reason that the approach is described as interpretative because 'a person's thoughts are not transparently available from, for example, interview transcripts, [so, the researcher] engages in the analytic process in order, hopefully, to be able to say something about the thinking' (Smith, 1996: 219).

A series of studies have illustrated the value of this approach for exploring the experience of illness. In an IPA study of the experience of living with diabetes Schur, Gamsu and Barley (1999) conducted interviews with eight young people, four male and four female. Their analysis of the interviews identified two broad super-ordinate themes labelled 'developing a relationship with diabetes' and 'managing threats from diabetes'. Box 16.2 provides a summary of the various sub-themes.

Box 16.2

Young person's perspective on living with diabetes

Developing a relationship with diabetes

The shock of diabetes

Emotional responses
Searching for an understanding (Why me?)

(Continued)

(Continued)

Learning to live with diabetes

Parental involvement
Sharing

Seeking an optimal relationship with diabetes

Acceptance
Finding a balance

Managing threats from diabetes

Intrapersonal threats

Distressing emotions
Fears in the present and future
Vulnerability

Self-protective strategies

Adaptive denial
Rosy view of the past
Control
Downward comparisons

Interpersonal threats

Difference
Stigma

Self-protective strategies

Development of an identity relatively independent of diabetes
Stigma management
Externalizing the problem
Rationalizing
Telling others

Source: Schur et al., 1999

In a comparable study, Kay, Davies, Gamsu and Jarman (2009) explored the experiences of young women living with Type 1 diabetes. Using IPA as their analytic frame they identified four main super-ordinate themes:

1 The relationship with the body: this theme was concerned with how the women viewed their bodies, especially the importance of weight and how diabetes impacted on their health;
2 Personal challenges: this theme was concerned with the impact of diabetes on their everyday lives;
3 Impact of relationship: this theme focused especially on the impact of diabetes on relationships;
4 Changing and adapting: this theme was concerned with how the young women managed the disease.

Considering these two studies it is apparent that there are certain similarities in how young people describe their experience of diabetes. They are particularly concerned with the impact of the disease on their lives and on their relationships and how they manage both of these. In both studies diabetes is perceived by the young people not as a fixed unchanging thing but an ongoing process with which they engage on a daily basis. The character of the experience of these young people depends upon who they are and the various supports available. It also depends upon broader societal expectations. For example, the young women in the second study were particularly concerned about the impact of the illness on their body image and interpersonal relationships.

Diabetes is a long-term condition and the accounts of the young people in these studies emphasized the importance of how they integrated the disease into their lives and their ongoing management of it. Other diseases are more life threatening and the experiences of those suffering from them are quite different. For example, Moore, Norman, Harris and Makris (2008) conducted an IPA study of a sample of women suffering from venous thromboembolic disease (VTE), a life-threatening condition. The women in their sample had received a diagnosis of inherited thrombophilia. The researchers identified three main themes in the interviews they conducted with these women:

1 Causal models: the women participants identified multi-causal models of VTE including surgery, stress and HRT;
2 Primary control efforts: a variety of self-protective behaviours (e.g. walking, compression tights) that reduced the risk of recurrence;
3 Secondary control efforts: this was concerned with the broader acceptance of having the disease.

Once again, the IPA revealed the ongoing phenomenological process involved in having a disease, in this case a life-threatening one. The illness representations were not fixed but dynamic. The women identified a complex model of causes of the disease and linked this to their everyday lives. They talked about the reassurance provided by having established a biological cause of the disease but the additional causes they identified meant that they could potentially exert some control over the disease. They also mentioned their anxiety of passing it onto their children but managed that anxiety by identifying other possible more controllable causes of the disease. The primary control strategies they mentioned were not single strategies but ongoing processes of maintaining some control over the disease and reducing the likelihood of recurrence. The third theme labelled secondary control was more an ongoing attitude which was in turn related to the broader social and religious beliefs of the women involved. A central theme in this study was the emphasis on the ongoing tension involved in having a life-threatening disease and still trying to lead a normal life.

Most IPA studies have used semi-structured interviews as their primary source of information about the lived experience of particular health problems. More recent studies have begun to explore additional sources of subjective information. An example is the study by Murray (2005) on the social meanings of prosthesis use. In this study three sources of information were used: semi-structured face-to-face interviews, e-mail interviews, and an analysis of the posts made on an Internet discussion group. The researcher then integrated the three sources of information. In doing so he was aware of the different character of the three datasets. Murray noted that 'the use of e-mail interview extracts allows the representation of temporal experiences, while the use of Listserv posts provides in a more direct way the social contexts in which the social meanings of prosthesis use arise while also supplementing the more "public" account of the one-on-one interview with the "private" accounts of persons with a common membership (see Cornwell, 1984)' (p. 430). From this detailed analysis of these different sources of information he identified four themes concerned with the social meaning of prosthesis use:

1 Prosthesis use and social rituals
2 Being a leper: reactions of others
3 Social meanings of concealment and disclosure
4 Feelings and experiences regarding romantic and sexual relationships.

Once again, it is apparent that the experience of prosthesis use was not a fixed event but an ongoing process which the IPA study revealed was part of the person's involvement in the social world. Thus having the prosthesis not only changed the way the person acts in the world but the way others act towards them. The IPA study provided a vivid description of this process which in turn the researcher interpreted. Murray drew especially on the work of Erving Goffman (1963) who described the process of stigmatization and how the person with a stigma develops a range of strategies to manage everyday social interaction. The study by Murray illustrates the value of using multiple sources of data to reveal the lived experience of people with a particular health problem.

IPA continues to attract an increasing amount of research. As a newly evolving approach it has also attracted discussion about its theoretical and methodological assumptions. For example, Willig (2001) noted that the concern with trying to describe cognitive or thinking processes may not be compatible with some forms of phenomenology which are concerned with non-propositional, pre-cognitive forms of knowledge. IPA is often compared with grounded theory (Glaser & Strauss, 1967) although that approach has a greater focus on method than on theory. Willig adds that grounded theory is more suitable for understanding social processes whereas the focus of IPA is on personal experiences. Admittedly, the distinction between these foci is not very clear as is apparent in the previously described studies.

An extensive review of the literature by Brocki and Wearden (2006) identified 55 articles using this approach with a further seven identified subsequently. They noted a series of methodological concerns including lack of clarity as regards the role of the researcher in data collection and analysis, the inconsistency in sample sizes in reported studies, and the role of theory in interpretation. The original developers are aware of these and other criticisms and keen to extend discussion about refining and further developing this approach (Smith, Flowers and Larkin, 2009).

Illness Narratives

Another phenomenological approach is that of narrative psychology. According to narrative psychologists (e.g. Sarbin, 1986) *narrative* construction is an intrinsic part of making sense of the world. The process of creating a narrative enables the person to give meaning to their constantly changing world. Before the narrative there is merely a disjointed sequence of events. In creating the narrative the person selects some pieces of information and ignores others and pieces a story together. Admittedly this process is not conducted in isolation but as part of a wider process of social engagement.

According to narrative psychology people generate stories about illness experiences (Murray, 1997). The construction of these narrative accounts enables the person to grasp its meaning and to begin to exert some control over it. The character of these stories varies depending upon a variety of factors such as previous experience and public repertoires. In terms of orientation, some stories may offer the prospect of advancement, while others are more pessimistic. In terms of emotional valence, some stories may convey excitement whereas others are more placid or depressing.

Research into illness narratives was initially taken up by medical sociologists and anthropologists. Frank (1993) suggested that the central point in any crisis narrative is an epiphany when the actors begin to reassess their position in the world. This can occur at any time during the course of an illness but subsequently the sick person sees the illness in a new light. It is at this stage that the illness story turns from a regressive narrative into a progressive narrative. Admittedly not all sick persons encounter such an epiphanous moment. As Frank (1993) stated: 'Insofar as changing your life is a historically defined project, so the general possibility of epiphanies is also socially constructed. To experience an epiphany requires a cultural milieu in which such experiences are at least possibilities, if not routine expectations' (p. 42).

Frank (1995) developed a three-part typology of illness narratives:

1 Restitution narrative: the participant minimizes the experience of illness, rather considering it a temporary interruption that will be overcome;
2 Chaos narrative: the ill person loses a sense of order in their life and is unable to develop a way of dealing with the illness experience;
3 Quest narrative: the illness is a challenge to be met.

Subsequently, Ezzy (2000) proposed an extension to this typology to take into consideration the temporal dimension:

1 Restitutive linear narratives in which the future is controlled through current actions
2 Chaotic linear narratives in which there is no prospect of exerting control
3 Polyphonic narratives in which the emphasis is on the present rather than the future which is portrayed as uncertain.

These typologies have attracted substantial interest although like all typologies they should not be considered definitive but rather loose characterizations.

Another sociologist, Michael Bury, characterized the onset of illness as a period of *biographical disruption*. This term was developed by Michael Bury (1982) to describe the experience of people diagnosed with rheumatoid arthritis (RA). The onset of this disease disrupted plans and hopes for the future. For these people their life-story no longer fit with their everyday experiences and it needed to be recast. This process of reworking the parameters of the self has been termed *narrative reconstruction* by Williams (1984). Again working with people suffering from RA, Williams identified a pattern in the casual reasoning adopted by these individuals. They were attempting to integrate RA into their life plans. According to Williams this process of narrative reconstruction helped the sufferers 'reconstitute and repair ruptures between body, self, and world by linking and interpreting different aspects of biography in order to realign present and past and self and society' (p. 197).

These concepts of biographical disruption and narrative reconstruction have increasingly been used by a wide range of health practitioners and researchers including health psychologists. An example is the work of Mathieson and Stam (1995). They conducted detailed interviews with a sample of women who had had breast cancer. Their analysis of these interviews identified three major concerns and activities themes in the participants' accounts:

1 Disrupted feelings of fit: those bodily changes and other events in the woman's life that threatens their identity;
2 Renegotiating identity: the realization that there is a stigma associated with cancer and they will have to renegotiate their identity;
3 Biographical work: this is particularly concerned with how the events around the cancer make up a more or less coherent theme among the other events in their lives.

In developing Bury's concept of biographical disruption, Mathieson and Stam described the biographical work engaged by the women in their study as the process of integrating the illness events into their larger narrative identities. A challenge faced by the cancer patients was that they felt rejected by their peers because of the social and moral stigma attached to cancer. They felt deprived of opportunities for conversations within which they could conduct this biographical work.

In a follow-up study Yaskowich and Stam (2003) described the role of cancer support groups as providing such an opportunity for biographical work. They conducted interviews with women who participated in support groups. Analysis of these interviews identified five preliminary categories that were labelled 'talking safely', 'demystifying the unknown', 'deciding', 'hoping', and 'finding a separate space'. These categories were then transformed into two broader categories: 'a unique and separate social space' and 'biographical work'. It was within the support groups that the women felt that they had the opportunity to engage in biographical work that was not available elsewhere. As one woman said: 'Now you're done it [the treatment], everybody's sick and tired of talking about it. You're fixed. It's over with … I don't want to be burdening [my husband] with it' (p. 732).

One feature of narrative psychology is the focus on the individual account of illness experience or on that of a small number of individuals. An example is the study by Gray, Fergus and Fitch (2005) on the narrative accounts of cancer provided by two Black men. Four in-depth interviews were conducted with each of the participants. Between interviews the research team reflected on their content and identified particular issues to be pursued in subsequent interviews. In analysing the accounts Gray et al. were partially guided by Frank's three-part narrative typology. However, they were aware that such typologies can 'simplify and potentially distort'. Although there were elements of the restitution narrative in their accounts it was more an ongoing process and as such more similar to Ezzy's restitutive linear narrative. In the content of their narratives the two men intertwined personal and societal factors that made their accounts unique rather than abstract.

Although the dominant approach within narrative psychology has been the semi-structured interviews there is a growing body of research that has explored written narratives of various sorts. An example is the work by McGowan, Luker, Creed and Chew (2007) in which they examined the accounts written by women with chronic pelvic pain, a disabling condition with unclear underlying pathophysiology and resistant to various forms of medical intervention. Following a newspaper article the researchers approached over 100 women who were interested in describing their experiences. Subsequently they received hand-written letters from 26 women and a further 6 e-mail letters. Analysis of these letters revealed that they all followed the same chronological structure from initial awareness, through seeking medical advice and then receiving various treatments. Further analysis revealed one major theme which was labelled 'pathways to disengagement' that encompassed the various factors that disrupted or impeded the flow of the diagnostic cycle. This pathway was a passive process that occurred when the women felt they just could not face continued engagement with a health system that denied their pain. Unlike some of the other illness narratives, this narrative account did not have any end. Rather the women continued to experience pain and were frustrated at the lack of recognition of that pain. There is a need for health care to develop strategies to help these women re-engage with the health system or offer alternative forms of management of the pain.

Another source of illness narratives is the published accounts of people who have experienced various health problems. These are written not only by established writers but also by those with limited experience of writing. They are written both by patients and a variety of health practitioners. The increased popularity of this genre of writing has given rise to a descriptive term – pathography. A number of health psychologists have become interested both in the content of these published accounts but also in the whole process of writing about illness.

Murray (2009) analysed the written accounts of a sample of women who had breast cancer. These accounts were organized into a similar storyline with a beginning, a middle and an end. The beginning was the period before cancer that was often characterized as a time of innocence. The middle of the story was the diagnosis and the subsequent medical treatment. The end was the period of reassessment of identity and reintegration into society. In closing their story the women frequently emphasized the positive features of having cancer – it had given them an opportunity to reassess their lives. It was also apparent that the women were aware of the therapeutic benefits in telling their stories. They explicitly referred to this process of sense making.

This self-consciousness of the writers about the potential value of telling one's story has contributed to the growth of creative writing and drama classes in hospitals and health centres (Murray, 2009). This growth in what is termed therapeutic writing is partly informed by the work of Pennebaker and Beall (1986) who reported evidence from experimental trials of the health benefits of short periods of writing. More recent reviews of the benefits of this so-called expressive writing suggest that the effect is not large (Frattaroli, 2006). However, research in this field is limited through its focus on short periods of controlled writing. There is a need to explore the value of the more extensive creative writing (Nicholls, 2009).

Within the social science a recent methodological development has been the growth of autoethnography which is a disciplined reflection on the researcher's own experiences. In some ways this is a return to some of the earliest forms of psychological research. As an example, let us consider a researcher's writing about their own illness. Willig (2009) reported her analysis of her own written accounts of the experience of having skin cancer. In this study she was explicitly guided by Heidigger's (1962) philosophical phenomenology. In particular, she was concerned with the concept of being 'thrown' into the world. According to Heidigger as humans we are thrown into life circumstances which are changing and of which we have to make sense and act. Admittedly, in everyday life we do not experience this feeling of 'thrownness' but every so often crises occur when we are forced to reflect upon our position. Willig took this as the starting point for a reflection on her skin cancer dairy.

She described how the process of writing helped her to make sense of this threat to her life. On initial diagnosis she noted how 'meaning-making – something which had always seemed more or less effortless, even playful at times – felt like hard physical labour involving my whole body in the struggle against the black whole of meaninglessness' (p. 183). In the following days she developed what she described as a 'serviceable narrative'. This was one based upon confronting her mortality head-on rather than trying to evade it. This narrative gave her 'a sense of peace born from accepting where [she] had been "thrown"' but it was not easy to maintain. However, it was a narrative that she pursued since 'integrating the possibility of death into life as it was lived in the here and now seemed to remove some of the horror surrounding the idea of terminal illness' (p. 185).

Fortunately, the treatment for Willig's skin cancer was successful. Now that it was over she reflected not simply on the content of her narrative-making but also on the idea that perhaps from an existential perspective meaning-making may not always be helpful. As she noted, 'attempts to find meaning (especially backward-looking meanings such as the search for a cause) can interfere with accepting that life is, and always will be, uncertain, unpredictable and (to a large extent) uncontrollable' (p. 189).

Comment

Overall, it is apparent that these different phenomenological approaches provide an insight into the processes by which the individual attempts to make sense of illness. These approaches are growing in popularity and sophistication. Unlike the cognitivist approach they are much more open-ended and aim to connect personal representations of illness with changing everyday experiences. They also draw upon different philosophical traditions.

DISCURSIVE APPROACHES

Illness Discourse

The discursive turn in psychology has highlighted a problem with cognitive and phenomenological approaches to the study of illness representations in that they are concerned with trying to infer something about inner mental worlds from a study of verbal reports. An alternative approach is to focus on the character of the **discourse** itself and the context within which it occurs rather than on the structure of inferred inner mental phenomena. Within this approach the communicative nature of language is the focus of attention rather than inferred underlying beliefs (Potter and Wetherell, 1987).

Two main orientations have been identified in contemporary discourse analysis – discursive psychology and Foucauldian discourse analysis (Willig, 2004; McKinlay & McVittie, 2008). The former places emphasis on unpacking the various discursive strategies such as 'footing' and 'disclaiming' and their functions within a particular discursive context. The focus of this approach is on what the discourse is doing. The latter more critical form focuses on the particular discursive resources available within a culture and the implications for those who live there. These resources enable us to construct and live in the world in particular ways. It has been argued that these two orientations should not be seen as distinct approaches but rather complementary (Wetherell, 1998). Individuals are both producers and the products of discourse. More critical psychologists are wary at the assumed autonomy of the individual actor and the ignorance of issues of politics and power by discursive psychologists (Parker, 1997). Here we consider both approaches in a little more detail.

Discursive Psychology

Discursive psychologists have been concerned with how people talk about illness in different contexts. Detailed analysis of this discourse has provided insight into how illness is constructed through everyday language. An early example of this approach is the study by Middleton (1996) in which he explored the talk in a parent group for children with chronic renal failure. He argued that this talk is more than 'a display of inner workings of minds' but is 'part of the process of making [their] health care experiences socially intelligible' (p. 244). Rather than breaking the talk down into elemental beliefs, he attempted to understand it as part of the process of making sense of illness within a social context. He stressed that an important component of such talk is that it contains many contradictory elements and expressions of uncertainty. These elements are not deficiencies but rather are seen as being 'used to establish common understandings concerning what it is to care for chronically ill children' (p. 257). Further, the talk is more than self-presentation that can be ironed out by careful assessment but rather part of the broader collective process of meaning making.

KEY STUDY A discursive psychology approach to illness narrative

The focus of this study is exploring the character of the talk about a particular health problem, myalgic encephaloyelitis (ME) which is frequently known as chronic fatigue syndrome (CFS). In this study the research focused on the conversation between Angela, who has the ME, and Joe (her husband). An extract of this is shown below with the interviewer identified as Mary. It shows the very detailed annotation of the interview transcript used by discourse analysts. For example, = indicates an overlap in the conversation (what discourse analysts term 'latched') while (.) indicates a very short gap in the conversation. Each line is numbered in the transcription for ease of reference.

21. Mary mm and how did it (.) can you remember much about how it started ? =
22. Joe = heh heh
23. (.)

24. Angela	it started off with =
25. Joe	= it started off with a sore throat =
26. Angela	= I had a sore throat and I had the very worst headache I've ever had in
27.	my life (.) it was one evening =
28. Joe	=go back to where we believe it was caught at the swimming baths in
29.	(town) =
30. Angela	= yeah =
31. Joe	= we'd been going down in the evening (.) swimming once a week (.)
32.	and er it was after one of our sessions =
33. Angela	= yeah we thought we'd picked it up =
34. Joe	= I went swimming one week (.) you didn't feel up to it (.) then the
35.	following week =
36. Angela	= *you* were alright weren't you? =
37. Joe	=yeah and this ties in because it's now known that ME is caused by
38.	er (.) an enterovirus which is a prime place to pick up an enterovirus is
39.	a swimming baths (.) it's also the classic (.) *used* to be the classic place
40.	to catch polio in the old days (.) hot summers (.) and I think with
41.	swimming (.) kids being in the bath all through the day (.) at the end of
42.	the day the water wasn't getting through the cleansing plant quick
43.	enough (.) I suspect if you'd gone first thing in the morning it would be
44.	absolutely spot clean (.) but er I suppose by the time we got there (.)
45.	I suppose the enteroviruses were still there (.) yeah (.) just unfortunate

Source: Horton-Salway, 2001

A widely cited study by Horton-Salway (2001) is featured in the Box above. The extract illustrates what Horton-Salway describes as 'scene-setting'. This is how the person explores the potential causes of the health problem. In the extract Angela is identifying the visit to the baths as the cause of the ME. Thus, Angela and Joe are stating that other factors were not important. Also, in this extract Joe clearly describes the biomedical character of the ME as something that has a definite physical cause (lines 37–38). Thus, the discourse analyst is showing how in their conversation Angela and Joe jointly construct a theory of ME. This study also details other aspects of the conversation. It details the various problems that the two individuals experience and highlight the particular challenges of a contested illness. This discourse analysis of the conversation shows the strategies used by the speakers, for example referring to another person to support a particular argument or attributing blame to another to support the central person as virtuous. Horton-Salway emphasizes that such strategies are not motivated by insincerity and self-presentation but are rather part and parcel of the social construction of illness in everyday conversation.

Another example of the use of discursive psychology is the study by Radtke and Van Mens-Verhulst (2001) of mothers with asthma. Interviews with a number of these women revealed the dominance of the traditional medical discourse to describe asthma. Further, they identified certain causes of the disease in their everyday lives but distinct from their role as mothers. In discussing an exemplar case the authors noted that by avoiding any suggestion of a link between her asthma symptoms and mothering allowed the woman to do two things: 'first she positioned herself as a competent mother despite living with asthma' and 'second, it justified her claim that her previous employment situation and problems with her extended family were unjust and harmful and thereby had contributed to her illness'. In interpreting these findings Radtke and Van Mens-Verhulst emphasize that the women are both producers and products of discourse. 'As producers of discourse, the women do not draw upon the cultural resources available to them in some straightforward way, but rather use them strategically to accomplish certain actions' (p. 381).

This strategic use of discourse in everyday social interaction was developed further by Radley and Billig (1996) in their detailed commentary on the discursive context within which talk about health and illness is generated. In particular they contrasted the different positionings of healthy and sick people: 'the healthy have much to say about their illness experience, while the sick are often at pains to show their "normality"' (p. 225). Since the interviewer is usually a healthy person, the sick person feels strongly 'the need to *legitimate* [their] position'. This emphasizes that the 'accounts are situated in a rhetorical context of potential justification and criticism' (p. 226). Although this commentary was aimed at qualitative interview research, a similar comment can be made about quantitative questionnaire studies of health and illness beliefs.

Other studies have explored the dominant discourses that we draw upon to construct our sense of particular health issues. Drawing upon the concept of *interpretative repertoire* (Potter and Wetherell, 1987: 139) Benveniste, Lecouteur and Hepworth (1999) explored lay theories of anorexia nervosa. Interviews with five men and five women in Australia revealed three dominant themes that were labelled as a socio-cultural discourse, a discourse of the individual and a discourse of femininity. Drawing upon the socio-cultural discourse enabled participants to attribute a source of blame for anorexia nervosa to factors external to the individual. Conversely, the individual discourse located the cause of anorexia within the individual. However, it is argued that both of these discourses are premised upon a humanist conception of the individual as an autonomous rational being. This separation of sociocultural factors from individual psychology maintains the idea that anorexia nervosa is a manifestation of psychopathology.

Foucauldian Discourse Analysis

The internalization of dominant discourses of health and illness can be considered part of disciplinary power by which social norms are accepted (Foucault, 1979). Deviation from such norms can cause severe distress to the individual concerned. An example is the case of hirsutism: a medical term used to describe an excess of hair on the female body. In Western society, women spend a substantial amount of money to remove such hair. A study of women who had self-perceived hirsutism found that the women had strongly internalized the dominant discourse around female bodily hair and adopted a range of personal strategies to reduce the associated distress (Keegan, Liao and Boyle, 2003). 'Through self-surveillance and correction to such norms, and the regulation of bodies through body practices such as depilitatory regimes, women are rendered less socially oriented and more focused on self-modification' (p. 338). A particular point of interest was the way removal of hair was perceived as 'looking-after', an example of how body regulation is seen as self-care rather than a process of gender control.

A similar study of women with bulimia (Burns & Gavey, 2004) revealed the importance of the dominant discourse of healthy weight. This interacted with the dominant discourse on female body shape. The authors argue that both 'bulimic' and 'healthy' female bodies are underwritten by 'normalizing discourses that derogate female fat and amplitude and that promote engaging in regulatory practices designed to promote a slender body'. They continue that by focusing on healthy weight rather than a broader concept of health, current health promotion campaigns are 'paradoxically implicated in the shaping and production of subjectivities, practices and bodies for some women in ways that are antithetical to an overt health message' (p. 562).

A particular feature of FDA is exploring how dominant ideas become embodied in the person. Thus FDA researchers are not simply investigating discourses as things in themselves but how they become material reality through a process of negotiation by the person. An example of this is the work by Willig and Paulson (2008) on older women's talk about their ageing bodies. They initially identified through a literature review four dominant discourses about the ageing body. These were:

1 A biological discourse that emphasizes the vulnerability of the ageing body through physical degeneration;
2 A social constructionist/historical and personal agency discourse that considers the tension between discourses of contextual determinism and personal agency;

3 A female beauty discourse that considers older women's talk about losing control of their appearance;
4 A feminist discourse that considers women's ageing bodies threatened by the male gaze in patriarchal society and by the beauty industry.

Considering these four 'expert' discourses Willig and Paulson conducted qualitative interviews with ten older women about their perceptions of their bodies. These interviews were subsequently analysed following the six stages developed by Willig (2001):

1 Highlighting the transcript for references to the body
2 Coding each section for wider cultural discourses
3 Specifying the action-orientation of each section of the text
4 Identifying the various subject positions
5 Considering the practical implications of each section of text
6 Identify the 'ways of being' made possible by each section of text.

This analysis contributed to a detailed understanding of how the women engaged with dominant discourses about the ageing body. An important feature was the tension within the older women's use of the dualist constructions of the ageing body. On the one hand the women could talk about their body as something separate which was in decline physically. On the other hand this separation of body and mind could be considered functional in that the women could exert their active mind to control these ageing bodies. Willig and Paulson concluded that this demonstrates how the cultural discourses of personal agency are as important as those of biological and contextual determinism in shaping the ageing body.

Overall, these discursive approaches argue that illness discourse is an active and social creation that reflects the attempts of the person or persons to make sense of a problematic situation. The character of the discourse is variable and needs to be considered with reference to the immediate and broader social context within which it is generated.

SOCIAL APPROACHES

Social Representations of Health and Illness

Although the various psychological approaches to lay representations of illness have considered the social context within which they are generated social representation theory places the social at the centre of the process of sense making. Unlike the other approaches which tend to focus more on individual experiences of illness **social representations** are concerned with the process by which representations are created in everyday social interaction. Social representation theory is concerned with both the content of these representations and how they operate to shape our engagement with the world. 'They do not represent simply "opinions about", "images of" or "attitudes towards", but "theories" or "branches of knowledge" in their own right, for the discovery and organization of reality' (Moscovici, 1973: xiv).

An increasing number of researchers have explored the character of social representations of illness. The early classic study was conducted by Claudine Herzlich (1973). From her interviews with a sample of French adults Herzlich concluded that a central concept in the popular definitions of health and illness is activity. For most lay people to be active means to be healthy while to be inactive means to be ill. Herzlich distinguished between three lay reactions to illness:

1 *Illness as destructive:* the experience of those actively involved in society.
2 *Illness as liberator:* the experience of those with excessive social obligations.
3 *Illness as an occupation:* the experience of those who accept illness and feel they must contribute to its alleviation.

Lay people are aware of these different reactions and not only adopt one or another of these strategies depending upon time and circumstance, but also characterize other individuals as belonging to a particular category.

The original formulation of SR theory emphasized the important role of science in shaping everyday common sense (Moscovici, 1984). More recent formulations have indicated a much more dynamic interaction between science and common sense (Joffe, 2002). In Western society, biomedicine is extremely important in shaping our understandings of health and illness. As Herzlich and Pierret (1987) stress: 'in our society the discourse of medicine about illness is so loud that it tends to drone out all others' (p. xi). The media plays a very important role in acting as a conduit of scientific medical ideas to the general public. As such, SR researchers are interested in both what lay people have to say about illness but also in how the media reports these ideas. The media help to transform scientific thinking into more everyday terms. In doing so they transform illness from something that is impersonal into something that is personal and is infused with particular cultural norms and values. Of course, since scientists are also lay people their language can also reflect these values.

An important characteristic of social representations is that they are not passive characteristics of the individual but part of the dialectical process of engagement between the individual and the social world. Moscovici (1984) refers to two particular processes, *anchoring* and *objectification,* which underlie the process of developing social representations. The first is the process whereby unfamiliar concepts are given meaning by connecting them with more familiar concepts, whereas the second is the process whereby a more abstract concept acquires meaning through association with more everyday phenomena.

Several researchers have used these concepts to explore popular views of particular illnesses. Joffe (1996) conducted detailed interviews about AIDS with a sample of young adults from London and from South Africa. She also conducted a content analysis of media campaigns. She notes that historically mass incurable illnesses have been anchored to the 'other'. In the case of AIDS this process is shown in the anchoring of that disease in the supposed aberrant behaviour of others. This process serves a protective function by distancing the person from the risk of contracting the disease. However, a certain amount of 'leakage' has occurred as it became apparent that AIDS could be spread via the blood supply and among heterosexuals. The process of objectification transforms an abstract concept into an image. Joffe (1996) noted that the media images of tombstones and coffins concretized the fear associated with AIDS.

Forming social representations helps to define a group and also to promote in-group solidarity and to defend group members from out-group threats. Consider the case of the Ebola virus that is deadly if contracted. Interviews conducted in Britain about this virus found that most lay people portrayed it as an African disease and that they are very unlikely to contract it. As one woman said: 'It just seemed like one of those mythical diseases, sort of thing, science fiction like thing, that happens in places like Africa and underdeveloped countries and doesn't come here' (Joffe and Haarhoff, 2002: 965). By clearly characterizing the disease in fantastical terms the lay public is symbolically protecting itself from this outside threat.

In a comparable study of representations of AIDS in Zambia (Joffe and Bettega, 2003) it was found young residents distanced themselves from the risk of the disease by representing it as originating in Western society and in deviant sexual and scientific practices. These findings highlighted the challenge of encouraging young people to take personal action to protect themselves against AIDS. Health campaigns designed to curtail the spread of AIDS would need to challenge these social representations.

SR theory is not just concerned with language but also with non-linguistic representations of phenomena such as illness. Joffe (2003) links this broader concern with the use of images and symbols to understand health and illness. For example, the ribbons used to convey support for particular diseases or the various metaphors that are associated with illness. The classic analyses by Sontag of the metaphors used to describe cancer (Sontag, 1978) and AIDS (Sontag, 1988) illustrate how difficult it is to talk and think about illness without reference to certain metaphors.

According to Joffe (1996) the potential for modifying social representations of disease is limited since they serve the function of preserving the status quo in a culture. They not only make the social world remain familiar and manageable but also maintain the dominance of certain ideas. Admittedly, certain organized groups within society can subvert these dominant ideas. The gay movement in Britain contributed to a reassessment of the dominant image of AIDS as belonging to a supposedly deviant minority group that in terms of religious beliefs were themselves to blame for contracting the disease (Markova and Wilkie, 1987). Instead, it was recharacterized as a disease that could affect heterosexual as well as gay individuals.

Other researchers have explored the potential of challenging the character of restrictive social representations of illness through various forms of social action. For example, Krause (2003) conducted a participant action research project with a group of individuals who had inflammatory bowel disease. Interviews were conducted with them before and after the participatory intervention. At the outset, the participants had a very negative social representation of the disease. The disease pervaded all aspects of their lives: family, work and social relations. Figure 16.2 provides a summary of the social representation of the disease before and after the participatory intervention. It shows how social representation theory is concerned with developing an understanding of the lay theories of illness and how these can change over time.

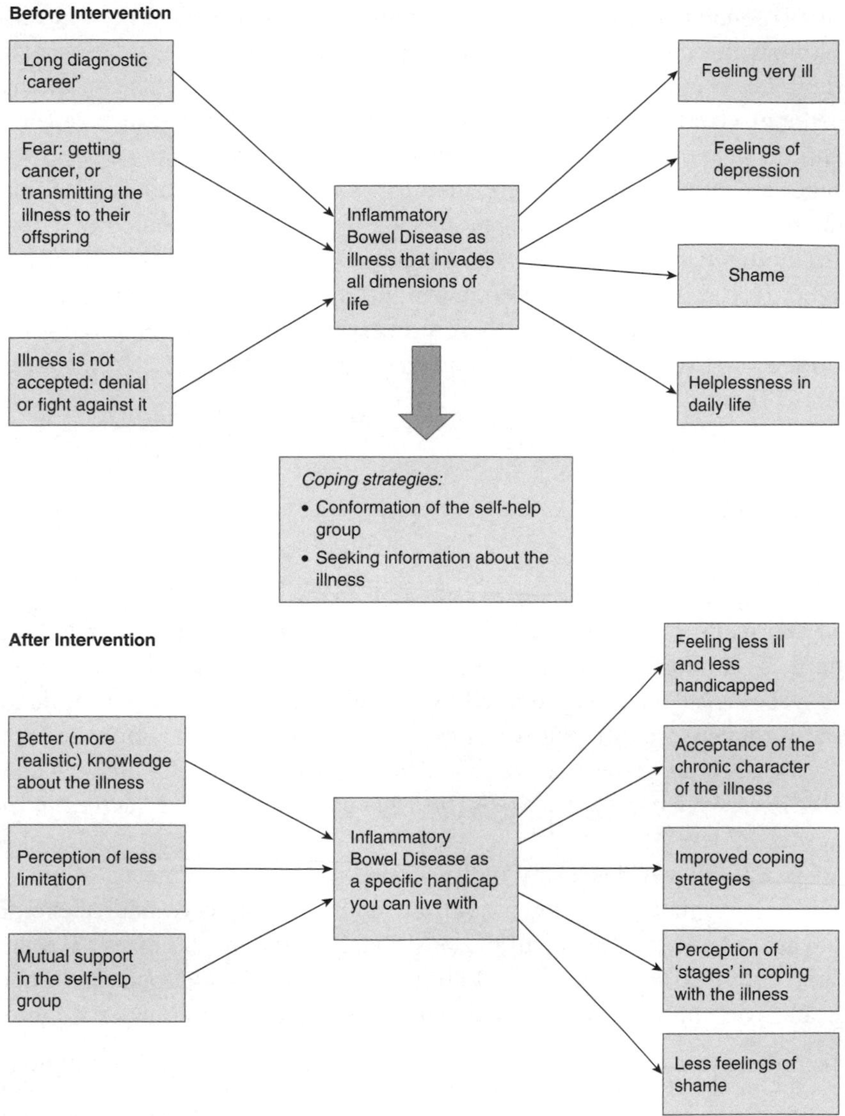

Figure 16.2 Social representations of inflammatory bowel disease

Media Representations

An important part of studies of social representations has been concerned with how particular phenomena are represented in the media. The initial study of Moscovici considered how psychoanalysis was represented in the Catholic and the Communist press in France in the 1950s. Today, the media is much more extensive. It can range from newspapers and television through to the Internet and zines. Public surveys have confirmed the extent of popular interaction with different forms of media. There is an obvious need to explore not only the character of illness representations in the various media but also how lay people engage with these representations and who sets the agenda in illness media production (Hodgetts & Chamberlain, 2006). Further, it is not just illness representations in themselves that are important but how they are constructed with reference to other social phenomena. For example, Nairn et al. (2006) have commented on how ethnic minorities and indigenous groups are popularly represented in a denigratory manner in the popular media. This in turn has implications for the health of the groups so portrayed. Recently, Estacio (2009) has highlighted the need for critical health psychologists to move from describing these processes to directly challenging them. Her study reported on a successful activist campaign to directly challenge media portrayal of Filipino workers.

CONCLUSIONS

The study of lay illness representations is a growing area within health psychology. Different theoretical and methodological approaches have guided research in this area. One way of integrating these different approaches to the study of illness beliefs is by considering the levels of psychological analysis proposed by Doise (1986). Doise suggested that a reason for the confusion between different social psychologists was that they operated at different levels of analysis. He suggested that we should distinguish between research which was conducted at the *intrapsychic* level of analysis from that which is conducted at the *interpersonal, group* and *societal* levels.

This classification provides a way of organizing research on representations of illness (Murray, 1993). At the intrapsychic level are both the cognitive and phenomenological approaches; at the interpersonal and positional levels are the discursive and narrative accounts while at the societal level are the social representational and Foucauldian discourse analytic approaches. The challenge is to explore the connection across these levels.

An example of the integration of the different levels was the study by Crossley (1999) who noted the connection between personal and cultural stories. Similarly Murray (2002) explored the connection between narrative and social representation theory. Detailed analysis of the three-fold typology of social representations of illness developed by Herzlich (1973) revealed their narrative structure. Conversely, narratives can also be explored at different levels of analysis (Murray, 2000). The challenge is to see the social and political in the personal accounts of illness and to explore the implications of this for strategies to improve health (Campbell, 2004b).

FUTURE RESEARCH

1 Illness representations evolve over time. There is a need for a greater understanding of their evolution.
2 Illness representations are connected with people's social world. Health psychologists need to be involved in mapping these connections within specific cultures.
3 Theoretically, health psychologists need to explore the conceptual connections between illness and health discourse.
4 The interconnectedness of illness discourse and bodily processes is still poorly understood. There is a need for a concerted programme of theoretical work in this area.
5 Lay representations of illness, or of groups of people, can have negative impact on the health of particular groups. Health psychology has a role in challenging these representations.

Summary

1 Psychologists have used a variety of theoretical perspectives to investigate lay representations of illness. The major approaches have been the cognitive, phenomenological, discursive and social perspectives.
2 Cognitive approaches have attempted to identify a limited number of dimensions of illness representations including identity, causes, time line, consequences' and control/cure. The cognitive approach has generated a substantial body of empirical research using various standardized measures.
3 The phenomenological approach is concerned with describing the subjective experiences of the individual patient. It is less concerned with identifying a limited number of illness dimensions but more with developing a sophisticated interpretative model. This approach prefers to use qualitative interviews to collect data.
4 Narrative psychology is a particular phenomenological approach which is concerned with the narrative character of people's accounts of illness.
5 Discourse analysis focuses on the character of the language used to talk about illness and the context within which it occurs rather than on the structure of inferred beliefs.
6 Social representation theory is concerned with the lay theories that underlie popular understandings of illness.

17

Illness and Personality

Ills of the body may be cured by physical remedies or by the power of the spirit acting through the soul.

Paracelsus

Outline

This chapter examines the influence of individual differences in personality and other psychological characteristics on susceptibility to illness. It begins with a brief history of the contrasting approaches of practitioners of orthodox and wholistic medicine. It goes on to consider Freud's work on hysteria and contemporary approaches to medically unexplained symptoms such as chronic fatigue syndrome. After an account of some of the ways in which Freud's theories became applied to organic illness by the psychosomatic schools of psychoanalysis, there is an analysis of the problems involved in investigating and explaining links between personality and physical illness. The chapter concludes with an assessment of contemporary research on personality and illness with particular reference to coronary heart disease and cancer.

ORTHODOX MEDICINE AND WHOLISTIC APPROACHES

Orthodox Western medicine has always been based on the belief that physical illness has physical causes and requires physical treatment. While there is increasing acceptance of the importance to be attached to health behaviours among the causes of illness, the assumption remains that the actual mechanisms are physical, including such things as viruses, bacteria, carcinogens, and genetic and physiological abnormalities. Partly as a result of DNA research and the influence of the pharmaceutical industry, this *physicalist* approach is increasingly being applied to psychological disorders, and conditions ranging from schizophrenia to mild cases of depression are commonly attributed to biochemical imbalances, often thought to be genetic. On the other hand, there are popular beliefs, supported to some extent by health psychologists, that people with certain kinds of personality may be particularly susceptible to heart disease or cancer and that psychological disturbances may be a cause of much physical illness. The research on stress and illness discussed in Chapter 12 is one aspect of this. Wholistic treatments and complementary therapies for physical diseases frequently have a large psychological component including stress management programmes, relaxation, breathing exercises and meditation. It is often claimed by proponents of such treatments that they are capable of correcting 'psychic' or 'energy' imbalances that have triggered the symptoms in the first place.

While wholistic approaches can be traced back at least as far as Plato (Bass, 2007), it is quite clearly shown in Roy Porter's history of medicine from its earliest origins to the present day (Porter, 1997), that most professional practitioners of medicine have taken a physicalist approach. In the history of Western medicine, the most influential doctrine has been the Hippocratic one, which dates back to the fifth century BCE and which presupposes that there is a physical basis for all disorders, whether physical or psychological. According to Galen (born AD129), a key figure in the Hippocratic tradition, psychological and physical disorders are both attributable to an imbalance of the four bodily humours: blood, phlegm, black bile and yellow bile. Little scope was left for psychological causation and this theory only really lost its hold on Western thinking in the 1850s. When Galen noted that *melancholy* women were more likely to get breast cancer than *sanguine* women he was not putting forward a psychological hypothesis. Although the psychological characteristics of melancholy correspond to some extent to the modern concept of depression, Galen took the view that breast cancer and melancholy were jointly attributable to humoral imbalance, in this case to an excess of black bile (see Table 1.1; also see Sontag, 2002).

As an indication of the grip these ideas had on medical thinking in Western Europe, the black bile theory of depression was still being articulated in 1836 by Johannes Freidreich, professor of psychiatry in Würzburg, together with the view that mania was caused by an excess of yellow bile, psychosis by an excess of blood, and dementia by an excess of phlegm (see Shorter, 1992). One feature of the doctrine of the four humours that even today finds its echo in psychological theory is Galen's description of the four *classical temperaments* (see Box 17.1).

Box 17.1

The four humours and modern personality theory

Anaximander (610–546 BCE) described the underlying condition of the universe as being boundless in time and space. The ancient Greeks believed that everything in the world was made of four elementary substances, Earth, Air, Fire and Water, in primary opposites. These supported the four bodily humours and temperaments described by Galen in the second century AD (see Chapter 1; Table 1.1). The temperaments characterized individuals possessing an excess of each of the four humours. The sanguine has an excess of blood, the choleric of yellow bile, the phlegmatic of phlegm and the melancholic of black bile. As descriptions of personality types they were still in use during the second half of the twentieth century. In his influential theory of personality the late Hans Eysenck proposed two basic dimensions of personality, extravert–introvert and stable–unstable, and developed a personality test to measure them. Both dimensions were assumed to be measurable along a continuum, with extreme examples towards each end and the average person in the middle. Although he considered the reduction of personality to four qualitatively different types to be an oversimplification, Eysenck (1970) pointed out that the classical temperaments do correspond quite closely with four extremes that can be identified using his personality test: the stable extravert (sanguine), unstable extravert (choleric), stable introvert (phlegmatic) and unstable introvert (melancholic), an interesting convergence of classical and contemporary personality theories.

The humoral theory was eventually abandoned following the rapid development of physiology in the nineteenth century, and notably the founding of the modern science of cellular pathology by Rudolf Virchow in Germany in the 1850s. This was the key that opened the door to our contemporary understanding of physical diseases. Since there were no obvious indications that cellular pathology could account for psychological disorders, the door was also open for the development of purely psychological explanations, particularly by Sigmund Freud. The historical dominance of the humoral theory and the modern ascendancy of organic medicine has not entirely inhibited speculation of the opposite kind, that psychological factors may play a part in causing physical diseases and influencing recovery. This is evident in the continuing widespread use of the concept of *stress-related disease.* A good historical example is provided by Dogen (1200–1253), the founder of the Soto school of Japanese Buddhism. Admonishing his pupils not to regard illness as a hindrance to performing their spiritual practices, he remarked:

> *I suspect that the occurrence of illness stems from the mind. If you lie to a hiccuping person and put him on the defensive, he gets so involved in explaining himself that his hiccups stop. Some years ago when I went to China, I suffered from diarrhoea while aboard ship. A violent storm arose, causing great confusion; before I knew it, my sickness was gone. This makes me think that if we concentrate on study and forget about other things, illness will not arise.*
> (Dogen's *Shobogenzo Zuimonki* quoted in Masunaga, 1972)

Sontag (2002) provides many European and North American examples. In England in the late sixteenth and seventeenth centuries it was widely believed that the happy man would not get plague. In 1871 the physician who treated Alexander Dumas for cancer wrote that, among the principal causes of cancer, were 'deep and sedentary study and pursuits, and feverish and anxious agitation of public life, the cares of ambition, frequent paroxysms of rage, violent grief'. At about the same time in England, one doctor advised patients that they could avoid cancer by being careful to bear the ills of life with equanimity; above all things, not to 'give way' to any grief. At this time also, tuberculosis (TB) was often thought to come from too much passion afflicting the reckless and sensual, or else to be a disease brought on by unrequited love. In fact TB was often called *consumption*, and hence the appearance in the English language of metaphors such as *consuming passion*.

FREUD, HYSTERIA AND MEDICALLY UNEXPLAINED SYMPTOMS

Freud and Hysteria

Having had a top quality orthodox medical education in the 1880s, Freud was not inclined to propose psychological explanations for organic disorders. His psycho-analytic theories, which were eventually to encompass the whole of human psychology, originated in the study of **hysteria**, symptoms which appeared to indicate serious neurological or other physical disorder, but for which there appeared to be no underlying physical cause (see Box 17.2). The medical theorists of ancient Greece first used the word hysteria to refer to anomalous physical complaints, which they believed occurred only in women. They regarded it as a gynæcological disorder caused by the womb moving away from its normal position. By the end of the nineteenth century, as a result of the pioneering work of Charcot, Breuer and Freud, it had become widely accepted that hysterical disorders are not restricted to women and that the causes are psychological rather than physiological. By using the newly discovered techniques of hypnosis, these pioneers were able to show that hysteria may be caused psychologically, but outside the awareness of the sufferer. Hysterical symptoms could be induced in any hypnotizable person by the use of hypnotic suggestion, and the symptoms of hypnotizable patients could often be relieved, unfortunately only temporarily, in this way. While this does not actually rule out the possibility that there is an organic basis to hysteria, it certainly made it a lot easier for Freud to put forward his bold psychological hypotheses. (For detailed accounts of this early work on hysteria and subsequent developments in the twentieth century, see Sulloway, 1980 and Shorter, 1992.)

Box 17.2

Hysteria: the case of Anna O

Psychological theories of hysteria first came to prominence as a result of the collaboration between Sigmund Freud and the Viennese physiologist Josef Breuer. From 1880 to 1882 Breuer treated a patient who became known as 'Anna O' and who proved to be of great importance in the history of psychoanalysis (see portrait below). Anna suffered from a spectacular range of hysterical and other symptoms, including paralysis and loss of sensation mainly on the right side of her body, disturbances of eye movements and vision, occasional deafness, multiple personality and loss of the ability to speak her native German. As a result of this last symptom, Breuer was obliged to talk to her in English over which she retained a perfect command. When she was asked to recall previous occurrences of each of her symptoms while under hypnosis, Anna invariably arrived at previously forgotten memories of distressing incidents that had occurred while she had nursed her dying father. As a result of this the symptom temporarily disappeared. For example, the paralysis of Anna's right arm disappeared after she recalled having had the hallucination of a large black snake while sitting at her father's bedside. Anna O's true identity was much later revealed to be Bertha Pappenheim and she went on to become a well-known feminist who campaigned on problems of single mothers, children in orphanages, prostitution and the white slave trade. Just how successful was her treatment for hysteria is still a matter of controversy and she herself remained ambivalent about the value of psychoanalysis, once remarking that it depends very much on the ability of the psychoanalyst whether it is a good instrument or a double-edged sword. For further details, see Sulloway (1980).

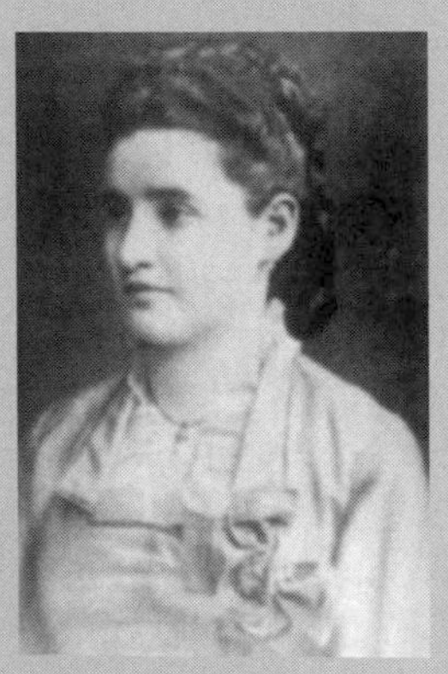

The term *hysteria* is not often used nowadays, having been largely replaced by **psychosomatic (or somatoform) disorder**, but it remains implicit in the new terminology that sufferers are somehow *somatizing* problems that are intrinsically psychological in nature. Freud found it difficult to convince his patients that they were not suffering from an organic disease and it is equally true today that sufferers from a variety of conditions are hostile to suggestions that these conditions may be psychological rather than organic in origin. Among the conditions that provoke controversy are **myalgic encephalomyelitis** (ME) or **chronic fatigue syndrome** (CFS), irritable bowel syndrome, repetitive strain injury, fibromyalgia, Gulf War syndrome, total allergy syndrome, migraine, and a variety of types of pain in the back, chest, abdomen, limbs and face. Arguments for believing that these are all contemporary forms of hysteria have been forcefully put by Shorter (1992) and Showalter (1997). On the other hand, there are many who share the views of the sufferers themselves that a failure to find an organic basis for a condition is not a convincing reason for asserting that one does not exist.

Medically Unexplained Symptoms

Bass (2007) notes that, perhaps in deference to patients' sensitivities with regard to suggestions of psychological causation, the currently fashionable terms replacing *psychosomatic disorders* are the relatively neutral *functional somatic symptoms and medically unexplained symptoms*. He points out that they account for nearly half of all primary care consultations and that only 10–15 per cent are subsequently shown to have an organic basis. The symptoms of apparently distinct syndromes such as chronic fatigue syndrome and irritable bowel syndrome are so great that it is debatable whether they can be fully clinically distinguished (Nimnuan et al., 2001). It is also widely accepted that cognitive behavioural therapy is the most effective treatment.

Brown (2004) reviews earlier explanations of medically unexplained symptoms and attempts to integrate them into a modern neuropsychological theory. The main earlier explanations, each of which he considers to be partially true, are based on the concepts of

1 *disassociation:* a loss of awareness, following traumatic experiences, of cognitive processes which are nevertheless still active;
2 *conversion:* the unconscious suppression (or *repression*) of traumatic memories which retain a neural energy which becomes *converted* into somatic symptoms that were either present at the time of the original trauma or represent it symbolically;
3 *somatization:* the tendency to experience or express psychological distress as the symptoms of physical illness.

He then presents a new integrative model that utilizes elements of each of these while locating his theory in modern conceptions of *attention, consciousness, control, personality, illness beliefs* and the *misattribution of symptoms*. He considers his model to be consistent with the use of cognitive behavioural therapy for treatment, but argues that it is also consistent with the use of psychodynamic psychotherapy, physiotherapy, occupational therapy and antidepressants, all treatments that are currently in use for medically unexplained symptoms.

PSYCHOSOMATIC MEDICINE AND ORGANIC ILLNESS

The rapid development of organic medicine from the 1850s led to a declining enthusiasm among medical practitioners for speculation about possible psychological causes of organic diseases. Freud was no exception. He insisted that psychoanalytic training should be restricted to those already qualified in medicine, on the grounds that only the medically trained psychoanalyst would have the skills necessary to decide whether or not a patient's symptoms needed to be investigated as indicating possible organic disorder. It was not until the period from the 1920s to the 1950s that Freud's theories were applied to physical illness by theorists who developed the *psychosomatic approach* in psychoanalysis.

A useful survey of this approach is given by Brown (1964). One of its most colourful representatives was George Groddeck, who believed that all illness is unconsciously motivated and has a meaning for the sufferer. Just as a hysterical pregnancy might be motivated by an unconscious wish to have a baby, so might a case of laryngitis be motivated by a desire not to speak. To take an extreme example, a heart attack might be viewed as an unconscious attempt to commit suicide. Another equally colourful representative was Wilhelm Reich, who believed, among many other extraordinary things, that repressed sexual feelings could cause a blocking of mysterious forms of organic energy leading to the development of cancer. Reich's cancer theories were pseudoscientific and absurd, but his idea that cancer may be caused by some block in the individual's normal flow of emotional energy has proved influential. The belief that psychological factors play an important part in the initial causation and subsequent disease course of cancer was widely held by many psychosomatic thinkers. By the mid-1950s when their influence was at its height, Leshan and Worthington (1956), reviewing research in this area for the *British Journal of Medical Psychology,* drew the following conclusions:

> *As one examines these papers, one is struck by the fact that there are consistent factors reported in studies that gathered material in different ways. There appear to be four separate threads that run through the literature. These are (1) the patient's loss of an important relationship prior to the development of the tumour; (2) the cancer patient's inability successfully to express hostile feelings and emotions; (3) the cancer patient's unresolved tension concerning a parental figure; (4) sexual disturbance.*

Views such as these are still widely held, although seldom by cancer specialists. They are often used to justify complementary therapies that aim to teach sufferers how to beat cancer by the power of the mind. This is all very well if they work, if psychological dispositions really do play a significant part in the causation and development of cancer. If not, as Sontag and others have pointed out, the propagation of these beliefs may be profoundly undesirable:

> *In Karl Menninger's more recent formulation: 'Illness is in part what the world has done to a victim, but in larger part it is what the victim has done with his world, and with himself…' Such preposterous and dangerous views manage to put the onus of the disease on the patient and not only weaken the patient's ability to understand the range of plausible medical treatment but also, implicitly, direct the patient away from such treatment.* (Sontag, 2002)

Of all the theorists in the psychosomatic tradition, the one who has contributed most to modern health psychology is Franz Alexander, the Chicago psychoanalyst who, in *Psychosomatic Medicine* (1950), combines psychoanalytic theory with hypotheses about physiological mechanisms, principally those involving the *autonomic nervous system* (ANS). He emphasizes the distinction between the *sympathetic* division of the ANS that, roughly speaking, controls emotional arousal and the fight-or-flight emergency reactions of the organism, and the *parasympathetic* division that, again roughly speaking, controls relaxation and the slowing down of functions activated by the sympathetic division. According to Alexander, sustained activity in either branch of the ANS without the counterbalancing effect of the other can have disease consequences. Excessive sympathetic activity contributes to cardiovascular disease, diabetes and rheumatoid arthritis, while excessive parasympathetic activity contributes to gastrointestinal disorders including dyspepsia, ulcers and colitis. Excessive sympathetic activity may occur as a consequence of prolonged stress (see Chapter 12), but Alexander also thought that some personalities may be predisposed to the excessive activation of one of the two branches of the ANS at the expense of the other.

Alexander's theories led to the development in contemporary health psychology of the distinction between the **Type A** and **Type B personalities** and their assumed differential susceptibility to cardiovascular disease, and to recent related work on hostility and cardiovascular disease. We will consider this work shortly but, before doing so, it is necessary to examine the logic underlying empirical research linking personality to physical disease and some of the pitfalls in its interpretation.

EXPLAINING LINKS BETWEEN PSYCHOLOGICAL STATES AND PHYSICAL ILLNESS

It is generally agreed today that the psychosomatic approach in psychoanalysis and the proponents of **psychosomatic medicine** failed to produce convincing evidence of causal connections between psychological characteristics and physical illness, or to demonstrate that their therapeutic interventions were effective (Holroyd & Coyne, 1987). They were criticized for much the same reasons that psychoanalysis has been criticized more generally (MacMillan, 1997). Their theories were highly speculative and relied on elaborate interpretations of clinical data rather than controlled statistical studies. They also suffered from the defect of being retrospective, seeking to 'explain' patients' illnesses as 'caused' by psychological characteristics already known to the clinician, rather than prospective, making predictions about future illness on the basis of present psychological assessments.

The period since the 1960s has seen the growth of a large empirical literature on the statistical relationship between personality, as assessed by a wide variety of standardized tests, and physical illness. These studies often derive their hypotheses from the earlier speculations of the psychosomatic approach but seek to rectify its defects by carefully analysing statistical evidence. There is, however, one major defect that cannot be overcome because it is intrinsic to this type of research. The evidence is obtained from correlational investigations rather than true experiments and, as a consequence, findings are open to a wide range of interpretations. Obviously no investigator can assign personalities at random to experimental participants and then study their subsequent proneness to illness. All that the investigator can do is to administer personality tests to the participants and obtain measures of their illness status. Statisticians constantly remind us that it is not possible to infer causation from correlation and, in the case of personality–illness correlations, it is possible to illustrate this by considering a range of important problems of interpretation. The issues are perennial problems in the health psychology literature and are essentially logical in nature. We have summarized these in Table 17.1.

These problems will now be considered in more detail.

Table 17.1 Problems of interpretation in research on personality and illness

Type of problem	Statement of the problem
Direction of causality	Cross-sectional studies are correlational and so there can be no certainty as to the direction of causality, as to what may be a cause and what may be an effect.
Background variables	Two variables (A and B) that are associated together may both be related to a third, background variable (C) that has not been measured and may not even be known to be relevant.
Self-reporting of illness	Health psychology research often relies upon self-reported illness that has not been verified by objective medical tests.
Dimensions of personality	The number of different personality variables to evaluate remains controversial.
Physiological mechanisms versus health behaviour	It is difficult to determine whether associations between personality and illness are mediated by physiological differences or health behaviour.

Direction of Causality

Psychological characteristics may be a cause of physical illness but they can also be a consequence of illness. This is a particular problem for cross-sectional studies that assess personality traits and illness status (present illness or illnesses experienced in the past) at the same time. For example, if patients with a history of coronary illness have higher scores on anxiety and depression than healthy controls, should we conclude that anxiety and depression are risk factors for coronary illness or that a history of coronary problems can cause people to become more anxious and depressed? Obviously the causal direction cannot be inferred from this type of study. The flaw may seem trivially obvious but it is surprising how many cross-sectional studies are to be found in the research literature on associations between personality and illness.

The problem cannot always be resolved by conducting prospective studies to investigate the extent to which the current personalities of healthy participants are predictive of future illness. The reason for this is that many major illnesses take a long time to develop and it is frequently the case that patients have experienced unusual and disturbing symptoms for some time before a diagnosis is given. It is therefore possible that psychological characteristics that appear to be a cause of subsequent illness are in fact a consequence of symptoms of developing illness occurring prior to diagnosis. Prospective studies are clearly far superior to cross-sectional studies but they do not necessarily eliminate the problem of the specification of causality.

Background Variables

A correlation may be found between two variables A and B when there is neither a direct effect of A on B, nor of B on A, but a third *background variable,* C, has an effect on both. Galen's explanation for the association he believed to exist between melancholy and breast cancer is a good illustration. Here an excess of black bile is the background variable that he hypothesized to be a cause of both melancholy and breast cancer. As a further illustration, suppose that some people have a history of childhood illness that leaves them constitutionally weak and prone to further illness. Suppose also that this history of childhood illness has had a deleterious effect on their personality development, perhaps by limiting their opportunities for social development. The inclusion of a number of such individuals in a sample along with constitutionally stronger individuals who have had a healthy childhood could produce a non-causal correlation in the sample between adult personality and adult proneness to illness, because both are influenced by childhood illness. Further examples of background variables, notably genetic predispositions, are discussed by Holroyd and Coyne (1987) and Suls and Rittenhouse (1990).

Self-Reporting of Illness

Stone and Costa (1990) and Cohen and Williamson (1991) point out that much health psychology research relies on self-reported illness rather than biologically verified disease. This does not only apply to minor ailments such as colds and flu. The diagnosis of angina pectoris, for example, is frequently based solely on patients' reports of chest pain. Stone and Costa argue that this reliance on self-reported illness is particularly unsatisfactory when considering research into links between personality and illness. They point out that there is extensive evidence that psychological distress is associated with somatic complaints but not with organic disease. Since many personality tests scores may be interpreted, at least to some extent, as measures of distress, it follows that correlations between test scores and self-reported illness may provide a false indication of a link between personality and disease when all that they really show is that neurotic individuals are the ones most likely to complain of being ill. However, it should not be assumed that any discrepancy between self-reported illness and biologically verified illness is necessarily an indication of neuroticism. Adler and Matthews (1994) note that there is evidence that perceived health predicts mortality independently of biological risk factors, leading them to conclude that self-reported health provides useful information over and above direct biological indications. The association between perceived health and mortality has now been confirmed by many studies, and Jylhä (2009) provides a detailed analysis of possible reasons for it.

Dimensions of Personality

Personality testing is not an exact science and there is little agreement as to what the basic dimensions of personality really are, or even whether the question is worth asking. Three influential theories have been those of Eysenck, who argued initially that there were only two dimensions, extraversion and neuroticism (see Box 17.1), and subsequently added a third, psychoticism; Cattell, who believed he had identified 16; and McCrae and Costa (2003) who settled for five. These so-called 'Big Five' personality traits, which have generated a considerable amount of recent research, consist of extraversion/introversion, agreeableness/antagonism, conscientiousness, neuroticism/emotional stability, and openness to experience.

A problem that arises in research using personality tests is that similar items can often be included in tests that are supposed to be measuring different traits so that, not surprisingly, scores for the same group of individuals given both tests may be highly intercorrelated. Consider some of the measures that are frequently used in research into the links between personality and illness. The individual who scores high on anxiety is also likely to score high on depression, neuroticism and **pessimistic explanatory style**, and correspondingly low on self-esteem, **self-efficacy**, **hardiness**, internal **locus of control** and **sense of coherence**. The common element that may run through all of these measures is probably best labelled, following Stone and Costa (1990), as *distress proneness*. Suls and Bunde (2005) discuss this issue in a detailed review of research linking anger/hostility, anxiety and depression with cardiovascular disease. They note that strong correlations exist between all three traits, which make it difficult to establish which of the associations with cardiovascular disease is of primary importance, or whether a more general trait of negative affectivity is the key variable.

Physiological Mechanisms Versus Health Behaviour

Psychological characteristics may be linked to illness, either by way of physiological variables with which they are associated, or more indirectly, by way of their relationship to health behaviour. The proponents of psychosomatic medicine, especially Franz Alexander, believed in the existence of physiological mechanisms linking personality to illness, often involving differences in the functioning of the sympathetic and parasympathetic divisions of the autonomic nervous system. Health psychologists who conduct research into the relationship between personality and illness are also primarily interested in physiological pathways. However, it is generally acknowledged that more prosaic explanations for correlations between personality and illness may be derived from the fact that personality differences are often associated with differences in health behaviour (Suls & Rittenhouse, 1990; Miller, Smith, Turner, Guijarro & Hallet, 1996; Stone & McCrae, 2007). Characteristics such as anxiety, depression, neuroticism and hostility have been variously shown to be associated with levels of smoking and alcohol consumption, diet and exercise, sleep disturbance, likelihood of seeking medical advice in the early stages of a disease and the likelihood of adhering to recommendations subsequently. Any of these variables, or some combination of them, could be invoked to account for an empirical correlation between personality and illness.

TYPE A PERSONALITY, HOSTILITY AND CORONARY HEART DISEASE

Type A and B Personality

Speculation about an association between the Type A and Type B personalities and coronary heart disease (CHD) has a history which dates back more than 50 years (Riska, 2000). The distinction between the two personalities was introduced in the mid-1950s by the cardiologists Meyer Friedman and Ray Rosenman, although, as we have already noted, their ideas can be traced back further to the work of Alexander in psychosomatic medicine. The Type A personality, thought to be at greater risk of CHD, is described as highly competitive and achievement oriented, not prepared to suffer fools gladly, always in a hurry and unable to bear delays and queues, hostile and aggressive, inclined to read, eat and drive very fast, and constantly thinking what to do next, even when supposedly listening to someone else. In contrast to this the Type B personality is relaxed, laid back, lethargic, even-tempered, amiable and philosophical about life, relatively slow in speech and action, and generally has enough time for everyone and everything. The Type A personality has much in common with Galen's choleric temperament, the Type B with the phlegmatic (see Box 17.1). It is well known that men are at greater risk of CHD than women, and Riska (2000) makes an interesting argument for the view that the concept of the Type A personality was an attempt to 'medicalize' and 'pathologize' traditional concepts of masculinity.

The key pioneering study of Type A personality and CHD was the Western Collaborative Group Study (WCGS) in which over 3000 Californian men, aged from 39 to 59 at entry, were followed up initially over a period of eight and a half years, and later extending over 22 years. When results were reported at the eight and a half year follow-up, it appeared that Type As were twice as likely compared with Type Bs to suffer from subsequent CHD. Of the sample 7 per cent developed some signs of CHD and two-thirds of these were Type As. This increased risk was apparent even when other risk factors assessed at entry, such as blood pressure and cigarette smoking, were statistically controlled for. Similar results were subsequently published from another large-scale study conducted in Framingham, Massachusetts, this time with both men and women in the sample and, by the early 1980s, it was confidently asserted that Type A characteristics were as much a risk factor for heart disease as high blood pressure, high cholesterol levels and smoking.

However, subsequent research failed to support these early findings. When Ragland and Brand (1988) conducted a 22-year follow-up of the WCGS, using CHD mortality as the crucially important measure, they failed to find any consistent evidence of an association. Much further research continued to be published up to the late 1980s, yielding few positive findings. Reviewing this evidence, Myrtek (2001) suggest that the modest number of positive findings that did exist were the result of over-reliance on angina as the measure of CHD. As we have already pointed out, this is an unreliable measure because it is frequently based solely on self-reported chest pain. Considering studies that adopted hard criteria, including mortality, Myrtek concludes that we can be confident that the Type A personality is not a risk factor for CHD.

Hostility

It can take a long time for a popular belief to fade away when there is a lack of evidence to support it. The extensive coverage still given to the Type A–CHD hypothesis by textbook writers is a good illustration of this. Researchers may be a little quicker to react as is indicated by the decline in publications in this field from the early 1990s. In fact it was largely replaced by an alternative hypothesis which was itself generated by the analysis of Type A–CHD research. This hypothesis is that hostility is the key dimension of personality that is associated with CHD.

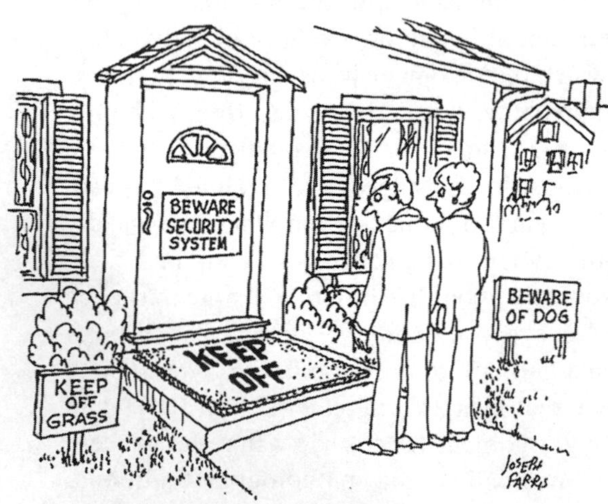

Reprinted by permission of www.cartoonstock.com

The Type A personality, as described briefly in the last section, contains a number of components that are not necessarily closely correlated. Measures of Type A and B personalities often included sub-components that could be separately analysed for their association with subsequent CHD. When this was done it emerged that there was only one component which did seem to have some predictive power, and this component was anger or hostility. Research into links between anger/hostility and CHD became as popular in the 1990s as Type A research had been in previous years, but unfortunately with a similar conclusion. By the end of the decade a number of reviews, including that of Myrtek (2001), found the studies to be of mixed quality, with inconsistent results. There was some evidence of a statistically significant but weak relationship for prospective studies of initially healthy individuals, but not for studies that have followed up patients already diagnosed with CHD.

In a curious mirroring of the breakdown of the Type A personality into sub-components, which led to hostility–CHD research, the hostility researchers themselves reacted to disappointing findings by breaking hostility down into separate components. These included cynicism, mistrust, verbal and physical aggressiveness, overt and experienced aggressiveness. It was proposed that more attention should be given to these sub-components in order to discover which are the most hazardous for health. However, Suls and Bunde (2005) noted that there is considerable overlap between measures of these sub-components of anger/hostility, with similar items being included in ostensibly different measures. Suls and Bunde also confirmed Myrtek's earlier conclusion that evidence of an association between hostility, however measured, and subsequent CHD suggests a weak relationship, possibly no more than a side effect of the correlation of hostility measures with anxiety and depression, characteristics which will now be considered because they appear to have a more substantial association with CHD.

ANXIETY, DEPRESSION, NEGATIVE AFFECT AND CORONARY HEART DISEASE

Much contemporary research on links between personality and illness is concerned with what might be termed positive and negative prevailing moods, or 'affectivity'. Researchers have often demonstrated that positive dispositions (e.g. optimism, high self-esteem, sense of coherence) are associated with good health, while negative dispositions (e.g. anxiety, depression, pessimistic explanatory style) are associated with poor health. However, these measures are frequently intercorrelated so that it is misleading to consider the research under separate headings for distinct dimensions of personality. It amounts to much the same thing to show, for example, that persons scoring high on a scale measuring depression have an increased risk of heart disease as it is to show that those scoring high on a scale measuring optimism have a reduced risk. It is also important to bear in mind that persons with negative dispositions are more likely than those with positive dispositions to report illness when not actually ill, and also to indulge in hazardous health behaviours, such as cigarette smoking and heavy drinking. With these cautions in mind we will now consider the research findings.

There have been a number of recent reviews that have concluded, on the basis of prospective studies, that there are substantial associations between both anxiety and depression and subsequent CHD (Hemingway & Marmot, 1999; Krantz & McCeney, 2002; Wulsin & Singal, 2003; Lett et al., 2004; Suls & Bunde, 2005). These associations have been found in studies of patients with clinically diagnosed distress and in general population studies. Anxiety seems to predict sudden cardiac death rather more than other types of CHD, and phobic, panic-like anxiety is a particularly strong predictor: Haines, Imeson and Meade (1987) found that sufferers were three times more at risk of sudden cardiac death over the next 7 years compared with non-sufferers. Kawachi et al. (1994) subsequently found similar results in a 2-year follow up of 33,999 initially healthy US male health professionals. The case study below gives a further example from a Taiwanese study together with mention of an important caution when interpreting research in this area.

Case Study

INTERNATIONAL CASE STUDY Panic disorder and heart attacks – data from Taiwan

Chen et al. (2009b) carried out a one-year follow-up investigation of 9641 Taiwanese patients who had been diagnosed with panic disorder compared with 28,923 matched control participants. Approximately 1 in 21 of the panic disorder patients suffered from *acute myocardial infarctions* (heart attacks) in the follow up period compared with 1 in 37 of the comparison cohort. The samples were matched for a number of relevant variables, but the possibility cannot be excluded that the panic disorders could have been provoked by cardiac symptoms preceding the heart attack, such as irregularities in heartbeats, rather than having a causal role.

Depression is predictive of a wider range of CHD than anxiety. In one UK study with 19,649 participants who were initially free of clinical manifestations of heart disease, Surtees et al. (2008) found, with an average follow-up period of 8.5 years, that those assessed as suffering from a major depressive disorder were 2.7 times more likely to die from ischemic heart disease over the follow-up period than those who did not, independently of age, sex, smoking, systolic blood pressure, cholesterol, physical activity, body mass index, diabetes, social class, heavy alcohol use, and antidepressant medication use. In a large prospective study of 96,376 post-menopausal women, Wassertheil-Smoller et al. (2004) report that depressive symptoms were substantially associated with death from cardiovascular disease after adjusting for age, race, education, income, diabetes, hypertension, smoking, cholesterol level, body mass index and physical activity.

These findings for anxiety and depression are impressive, but they should be considered alongside our earlier discussion of problems in interpreting personality–illness correlations. Hemingway and Marmot (1999) point out that these problems are particularly acute in this area. Anxiety and depression are certainly consequences of CHD as well as possible causes of it. Furthermore, symptoms of incipient CHD, such as breathlessness and chest pains, may occur for years prior to diagnosis, and lead in turn to experienced anxiety and depression. In this way, prospective studies could give the impression that anxiety and depression are causes of CHD when in fact the direction of causality is the other way round.

As Miller et al. (2009) point out, one practically useful way of resolving some of the methodological problems in interpreting findings in this area would be a robust demonstration that interventions designed to reduce anxiety and depression in patients suffering from CHD could produce an improved prognosis. Unfortunately the two most substantial trials which have been conducted so far, each targeting depression and with more than 2000 participants, showed no effect of interventions. Berkman et al. (2003) evaluated a programme that included cognitive behaviour therapy supplemented with antidepressants for the more severely depressed patients; van Melle et al. (2007) evaluated an intervention consisting simply of treatment with antidepressants. Neither study found any evidence of an improvement in event-free survival for the intervention groups compared with controls.

Further recent studies indicate that the relationship between emotional distress and illness is not restricted to heart disease. Mykletun et al. (2007) examined data from a population-based health study of 61,349 participants. With a mean follow-up of 4.4 years, they found that depression was equally associated with all disease-related causes of death, not just CHD. They did not find any evidence of an association with anxiety. On the other hand, Grossardt et al. (2009), in a follow-up of 7080 participants originally tested between 1962 and 1965, found that pessimistic, anxious and depressive personality traits were each predictive of all-cause mortality. Further research is needed to clarify reasons for the differences between the findings of the two studies. However, they both suggest that the association between psychological distress and disease-related death extends beyond CHD.

FURTHER STUDIES OF LINKS BETWEEN PERSONALITY AND ILLNESS

Depression and Cancer

The widely held belief that depression is an important factor in the onset and subsequent development of cancer has received little support from research. Adler and Matthews (1994) reviewed three large-scale prospective studies of the relationship between depression and both the incidence of and mortality from cancer. In these studies, initially healthy samples of up to 9000 were followed up over periods ranging from 10 to 20 years and no associations were found between depression and either cancer onset or mortality. Since then, two large-scale studies have produced conflicting results. Penninx et al. (1998) carried out a prospective study of 1708 men and 3117 women aged 71 and over. They found a significantly increased incidence of cancer for those who were diagnosed as suffering from chronic depression, indicated by repeated assessments of symptoms over 6 years. On the other hand, Whooley and Browner (1998) undertook a prospective study over 6 years of 7519 women aged 67 or over and analysed the relationship between depression and subsequent mortality from (a) cancer (b) cardiovascular disease and (c) all other diseases. They found no relationship between depression and cancer but a strong relationship with both cardiovascular disease and all other diseases.

Negative findings have also been reported from follow-up studies of patients who have been treated for cancer. For example, Barraclough, Pinder, Cruddas, Osmand, Taylor and Perry (1992) followed up 204 patients who had received surgery for breast cancer over 42 months after surgery. They used a detailed interview schedule, which included the assessment of prolonged major depression before surgery and during the follow-up period. They found no relationship at all between depression and relapse. Relapse was also unrelated to stress, including bereavement, long-term social difficulties and lack of a confiding relationship.

Coyne et al. (2007) note the persistence of the belief that psychotherapy promotes survival in people with cancer in the face of contradictory findings. They provide a systematic critical review of the relevant literature and conclude:

> *No randomized clinical trial designed with survival as a primary endpoint and in which psychotherapy was not confounded with medical care has yielded a positive effect. Among the implications of the review is that an adequately powered study examining effects of psychotherapy on survival after a diagnosis of cancer would require resources that are not justified by the strength of the available evidence.*

We reach a similar conclusion in reviewing the literature from the field of psycho-oncology in Chapter 20.

Conscientiousness and Longevity

Conscientiousness is one of the five factors of personality proposed by McCrae and Costa (2003) in their influential theory that was originally developed in 1985. A considerable amount of recent research has confirmed that this characteristic is associated with longevity. In a meta-analysis that pooled the results of 20 independent samples, Kern and Friedman (2008) found a modest but significant correlation of 0.11. A similar finding for men, but not for women, is reported by Taylor et al. (2009) in an analysis of all-cause mortality in a sample of 1592 Scottish men and women aged from 55 to 74 when recruited in 1987 and 1988. They found an association with longevity of about the same size also for openness, another of the five factors, again for men but not for women. As regards conscientiousness, the most plausible explanation for the findings is the influence of health behaviour. Bogg and Roberts (2004) pooled the results from 194 studies that incorporated measures of conscientiousness-related traits and assessments of any of the leading behavioural contributors to mortality (tobacco use, diet and activity patterns, excessive alcohol use, violence, risky sexual behaviour, risky driving, suicide, and drug use). They found that conscientiousness-related traits were negatively related to all risky health-related behaviours and positively related to all beneficial health-related behaviours.

Sense of Coherence, Locus of Control and Self-Efficacy

Sense of coherence (Antonovsky, 1979) is described as the ability to perceive one's world as meaningful and manageable. Surtees, Wainwright, Luben, Khaw and Day (2003) carried out a prospective study over six years of the relationship between sense of coherence and mortality from all causes for a UK sample of 20,579 participants aged 41–80 years. They found that a strong sense of coherence was associated with a 30 per cent reduction in mortality from all causes and also more specifically for cardiovascular disease. The explanation for this probably lies in the fact that sense of coherence is inversely correlated with anxiety and depression. In a study conducted in Finland of 4642 men and women aged from 25 to 74, Konttinen, Haukkala and Uutela (2008) found inverse correlations of 0.62 between sense of coherence and depression for both men and women; the inverse correlations between sense of coherence and anxiety were 0.57 for men and 0.54 for women. It follows that the findings of Surtees et al. could be basically the same as the positive correlations already discussed between anxiety and depression and both cardiovascular disease and all-cause mortality.

Another personality variable that has been of interest to health psychologists over the last 20 years is the notion of locus of control. Wallston, Wallston and DeVellis (1978) who developed the **Multidimensional Health Locus of Control (MHLC) Scale** applied this concept to health beliefs. This questionnaire has three sub-scales measuring the extent to which people attribute their state of health to their own behaviour (internal locus), and/or external factors including both powerful others, especially medical professionals, and chance or fate. The internal locus of control scale has much in common with the concept of self-efficacy (Bandura, 1977). In both cases the main focus of research interest has been not so much to investigate direct links with physical health, but rather to show that they are predictive of the adoption of positive health behaviours and the avoidance of negative ones.

In a detailed review of research on the topic, Norman and Bennett (1996) found that the results were mixed, and they concluded that the relationship between locus of control and health behaviour is a weak one, a conclusion that was confirmed by a large-scale study of a representative sample of 11,632 people who completed the MHLC in Wales (Norman, Bennett, Smith & Murphy, 1998). In this study, all three health locus of control dimensions were found to correlate significantly with a health behaviour index, with those engaging in more positive health behaviours scoring higher on the internal dimension ($r = 0.05$), lower on powerful others ($r = 0.09$) and lower on chance ($r = 0.16$). These are low correlations indicating a weak predictive relationship and leaving more than 95 per cent of the variance in health behaviour unaccounted for. Self-efficacy appears to be a rather better predictor of health behaviour and is perhaps the best predictor available (Schwarzer, 1992).

FUTURE RESEARCH

1 Studies to assess the role of psychological factors in medically unexplained conditions, such as chronic fatigue syndrome, including empirical testing of recent neuropsychological theories.
2 Research to clarify the structure of personality with particular reference to health, in order to reduce or eliminate the problem of overlapping measures.
3 Investigations to distinguish between personality variables that are associated with biologically verified illness, as distinct from those that are associated only with self-reported illness.
4 Studies to establish which dimensions of personality are directly associated with health-relevant physiological variables, and to distinguish them from those that are primarily associated with health behaviours.
5 Outcome studies to assess the effectiveness of interventions designed to modify psychological characteristics that are suspected of being health hazardous. It would be particularly valuable to assess whether interventions can improve the prognosis for those already diagnosed as suffering from organic disease. In the case of anxiety and depression, interventions would obviously be worthwhile if they relieve these conditions, whether or not they influence health outcomes.
6 Where personality variables are linked primarily to health behaviours, it would be useful to establish whether interventions designed to modify health behaviour (e.g. smoking cessation programmes) could be more effective if they took account of personality assessments of participants.

Summary

1 From the Ancient Greeks to modern times orthodox medical practitioners have usually believed that there is a physical basis to all illness, including psychological disorders. In contrast to this, there has also been a wholistic tradition, which has placed an emphasis on the role of psychological factors.
2 The modern history of psychological explanations for physical symptoms begins with Freud's theories of hysteria, physical symptoms of illness for which no organic basis could be discovered. These conditions are often referred to nowadays as 'medically unexplained symptoms', and recent theories about them have drawn on neuropsychological research and theories.
3 The psychosomatic approach was developed by psychoanalysts who extended Freud's theories of hysteria to provide psychological explanations for the causation of organic disorders such as heart disease and cancer.
4 Proponents of the psychosomatic approach generally failed to produce convincing evidence in support of their hypotheses. However, the theories of Franz Alexander on the physiological mechanisms that could underlie the relationship between the psychology of the individual and organic disease have led to modern conceptions of the Type A personality, hostility and stress as contributors to coronary heart disease (CHD).

5 Health psychologists have found it difficult to determine whether personality is associated with susceptibility to physical disease directly through physiological mechanisms, indirectly by way of health behaviour, or whether the data are best explained by statistical artefacts and flaws in the design of the studies from which they are obtained.
6 Early indications that the Type A personality is a risk factor for CHD were not confirmed by later studies. Attention then shifted to hostility but this variable now seems only to be a weak predictor.
7 Anxiety, especially phobic panic-like anxiety, and depression are both associated with an increased risk of CHD, although a number of different interpretations of these associations are possible.
8 There is little clear-cut evidence to support the view that personality variables are associated with risk of cancer or of relapse following treatment. Interventions based on treatment for depression have not been shown to improve the survival chances of cancer sufferers.
9 There is some recent evidence that conscientiousness and sense of coherence are associated with reduced risk of CHD and all-cause mortality.
10 Internal locus of control is only weakly associated with positive health behaviours. Self-efficacy shows an overall stronger relationship.

18

Medicine Taking: Adherence and Resistance

In our society the discourse of medicine about illness is so loud that it tends to drone out all the others. Caught between their undecipherable physical experience and the ordered and dominating language of science, today's sufferers are often at a loss to know whether they can speak, to whom they can speak, and how they can speak

(Herzlich & Pierret, 1987)

Outline

Adherence and compliance are terms used to describe the extent to which patients adhere or comply with recommended treatment regimens. It is one of the most widely researched forms of health-related behaviour. The assumptions underlying the term compliance imply an authoritarian stance on the part of the physician or other health professional that is challenged by recent changes within health-care systems. This chapter considers the extent and character of treatment non-adherence and the issue of medical error. It also considers the patient-centred formulation of health care that focuses on shared decision-making and patient empowerment.

WHAT IS ADHERENCE?

Character of Adherence

The prescription of medicines is the most common form of medical treatment. Indeed, the terms for the profession and the form of treatment are inter-changeable. However, a challenge faced by medicine is that most patients do not fully comply with the prescribed medication. This non-compliance can take various forms including not having prescriptions filled, not taking the correct dosage, not taking the medicine at the correct times, and stopping the medication before the course of treatment is completed. This incomplete medicine taking has attracted a massive research effort and given rise to a range of competing claims.

The terms used to describe the process have changed over the years. Initially the most popular descriptive term was **compliance** which referred to the extent to which the patient passively accepted the physicians' instructions on medicine taking. With the growing challenge to the power of medicine the term that became more popular is **adherence** which was considered a more neutral expression. More recently, the term **concordance** has been introduced since it was felt that this implied a more cooperative relationship between the physician and the patient. In this chapter we will start with the popular term adherence and then consider some more critical options.

Extent of Adherence

The extent of adherence varies across the different forms of recommended medication-related behaviours. In general, most people do not adhere to specific medical or health-care directives – at least not fully. While non-adherence would seem to be the norm, its extent varies. It has been estimated that 50–75 per cent of patients do not adhere to medical advice (Wertheimer and Santella, 2003). Some further estimates include:

- 14–21 per cent of patients do not fill their prescriptions;
- 60 per cent of all patients cannot identify their own medication;
- 30–50 per cent of all patients ignore or compromise medication instructions;
- 12–20 per cent of patients take other people's medication;

From a medical treatment perspective this reflects a major failure in the system. There have been attempts to document the negative impact of non-adherence. For example, Wertheimer and Santella (2003) estimated that each year in the USA:

- Approximately 125,000 people with treatable ailments die of inappropriate medication usage;
- Approximately one quarter of nursing home admissions are due to inappropriate medication usage;
- Hospital costs due to medication non-adherence are $8.5 billion.

Certain forms of non-adherence are potentially more dangerous than others. One common health problem that has a high rate of non-adherence is asthma. Despite the large number of drug education programmes the proportion of people with asthma who do not comply with the recommended treatment remains high (Bender et al., 1998). In the UK, the Office for Health Economics estimated that management of asthma cost the NHS almost £900 million in 2001. It has been suggested that a large proportion of this cost could be eliminated if adherence with medication was improved (Bender et al., 1998).

This low rate of adherence has attracted a massive research effort to identify what factors are associated with the process and how it can be enhanced. In an extensive review of the research literature Vermeire, Hearnshaw, van Royen and Denekens (2001) concluded there has been limited consistent success in identifying factors that predict adherence due to a lack of concern with the patient's perspective and a preference for quantitative methods. We will start by summarizing some of the evidence from the more quantitative research before considering alternative approaches.

FACTORS ASSOCIATED WITH NON-ADHERENCE

Patient Characteristics

There has been some success in identifying the social and personal characteristics of the non-adherent patient. In general, the less social support and the more socially isolated the patients are, the less likely they are to follow medical directives. For example, in a study of treatment adherence in an outpatient clinic for people with tuberculosis, it was found that homelessness was the only factor that predicted non-completion of therapy (Brainard et al., 1997). Further, individuals who came from unstable families were also found to be less compliant with medical treatment (Bender et al., 1998). A study of adherence among diabetes patients found that adherence to medication was associated with higher levels of social support (Garay-Sevilla et al., 1995).

There has been much effort to identify the so-called 'non-compliant' personality. However, like much personality research in general, this effort has met with limited success. In reviewing the evidence, Hulka (1979) found no consistent relationship between age, sex,

Table 18.1 Patient characteristics associated with adherence

Social characteristics	Personal characteristics	Health beliefs
Characteristics of individual's social situation	Demographics Sensory disabilities	Inappropriate or conflicting health beliefs
Lack of social supports Family instability or disharmony	Type and severity of psychiatric disorder	Competing socio-cultural and ethnic folk concepts of disease and treatment
Parent's expectations and attitudes toward treatment	Forgetfulness Lack of understanding	Implicit model of illness
Residential instability		
Environment that supports non-adherent behaviour		
Competing or conflicting demands		
Lack of resources		

Source: Meichenbaum and Turk, 1987: 43

marital status, education, number of people in the household, social class and adherence. Admittedly, this is not to deny that specific groups of patients may be resistant to accepting certain types of treatment. For example, certain cognitive deficits or emotional upsets may reduce adherence. There is also evidence that people with a range of psychological problems are less likely to adhere to treatment (e.g. Christiannse et al., 1989). Table 18.1 summarizes some of the patient characteristics associated with adherence.

It has been argued that the more the prescribed medication accords with the patients' belief systems, the more likely they are to comply with the treatment. In an attempt to coordinate this research beyond the extensive listings of variables, some investigators have turned to the popular social cognition models. Probably the most frequently used such model has been the **Health Belief Model (HBM)**. Indeed, this model was originally formulated to explain compliance with medical recommendations (Becker & Mainman, 1975). According to the HBM, the extent to which a person complies or adheres with certain medication advice depends upon perceived disease severity, susceptibility to the disease, benefits of the treatment recommended and barriers to following the treatment (see also Chapter 13).

Varying degrees of support have been found for this model. For example, Masek (1982) found that the more the patients perceive their condition to be serious, the more likely they will be to comply with the recommended treatment. However, Glasgow, Hampson, Strycker, and Ruggiero (1997) found that perceived seriousness of diabetes was not predictive of adherence. In a study of drug therapy defaulting, Fincham and Wertheimer (1985) found that belief in the benefits of medical care and low barriers to care predicted high adherence. Glasgow et al. (1997) found that the perceived effectiveness of the treatment was a better predictor of adherence in diabetes than the perceived barriers.

Social learning theory has also been used with varying degrees of success to explain non-adherence. Tillotson and Smith (1996) found that although internal **locus of control** predicted adherence to a weight-control programme for patients with diabetes, its importance was small and depended on the degree of social support. In a study of patients with rheumatoid arthritis Beck et al. (1988) found that patients' predictions concerning their adherence (**self-efficacy** expectations) with treatment predicted actual adherence. There has been a growing literature on adherence to HIV antiretroviral treatments. Some of these have found support for some of the social-cognitive dimensions. For example, a study in New York found that self-efficacy for adherence to HIV treatment significantly predicted adherence (Halkitis, Kutnick & Slater, 2005). However, this relationship may have been complicated by the role of recreational drugs which are common among individuals who are HIV positive and which in turn are associated with poorer adherence and also with avoidant coping. This led the authors to conclude that there is a need to consider the complex relationship between intrapsychic and socio-cultural realities in order to explain HIV treatment adherence.

The social cognition models of adherence describe the beliefs that are associated with or predict adherence. These models can be criticized on both empirical and theoretical grounds. On empirical grounds the major problem is that the beliefs have been found to predict only a small proportion of the variance of adherence behaviour. Theoretically, the major problem is that these models reify the phenomenon. As such it characterizes the behaviour as fixed and abstracted from the changing social relations and the broader social context within which adherence occurs (see Chapter 6). Treatment is not usually a one-off event but extends over a period of time. In the case of chronic illness this period can be a lifetime. To understand adherence fully therefore requires an understanding of the social context and how the patient integrates the treatment into his/her everyday life.

Disease Characteristics

Certain disease characteristics have been found to be associated with adherence. Perhaps the most frequently mentioned disease characteristics are the severity of the disease and visibility of the symptoms. The relationship with disease severity would appear not to be linear. A number of studies have found that patients with asymptomatic chronic diseases frequently do not comply with treatment (e.g. Miller, 1997). When the symptoms are obvious and unwanted, the person is more likely to comply with treatment that offers a promise of removing them. However, when the prognosis is poor there is evidence that the rate of adherence is reduced. For example, Dolgin et al. (1986) found adherence lower in those cancer patients whose survival prospects were poor.

Treatment Factors

There are a large number of treatment factors associated with adherence. These are summarized in Table 18.2 under four broad temporal headings. Before the patient is actually prescribed a treatment, s/he has to obtain an appointment with the physician. The character of this process prepares or sets the scene for the physician's recommendations. Lengthy or inconvenient waiting times can lead to considerable frustration and an unwillingness to comply.

Table 18.2 Treatment factors associated with non-adherence

Preparation for treatment	Immediate character of treatment	Administration of treatment	Consequences of treatment
Characteristics of treatment setting	Characteristics of treatment recommendations	Inadequate supervision by professionals	Medication side effects
Long waiting time	Complexity of treatment regimen	Absence of continuity of care	Social side effects
Long time elapsed between referral and appointment	Duration of treatment regimen	Failure of parents to supervise drug administration	
Timing of referral	Degree of behavioural change		
Absence of individual appointment times	Inconvenience		
Lack of cohesiveness of treatment delivery systems	Expense		
Inconvenience associated with operation of clinics	Characteristics of medicine		
Poor reputation of treatment facility	Inadequate labels		
	Awkward container design		

Source: Meichenbaum & Turk, 1987, p. 43

The more complicated the treatment prescribed, the less likely the patient is to comply fully. Admittedly, there have been attempts to simplify treatment regimens by providing patients with detailed information. However, the evidence suggests that adherence is still poor. One reason is information overload (Meichenbaum and Turk, 1987). In an attempt to cope with a very complicated treatment regimen the patient simply gets confused or ignores much of the information. Although physicians may explain the treatment, patients frequently do not understand or forget the instructions provided. Ley (1979) found that patients forget at least one third of the information given by their physician. A variety of factors influences understanding. Basically, the more extensive and complex the instructions given, the less likely the patient is to recall it subsequently.

Besides complexity, an important treatment characteristic is the actual length of the treatment regimen. Adherence declines with an increase in the number of medications or doses and with the length of recommended treatment (Hulka, Cassel & Kupper, 1976). Sackett and Snow (1979) estimated that adherence with long-term therapy declines to approximately 50 per cent, irrespective of illness or setting. Masur (1981) suggests that it is not the length of treatment that is the reason for this decline in adherence but rather the absence of symptoms.

Long-term therapy is often recommended for chronic medical conditions which have few symptoms or for which there is no definite improvement in symptoms as a result of medication. In these cases the patient has no feedback on the benefits of medication. This lack of feedback undermines any motivation to comply with the medication. Leventhal et al. (1992) found that when patients with hypertension were able to identify symptoms of their disease that were controlled by medication they were more likely to comply with it.

The actual character of the treatment is also important. For example, some people with asthma do not like taking inhaled medication while others do not follow the correct inhalation procedure, thus reducing overall adherence (McFadden, 1995). Understanding how the patient feels about a particular procedure or treatment is a necessary step in improving adherence.

It would perhaps be expected that those drugs with few *physical side effects* would be associated with higher adherence. It would seem that the social side effects, in terms of stigma, are just as important (see section on empowerment). A related factor is the extent to which the treatment disrupts the patient's everyday life.

Interpersonal Factors

The character of the physician–patient relationship has been at the centre of research into adherence. Physician styles in physician–patient communication have been classified as either '**patient-centred**' or '**authoritarian**' (see Chapter 11). The patient-centred or affiliative style is designed to promote a positive relationship and includes behaviours such as interest, friendliness and empathy. The authoritarian or control-oriented style is designed to maintain the physician's control in the interaction. Not surprisingly, patients prefer those physicians who adopt the more affiliative style (Buller and Buller, 1987). Various related styles of physician interaction have been associated with adherence. In behavioural terms the physician keeps good eye contact, smiles a lot and leans in towards the patient – all behaviours which are interpreted as demonstrating interest and consideration. Hall, Roter and Katz (1988) found in their meta-analysis of 41 studies that patient satisfaction was associated with perceived interpersonal competence, social conversation and better communication as well as more information and technical competence.

Several studies have found an association between physician job satisfaction and aspects of adherence. Cecil and Killeen (1997) found that patients were more satisfied with those physicians who exhibited less dominance by encouraging them to express their ideas, concerns and expectations. A related factor is the physician's sense of security. Since many conditions are resistant to standard medical interventions many physicians can experience a sense of inadequacy. This, in turn, could lead to reduced job satisfaction and more conflict with patients. Indeed, when general practitioners receive complaints from their patients, they initially feel out of control, and may experience feelings of shock, panic and indignation (Jain and Ogden, 1999).

Physicians and patients have a different view of health and illness. For example, St. Claire et al. (1996) compared the definitions of health provided by a sample of family physicians and those provided by a sample of patients with asthma. Whereas the former defined health in terms of absence of disease, the latter referred to 'being able', 'taking action' and 'physical well-being'. The more understanding the physician of the patient's belief system, the more compliant the patient is. For example, Ruiz and Ruiz (1983) found that Hispanic patients tend to comply more when their physician is more understanding of their cultural norms and practices.

An important although less explored factor is the physician's view of the patient. This factor overlaps with the physician's understanding of the patient's health beliefs and suggests that when the physician has a positive view of the patient then s/he will adopt a much more affiliative style of communication. This helps to explain the well-established social class effect that upper and middle-class patients receive more information and attention from physicians. For example, Taira et al. (1997) conducted a large survey of state employees in Massachusetts. According to the responses physicians were more likely to discuss healthy lifestyle issues such as diet and exercise with high-income patients but they discussed smoking more with low-income patients. Physicians frequently report more frustration with and less interest in lower and working-class patients (Hall et al., 1988).

An interesting additional factor is the effect of a physician's 'tactile contact' with the patient. In a recent study in France (Gueguen & Vion, 2009) a group of physicians were instructed to lightly touch their patients when giving advice on medication. It was found that compared with a control group of patients the 'touched' patients were significantly more likely to consume more of the prescribed tablets. This effect was apparent seven days after the consultation. It was suggested that this effect may be due to those physicians who lightly touched their patients being perceived as more competent. However, in view of the potential misinterpretation of touch there is a need to advise caution in applying these findings particularly in societies where there are clear professional restrictions on tactile behaviour towards patients.

Social and Organizational Setting

The medical consultation takes place in a social setting. Meichenbaum and Turk (1987) identified 10 setting characteristics potentially associated with non-adherence. Adherence is greater when the referral to a specialist is seen as part of the assessment rather than as a last resort, when care involves follow-up and is personalized, when appointments are individualized and waiting times are reduced, when treatment is available on site, when treatment is carefully supervised through home visits, special nursing care, etc., when there are good links between inpatient and outpatient services and when staff have a very positive attitude toward the treatment. In particular with long-term therapy, there is evidence that regular follow-up by the physician increases adherence (Bond and Monson, 1984).

It is not just the immediate medical context but also the local social context, in terms of family and friends, which is important. If family members remind and assist the patient concerning their medication it would only be expected that the patient would be more compliant. Indeed, it has been suggested that the patient's partner's views of the medication prescribed is the most important factor in explaining adherence. In a meta-analysis of 122 studies on the impact of social support DiMatteo (2004) found that practical support had a high correlation with adherence. He also found that adherence was higher in cohesive families and lower in families in conflict. This concern with social context requires consideration of the broader socio-political context that conditions the character of health care and of adherence.

ALTERNATIVES TO ADHERENCE

While the extensive quantitative literature on non-adherence has provided some insight into the character of the phenomenon, it has not contributed to its reduction (Vermiere et al., 2001). One of the main reasons for this lack of progress is that the majority of adherence research has been based upon a static model of the phenomenon that ignores the broader social context of health care and the dynamic nature of health and illness behaviour. An alternative more social and psychological approach requires an understanding of the role of medicine in our society and of the actual lived experience of illness and of managing illness.

Modern Medicine

In Western society medicine has been based upon power and authority. Since it is founded on the assumption that it has the monopoly on truth, it follows that patient non-adherence is a result of ignorance and/or deviance. Thus it is not surprising that Trostle (1998) describes the literature on compliance as 'a literature about power and control' (p. 1299). He argues that the increasing research interest in medical compliance is a reflection of 'a concern for market control combined with a concern for therapeutic power' (p. 1301). However, this very concern with maintaining power may carry with it an equal and opposite reaction evidenced by a reluctance of patients to comply.

According to **reactance theory** (Brehm, 1966), individuals believe they have the right to control their own behaviour. When this right is threatened they react and attempt to regain control over that behaviour and to prevent the loss of other freedoms. Basically, people do not like being pushed around and will attempt to subvert attempts to do so. In a revision of the original theory, Brehm and Brehm (1981) defined the concept of freedom as equivalent to that of control. People like to feel in control of their lives. Any attempt to reduce the sense of control over specific areas of our lives is a threat to the sense of freedom and is generally resisted.

The theory of psychological reactance has been used as an explanatory framework for non-compliance. The more extensive and complex the treatment prescribed, the greater the threat to perceived freedom (Fogarty, 1997). Admittedly, this threat would be accepted if there was an indication that it was worthwhile. However, the very complexity of some regimens may sensitize the patient to additional threats to their freedom such that patients may become resistant to additional demands. Non-compliance can thus be interpreted as a means of resisting medical dominance.

Admittedly, not all patients are critical of the traditional authoritarian stance of the physician or feel the need to resist or not comply. Some people are more accepting of authority than others. In recent years there has been more public opposition to the idea of the all-powerful doctor and demands for greater control over health care. Despite this apparent change in public attitudes, several researchers have found that many people are reluctant to adopt a more resisting, consumerist attitude. Haug and Lavin (1983) found that while younger and more educated patients are more consumerist in their attitude regarding their role in the doctor–patient encounter, older patients are more accepting and accommodating.

Lupton (1997) investigated the impact of the supposed cultural shift on the attitudes of patients in Australia. She argued that contemporary popular advice is that the patient should adopt an active consumerist attitude to health care. In her interviews with a sample of patients, Lupton found a more mixed picture. Many of the patients, especially the older ones, still preferred the passive patient role. Admittedly, they accepted that the traditional authoritarian image of the doctor had been challenged over the past generation as a result of publicity about medical negligence and sexual harassment. This resulted in ambivalence about the doctor and a tension between adopting the consumerist or passive patient role. Thus while some patients would demand a more active role in their treatment and would be frustrated if they were denied it, many patients still preferred to adopt the traditional passive patient role.

The more consumerist stance of certain patients is not always welcomed by physicians. Although several studies have shown that patients generally express a desire for information about their condition, many physicians are reluctant to disclose much information. In his study, West (1984) found that physicians often ignored patients' requests for information. Indeed it was found that patients' requests for more information were often met by challenges to their intelligence.

Role of the Physician

Trostle (1998) suggested that 'the last decade's preoccupation with adherence is a consequence of the declining authority of the [medical] profession' (p. 1303). In traditional non-Western societies the physician maintains the dominant role and the patient is more inclined to adopt a compliant stance. For example, Matsumoto et al. (1995) found that first generation Japanese–Americans were much more likely to report a willingness to comply than their second-generation peers. Conversely, in Western society the demand for greater control over one's life conflicts with the traditional passive role and leads to greater resistance to medical advice.

Another feature of medical dominance is the power of the physician to define sickness. It is often assumed that the doctor typically makes the correct diagnosis and prescribes appropriate treatment. This is the ideal medical model. Thus non-adherence is the patient's fault. However, the evidence suggests that there are many sources of error on the part of the physician. For example, patients frequently attend with a variety of psychosocial problems, but the physician often ignores these. Bertakis, Roter and Putnam (1991) estimated that as many as 85 per cent of patients who come to see their family doctor have some degree of psychological distress. As Mishler (1984) has emphasized, scientific medical discourse does not contain language to handle these issues so the physician prefers to focus concern on biomedical matters which may be of limited concern to the patient.

In a large study conducted over 11 sites in the USA, Bertakis et al. (1991) analysed the verbal content of 550 physician–patient interviews. They found that physician questions about biomedical topics were negatively related to patient satisfaction while physician questions about psychosocial topics were positively associated with patient satisfaction. In addition, those patients whose physician dominated the interview reported less satisfaction. Bertakis et al. concluded that 'patients are most satisfied by interviews that encourage them to talk about psychosocial issues in an atmosphere that is characterized by the absence of physician domination'.

However, Waitzkin (1989) argues that the exclusion of discussion of the social context of health complaints is a 'fundamental feature of medical language … a basic part of what medicine is in our society' (p. 232). Not only does medical language ignore these social issues but also medical treatment does not address these social issues. He suggests a redirection for medicine: 'by suggesting collective action as a meaningful option, medical professionals might begin to overcome the impact that its exclusion exerts'. To do this it needs to recognize the 'limits of medicine's role and the importance of building links to other forms of praxis that seek to change the social context of medical encounters' (p. 237).

The movement towards patient-centred models of medical treatment indicates that the medical profession is well aware of the growing criticism. So too are pharmacists who play a central role in dispensing medication. A report by the Royal Pharmaceutical Society of Great Britain (1997) called for a new approach to patient care. In a commentary on the report, Marinker (1997) noted that 'compliance may have been appropriate within a welfare state rooted in the values and thinking of society in the 1930s, when services were driven by benign paternalism and the practice of patients trusting their doctors' (p. 7082). The alternative that the report proposed was *concordance* which is a model of the doctor–patient relationship based upon mutual respect (Vermeire et al, 2001). Marinker (1997) concluded: 'The price of compliance was dependency – it belongs to an older world. The price of concordance will be greater responsibility' for both the doctor and the patient. While this vision of shared responsibility seems commendable, as we shall discuss subsequently, it also holds the potential of medical neglect.

Overall, there is much evidence to suggest that non-adherence is an integral component of the contemporary medical-dominated health-care system. To reduce non-adherence thus requires a reassessment of this system. It also requires an understanding of what it means to the patient to be ill.

LIVED EXPERIENCE OF CHRONIC ILLNESS

The extent to which people, especially those with chronic illness, comply with recommended treatment is enmeshed in their experience of living with illness. Adherence is not a fixed event but a changing process. An increasing number of qualitative studies of illness help us to understand the processes by which people make sense of the prescribed treatment regimens. Some of these processes are considered here.

Self-Regulation

Individuals with chronic illness actively monitor and adjust their medication on an ongoing basis. It is not that they are recklessly ignoring professional advice but rather they are carefully regulating it according to a variety of factors. This is illustrated in the study conducted by Conrad (1985). Over a three-year period he conducted interviews with 80 individuals who had epilepsy about their life experiences with the disease. He noted that the individuals developed a personal 'medication practice' which best fitted with their self-image and their lifestyle. The patients realized the benefits of medication for seizure control and frequently stated that the medication helped them be more 'normal'. However, simultaneously the medication was seen as a daily reminder that they had epilepsy. They felt that reducing the medication was evidence that they were 'getting better'. Side effects were a frequently given justification for not complying with the recommended treatment. However, although side effects were mentioned they rarely referred to bodily side effects. Rather, they referred to social side effects. If the people with epilepsy felt that the medication was impairing their ability to handle routine social activities, they modified the medication to reduce this impact.

Box 18.1 summarizes four reasons that Conrad suggested underlie individuals' preference to **self-regulate** the treatment rather than comply fully with the recommended regimen. These illustrate how non-adherence is a rational process whereby the individual carefully adjusts the medication to maximize its impact.

Box 18.1

Reasons for self-regulation of medication

- Testing: the way patients test the impact of varying dosages.
- Controlling dependence: the way patients assert to themselves and others that they are not dependent on the prescribed medication.
- Destigmatization: an attempt to reject the illness label and to be 'normal'.
- Practical practice: the way patients modified their dosage so as to reduce the risk of seizures, e.g. increasing the dosage in high stress situations.

Source: Conrad, 1985: 34–5

People carefully monitor the impact of prescribed medication and adjust the dosage accordingly. They do not simply follow the standardized instructions provided by the physician but rather adjust them to suit their own personal needs. This is illustrated in a study by Hunter, O'Dea and Britten (1997) who looked at middle-aged women's usage of hormone replacement therapy (HRT). They interviewed 45 women and identified three broad themes within which the women talked about HRT:

1 *Hot flushes and night sweats*: the women would not take the medication when there were no symptoms, e.g. one woman said: 'I have no extraordinary symptoms, therefore I have no need of HRT' (p. 1544).
2 *Doctors' opinions and behaviour:* the women listened carefully to their doctor's advice and decided whether or not to take HRT, e.g. one woman said: 'I came to the doctor and had a discussion. I felt that I weighed up the advantages and disadvantages' (p. 1544).
3 *Taking hormones or medication for a 'natural' process*: the women were reluctant to take medication for something that they felt was natural. They sometimes referred to a similar concern with taking the contraceptive pill, e.g. 'I might consider it if I was suffering from symptoms which I felt I could not put up with. I'm a bit wary. I never really wanted to go on the pill because I'm always a bit wary of interfering with nature' (p. 1545).

This study illustrates that the patient's attitude to the recommended treatment is interwoven with their attitude to the illness and their attitude to their physician.

The **Self-Regulatory Model of Illness** developed by Leventhal and Cameron (1987) provides a framework to explore patients' medication beliefs (see Chapter 16). This model considers health-related decisions as dynamic rather than static. According to the model whether a person adopts a certain coping procedure (e.g. adherence with medication) depends upon perception of illness threat and the perceived efficacy of the coping strategy. According to the model, concrete symptom experience is important in formulating both representations of the disease and in monitoring medication efficacy. Thus, a perceived lack of evidence of the disease or of the efficacy of the medication would encourage non-adherence. For Leventhal, the patient can best be considered as an active problem-solver.

An extension of this approach was developed by Horne and Weinman (1999). They developed a measure of medication beliefs that distinguished between the perceived benefits and harms of the medication. They found that patients' beliefs about the efficacy and necessity of medication were tempered by concerns about the potential for harm. A study of patients with chronic illness found that there was a strong relationship between perceived necessity of the medication and reported adherence to the treatment (Horne and Weinman, 1999). In an extension of this work with individuals who had asthma it was found that there was a relationship between illness perceptions (see Chapter 16), medication beliefs and adherence (Horne and Weinman, 2002). Those individuals with strong medication necessity beliefs also perceived asthma as having a lengthy time line and that its consequences were serious. A statistical model found that treatment concerns and necessity and illness consequences were significant predictors of reported medication adherence.

A study using the Beliefs about Medicines Questionnaire (BMQ; Horne and Weinman, 1999) found further supporting evidence of the importance of the patients' medication beliefs. The study considered medication adherence among individuals suffering from chronic arthritis (Treharne, Lyons & Kitas, 2004). It found that those who perceived their medications as being more necessary and those who perceived medications as not being overused were more adherent to the prescribed medication.

Similar findings were found in a study of non-pharmacological treatment for dizziness (Yardley, Sharples, Beech & Lewith, 2001). In this study patients were interviewed about the treatment. It was found that those patients who did not adhere to the recommended treatment attributed their symptoms to causes inconsistent with the rationale for the therapy. However, some other patients who did adhere also attributed inconsistent causes but emphasized trust in their physician or a willingness to try anything that might help. These patients reported an improvement in symptoms during the treatment period although they were hesitant about attributing the cause of this to the treatment. Yardley et al. concluded that while this study provided some evidence for Leventhal's illness regulation model there were also inconsistencies. It was suggested that these might be explained by considering the role of the therapist. They concluded that their findings 'highlight the reciprocal interactions between subjective experiences of bodily symptoms, abstract images of illness and treatment and social interactions between patient and therapist – in other words between the "material" (i.e. concrete, embodied) and the discursive (i.e. symbolic, socioculturally mediated) aspects of health care' (Yardley, 1997). Together these findings would extend the illness regulation model to include the discursive and social context within which the illness and the treatment are situated.

Finally, a recent study of adherence to complementary therapies developed a dynamic extended model of treatment and illness representations (Bishop, Yardley & Lewith,

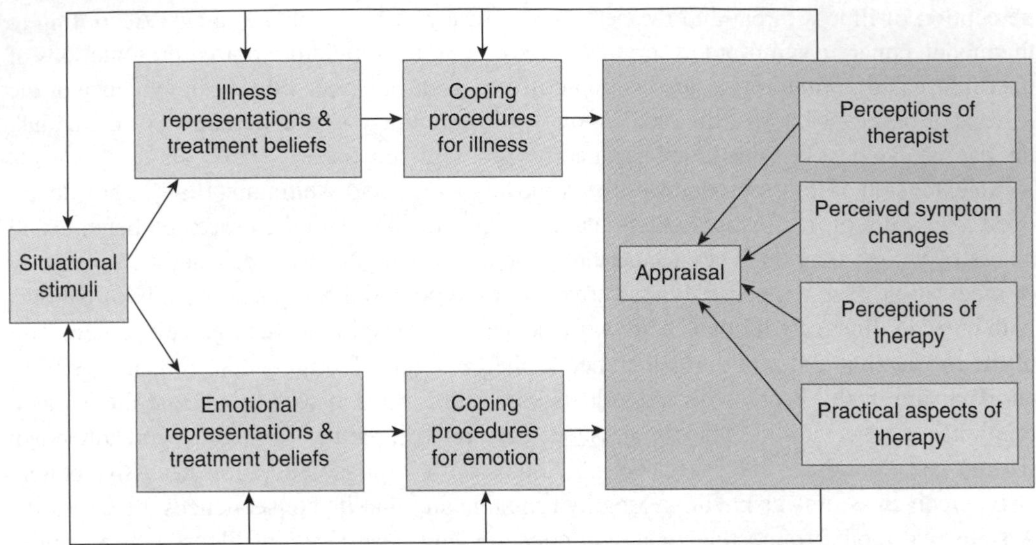

Figure 18.1 Dynamic extended model of treatment and illness representations
Source: Bishop et al., 2008: 703

2008). Figure 18.1 shows that this model conceives of the patient as being involved in an ongoing review of the treatment to assess its effectiveness and the value of continued treatment. Using this model to test adherence to complementary therapies it was found that positive perceptions of one's therapist as well as a belief that the illness was not caused by mental factors predicted adherence to appointments. In addition, beliefs about the value of holistic health and difficulty attending appointments predicted adherence to remedies prescribed.

Fear of Medication

From the physician's perspective, non-adherence can seem a foolhardy process. However, to the layperson non-adherence can be perceived as a means of reducing a variety of fears. This is illustrated in the findings of a study conducted by Donovan and Blake (1992). They investigated the extent to which a sample of people with various forms of arthritis complied with the recommended treatment. The study involved interviews and observations of 44 patients over a period of several years. They found that about half the patients did not follow the prescribed treatment. Detailed questioning of these patients revealed that they were carefully considering the implications of this non-adherence. It was not just a matter of obeying instructions or not – they were experimenting with dosages and timing. They were reluctant to follow the prescribed treatment for these reasons:

- fear of side-effects;
- fear of dependency;
- fear of reduced effectiveness;
- did not fit with lifestyle;
- drugs as a sign of weakness;
- drugs do not fit with health beliefs.

Similarly, Britten (1994) in her study of lay people's perceptions of medicines found that many people have a range of fears and anxieties about medication. This was especially the case among those people who reported that they often did not comply with prescribed medication. In her discussion, Britten comments on the physicians' urge to prescribe and suggests they should consider other options to medication.

In the development of the Beliefs about Medicines Questionnaire, Horne (1997) distinguished between General Overuse (beliefs that medicines in general are overused by doctors) and General Harm (beliefs that medicines in general are harmful addictive poisons). These two beliefs were found to be closely related. Subsequent work found that in a sample of British students, males, those with less experience of medication and those from an Asian background had a stronger belief in the General Harm of medicines (Horne, Graupner, Frost, Weinman, Wright & Hankins, 2004). This would indicate that medication beliefs are closely intertwined with gender and cultural identity and with experience of medication.

Identity Control

Medication adherence is also tied to the extent to which the patient accepts that s/he has an illness and wishes to control it. This is illustrated in the study by Adams, Pill and Jones (1997). They conducted detailed interviews with a sample of asthma sufferers registered with a general practice in South Wales. Analysis of these interviews revealed that the extent to which the individuals complied with the recommended treatment (daily use of a curative and a prophylactic inhaler) was intimately bound up with how they defined themselves and their attitude to the illness. Three groups of patients, each with a particular pattern of medication, were identified:

1 *Deniers/distancers:* these were the individuals who argued that despite the medical diagnosis they did not have asthma but rather just 'bad chests'. They would fall into Goffman's (1963) 'discreditable' category and took steps to ensure that others were not aware of their diagnosis. They generally had a negative view of people with asthma (e.g. 'weakling' or 'wimp') and wished to avoid such a label. Although they took reliever medication when necessary, they were reluctant to take prophylactic medication regularly. While the former helped their 'bad chest', the latter was a symbol that they were 'asthmatic'.
2 *Accepters:* these individuals reluctantly accepted that they had asthma. They also held a variety of negative associations of people with asthma. They emphasized that they were

not stereotypical asthmatic people but rather more like certain individuals who were able to achieve despite having asthma, e.g. certain athletes. They defined asthma as a 'condition' that needed to be controlled. As such they not only took the reliever medication but also the prophylactic medication. However, these individuals emphasized that although they took their medication regularly they were not dependent on their doctor. Rather, they were proud that they controlled their asthma themselves, using the drugs, with limited contact with their physician.

3 *Pragmatists:* these individuals did not fall neatly into the previous two categories although they were closer to the accepters. All of them accepted that they had asthma but their notions of asthma and medication usage were somewhat idiosyncratic. Unlike the secrecy of the deniers and the public stance of the accepters this group adopted a more pragmatic attitude and practiced what Adams et al. described as a strategic policy of disclosure. This was related to their self-medication practices to which they adopted a pragmatic stance.

Meaning of Illness

Within the phenomenological and narrative literature there has been substantial discussion on the role of perceived meaning. For example, within narrative psychology it has been argued that the creation of a narrative account helps bring order and meaning to events that are confusing (Murray, 2008; also see Chapter 16). There is a substantial research literature on the perceived meaning of illness. In a study of published accounts of breast cancer it was shown that many women search for meaning in their disease (Murray, 2009). It has been argued that greater narrative coherence is associated with feelings of well-being (Baerger & McAdams, 1999). It is possible that it is also linked to treatment adherence.

Recent research on writing has suggested that the process of writing can provide an opportunity for people to clarify the meaning of events in their lives. In a study by Westling, Garcia and Mann (2007) women with HIV were asked to participate in a regular writing task over one month. Analysis of what they had written found that those women who, during the writing task, had found some personal meaning in having HIV were more likely to have greater adherence to the medication prescribed at the end of the project. In this case discovery of meaning was defined as 'a major shift in values, priorities, or perspectives'. There is ongoing discussion about what is going on in such writing activities (Nicholls, 2007). The growth of creative writing classes in health-care settings provides an opportunity for further research.

RESISTANCE TO MEDICINE TAKING

A common feature in qualitative research into medicine taking is the active role of the patient in assessing the value of the prescribed medication and deciding to what extent they should

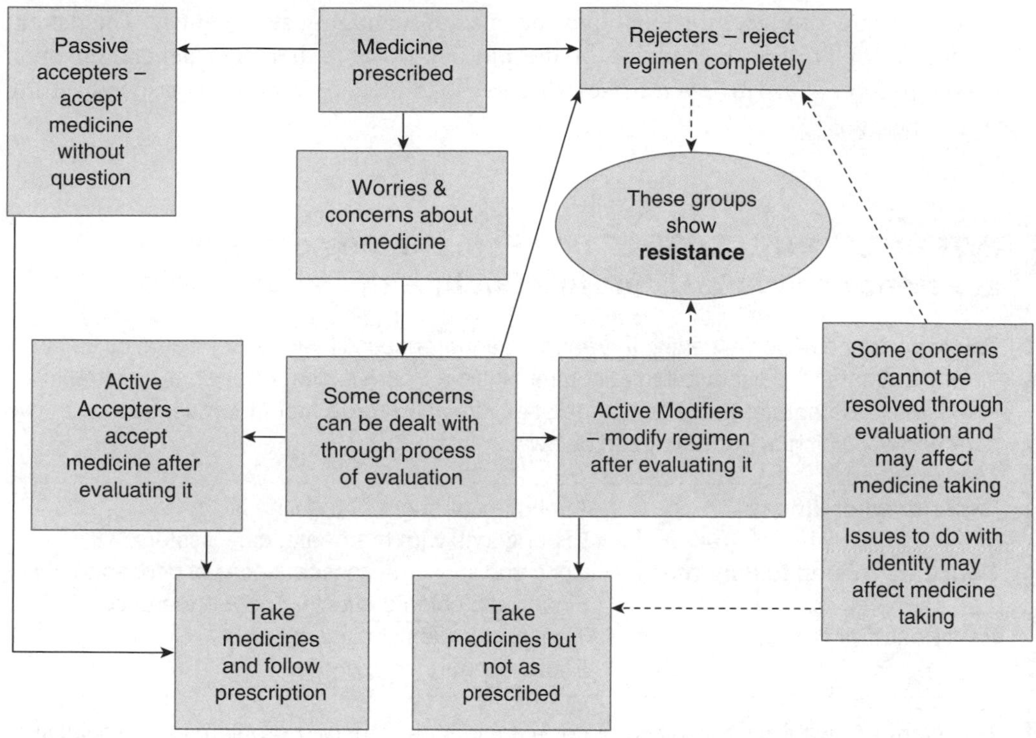

Figure 18.2 Model of medicine taking
Source: Pound et al., 2005: 139

accept or resist it. In an extensive review of the qualitative research Pound et al. (2005) concluded that 'the urge to evaluate suggests widespread caution about taking medicines as well as distrust in the information given about medicines' (p. 149).

They developed a model of medicine-taking that highlighted the active role of the patient in decision making. Figure 18.2 shows that people will resist medication for a variety of reasons especially concern about adverse drug reactions. They conclude that if the term resistance sounds strong 'it should be remembered that the huge literature on "non-compliance" only exists because so many people have continued to resist taking medicines in the face of sustained advice, interventions and admonishments' (p. 152).

Social Support

These studies illustrate that the extent of adherence with the recommended treatment is intertwined not only with the character of the disease but also with the patient's self-definition and the perceived meaning of the illness. Adherence or non-adherence is not only a means of managing symptoms but also of managing self-identity. The patient does not simply follow the advice of the physician but rather acts depending upon how s/he interprets it. However, these processes take place in a particular social setting (see Box below).

Case Study

INTERNATIONAL CASE STUDY Explanations of treatment adherence among patients in a South African community

The importance of social setting in treatment adherence is illustrated in a qualitative study among patients in a disadvantaged community in a South Africa. After analysing the interviews with a sample of patients, Kagee et al. identified three main themes, each with two sub-themes, which are summarized below:

Experience of illness	Attribution of origin of the illness
	Experiences with the health care system
Concerns related to adherence	Concerns about the consequences of poor adherence
	Financial problems affecting poor adherence
Psychosocial issues	Transport issues
	Social support

This study shows the importance of social factors as transport problems and social support within these themes. The authors conclude that 'treatment adherence is not simply an individual volitional act that conforms to rational and objective logic' (p. 457). Rather it is an active psychological process which is enmeshed in a broader socio-cultural context.

Source: Kagee, Le Roux & Dick, 2007

MEDICAL ERROR

The desire of patients to evaluate the impact of the medication prescribed on their health is supported by the evidence on the extent of medical error. The term **iatrogenesis** was developed by Ivan Illich (1976) to describe health problems that are caused by medicine. While this term applies to the overall negative effects of the medical system, a particular issue is the extent of preventable **medical error**. Over the past ten years there has been increasing awareness of the extent of medical error. In 2000 the US Institute of Medicine (IOM, 2000) published a report summarizing the growing evidence of the risk to the health of patients due to medical error. This report highlighted two studies – one in Colorado and Utah and the other one in New York (Brennan et al., 1991) – that found that adverse events occurred in 2.9 per cent and 3.7 per cent of hospitalizations, respectively.

Extrapolating to the whole of the USA the report estimated that 44,000 to 98,000 Americans die each year as a result of medical error. That is more than die each year from motor-vehicle accidents, breast cancer or AIDS.

Since the publication of the IOM report, other countries have produced similar reports. For example, in 2001 the UK Chief Medical Officer produced a report entitled *An Organisation with a Memory* (DOH, 2000a) and a subsequent action report detailing specific recommendations (DOH, 2001). This was followed by a report by the UK Chief Pharmaceutical Officer (Smith, 2004). These reports also referred to the high rate of adverse medical events. They highlighted one British study (Vincent et al., 2001) that found that 10 per cent of patients admitted to two London teaching hospitals had experienced an adverse event, of which half were preventable. It was estimated that such adverse events generated up to £2 billion in additional costs to the NHS (DOH, 2000a). A recent survey conducted by the Health Foundation (2004) in the UK estimated that as many as 40,000 deaths a year were due to medical error.

Smith (2004) estimated that 10–20 per cent of adverse medical events are due to medication errors. In a study of 550,000 prescriptions written by GPs in Britain pharmacists identified and averted 54 potentially harmful cases (0.01 per cent) (Greene, 1995). However, a large proportion of errors go undetected or unreported. For this reason Smith proposed a medication error iceberg to describe the situation. At the tip were those errors that cause actual damage and are reported. But then there are the unreported errors that include errors identified with potential to cause harm (near-misses), errors identified but considered insignificant, potential errors and unnoticed actual errors. Together, this indicates the extent of the problem is much greater than appears from initial figures.

Explanations for Medical Error

Explanations of medical error frequently distinguish between the person and systems approaches (Reason, 2000). The person approach focuses on the individual and leads to the so-called 'name, blame and shame' approach to error management. The alternative systems approach considers the broader context within which errors occur. It emphasizes the importance of organizational change in order to reduce the risk of error. A summary of the person and system explanations of medical error is provided in Figure 18.3.

In hospitals it is junior physicians who do most of the prescribing. They are the ones with least knowledge and also the ones who make the most prescribing errors (Lesar et al., 1997). Wu et al. (1991) surveyed junior hospital physicians in internal medicine training programmes. They found that 45 per cent reported making at least one error, 31 per cent of which resulted in a patient's death.

Weingart, Wilson, Gibberd and Harrison (2000) in their review of medical error identified a series of potential risk factors. These included:

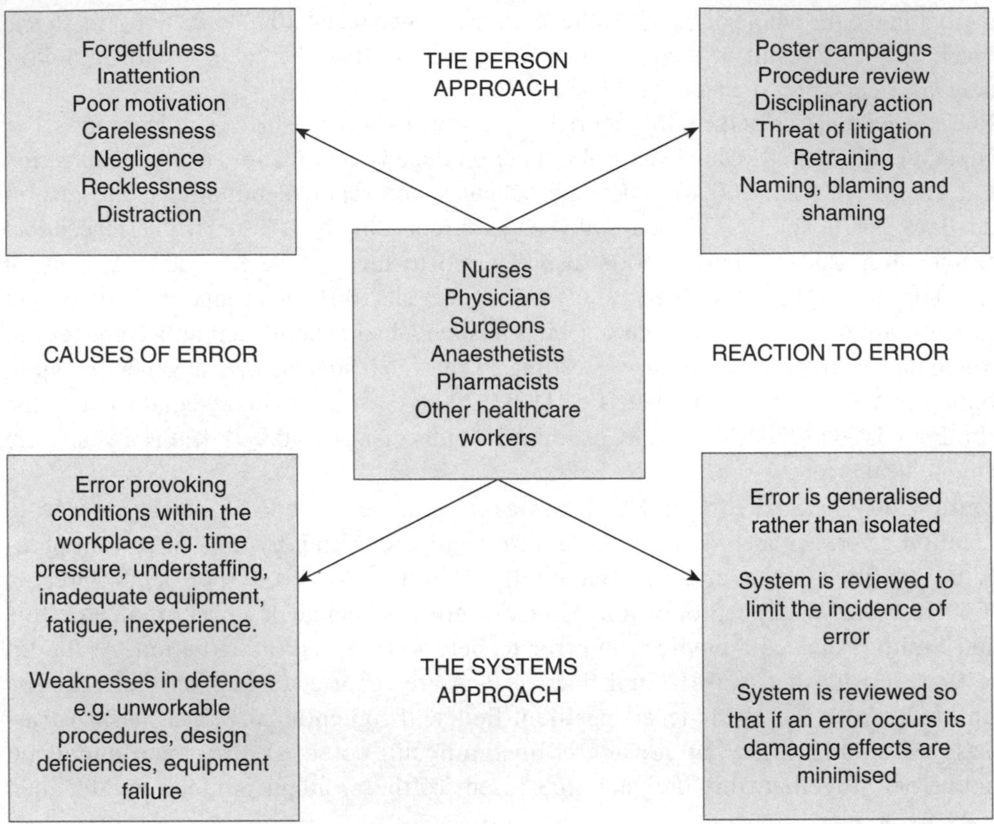

Figure 18.3 Person and system approaches to medication error

- Age of patient: older patients are more at risk
- Type of intervention: certain types of surgery are particularly risky
- Emergency room usage
- Lengthy medical care
- Intensive medical care

They concluded 'unless we make substantial changes to the organisation and delivery of medical care, all patients – particularly the most vulnerable – will continue to bear the burden of medical error' (p. 776).

An important factor overall is the character of the physician–patient relationship. A survey of American physicians and members of the general public (Blendon et al., 2002) found that they agreed on two possible causes of medical error: shortage of nurses (53 per cent physicians vs. 65 per cent of the public) and overwork, stress and fatigue of health providers (50 per cent vs. 70 per cent). In addition, 72 per cent of the public referred to too little time with their physician and 67 per cent referred to health-care professionals not working as a team or not communicating.

In a national survey of residents (junior hospital doctors) in the Netherlands (sample of over 2000 with 41 per cent response rate) it was found that 94 per cent reported that they had made one or more mistakes that did not have negative consequences for the patient. However, more than half (56 per cent) reported that they had made at least one mistake that had a negative consequence for the patient (Prins et al., 2009). The strongest predictors of self-reported errors were emotional exhaustion and depersonalization. In addition, burnout was more predictive of perceived errors due to lack of time than errors due to judgement/inexperience. They concluded that there was a need for greater supervision and emotional support for junior doctors.

Medical Silence

One common problem raised by all of the recent reports has been that of medical silence: the reluctance of health professionals, in particular physicians, to report errors. In a survey of physicians conducted in five countries (Australia, New Zealand, Canada, US and UK) a large proportion reported that they felt discouraged from reporting or that they were not encouraged to report (Blendon et al., 2002). The proportion was over 60 per cent in Australia and about 30 per cent in the UK. This contrasts with the large proportion of patients and the general public who would prefer reporting of medical errors (Gallagher, Waterman, Ebers, Fraser & Levinson, 2003).

The DOH (2000a) identified several reasons for this reluctance to report on the part of medical personnel. These included:

- Lack of awareness that an error has occurred
- Lack of awareness of the need to report, what to report and why
- Perception that the patient is unharmed by the error
- Fear of disciplinary action or litigation, for self or colleagues
- Lack of familiarity with reporting mechanisms
- Loss of self-esteem
- Staff feeling they are too busy to report
- Lack of feedback when errors are reported.

The IOM (2000) report expressed alarm that despite the high rate of error 'silence surrounds this issue. For the most part, consumers believe they are protected' (p. 3). It continued: 'The goal of this report is to break this cycle of inaction. The status quo is not acceptable and cannot be tolerated any longer. Despite the cost pressures, liability constraints, resistance to change and other seemingly insurmountable barriers, it is simply not acceptable for patients to be harmed by the same health care system that is supposed to offer healing and comfort' (p. 3). This reluctance on the part of physicians to report has led to the establishment of mandatory reporting systems in many countries.

However, the reluctance of the physician to report also reflects their power and status in society and the reticence of the public and the patient to question medical authority. Thus implicit within any model to reduce medical error and to improve patient safety is the challenge of increasing public and patient involvement and control of health care.

PATIENT EMPOWERMENT

Rather than attempting to control the patient, an approach that is implicit within models of compliance, empowerment attempts to increase patient autonomy and self-control. The empowerment approach is derived from the work of community educators and psychologists and is defined as the process whereby 'people gain mastery over their lives' (Rappaport, 1987). Instead of imposing the views of the expert health professional, empowerment seeks to enhance the patients' self-understanding and the potential of self-care (Feste & Anderson, 1995).

The focus of this approach is the enhancement of the strengths and potential of the patient. Through dialogue the health professional seeks to understand the needs of the patient. Skelton (1997) suggests that the aim of patient education within this model is to 'blur' the boundaries between professional-as-teacher and patient-as-learner. Instead of the professional's health knowledge being considered paramount, the patient's lay health beliefs and knowledge is considered of equal or greater value. A central component of this understanding is the opportunity for patients to tell their stories. In describing this process Hunter (1991) notes that 'medicine has the power not only to rewrite the patient's story of illness but also to replot its course' (p. 139). Dependent upon the story that is handed back the patient will assess its relevance to their lives. As Hunter (1991) continues: 'if the two are widely disparate and the physician fails to recognize the distance between them, the interaction founders. The medicine will go untaken, the consultation unsought, the prescription unfilled' (p. 142).

Desire for Control

Patient empowerment can aim to involve the patient more in health care through attention to patient needs or it can increase the patients' awareness of the broader social and political factors that adversely affect their health status. Admittedly, as Lupton (1997) found, not all patients wish to be actively involved in their personal health care or in taking broader collective action.

Desire for control can be conceptualized along three dimensions (Auerbach, 2001):

- Cognitive/Informational control is concerned with processing relevant information and thereby reducing ambiguity and leading to an enhanced sense of control over the particular situation. In the case of health care this involves obtaining and reviewing information about the health problem and the proposed treatment;
- Decisional control refers to the opportunity for reviewing and selecting preferences for treatment;
- Behavioural control involves direct action whereby the individual is involved in changing the situation. It implies that the patient has the opportunity to select and guide the actual treatment.

There is substantial evidence that patients desire information about their health (Auerbach & Pegg, 2002), younger more educated patients having a greater desire for such information. In the case of decisional control, the evidence is more equivocal with many patients indicating that they would prefer physician control or at best some form of joint or collaborative control. A variety of factors influence this preference: 1) less desire for control when the disease is serious, 2) less desire for control among older patients, 3) less desire for control among patients with lower education. In concluding his review, Auerbach (2001) concluded: 'if there is a predisposition on the part of patients to want to assume control, it is strongly influenced by their appraisal of whether they think involvement on their part will positively influence the outcome of their situation' (p. 197).

Critical Approach to Empowerment

Many health-care providers have enthusiastically endorsed the idea of empowerment. However, there is a need for some caution as regards why this idea has become so popular and its implications for patient care. Although most physicians prefer to adopt the dominant role in patient care (Beisecker et al., 1996) there is increasing evidence that many are promoting greater control by the patient (e.g. Coulter, 1999). Indeed, this orientation connects with the identification of the patient as responsible in some way for both their illness and their treatment. This is particularly the case in those illnesses associated with lifestyle practices such as smoking, diet and exercise, but also with chronic diseases.

This critical approach to patient empowerment considers it part of the extended biopsychosocial model (Salmon & Hall, 2003). This model extends the traditional dualistic approach to the body by identifying psychosocial factors as aetologic agents of disease. This in turn leads to concern with promoting increased control and various coping strategies as ways of patient empowerment. Implicit in this discourse is the transformation of the patient from a passive sufferer to an active manager of their own suffering 'from which it is a small step to locating with the patient the moral responsibility to become well' (Salmon & Hall, 2003: 1973). This provides the physician with the opportunity to evade responsibility for treatment of those problems for which they have limited insight (e.g. chronic illness and mental illness). Thus the language of empowerment can serve the physician's interests rather than those of the patient. It can also absolve the physician of responsibility for certain medical errors.

A graphic illustration of the negative impact of empowerment is the enthusiasm of many physicians to promote the so-called 'fighting spirit' attitude among cancer patients. Initial research by Greer, Morris and Pettingale (1979) had suggested that patients with this attitude had better survival prospects. Many patients report that their clinicians encourage them to be positive and to fight (e.g. Byrne et al., 2002). Unfortunately, such encouragement can be disempowering as the patient feels depressed because s/he cannot control the disease. In our review of the evidence, there is little empirical support that personality or coping strategies improve the prospects of survival (see Chapters 17 and 20).

Another example of this disempowering advice is the case of 'patient-controlled analgesia' (PCA) which is a strategy designed to provide post-operative patients with control over their analgesia. However, in interviews with the patients it was found that PCA did not give them control over their pain. Rather, they liked PCA because it freed them of the need to exercise control by 'bothering' nurses with requests for analgesia (Taylor et al., 1996). In a comparison study that involved teaching post-operative patients to feel in control of their recovery it was found that patients interpreted the programme as a request not to annoy the staff. Together these studies question the practice of strategies designed to empower patients.

Kugelmann (1997) develops a similar critique in his review of the growth of the gate control model of pain. He notes that an important component of this and other biopsychosocial models is the insistence on personal responsibility for pain management. The alternative to assuming responsibility is learned helplessness and passivity. While the patient is expected to assume responsibility 'they should not expect, however, that the professionals should relinquish their salaries or expertise' (p. 61). Kugelmann also connects his critique with the ignorance of social problems. 'If pain is truly epidemic today, then something is terribly wrong, not only with patients, or inadequate pain technologies, but with the social matrix that produces suffering. To tempt people to be co-managers in such a social world only deepens our true helplessness' (p. 62).

Other researchers have questioned the whole movement towards promoting empowerment. As Lord and McKillop Farlow (1990) note: 'people mistakenly talk about "empowering families" or "empowering professionals" as if empowerment is something one person does to another' (p. 2). Powers (2003) argues that rather than challenging the traditional medical paternalism, 'empowerment equals paternalism' (p. 229). Within a capitalist state this promotion of empowerment has a hidden agenda:

1 It allows health-care disciplines to reframe questions regarding oppression to questions regarding free individual choices among predetermined alternatives in the context of a belief in natural rights;
2 It allows the health-care provider to assign blame when the strategy fails, i.e. when the patient chooses the 'wrong' option;
3 It makes health education a technology of the self, a way to get people to think they are taking charge of their own health and exercising their rights instead of being dependent.

The move toward empowerment is especially directed at those people who do not conform to mainstream values and practices rather than attempting to promote broader changes in social structures. The physician and other health professionals can now continue to disparage the most deprived and marginalized not for their non-compliance but rather for their refusal to accept responsibility for self-management.

These criticisms are a challenge and highlight the need for health psychology to adopt a broad critical perspective such that it does not simply continue to be another agent of health-care oppression in the guise of a more critical language.

FUTURE RESEARCH

1 New medical procedures and drugs are constantly being developed. While these can be efficacious in the controlled clinical trial setting, there is an ongoing need to assess the problems involved in their adoption in the community.
2 Different health problems require different forms of treatment. Research needs to consider the appropriateness of different interventions.
3 Similarly, not everyone will accept certain procedures. Further research is needed to explore the meaning of different treatments to different populations.
4 As attitudes to health care change, research needs to address the changing needs of different client groups and how these can best be addressed.
5 Research needs to address how best to involve people more directly in all aspects of their health care.

Summary

1 Adherence refers to the extent to which the patient follows the prescribed treatment regimen.
2 A wide range of social and psychological factors has been found to be associated with non-adherence. These factors are associated with the characteristics of the patients, the

(Continued)

(Continued)

disorders they have, the treatments they are given, and the relationships they have with their physicians and organizational factors.

3 An alternative approach is to consider the impact on patient behaviour of the socio-political role of the physician and the meaning of the health problem and of the prescribed medication for the patient.

4 Medical error leads to a wide range of health problems. Explanations of medical error include both person and system factors. Medical silence has traditionally concealed the extent of medical error.

5 Patient empowerment aims to involve patients in health care through listening to their needs not as recipients but as active partners in the process of health care.

6 Patient empowerment conversely can centre responsibility for illness management on the patient and absolve the physician and health professional from responsibilities.

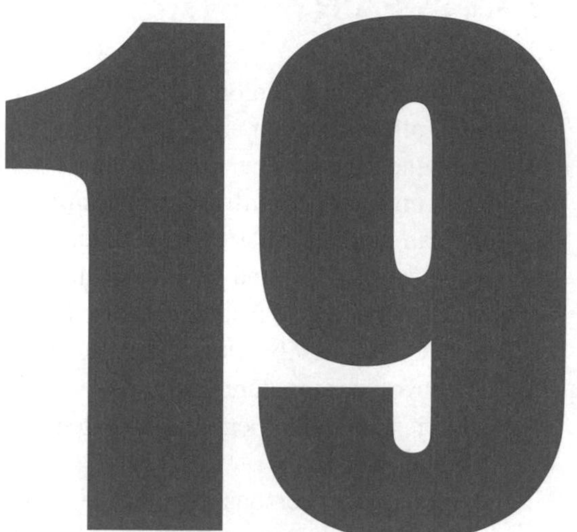

Pain[1]

Prolonged pain, even if not particularly severe, tends to take the joy out of life.

Finkelstein and French, 1993: 36

Outline

This chapter discusses the nature of pain and the distinction between acute and chronic pain. The focus is chronic pain. We discuss the major theories, including direct line of transmission theories and multidimensional gate control theory, which acknowledges psychological influences. A range of psychosocial factors implicated in the mediation of the pain experience are considered. We summarize pain assessment methods. Finally, we explore the issue of pain management using psychological techniques.

[1]An earlier draft of this chapter published in the Second Edition was written by Cailine Woodall.

WHAT IS PAIN?

Pain evolved as a biological safety mechanism to warn us when something is physically wrong, allowing us to take appropriate action to alleviate the problem. It is a highly adaptive phenomenon. The importance of this mechanism can be seen when cases of congenital universal insensitivity to pain (CUIP) are considered. One such case was a young Canadian woman, Miss C, who never experienced pain. She suffered repeated injuries (e.g. third degree burns) and severe medical problems from not making positional adjustments normally evoked by discomfort or pain (e.g. pathological abnormalities in knees, hips and spine). Consequently, Miss C died aged just 29 (see Melzack and Wall, 1982). Most cases of CUIP involve premature death.

Pain is a uniquely personal experience, which has been defined in many ways, including:

- An aversive, personal, subjective experience, influenced by cultural learning, the meaning of the situation, attention and other psychological variables, which disrupts ongoing behaviour and motivates the individual to attempt to stop the pain (Melzack & Wall, 1988).
- Whatever the person experiencing it says it is, existing whenever the experiencing person says it does (McCaffery & Thorpe, 1988).
- It is an unpleasant sensory and emotional experience associated with actual or potential tissue damage, or described in terms of such damage (Merskey, 1996).

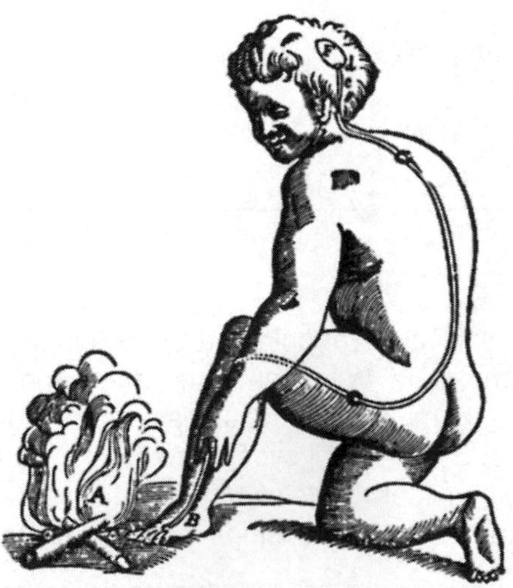

Figure 19.1 The pain pathway in René Descartes' *Traite de l'homme* (1664). *This specificity view of pain has been replaced with more complex theories*

Such definitions highlight the subjective, emotional and multidimensional nature of pain experience. Pain has been further classified as either acute or chronic, differentiated only by duration (acute being under and chronic over six months). The six-month cut-off is arbitrary and other suggested cut-off points of 30 days, three months or twelve months.

The International Association for the Study of Pain (IASP) published pain terminology in 1994 and in slightly revised form in 2007 (IASP, 2010). Changes were made to definitions of Central Pain: 'pain initiated or caused by a primary lesion or dysfunction in the central nervous system'; and Hyperpathia: 'a painful syndrome characterized by an abnormally painful reaction to a stimulus, especially a repetitive stimulus, as well as an increased threshold'. Two new forms were added: Neuropathic Pain: 'pain initiated or caused by a primary lesion or dysfunction in the nervous system'; and Peripheral Neuropathic Pain: 'Pain initiated or caused by a primary lesion or dysfunction in the peripheral nervous system' (IASP, 2010).

Acute pain is a useful biological response provoked by injury or disease (e.g. broken leg, appendicitis), which is of limited duration (IASP, 2010). It tends to be amenable to pharmacological treatment. **Chronic** pain is described as pain persisting for six months or more and tends not to respond to pharmacological treatment.

Further definitional distinctions include:

- malignant (associated with progressive illness e.g. cancer);
- benign (not associated with progressive illness e.g. lower back pain);
- progressive (becomes worse over time e.g. arthritis);
- intractable (resistant to treatment e.g. lower back pain);
- intermittent (pain that fluctuates over time and in intensity e.g. fibromyalgia);
- recurrent (acute pain occurring periodically e.g. migraine);
- organic (involving observable tissue damage e.g. arthritis);
- psychogenic (absence of demonstrable pathology e.g. fibromyalgia);
- referred (pain originating in one body area which is perceived as originating from another e.g. perceiving an earache that in fact originates from a bad tooth).

Responses to acute pain that are adaptive will often be maladaptive in response to chronic pain.

Pain is a complex, multidimensional phenomenon with physiological (aetiology), sensory (intensity, quality), affective (emotional response), cognitive (thoughts about the experience) and behavioural (e.g. grimacing, avoidance) components. It can affect anyone at any time, often involving all aspects of a person's life including physical, psychological and emotional states, disrupting daily activities, work, finances, social, marital and family life and relationships (e.g. Marcus, 2000). In addition to the association between many chronic illnesses and pain (e.g. cancer, HIV/AIDS, sickle-cell anaemia), particular groups appear more likely to experience chronic pain, especially the elderly and many disabled people even in the absence of illness (e.g. pain from braces or harnesses).

A different concept of pain, so-called 'psychological pain', is often used in everyday discourse. Kugelmann's (2000) analysis of 42 pain narratives suggested that psychological and physical pain have similar phenomenological structures. Both kinds of pain are 'felt bodily performances that entail at least temporarily a disabling of a potentiality for action' (Kugelmann, 2000: 305). Pain is a performance of affliction of a person in a social situation suggesting that pain can affect any aspect of existence, not only the physical body. However, in the rest of this chapter, we discuss the conventional concept of physical pain.

THE COST OF PAIN

Pain inflicts significant costs on individuals, their families, the health services and society in general. It is the most commonly cited reason for which patients seek medical help. It is estimated that 80 per cent of all doctor consultations in the USA and around 40 per cent in the UK relate to pain. Pain is associated with extended hospital stays, lost working days and increased take-up of benefits. The resultant economic costs are very high. Back pain is the most common chronic pain condition. In 1998, it was estimated that in the UK back pain had a prevalence rate of 37 per cent (or 17.5 million individuals), equating to direct costs for care and treatment of £31.63 billion and indirect costs as lost production and informal care of £310.67 billion (Maniadakis & Gray, 2000).

Fortner et al. (2003) surveyed 373 cancer outpatients about direct costs resulting from pain-related hospitalizations, emergency department visits, physician office visits, and use of analgesic medications and indirect costs related to pain-related transportation, complementary therapies to improve pain management, educational materials, over-the–counter medication, domestic support and childcare. Sixty-nine per cent experienced direct medical costs due to pain, resulting in an average total cost of US$ 825/month per patient. Fifty-seven per cent reported at least one indirect pain-related expense for an average indirect cost of US$ 61/month per patient.

The cost of pain in terms of human suffering is also high. Pain statistics are likely to under-represent the problem as many people endure significant levels of pain without seeking help. Pain is often the most distressing and debilitating aspect of chronic illness. Its effects on quality of life can be devastating to the individual and their significant others, including distress, loss of function, relationship problems, social, financial and employment difficulties and stigma. The emotional toll of severe chronic pain should not be underestimated. It is estimated that around 50 per cent of severe chronic pain patients consider suicide. This association is mediated by depression. Similarly, the experience of unremitting pain in cancer patients has been reported as the most common reason underlying requests for physician-assisted dying.

THEORIES OF PAIN

The specific mechanisms for the transmission and perception of pain are not well understood, although our knowledge is expanding. Several prominent theories of pain have been proposed including specificity theory, pattern theory and gate control theory. Both specificity theory and pattern theory view pain as a sensory experience.

Specificity Theory

Specificity theory suggested by Descartes in 1664 (Figure 19.1) and taken up by Von Frey in 1894 describes a direct causal relationship between pain stimulus and pain experience. Stimulation of specific pain receptors (nociceptors) throughout the body sends impulses along specific pain pathways (A-delta fibres and C-fibres) through the spinal cord to specific areas of the sensory cortex of the brain. Stimulus intensity correlates with pain intensity, with higher stimulus intensity and pain pathway activation resulting in a more intense pain experience. Failure to identify a specific cortical location for pain, realization that pain fibres do not respond exclusively to pain but also to pressure and temperature, and the disproportional relationship between stimulus intensity and reported pain intensity (e.g. injured soldiers reporting little pain while similarly injured civilians requiring substantial medication) led to specificity theory losing favour.

Pattern Theory

Pattern theorists proposed that stimulation of nociceptors produces a pattern of impulses that are summated in the dorsal horn of the spinal cord. Only if the level of the summated output exceeds a certain threshold is pain information transmitted onwards to the cortex resulting in pain perception. Evidence of deferred pain perception (e.g. soldiers not perceiving pain until the battle is over), intact pain transmission systems where pain is perceived without (ongoing) injury (e.g. phantom limb) and injury without pain perception (e.g. CUIP) raised questions concerning the comprehensiveness of pattern theories. In addition, there was growing evidence for a mediating role for psychosocial factors in the experience of pain, including cross-cultural differences in pain perception and expression.

Gate Control Theory

Conscious experience, whether pain or otherwise, is derived from a complex array of afferent information arriving via sensory transducers alloyed with cognitive and emotional information about the context, history and future implications of the stimulus environment. The growing body of evidence contradicting direct line of transmission theories culminated in the development of the **gate control theory** (GCT; Melzack and Wall, 1982). The GCT views pain as a multidimensional, subjective experience of perception in which ascending physiological inputs and descending psychological inputs are equally involved. GCT posits that there is a gating mechanism in the dorsal horn of the spinal cord that permits or inhibits the transmission of pain impulses (see Figure 19.2).

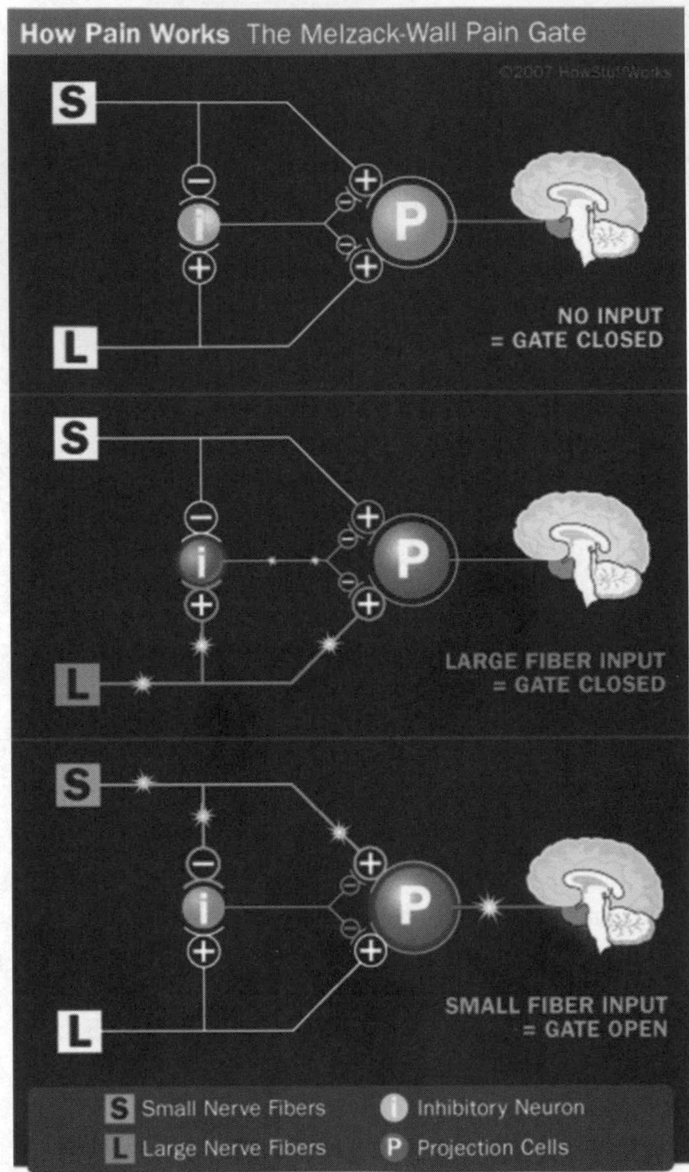

Figure 19.2 The Melzack–Wall Gate Control Theory of pain

The **dorsal horn** receives inputs from nociceptors which it projects to the brain via a neural gate. The dorsal horn also receives information from the brain about the psychological and emotional state of the individual. This information can act as an inhibitory control that closes the neural gate preventing the transmission of the nociceptive impulses and thus modifying the perception of pain. The mechanism operates based on the relative activity of the peripheral nociceptor fibres and the descending cortical fibres. Pain impulses must reach conscious awareness before pain is experienced. If awareness can be prevented, the experience of pain is decreased, eliminated or deferred.

GCT is the most influential theory of pain and continues to inform theoretical and empirical work. GCT offered substantial explanatory power, acknowledging a role for descending control and psychological, social and behavioural factors. However, the theory has received criticism, the most significant being the absence of direct evidence of a 'gate' in the spinal cord. Also, the gate control theory is not able to explain several chronic pain problems, such as phantom limb pain. Melzack (1999) updated the theory describing a neuromatrix, in place of the gate. The neuromatrix theory proposes that pain is a multidimensional experience produced by characteristic 'neurosignature' patterns of nerve impulses generated by a widely distributed neural network – the 'body-self neuromatrix' – in the brain. These neurosignatures may be triggered by sensory inputs or can be generated independently of them. Pain is produced by a 'widely distributed neural network in the brain rather than directly by sensory input evoked by injury, inflammation or other pathology' (Melzack, 1999: 880). Pain is the result of the output from this neural network programme, which is determined by sensory, cognitive, affective, experiential and genetic influences. Mapping the neural networks proposed by Melzack, and development of treatment approaches based on the theory, will determine the theory's potential to further our understanding of pain.

NEURAL CORRELATES OF PAIN

What is the evidence for the kind of 'widely distributed neural networks in the brain' that Melzack and others believe must help to explain the subjective experience of pain? Are the differences in self-reported pain associated with measurable neural differences? Experience of a specific stimulus is unique to a given individual. Thus, how can a third-person observer appreciate the first-person experience of another individual? Coghill, McHaffie and Yen (2003) used psychophysical ratings to define pain sensitivity and functional magnetic resonance imaging (fMRI) to assess brain activity. They found positive evidence that individuals who were more sensitive to pain stimuli exhibited more frequent and more robust pain-induced activation of the primary somatosensory cortex, anterior cingulate cortex, and prefrontal cortex than did insensitive individuals. Coghill et al. have identified objective neural correlates of subjective differences, validating the use of self-reported pain from introspection as a method of communicating a first-person experience.

KEY STUDY How can we know when another person really experiences pain?

First-person introspection is necessary for communicating pain experience to a third-person observer. The study by Coghill et al. identified the neural correlates of an individual's subjective experience of pain. Seventeen healthy volunteers (8 women and 9 men of mean age 26) participated in a psychophysical and fMRI study of individual differences in pain sensitivity. Thermal stimuli were delivered and assessed with a 10-unit mechanical VAS for pain intensity. Thirty-two stimuli (35°C, 43–49°C, 5-s duration) were applied to their non-dominant ventral forearm. Each participant underwent functional imaging during thermal stimulation of the skin of the right lower leg. For painful stimulation, five 30-s duration epochs of 49°C stimulation were interleaved with six 30-s duration epochs of 35°C stimulation. At the end of each 330-s series, participants provided a rating of pain intensity. Participants were assigned to a high- (mean VAS rating = 7.43), moderate- (mean VAS rating = 4.44), or low-sensitivity (mean VAS rating = 2.43) sub-group. To identify brain regions that were activated more frequently in the high-sensitivity individuals, the frequency map of the low-sensitivity group was subtracted from that of the high-sensitivity group.

Cortical regions involved in sensation, attention, and affect were activated more frequently in pain sensitive individuals than in those who were insensitive. The most robust difference between high-sensitivity and low-sensitivity sub-groups was located within a portion of the anterior cingulate cortex, where 6/6 of the highly sensitive volunteers, but none of the insensitive volunteers, displayed statistically significant activation (Figure 19.3). This study shows that individuals with similar subjective reports of pain evoke similar patterns of activation magnitude suggesting that people can accurately represent their conscious experience via introspection.

Source: Coghill et al., (2003)

PSYCHOLOGICAL ASPECTS OF PAIN

Many psychosocial factors have been investigated in relation to pain and these appear to exert independent effects on the experience of pain. The most significant determinant of pain chronicity appears to be the level of impact on activities of daily living, the functional disability associated with the pain. While the role of psychological factors in the experience of pain is now generally accepted, discussion of psychological inputs to pain is likely to provoke passionate responses and/or denials from sufferers, who fear invalidation of their very real experiences as 'all in the mind'. Health professionals need to be sensitive to this fear and

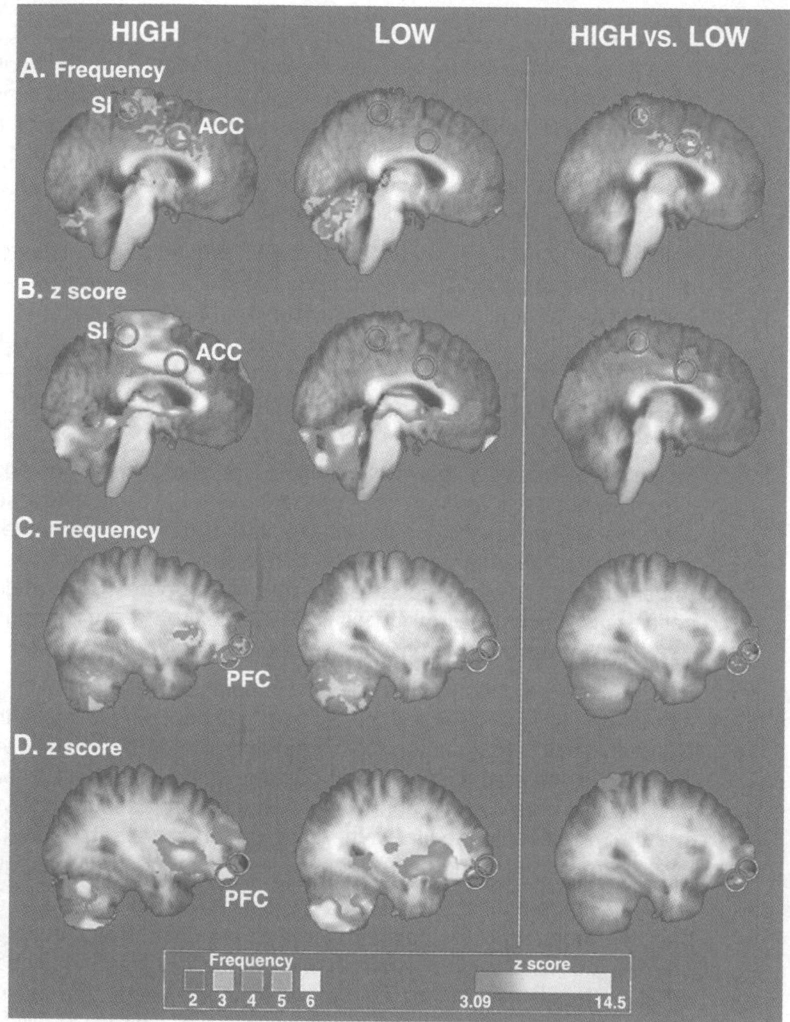

Figure 19.3 Brain regions displaying different frequencies of activation between high- and low-sensitivity sub-groups. Circles are centred on regions where the peak differences between groups were located. Shades in A and C correspond to the number of individuals displaying statistically significant activation

Source: Coghill et al., 2003: Figure 2; Reproduced with permission

present psychological issues skillfully, in ways that cannot be interpreted as invalidating the experience of the individual. Eccleston (2001) provided helpful guidelines for the clinical care of a patient with pain (see Table 19.1).

Table 19.1 Using psychological factors in clinical practice

Vigilance to pain	Patients are distracted by the pain and are urged to react. Pain patients will have impaired concentration as they are being interrupted constantly by an aversive stimulus. Keep all communications clear and brief. Repeat key points often. Expect patients to talk about the pain often, as it is being brought repeatedly into attentional focus for them. This is not a sign of a somatization disorder or hypochondria.
Avoidance	Patients will naturally avoid pain and painful procedures. Be aware that this will occur and plan for it. Painful treatments will be avoided and patients will compensate for any disability caused by avoidance (e.g. shifted body weight distribution). If a habitual pattern of avoidance develops, this may lead to chronic pain. Patients must be given an understanding that pain does not necessarily equal damage. A credible medical authority must deliver this message.
Anger	Patients with pain may shout at you, abuse you and generally be hostile to you. If they are hostile to you they have probably been hostile to everyone. Most often this will have nothing to do with you, and you will need to understand that anger normally means extreme frustration, distress and possibly depression. Anger functions to push people away and isolate a person. The angry pain patient is therefore less likely to have received or heard any information about their problems and be more confused than the non-angry patient.
Involve the patient	First, assess the patient's normal way of coping with pain by simply asking how he or she has coped with predictable pain, such as a visit to the dentist. Secondly, match your strategy to the patient's preference. If the patient needs information, inform them how much pain they may expect to feel, what it may feel like and, critically, for how long (if this information is known). Always slightly overestimate the time rather than underestimate it. Finally, if possible, involve the patient in the delivery of any pain management strategy.
Make sense of the pain	Always ask the patient what they know and fear about the cause of the pain, the meaning of the pain and the time course of the pain. Expect the unexpected. What makes sense to one person is nonsense to another. What matters is that it is their understanding, not yours, that will inform their behaviour. Uncertain diagnoses or unknown diagnoses will lead to increased vigilance to pain and increased symptom reporting.
Consistency	Develop a consistent approach to clinical information, patient instruction and patient involvement within pain management. Practice should be consistent for each patient and from each member of the pain team, over time.

Source: Eccleston, 2001; Reproduced with permission

Cognitions

Cognitions influence and interact with our emotions and behaviour. An individual's cognitions influence the experience of pain, particularly the appraisal of situations for their significance and meaning (e.g. association of pain and sexual pleasure for masochists). Three aspects of cognition that have received attention in relation to pain are attention, dysfunctional thinking and coping styles.

Increased attention to pain has been associated with increased pain perception. Pain may demand attention, reducing the ability to focus on other competing activities and therefore increasing pain perception. This may explain why distraction techniques are useful in combating pain. However, the role of attention may differ for acute and chronic pain. In acute pain, taking attention away from pain (e.g. via distraction) appears to be associated with reduced anxiety and depression whereas it has an opposite effect for chronic pain patients, for whom attending to rather than avoiding the pain may be more adaptive.

Dysfunctional thoughts, attitudes and beliefs about pain are automatic patterns of thinking that block the attainment of an individual's goals (e.g. participating in work or social activity). A major form of dysfunctional thinking that influences the pain experience is **catastrophizing** (e.g. it's hopeless, pain has ruined my life, I can't cope, it will never get better). Catastrophic thinking has been found to increase likelihood of chronicity, level of perceived intensity and disability and even to have a small association with pain onset (e.g. Crombez et al., 2003). Other dysfunctional thoughts include negative mental bias, discounting the positive, fortune telling and magnification.

Cognitive coping styles are strategies an individual uses to attempt to deal with their pain. They can be divided into active and passive coping. Both can be functional or dysfunctional. Active coping might include keeping oneself busy or taking recreational drugs, which could easily become dysfunctional. Passive coping might include resting, which would be useful in the early stages of pain but could become dysfunctional if continued for too long. In general, active coping styles have been found to be associated with improved coping, reduced pain intensity and improved recovery rates. However, McCracken and Eccleston (2003) suggest that acceptance of pain and its incorporation into one's sense of self appears to be an adaptive cognitive technique for chronic pain. Specific coping techniques are detailed below under pain management.

Self-Efficacy

Self-efficacy beliefs (Bandura, 1977) have been identified as a significant component of cognition and refer to an individual's beliefs about how well they can handle a given situation. A relationship between an individual's self-efficacy beliefs about their ability to manage pain, whether acute, chronic or experimentally induced, has been found (e.g. Brekke, Hjortland & Kvien, 2003). Low self-efficacy beliefs have been associated with higher chronic pain-related disability levels, as well as with depression, although the associations are insufficient to eliminate the strong influence of pain intensity. Self-efficacy beliefs may also relate to a second cognitive component that has been associated with pain – **perceived control**.

Perceived Control

Both cognitive control (e.g. ability to distract thoughts from the pain) and behavioural control (e.g. being able to remove pain-inducing stimuli) have been found to influence pain experience. Bowers (1968) showed that individuals endure more pain when they control the pain-stimulus on/off switch than when it is controlled by someone else. This concept relates to the development of patient controlled (or self-administered) analgesia (PCA), in the management of post-operative pain and in palliative care. PCA resulted in patients administering less analgesic morphine than when it was controlled and administered by nurses or through continuous infusion. PCA appears to result in better pain management, less opiate use and earlier discharge from hospital than intramuscular therapy (Royal College of Surgeons and Anaesthetists, 1990).

Rotter's (1966) theory of locus of control (LOC) has also been applied to the concept of pain. Individuals with an internal locus of control believe that what happens to them is under their own control, while those with an external LOC believe that what happens is due to chance, fate or powerful others.

Previous Experience and Conditioning

Previous experience of pain is a significant factor in current pain experience. Both classical and operant **conditioning** have been implicated in the etiology of chronic pain via the association of behaviour and pain. In classical conditioning theory a particular situation or environment may become associated with pain (e.g. the dentist) and therefore provoke increased anxiety and pain perception. Jamner and Tursky (1987) report that even the words used by migraine sufferers to describe their pain appear to reinforce the experience by provoking stronger physiological responses than non-pain words. In operant conditioning theory, pain stimuli are perceived as a sensation and an unpleasant affect that generally evokes responses like grimacing or limping demonstrating the person is in pain. Pain behaviours become conditioned responses through positive (e.g. attention, medication, time off work) and negative (e.g. disapproval of others, loss of earnings) reinforcements. Pain behaviours may be functional and appropriate (e.g. removing hand from a burning source of heat), or they may be less functional and therefore pain maintaining (e.g. avoidance, alcohol).

Secondary Gains

The role of secondary gains in the development and maintenance of pain and illness behaviours has been described. Secondary gain relates to social rewards accruing from the demonstration of pain behaviours (e.g. receiving attention, financial benefits, time off work). These secondary gains are thought to reinforce pain behaviours and thus maintain the condition. For example, receipt of financial disability compensations has been associated with slower return to work and increased pain. However, this may actually reflect that those in receipt of compensation can allow themselves appropriate time to recover and says nothing about the quality of life of those who returned to work earlier. For many individuals, pain results in the loss of jobs, social contact, leisure activities, valued identities, reduced incomes and concomitant reduced standard of living. Such losses are very real and distressing and are often associated with substantial hardships, lowered mood and loss of self-esteem, unlikely to be outweighed by incidental benefits.

Personality

It has been suggested that there is a 'pain-prone personality' (Engel, 1959) and that psychological factors are the primary contributor to the pain experience for pain-prone individuals. Features of the pain-prone personality include continual episodes of varying chronic pain, high neurotic symptoms (guilt feelings, anxiety, depression and hypochondria). Generally, empirical support for the pain-prone personality has not been forthcoming and it has been suggested that the higher scores for particular personality factors (i.e. neurotic triad) may be a consequence rather than a cause of long-term pain.

Mood

The most common moods that have been associated with pain are anxiety and depression. Where these moods are present pain appears to be increased. It has been reported that acute pain increases anxiety but once pain is decreased through treatment the anxiety also decreases, which can cause further decreases in the pain, a cycle of pain reduction. Alternatively, chronic pain remains unalleviated by treatment and therefore anxiety increases which can further increase the pain, creating a cycle of pain increase. Research has shown that anxiety increases pain perception in children with migraine and people with back pain and pelvic pain (McGowan, Clark-Carter & Pitts, 1998).

Anxiety is normally a result of fear. Pain-related fear can be specific or general (e.g. the pain is going to get worse or what will the future be like). The fear-avoidance model of pain suggests that fear of pain amplifies perception and leads to pain avoidance behaviours in some people, especially those with a propensity to catastrophic thinking (Vlaeyen & Linton, 2000). This cycle results in pain experience and behaviours becoming separated from pain sensation through exaggerated pain perception. A prospective study by Klenerman et al. (1995) found fear-avoidance variables correctly predicted future outcome in 66 per cent of patients. A more recent prospective study (Linton, Buer, Vlaeyen & Hellsing, 2000) also found that higher baseline scores for fear avoidance in a non-pain population were associated with double the likelihood of reporting back pain in the following year and a significantly increased risk of reduced physical functioning.

People who experience severe and persistent pain often have feelings of hopelessness, helplessness and despair. Depression is commonly associated with pain and may even have a causal role in the development of chronic pain. Others have argued that depression is most likely the consequence of experiencing protracted pain, supported by the fact that any effective treatment leads to mood improvements. One prospective study on depression and chronic pain suggests that the relationship between the two may not be unidirectional (Magni, Moreschi, Rigatti-Luchini & Merskey, 1994). There are many overlaps between depression and pain including the central involvement of the same neurotransmitters, serotonin, norepinephrine, substance P and corticotrophin-releasing factor (Campbell, Clauw & Keefe, 2003).

While correlations between mood states and pain have been found, the causal direction and the nature of the relationships remains unclear. Most recent work appears to indicate that negative mood states are an outcome of chronic pain rather than a cause.

ASSESSMENT

Pain **assessment** is not a simple process. Part of the problem is the inherent difficulty in trying to describe a uniquely individual experience to another person. Assessment is crucial to the understanding and treatment of pain including its underlying mechanisms and mediating factors, as well as the development of effective treatment programmes.

Assessments are mostly undertaken for medical, research or compensation claim purposes and the purpose will influence the type of assessment used. Assessment measures may include intensity, psychological and functional effects and pain behaviours. Assessment methods can generally be grouped under one of four categories: physiological measures, pain questionnaires, mood assessment questionnaires and observations (direct observations or self-observations).

Pain questionnaires typically present commonly used descriptive words (for aspects of pain or mood) that the individual uses to rate their current experience. The words may be presented in rating scales or descriptive lists. The McGill Pain Questionnaire (MPQ) (Melzack, 1975) is the best known and most frequently used questionnaire (see Box 19.1).

Box 19.1

The McGill Pain Questionnaire (Melzack, 1975)

To use the questionnaire, circle the words that describe your pain but do not circle more than one word in a group. Then when you have that done, go back and circle the three words in groups 1–10 that most convey your pain response. Pick the two words in groups 11–15 that do the same thing. Then pick one word in group 16. Finally, pick 1 word in groups 17–20. At the end you should have seven words that you can take to your doctor that will help describe both the quality of your pain and the intensity of it.

Group 1	Flickering, Pulsing, Quivering, Throbbing, Beating, Pounding
Group 2	Jumping, Flashing, Shooting
Group 3	Pricking, Boring, Drilling, Stabbing
Group 4	Sharp, Gritting, Lacerating
Group 5	Pinching, Pressing, Gnawing, Cramping, Crushing
Group 6	Tugging, Pulling, Wrenching
Group 7	Hot, Burning, Scalding, Searing
Group 8	Tingling, Itching, Smarting, Stinging
Group 9	Dull, Sore, Hurting, Aching, Heavy
Group 10	Tender, Taut (tight), Rasping, Splitting
Group 11	Tiring, Exhausting
Group 12	Sickening, Suffocating
Group 13	Fearful, Frightful, Terrifying
Group 14	Punishing, Grueling, Cruel, Vicious, Killing
Group 15	Wretched, Binding
Group 16	Annoying, Troublesome, Miserable, Intense, Unbearable
Group 17	Spreading, Radiating, Penetrating, Piercing
Group 18	Tight, Numb, Squeezing, Drawing, Tearing
Group 19	Cool, Cold, Freezing
Group 20	Nagging, Nauseating, Agonizing, Dreadful, Torturing

Source: Melzack (1975) Reproduced by permission

Table 19.2 summarizes some of the common measures that have been described in the literature. Medical examinations form the backbone of clinical pain assessments and include joint mobility and heart rate. Other physiological measures attempt to measure objective physical responses to pain. For example, EEGs measure electrical activity in the brain and EEG spikes have been shown to correlate with intensity of pain stimuli, presence of analgesics and subjective reports of pain (Chapman, Casey, Dubner, Foley, Gracely & Reading, 1985). Much of the work using physiological measures comes from the experimental rather than clinical paradigm and results have been inconsistent across differing levels of reported pain. It has been suggested that such measures are more useful for assessing emotional responses to pain than pain itself (Chapman et al., 1985). Other questionnaire scales including verbal rating, box and visual analog scales are shown below. Questionnaires may use a number of scales along with body outlines (mark the body matching where you experience pain) and other techniques.

- *Verbal Rating Scale:*

No pain   Mild pain   Moderate pain   Severe pain   Excruciating pain
Place mark above the words that best indicate your present level of pain
Mark one point somewhere along the line to show how strong your pain is

Table 19.2 Summary of common pain assessment measures

Physiological measures	Questionnaires assessing pain	Questionnaires assessing mood	Observations – direct or self
Medical examination including pain sites, joint mobility, history etc.	Minnesota Multiphasic Personality Inventory (MMPI) (Dahlstrom & Welsh, 1960)	Beck's depression inventory (Beck, 1972)	Activity levels
Muscle tension-electromyography (EMG)	McGill Pain Questionnaire (MPQ) (Melzack, 1975)	Hospital Anxiety and Depression Scale (Zigmond & Snaith, 1983)	Standing and sitting time (uptime and downtime)
Heart rate	Multidimensional pain inventory (MPI) (Kearns, Turk & Rudy, 1985)	Well-being Questionnaire (Pincus, Griffith, Isenberg & Pearce, 1997)	Sleep patterns
Hyperventilation	Sickness Impact Profile (SIP) (Follick, Smith & Ahern, 1985)		Sexual activity
Galvanic skin response	Survey of Pain Attitudes (Jensen, Karoly, Huger, 1987)		Medication requests and usage
Electroencephalograph (EEG)	Pain Information and Beliefs Questionnaire (Shutty, DeGood, and Tuttle, 1990)		Appetite and eating
Pedometer	Bio-behavioural Pain Profile (Dalton, Feuerstein, Carlson and Roghman, 1994)		Normal household activities
EEG			Leisure activities

Other questionnaire scales including verbal rating, box and visual analog scales are shown opposite. Questionnaires may use a number of scales along with body outlines (mark the body matching where you experience pain) and other techniques.

Visual analogue scales (VAS) may be the most appropriate for use with diverse cultural groups, children, the elderly and people with communication difficulties. They are easy to use

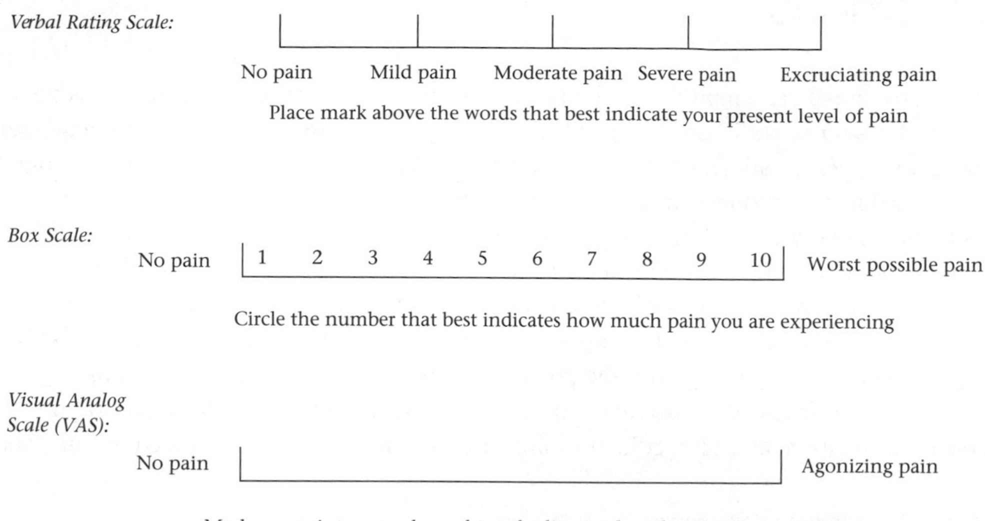

(e.g. in diaries or logs). However, direct and self-observations have drawbacks. Direct observations can never elicit unbiased data, being influenced by the setting in which they occur (e.g. clinical setting, home), the purpose of the assessment (e.g. benefit claim versus treatment assessment) and assessor characteristics (e.g. gender, ethnicity). Similarly, self-observations (e.g. pain diaries) may be inaccurate or overly subjective. An alternate approach is to use interviews that attempt to assess all aspects of the pain experience including a full pain history, assessing emotional adjustment and pre- and post-pain lifestyle. Effective pain assessment must be multidimensional including physiological, medical, sensory, behavioural, affective and evaluative information.

Issues in Assessment

Many assessment instruments are insensitive to age, disability and culture. For groups who have communication difficulties, due to age, language problems, sensory or cognitive deficits, assessment may require extended assessment time to enable rapport building. Herr, Bjoro and Decker (2006) found that there is no standardized tool based on non-verbal/behavioural pain indicators in English that can be recommended for clinical practice. It is therefore necessary to rely on the reports of significant others (e.g. carer, interpreter), which has additional challenges of perception, interpretation and motivation. More work is required to address issues around the impact of situational context and assessor characteristics on the assessment process. Further investigation is needed of the influence of assessment, including the impact of compensation claim assessments, and of the need to prove the existence of pain and how it restricts the sufferer's daily activities.

INTERVENTIONS

Before the complex and multidimensional nature of pain had been accepted, pain was treated through the administration of analgesic drugs, surgery and rest. Today pain management programmes seek to address the pain experience utilizing pharmacological, psychological and physical interventions, with considerable emphasis on psychology. The historical aim of pain management was to eliminate pain. More recently the aims have shifted to modifying pain perception, improving coping ability, increasing functional ability, decreasing drug reliance and distress. Many commonly used pain management strategies are listed in Table 19.3.

Whether prescribed by health professionals or independently adopted by the individual, any pain management strategy has the potential to improve the situation (e.g. numbing pain sensations with drugs or improving mood with aromatherapy). Equally any strategy can worsen the situation, as with medication side effects or lowered mood induced by substance

Table 19.3 Common pain management strategies

Multidisciplinary pain management centres/programmes				
Cognitive Behavioural Therapy (CBT)				
Behavioural	Cognitive	Pharmacological	Physical	Other
Operant conditioning	Cognitive restructuring	Non-opioid analgesics:	Surgical	Hypnosis
Contingency management	Cognitive coping skills training e.g. distraction	Paracetamol NSAIDS (e.g. ibuprofen, aspirin)	Transcutaneous electrical nerve stimulation (TENS)	Other alternative therapies e.g. REIKI, Chinese medicine, music therapy
Graded exercise	Acceptance	Opioid analgesics: Morphine & derivatives (e.g. codeine)	Acupuncture Physiotherapy Heat and Cold	Support groups
Biofeedback	Imagery	Local anaesthetics	Vibration Massage Aromatherapy	Internet advice
Autogenic training	Meditation & prayer	Indirect action drugs (e.g. sedatives, anti depressants, tranquillizers)	Spinal cord stimulation	Self-help books
Relaxation	Information	Placebos	Reflexology	Spiritual including prayer
Progressive muscle relaxation	Stress management	Self medications: (e.g. cannabis, alcohol) heroine)	Mobility enhancing exercise	

abuse. It is important that an individual's own attempts at self-management are respected and that health professionals work in partnership with the individual to identify the optimum programme for that individual.

Behavioural Strategies

Most behavioural strategies are based upon operant learning processes, like using operant conditioning in which pain behaviours are ignored (negative reinforcement) and improved activity is praised (positive reinforcement). Conditioning was integral to contingency management. A typical 2–6 week inpatient programme consists of nursing staff ignoring medication requests, reinforcing targeted 'well' behaviours, introducing or increasing exercise quotas, and employing a fixed-schedule 'pain cocktail'. The pain cocktail delivers medication within a strong tasting masking fluid that allowed medication dosages to be reduced without the patient noticing. While such programmes have had good (even dramatic) short-term results, they have been less successful in maintaining such gains, possibly due to non-generalization outside the hospital environment. It is rare for programmes today to focus solely on conditioning methods.

Graded exercise strategies involve setting a starting level of activity that the person can manage and then developing a schedule to gradually increase the length of time and intensity of the exercise. The schedule allows the person to gain the confidence to handle each new level before the next increment.

Cognitive Strategies

Cognitive strategies work on the principle that our cognitions (thoughts, beliefs, etc.) are responsible for the consequences of events, not the event itself, and if these cognitions can be changed the consequence(s) will also change. In relation to pain management, cognitive strategies aim to help the individual identify and understand their cognitions and their connection with their experience of pain and then change negative cognitions to improve it. This includes teaching individuals to identify and challenge distorted thinking (e.g. catastrophizing), a process known as cognitive restructuring, an active coping technique that promotes the internal attribution of positive changes.

Training in cognitive coping skills has generally been found to be beneficial to pain patients. For example, Gil, Carson, Sedway, Porter, Wilson Schaeffer and Orringer (2000) found enhanced pain coping in patients with sickle-cell disease following brief coping skills training. Distraction and positive self-talk are just two examples from the repertoire of coping skills. Distraction techniques involve deliberately shifting attention away from pain to non-painful stimuli in the immediate environment or to some stimuli of interest (e.g. watching television). Redirecting attention may be more effective in relation to acute pain as it appears to reduce the perception of pain at least only for as long as the person remains distracted. Positive self-talk teaches the individual to use positive self-statements when thinking about their pain (e.g. I cope well with my pain). The beneficial effect of positive self-talk may relate to resultant boosts in self-esteem and self-efficacy. Sanders, Labott, Molokie,

Shelby and Desimone (2010) investigated pain, coping and health care utilization in younger and older adults with sickle-cell disease. Older patients attended an outpatient clinic, while younger patients tended to go to the Emergency Department. Younger patients were more likely to try to ignore their pain, or use heat, cold or massage. Older patients were more likely to pray and hope indicating that coping with sickle-cell disease differs according to age.

While coping strategies can be helpful, there is growing evidence that pain control efforts directed at uncontrollable pain can come to dominate an individual's life and distance them from important and valued aspects of their lives like family, friends and work. McCracken, Carson, Eccleston and Keefe (2004) describe acceptance as an acknowledgement of reality (i.e. pain is present, persistent and not easily controlled) and a willingness to persist in valued activities in spite of pain-related sensations, thoughts and related feelings. They found pain acceptance was associated with better work status, lower reports of pain and lower pain-related anxiety, avoidance behaviour, depression and disability, independent of pain intensity. Treatment approaches that incorporate acceptance have shown positive results (e.g. mindfulness meditation). However, further studies are needed to confirm these results and to identify when and for whom they are most likely to be of benefit.

Morley, Eccleston and Williams (1999) carried out a meta-analysis of 25 randomized controlled trials of CBT and behaviour therapy for chronic pain in adults, excluding headache. The review compared CBT with waiting list and alternative treatment control conditions. CBT showed significant and fairly large effect sizes on pain measures greater than alternative active treatments for pain experience, cognitive coping and appraisal (positive coping measures), and reduced behavioural expression of pain. Tatrow and Montgomery (2006) reviewed cognitive behavioural therapy techniques for distress and pain in breast cancer patients in a meta-analysis of 20 studies using CBT techniques with breast cancer patients. The results showed that CBT techniques have a significant impact on distress and pain with 62 and 69 per cent of breast cancer patients in the CBT groups reporting less distress and less pain respectively, relative to the control groups. The findings support the use of CBT administered individually to manage distress and pain in breast cancer patients.

Imagery

Imagery involves forming and maintaining pleasant, calming or coping images in the mind. In guided imagery attention is guided away from an undesirable sensation or mood (e.g. pain) by another person who verbally describes the image while the patient relaxes. Most imagery involves relaxation and employs images of a peaceful, safe, pain-free place, which the individual focuses upon while relaxing. The person may also be guided to visualize energy flowing into their body and pain flowing out. Alternatively, confrontational imagery may be employed, for example visualizing white blood cells as an army attacking the source of pain (e.g. a tumour). Imagery has been found to be effective for the treatment of pain. The benefits of imagery may relate to relaxation, distraction effects and an active stance increasing feelings of self-efficacy. As imagery generally involves elements of relaxation it is unclear what unique and independent effects it has. Syrjala, Donaldson, Davis, Kippes and

Carr (1995) compared relaxation and imagery with cognitive-behavioural training to reduce pain during cancer-treatment in a controlled clinical-trial. Results confirmed that patients who received either relaxation and imagery alone or patients who received the package of cognitive-behavioural coping skills reported less pain than patients in general. Adding cognitive-behavioural skills to the relaxation with imagery did not further improve pain relief.

Meditation also frequently forms part of relaxation training and involves the individual focusing their attention on a simple stimulus, like a monosyllable word repeated slowly and continuously (aloud or in their head), to the exclusion of all other stimuli. Mindfulness-meditation involves focusing attention on the moment-to-moment reality, including the self in each moment, in a non-reactive, non-judgemental way, attending to and accepting all aspects of the current experience. Early work on mindfulness-meditation looked at chronic pain and found positive benefits including lower back pain reports and less medication usage. However, more recent work has not looked at pain, so further studies are needed. Prayer is another common coping strategy patients have reported to be helpful in response to pain, including headaches, neck-pain and back pain (McCaffery, Eisenberg, Legedza, Davis & Phillips, 2004). Both meditation and prayer inherently involve some distraction and possibly aspects of relaxation, although this is far from consistent.

Information provision has been shown to reduce pain reports and intensity, possibly by alleviating the fear and anxiety of not knowing what to expect for acute and post-operative pain (Williams, Golding, Phillips & Towell, 2004). The widespread interest in self-help literature, Internet information and support groups may be indicative of the desire of people in pain to understand their experience, what to expect and potential treatment options.

Cognitive Behavioural Therapy

Cognitive-behavioural therapy (CBT) utilizes the full range of cognitive and behavioural techniques already described in individualized programmes that emphasize relapse prevention strategies. Stress management training is often included due to the significant levels of stress implicated in the generation and exacerbation of pain. The literature on CBT and pain suggests it shows considerable promise as an effective treatment for pain in adults (Eccleston, Morley, Williams, Yorke & Mastroyannopoulou, 2002). It forms the major component of most current pain management programmes. Improved mood, affect, function and coping have been associated with CBT in up to 85 per cent of pain patients. While there is some support for the efficacy of CBT for the control of headache pain in children, there is a paucity of research relating to other pain conditions in children, as well as CBT for pain in the elderly and people with intellectual or communication difficulties, probably as it may be assumed not to be an appropriate treatment option for these groups.

Pharmacological Strategies

Various analgesics and anaesthetics are prescribed for the treatment of pain. Anaesthetics (local or central) are used to numb the sensation of pain. The identification of endogenous opioid mechanisms have confirmed the status of opioid analgesics as an effective pain treatment. However, the associated perceived high risk of addiction has resulted in their use being restricted to severe pain cases like cancer, a perception challenged by the findings from studies of patient-controlled analgesia and low dose opioid treatment that suggest the risk of addiction may not be very high (e.g. Urban, France, Steinberger, Scott & Maltbre, 1986). Non-opioid analgesics, NSAIDs (non-steroidal anti-inflammatory drugs) and drugs that control pain indirectly (e.g. antidepressants, sedatives) are commonly used. Drugs with indirect effects may be beneficial due to their action on higher brain regions, modulating the downward transmission of pain, or due to their modulating effects on negative mood states.

Another aspect relating to drugs is the placebo effect. It has been shown that substantial pain relief occurs in about 50 per cent of patients when they are treated with an inert compound rather than the drug they are expecting, often equalling the relief felt by those receiving the actual medication (Melzack & Wall, 1982). The effect is strongest with high doses, when it is injected and depends upon the individual believing they are receiving a pain-relieving substance. The effect rapidly declines with repeated use.

In addition to prescribed drug treatments many individuals self-medicate with recreational drugs like alcohol and cannabis to alleviate their pain. However, there is considerable anecdotal evidence for cannabis as an effective pain control treatment, and an endogenous cannabinoid pain control system has now been identified. This system functions as a parallel but distinct mechanism from the opioid system in modulating pain (Iversen & Chapman, 2002). Cannabinoids have been authorized for the treatment of pain and other conditions in a number of countries, including the Netherlands, the USA and the UK. While current research may result in new cannabinoid-based NSAID-like treatments in the future, problems with the restricted range of dosages that allow pain control before producing psychotropic effects and concerns about the incidental condoning of recreational cannabis use mean this is far from being certain. The informal use of cannabis for pain control and its interaction with other pain control strategies warrants further investigation.

Physical Strategies

Surgical control of pain mainly involved cutting the pain fibres to stop pain signal transmission. However, it provided only short-term results and the risks associated with surgery mean it is no longer viewed as a viable treatment option (Melzack & Wall, 1982).

Physiotherapy may be used to increase mobility and correct maladjusted posture, encourage exercise and movement (often despite pain), and education. In addition individuals may be taught safe ways to function (e.g. stand up, sit down, lift objects). Physiotherapy is about maintaining mobility, increasing function and helping the individual manage their lives (e.g. Eccleston & Eccleston, 2004).

Many physical strategies involve some form of sensory control employing variations of counter-stimulation. Counter-stimulation is a frequently used natural response to pain (e.g. squeezing hard on an area of pain), that provides temporary pain relief. Sensory techniques work on the same basis, like the stimulation of nerves under the skin in TENS treatment (e.g. Chesterton, Foster, Wright, Baxter & Barlas, 2003). Such techniques appear more beneficial for acute pain but show less consistent results for chronic pain (e.g. Köke et al., 2004).

A recent additional strategy is the promotion of mobility enhancing exercise to help retain and improve physical function and prevent lack of mobility from exacerbating pain problems. General practitioners can now refer pain patients to specialist rehabilitation classes at local fitness centres, which has shown some success for older people with musculo-skeletal disorders (Avlund, Osler, Damsgaard, Christensen & Schroll, 2000).

Other Strategies and Approaches

There are many other strategies and alternative therapies that individuals use in their efforts to deal with their pain. Acupuncture has been around for centuries and while the mechanisms by which it produces beneficial effects are not well understood it does appear to exert substantial analgesic effects (World Health Organization, 2003). This may derive from the incidental involvement of counter-stimulation, placebo effects, distraction and relaxation, as well as the release of natural pain-relieving endorphins.

There is evidence that hypnosis has beneficial effects for the treatment of acute (e.g. childbirth) and chronic pain (e.g. cancer-related) conditions. Hypnosis involves relaxation, assurances of pain reduction, distraction, and cognitive restructuring (via guided imagery), and may include an altered state of consciousness (Marks et al., 1989). However, it is still uncertain whether hypnosis works over and above its effect on outcome expectancy (a placebo effect). Jensen and Patterson (2006) systematically reviewed controlled trials of hypnotic treatment of chronic pain. The findings indicated that hypnotic analgesia is capable of producing significantly greater decreases in pain relative to no-treatment and non-hypnotic interventions such as medication management, physical therapy, and education/advice. However, the authors concluded that the effects of self-hypnosis training on chronic pain are similar to those from progressive muscle relaxation and autogenic training. No published study had, by the time of Jensen and Patterson's review, compared hypnosis to an equally believable placebo or minimally effective pain treatment. This gap in methodology means that there are no definite conclusions concerning whether hypnotic analgesia treatment is specifically effective beyond its effects on patient expectancy. Other findings suggested that hypnotic responsivity and the ability to experience vivid images are associated with treatment outcome in hypnosis, progressive relaxation, and autogenic training treatments.

Crawford, Gur, Skolnick, Gur and Benson (1993) studied the effects of hypnosis on regional cerebral blood-flow during ischemic pain with and without hypnotic analgesia. Using Xe-133 regional cerebral blood flow (CBF) imaging, two male groups with high and low hypnotic susceptibility were compared in waking and after hypnotic induction. During hypnotic analgesia, highly hypnotizable persons showed CBF increase over the somatosensory cortex, while low-hypnotizable persons showed decreases. These findings are important in showing that hypnotic susceptibility has a cortical component which can act as a marker of hypnotic analgesia.

Individuals frequently use complementary or alternative therapies (e.g. aromatherapy, Chinese medicine) to combat pain and there is growing support for the belief that they help chronic pain control (e.g. National Institutes of Health, 1997). Again the mechanisms are not well understood and may derive from placebo effects, relaxation, distraction or improved self-efficacy from active coping. Bardia, Barton, Prokop, Bauer and Moynihan (2006) reviewed complementary and alternative medicine therapies for the relief of cancer pain. Eighteen RCTs were identified of which eight were poor, three intermediate, and seven high quality studies with 1499 patients. The median sample size was only 53 patients, and the median intervention duration only 45 days. These figures show that the RCTs were very small-scale in both numbers of participants and duration. The authors reported that: 'Hypnosis, imagery, support groups, acupuncture, and healing touch seem promising, particularly in the short term, but none can be recommended because of a paucity of rigorous trials. Future research should focus on methodologically strong RCTs to determine potential efficacy of these CAM interventions' (Bardia, Barton, Prokop, Bauer & Moynihan, 2006: 5457). Similarly self-help information, support groups and Internet use for information and advice may be of value in pain management, but need further investigation.

The widespread use of alternative strategies may reflect dissatisfaction with mainstream approaches. It is important that such strategies are evaluated independently and in conjunction with traditional approaches.

Airaksinen et al. (2006), in European guidelines for the management of chronic low back pain (CLBP), recommended the assessment of work-related factors, psychosocial distress, depressive mood, severity of pain and functional impact, prior episodes of LBP, extreme symptom reporting and patient expectations in the assessment of patients with non-specific CLBP. Conservative treatments included: CBT, supervised exercise therapy, brief educational interventions, and multidisciplinary (bio-psycho-social) treatment. However, the use of acupuncture, physical therapies (heat/cold, traction, laser, ultrasound, short wave, interferential, massage, corsets) and TENS could not be recommended. The most promising approach was judged to be cognitive-behavioural interventions encouraging activity/exercise.

Multidisciplinary Pain Management

Originally run as inpatient programmes, today pain management programmes tend to be run on an outpatient basis in specialist pain management centres. Multidisciplinary teams may include doctors, nurses, physiotherapists, psychologists, psychiatrists, occupational therapists and counsellors, and provide a range of management techniques underpinned by CBT. Individual programmes are developed that aim to improve the individual's quality of life by reducing pain (as far as possible), increasing activity and coping, restoring function, promoting self-efficacy and self-management. The patient receives a full assessment, education, skills training, exercise schedules, relapse prevention and family work. Multidisciplinary rehabilitation programmes represent the most comprehensive approach to date, by targeting the individual's specific pain experience and tailoring appropriate treatment combinations.

Flor, Fydrich and Turk (1992) evaluated the efficacy of 65 studies of multidisciplinary pain treatments for chronic back pain. Multidisciplinary treatments for chronic pain were found to be superior to no treatment, waiting list controls, as well as single-discipline treatments such as medical treatment or physical therapy. The beneficial effects included improvements in pain, mood and behavioural variables such as return to work or use of the health-care system. However, the quality of the study designs and study descriptions was marginal and so caution is necessary in interpreting these findings.

Treatment Issues

Pain management can be a particularly controversial issue. Evidence suggests that in many circumstances pain is under-treated. Some of the reasons for this include inadequate assessment, focus on underlying pathologies, negative stereotypes and erroneous assumptions about certain population groups, addiction fears, the inappropriateness of non-pharmacological treatments and patients' inability to verbalize pain information or requests for medication (e.g. Greenwald, Narcessian & Pomeranz, 1999). Many medical professionals have their own benchmarks concerning acceptable pain behaviour and medication levels for different conditions. It has also been shown that many prejudices and misconceptions operate in the treatment of pain patients, with various populations (e.g. children, people with communication difficulties and the elderly) being under-treated for pain (Todd, Deaton, DAdamo & Goe, 2000). For example, sickle-cell patients are often assumed to be drug addicts and their pain outcries to be drug-seeking behaviour, resulting in inadequate medication being administered. Similarly, pain has only recently been recognized as part of the symptom repertoire of HIV/AIDs and therefore up to 85 per cent of people with HIV/AIDs receive inadequate pain management (Marcus et al., 2000).

Karus et al. (2005) investigated patients' reports of symptoms and their treatment at three palliative care projects servicing individuals with HIV/AIDS in Alabama, Baltimore and New York City. Pain, lack of energy, and worry were reported by a majority of patients at all sites, often with a high level of associated distress. However only four symptoms (pain, nausea, difficulty swallowing, and mouth sores) were being treated in half or more of patients at all sites.

Pain is sometimes deemed to be psychogenic, resulting from emotional, motivational or personality problems. However, the distinction between organic and psychogenic pain may have little practical value. A number of diseases where historically pain was not thought to be a valid symptom have subsequently had a physiological basis for pain identified including multiple sclerosis and HIV/AIDs (e.g. Marcus et al., 2000), so some pain designated 'psychogenic' may relate to as yet undetected or unidentified organic pathology. Health psychologists must endeavour to promote the sensitive and respectful care of individuals reporting pain in terms of research, intervention development and treatment.

FUTURE RESEARCH

1 Further work to map the neuromatrix proposed by Melzack is required, along with the development of new treatment approaches based on this mapping theory. One way of testing the theory is to develop a new intervention based on the theory and to show that the intervention is effective.
2 Long-term, prospective studies are required to further elucidate the relationships between various psychosocial factors and pain, particularly the relative weights of their influence and the identification of relatively homogeneous sub-groups within the chronic pain patient population.
3 Additional research regarding the pain experience of under-represented groups especially those who are verbally challenged (e.g. babies, older people, people with disabilities, people with a diagnosis of dementia), including development of improved measurement instruments and assessing the efficacy of CBT in these groups.
4 The influence of social factors (e.g. SES, poverty, discrimination) on the treatment of pain should be a significant research focus, particularly for groups who disproportionately experience inadequate pain treatment.

Summary

1 Early pain theories proposed that pain was a sensation that involved a direct line of transmission from the pain stimulus to the brain.
2 The growing body of evidence for the psychological mediation of pain saw the development of the gate control theory, which acknowledged psychosocial influences.
3 The body of research suggests that pain is a complex and multidimensional phenomenon that includes biological, psychological and behavioural components.
4 Recent neuropsychological studies have demonstrated cortical correlates of experienced pain.
5 Many psychological variables that influence the pain experience have been examined including cognitions, self-efficacy, perceived control, prior experience, conditioning, secondary gains, personality and mood.
6 Particular groups appear to be under-represented in the pain literature including ethnic minorities, children, the elderly, some disabled people and people with certain medical conditions (e.g. dementia, HIV and CFS).
7 Assessment of pain is difficult and various techniques are used singly or in combination (e.g. medical examinations, observations, questionnaires, diaries and logs, and interviews).
8 A wide variety of pain management strategies exist. Currently, the most successful approach appears to be programmes that combine cognitive behaviour therapies and traditional medical therapies.
9 The assessment and treatment of pain, particularly chronic pain, can be influenced by misconceptions about specific patient groups including ethnic minorities, children, the elderly, some disabled people, and people with rare medical conditions.
10 Health psychologists can make a significant contribution in promoting sensitive and respectful research and treatment for people experiencing long-standing painful conditions.

20 Cancer and Chronic Diseases[1]

Chronic diseases – such as heart disease, cancer, and diabetes – are the leading causes of death and disability. Adopting healthy behaviors such as eating nutritious foods, being physically active, and avoiding tobacco use can prevent or control the devastating effects of these diseases

US Centers for Disease Control and Prevention, 2005

Outline

In this chapter we consider three life-threatening and disabling diseases: cancer, coronary heart disease and HIV/AIDS. In each case we consider five issues: 'What is xx?'; 'Interventions for xx'; 'Living with xx'; 'Adaptation to xx'; and 'Caring for someone with xx'. The contribution of psychosocial interventions for patients suffering from these conditions has been evaluated in systematic reviews. The evidence suggests that psychosocial interventions have not yet demonstrated their full potential. The quality of evaluation research with psychosocial interventions has generally been rather poor and the findings inconclusive. We suggest further research to strengthen psychological understanding of treatment and care for these conditions.

[1]Authors' note: An earlier version of this chapter in the second edition was written in collaboration with Catherine M. Sykes.

GENERAL ISSUES

Chronic illness and cancer have replaced acute illness as the predominant disease pattern in developed countries over the past 50 years. Greatly improved longevity has meant an increased **burden of disease** caused by cancer and chronic conditions such as heart disease, stroke, AIDS, back pain, diabetes and dementia. As life expectancy of the human population increases, so does the prevalence of diseases of older age. A large proportion of the global burden of disease is caused by a **toxic environment** that encourages health-aversive behaviours and choices. As we saw in Chapter 1, the major risks of underweight (developing countries), overweight and obesity (developed countries), unsafe sex, high blood pressure, alcohol and tobacco (everywhere) account for 30 per cent of the global disease burden. All are consequences of human behaviour within the toxic environment, which are creating a significant proportion of ill-health and suffering in the world.

Over 60 per cent of people in developed countries live to at least 70 years of age, compared with only about 30 per cent in developing countries. Of the 45 million deaths among adults worldwide in 2002, 32 million were caused by non-communicable diseases. HIV/AIDS has become the leading cause of mortality among adults aged 15–59 years. Unipolar depressive disorders are the leading cause of disablement for females.

Chronic illnesses most often strike in middle and older age and, while they can be fatal, most people with a chronic illness live for many years with the condition. As a consequence cardiovascular and coronary heart disease and HIV/AIDS are significant causes of disablement (see Chapter 1 for figures).

The evidence suggests that personality is a poor predictor of the development of disease (Chapter 12). Health-aversive behaviours, and genetic factors, are the primary determinants of many chronic illnesses. The focus of this chapter will be on the psychological aspects of disease management. Management of fatal or chronic diseases is a principal feature in the lives of 10–15 per cent of the population. This informal care occurs almost invisibly with little recognition or financial support from society at large.

People with different serious chronic illnesses have similar concerns and needs (World Health Organization, 2004). Chronic illness typically involves restrictions on activities of daily living, increases in pain, fatigue, depression and anxiety. Patients must cope with ongoing symptoms, their ambiguity, the life threat involved, and the requirements of treatment. Maintaining effective relationships with health-service personnel and family and friends requires many adaptations (Stanton & Revenson, 2005) and adjustments in lifestyle. Uncertainties over prognosis can cause a great deal of worry and fear. In cancer prognosis can often be predicted, as there is a short period of evident decline, but in CHD people tend to live with greater disability for longer time, but die suddenly with little warning after a rapid deterioration (World Health Organization, 2004). In all life-threatening conditions, family members can experience emotional, economic and social challenges.

Sontag (1978) pointed out that illnesses are often constructed metaphorically, a tendency that needs to be guarded against for the unwanted surplus meanings such metaphors often carry. Sontag stated: 'The most truthful way of regarding illness – and the healthiest way of being ill – is one most purified of, most resistant to, metaphoric thinking' (p. 25). For example, cancer is viewed as a disease of repression, of inhibited passion. The sufferer is a suppressor of emotion, which after many years emerges from the unconscious self as malignant growth. In Chapter 17 we concluded that empirical support for the psychosomatic position does not exist. Sontag believed that when the aetiology and treatment of a disease is more fully understood, the metaphorical connotations will fade. However, metaphorical thinking can be useful in coping but it carries the danger that victims and families may blame themselves which may engender hopelessness, and increase feelings of stigmatization.

Petrie and Revenson (2005) identified three developments in psychological interventions for chronic illness:

1 Psychological interventions are becoming more theory-based and sophisticated in the behavioural targets they are seeking to alter. Successful interventions are typically based on a model of behaviour change and analyse the key issues that the intervention is aimed to resolve.
2 An increased awareness of sub-populations for whom the intervention may be more efficacious.
3 An increasingly sharp focus on possible biobehavioural and psychosocial mechanisms.

A fourth development has been recent research on possible psychosocial associations with the incidence of disease. Some studies have linked psychosocial factors with the incidence of disease. Chida and Steptoe (2008) systematically reviewed prospective observational studies of positive psychological well-being and mortality.

The authors identified 35 studies of mortality in initially healthy populations and 35 studies in disease populations. Positive psychological well-being was associated with reduced mortality in both populations. Positive affect (e.g., emotional well-being, positive mood, joy, happiness, vigour, energy) and positive dispositions (e.g., life satisfaction, hopefulness, optimism, sense of humour) were found to be associated with reduced mortality in the healthy population. Positive psychological well-being was associated with reduced cardiovascular mortality in healthy population studies, and with reduced death rates in patients with renal failure and with human immunodeficiency virus-infection. The authors concluded that 'positive psychological well-being has a favorable effect on survival in both healthy and diseased populations' (Chida & Steptoe, 2008: 741).

In a similar study, Chida, Hamer, Wardle and Steptoe (2008) investigated whether stress-related psychosocial factors contribute to cancer incidence and survival. The authors evaluated longitudinal associations between stress and cancer in 165 studies. The results suggested that stress-related psychosocial factors are associated with higher cancer incidence in initially healthy populations while poorer survival tends to be the case in more stressed patients with a diagnosis of cancer. 'Stress-prone personality', unfavourable coping styles, negative emotional responses or poor quality of life were related to higher cancer incidence, poorer cancer survival and higher cancer mortality. Site-specific analyses indicate that psychosocial factors are associated with a higher incidence of lung cancer and poorer survival in patients with breast, lung, head and neck, hepatobiliary, and lymphoid or hematopoietic cancers. Chida et al. concluded that the analyses suggest that stress-related psychosocial factors have an adverse effect on cancer incidence and survival.

The results of both reviews should be interpreted with caution. In both, the authors found evidence of publication bias, the tendency for journals to publish positive findings and reject studies reporting negative findings. Further carefully controlled prospective research is required to unravel the many background factors that might be confounded in producing these empirical associations between stress, personality and illness. Chapter 17 discusses research on links between illness and personality in more depth and detail.

Taylor et al. (2007) carried out a prospective study of the extent to which perceived discrimination may contribute to somatic disease. The authors examined the association between perceived discrimination and breast cancer incidence in Black women. In 1997, participants had completed questions on 'everyday' discrimination (e.g., being treated as dishonest) and major experiences of unfair treatment due to race (job, housing and police). From 1997 to 2003, 593 breast cancer cases were ascertained. Weak positive associations were evident between cancer incidence and discrimination which appeared stronger among younger women. Women under 50 years who reported frequent everyday discrimination were at higher risk than were women who reported infrequent experiences. The incidence rate ratio was 1.32 (95 per cent confidence interval: 1.03, 1.70) for those who reported discrimination on the job and 1.48 (95 per cent confidence interval: 1.01, 2.16) for those who reported discrimination in relation to housing, job and police relative to those who reported none. The findings suggest that experiences of perceived racism are associated with increased incidence of breast cancer among US Black women, particularly younger Black women.

In the next three sections we review psychosocial aspects and interventions relevant to people diagnosed with cancer, CHD and HIV/AIDS respectively. Table 20.1 compares and contrasts these three conditions in terms of some of the key features of these life-threatening conditions.

CANCER

The study of the psychological aspects of cancer care and treatment is referred to as '**psycho-oncology**'. Psycho-oncology is concerned with (1) the psychological responses of patients, families and caregivers to cancer at all stages of the disease, and (2) the psychosocial

Table 20.1 Comparison of three life-threatening conditions

Feature	Cancer	CHD	HIV/AIDS
Preventable	In part	In part	100%
Behavioural risk factors	Smoking, diet, drinking	Diet, smoking, drinking	Unsafe sex
Stigma	Strong	Some	Severe
Onset	Mixed	Slow	Slow
Treatable	Mixed	Mixed	HAART shows good outcomes, but is expensive and so not universally available
Prognosis	Mixed	Good	Good, with HAART, not otherwise

factors that may influence the disease process. Unfortunately many cancer patients remain untreated owing to **stigmatization** and lack of resources to diagnose, treat and support. Cancer causes anxiety and depression in more than one-third of patients and often affects the sufferer's family emotionally, socially and economically. Inequalities in cancer treatment and care occur across different regions and social groups.

What is Cancer?

'Cancer' is an umbrella term for more than 100 different but related diseases. Cancer occurs when cells become abnormal and keep dividing and forming more cells without any internal control or order. Normally, cells divide to produce more when the body needs them to remain healthy. However if cells keep dividing when new cells are not needed, a mass of extra tissue known as a **tumour** or neoplasm forms, which can be benign or malignant. Benign tumours are not cancerous and, usually, can be removed and when removed, in most cases, do not reform. Cells from benign tumours also do not spread to other parts of the body and so benign tumours are rarely life-threatening. In the case of malignant tumours, cancer cells can invade and damage nearby tissues and organs. They can also break away from a malignant tumour and enter the bloodstream or the lymphatic system forming new tumours or **metastasis** in other parts of the body. This process is described in more detail in Figure 20.1.

Risk factors for cancer are:

- growing older
- tobacco
- sunlight, sunlamps and tanning machines, i.e. ultraviolet (UV) radiation
- ionizing radiation, e.g. radioactive fallout, radon gas, x-rays

- certain chemicals and other substances, e.g. asbestos, benzene, benzidine, cadmium, nickel or vinyl chloride
- some bacteria (e.g. helicobacter pylori) and viruses (e.g. hepatitis B virus, human papilloma virus, human immunodeficiency virus, and others)
- certain hormones
- family history of cancer
- alcohol
- poor diet, lack of physical activity, or being overweight

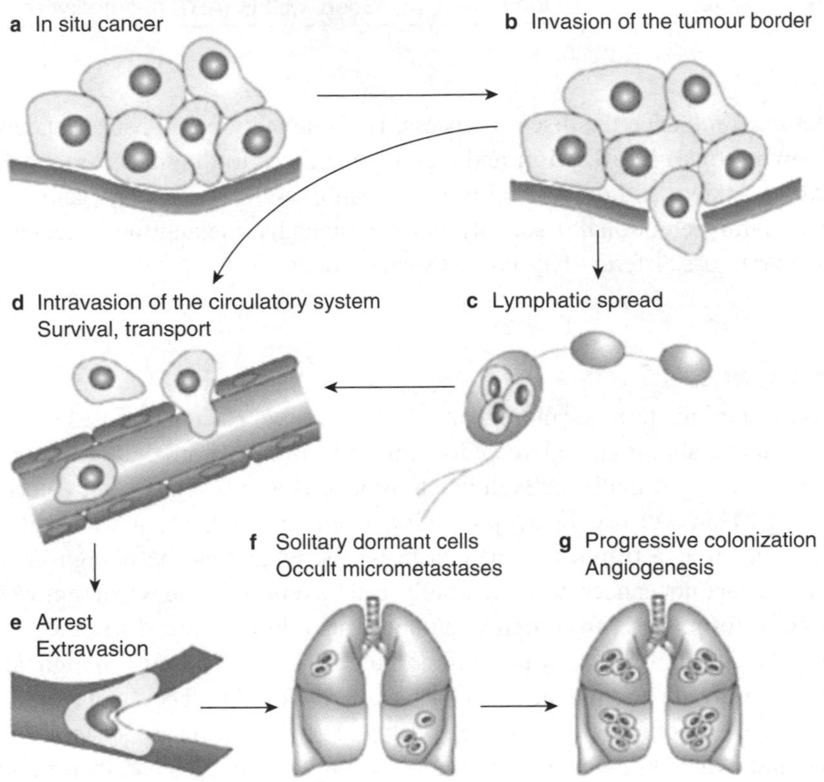

Figure 20.1 A schematic of cancer and the metastatic process: (a) an *in situ* cancer surrounded by an intact basement membrane; (b) invasion requires reversible changes in cell–cell and cell–extracellular-matrix adherence. Metastasizing cells can (c) enter via the lymphatics, or (d) directly enter the circulation; (e) survival and arrest of tumour cells, and extravasion of the circulatory system; (f) metastatic colonization of the distant site progresses through single cells and (g) progressively growing, angiogenic metastases

Source: Steeg (2003); Reproduced with permission

Interventions for Cancer

The purpose of treatment can be to cure the cancer, control it or treat its symptoms. The type of treatment depends on the type of cancer, the stage of the cancer, and individual factors such as age, health status and the personal preferences of the patient and his/her family. The patient needs to be made to feel comfortable enough ('empowered') to discuss with the care team which treatment choices are most suitable and acceptable. The four major treatments for cancer are surgery, radiation, chemotherapy and biological therapies such as hormone therapies (e.g. tamoxifen) and transplant options (e.g. with stem cell therapy or bone marrow).

Psychosocial interventions for patients diagnosed with cancer include:

- counselling;
- psychotherapy;
- behaviour therapy (e.g. systematic desensitization);
- cognitive behavioural therapy;
- pain control techniques (see Chapter 19);
- biofeedback;
- relaxation;
- hypnosis;
- guided imagery;
- music therapy;
- art therapy;
- group support;
- complementary therapies;
- yoga and meditation.

Objective evidence of efficacy is not generally strong. Reviews in the 1990s focusing on the four main psychosocial interventions – behavioural therapy (including relaxation, biofeedback and hypnosis); educational therapy (including training in coping skills and providing information to enhance a patient's sense of control); psychotherapy (including counselling); and support groups (which help patients to express their emotions) indicated some limited evidence of efficacy. One encouraging line was a reduction in the side effects of chemotherapy after biofeedback and relaxation therapy and a reduction in pain, less mood disturbance, and fewer maladaptive coping responses after supportive group therapy. Some researchers even claimed that their interventions extended their patients' survival but the evidence for this claim is weak or non-existent.

Meyer and Mark (1995) carried out a meta-analysis of 62 studies that had compared treatment and control groups for different kinds of psychosocial, behavioural and psychoeducational interventions. They found significant beneficial effect sizes ranging from 0.19 to 0.28. Fifteen years after this review, the position is by no means clear as there have been conflicting results from systematic reviews and the picture does not look as encouraging as it did back then. The results from the most recent systematic reviews often do not match the enthusiasm and good intentions of therapists and psycho-oncologists. Unfortunately the quality of evaluation research has been rather poor with small samples, poor designs and weak effects. This situation must be corrected.

Edwards et al. (2004) reported a systematic review of psychological interventions for women with metastatic breast cancer. This study assessed the effects of psychological interventions (educational, individual cognitive behavioural or psychotherapeutic, or group support) on psychological and survival outcomes for women with metastatic breast cancer. Five studies showed very limited evidence of short-term benefit arising from these interventions which was not sustained at long-term follow-up. The effects of the interventions on survival were not statistically significant.

Chow, Tsao and Harth (2004) carried out a meta-analysis to investigate whether psychosocial intervention improves survival in cancer. Eight randomized trials with 1062 patients published between 1966 and June 2002 were identified. One- and four-year survival rates were evaluated but these showed no statistically significant difference in the overall survival rates, suggesting again that psychosocial intervention does not lengthen survival.

Fellowes, Barnes and Wilkinson (2004) carried out a systematic review of aromatherapy and massage with patients with cancer. The reviewers investigated whether these therapies decrease anxiety and depression, lessen symptom distress and/or improve patients' quality of life. Four trials (207 patients) measuring anxiety detected a reduction in anxiety of 19–32 per cent. The evidence for any impact on depression was variable with only one trial finding any significant difference in this symptom. However, three studies (117 patients) found a reduction in pain following intervention, and two (71 patients) found a reduction in nausea.

It is clear from the above review that the quality of research in this field is poor. Unless this situation is corrected, it is unlikely that psycho-oncology will reach its full potential. Large-scale evaluations with longer-term follow-up are needed.

Living with Cancer

In spite of the negative results concerning long-term benefits, there are several aspects of cancer experience that psychological expertise can help to understand, e.g. pain, fatigue, depression and anxiety. Incidence estimates for pain range from 14 per cent to 100 per cent, for depression, from 1 per cent to 42 per cent, and for fatigue, from 4 per cent to 91 per cent. The lack of consistency across studies suggests that measurement, conceptual and methodological issues remain unsolved.

Miovic and Block (2007) review evidence that around 50 per cent of patients with advanced cancer meet the criteria for a psychiatric disorder, the most common being adjustment disorders (11–35 per cent) and major depression (5–26 per cent). Most clinical assessments of pain, depression and fatigue rely on self-report. A variety of assessment tools is available. The Hospital Anxiety and Depression Scale (HADS) and the EORTC OLQ-C30 have both shown promise for screening treatable unmet needs in patients attending routinely for radiotherapy. However, few instruments exist for children and adolescents, older adults, individuals with cognitive impairments, and individuals from different ethnic and cultural groups. There is also relatively little research on the role played by informal carers in the management of symptoms. The most commonly described strategy for improving symptom management involves regular assessment using visual analogue or numerical scales, followed by quality of life (QoL) improvement interventions. Studies on efficacy of interventions on QoL have found positive results.

Rehse and Pukrop (2003) meta-analysed controlled studies of psychosocial interventions on QoL. The overall effect size was 0.31. The most important moderating variable was duration of psychosocial intervention with treatments lasting more than 12 weeks being more effective than shorter interventions. Uitterhoeve et al. (2004) also reviewed psychosocial interventions for improving QoL of advanced cancer patients. Twelve trials evaluating behaviour therapy found positive effects on one or more indicators of QoL, for example, depression. These two systematic reviews are consistent in showing significant benefits from behavioural and psychosocial interventions for cancer patients' QoL.

Eysenbach (2003) explored the impact of the Internet on cancer outcomes. Eysenbach distinguished four areas of Internet use: communication (electronic mail), community (virtual support groups), content (health information on the World Wide Web), and e-commerce. He claimed that over 12.5 million health-related computer searches were being conducted each day on the World Wide Web. Eysenbach estimated that, in the developed world, 39 per cent of cancer patients were using the Internet, and approximately 2.3 million persons living with cancer worldwide were online. For more discussion of the Internet and health communication, see Kreps (2003).

Adaptation to Cancer

A variety of factors have been associated with adaptation to cancer patients, partners and families, and the interactions between the patients and their families. A large amount of research has studied coping styles such as fighting spirit, helplessness/hopelessness, denial and avoidance. This topic has led to mixed and inconsistent findings. Watson, Haviland, Greer, Davidson and Bliss (1999) studied the influence of psychological responses on survival in women with early-stage breast cancer. Psychological response was measured by the mental adjustment to cancer (MAC) scale, the Courtauld Emotional Control (CEC) scale, and the HAD scale 4–12 weeks and 12 months after diagnosis. The women were followed up for at least five years. There was a significantly increased risk of death from all causes by five years in women with high scores on depression, helplessness and hopelessness. No significant results were found for 'fighting spirit'.

Petticrew et al. (2002) reviewed evidence on psychological coping in relation to survival and recurrence in people with cancer. However, the results from Watson et al. (1999) were excluded. The majority of studies that had investigated fighting spirit (10 studies) or helplessness/hopelessness (12 studies) found no significant associations with survival or recurrence. Positive findings were confined to small studies, indicating a potential publication bias. Little consistent evidence was available that coping styles play a part in survival or recurrence. Watson, Davidson-Homewood, Haviland and Bliss (2003) contested the fairness of this review.

Laubmeier, Zakowski and Bair (2004) studied the role of 'spirituality' which may well be related to emotional well-being and QoL. Spirituality, particularly the existential component, was associated with less distress and better quality of life, regardless of life threat.

Cunningham and Watson (2004) carried out an interview study on how psychological therapy may prolong survival in metastatic cancer patients. They interviewed 10 medically incurable cancer patients who had outlived their prognoses from 2.2 to 12.5 years. Common themes were:

- 'authenticity', a clear understanding of what was important in one's life;
- 'autonomy', the perceived freedom to shape life around what was valued;
- 'acceptance', a perceived change towards enhanced self-esteem, greater tolerance for and emotional closeness to others, and a more peaceful and joyous affective experience.

Cunningham and Watson (2004) stated 'survivors' displayed a higher degree of early involvement in their psychological self-help than did their non-surviving peers, suggesting that healing may be assisted by a 'greater authenticity of thought and action'.

Vance and Eiser (2004) systematically reviewed studies of the effects of parents' behaviour on children's cancer coping. Parents who criticized, or apologized, had more distressed children. Parents who were permissive had more problems with adherence. Longitudinal studies to determine how parenting behaviours affect longer-term child adjustment are recommended.

Labay and Walco (2004) studied empathy in the psychological adjustment in siblings. Participants were 29 siblings and 14 children with acute lymphoblastic leukaemia, myelocytic leukaemia, or non-Hodgkin's lymphoma. Siblings did not exhibit increased rates of behaviour problems, but displayed more social and academic difficulties. However empathy was found to be a significant predictor of externalizing problems. Cancer knowledge was not related to adjustment, but was associated with empathy. Empathy may play an important role in sibling adjustment following diagnosis.

Manne, Sherman, Ross, Ostroff, Heyman and Fox (2004) studied couples' support-related communication, psychological distress, and relationship satisfaction among women with early stage breast cancer. For the study, 148 completed a videotaped discussion of a cancer-related issue and a general issue and measures of psychological distress and relationship satisfaction. During cancer-issue discussions, patients reported less distress when partners responded to disclosures with reciprocal self-disclosure and humour and when partners were less likely to propose solutions. Results suggest partner responses play a role in women's adaptation to breast cancer.

Cancer survival varies by socio-economic status (SES). These differences are often attributed to differences in the stage of disease at diagnosis, those with higher SES having better access to services. Woods, Rachet and Coleman (2006) investigated the origins of socio-economic inequalities in cancer survival in studies published since 1995. They again found an association between socio-economic status and cancer survival. However, Woods et al. suggest there arc at least possible explanations: stage at diagnosis, and differential treatment between social groups.

Deimling, Bowman, Sterns, Wagner and Kahana (2006) studied cancer-related health worries and psychological distress among older adult, long-term cancer survivors (5 years+). Deimling et al. found that almost one-third of survivors continued to report worries about recurrence, second cancer, and potential cancer symptoms. Such worries were a significant predictor of depression and anxiety. Race was also a significant predictor, with African–Americans reporting fewer cancer-related health worries. More symptoms during treatment was also a predictor of having more cancer-related health worries. However, dispositional optimism/pessimism was the most consistent predictor of psychosocial distress with more optimistic individuals reporting fewer cancer-related health worries, and lower levels of both anxiety and depression.

Caring for Someone with Cancer

The stress experienced by family members can often be high. The condition can create emotional turmoil with fear, anxiety, stigma, depression, hopelessness, fatigue, pain and insomnia all entering the relationship at various stages. The social support provided by the immediate family and friends can be a key factor in promoting the patient's adaptation and QoL. The so-called 'carer burden' can be high, and interventions are available to support the informal carer.

Problems are likely to become particularly challenging if the patient moves into palliative care. It is understandable that most patients want to be at home during their final illness. Informal carers are vital to the support of patients at home but often have unmet needs. Anxiety, depression and feelings of isolation are common, particularly after the patient's death. In certain cases, the death of a loved one may be described 'as a blessed relief'. Ramirez, Addington-Hall and Richards (1998) report that approximately one-third of cancer patients in the UK receive care from one close relative only, while about half are cared for by two or three relatives, typically a spouse and an adult child. Approximately two-thirds of cancer patients and a third of non-cancer patients typically receive some kind of formal home nursing.

Kroenke, Kubzansky, Schernhammer, Holmes and Kawachi (2006) prospectively investigated the role of social networks, social support, and survival after breast cancer diagnosis. Participants were 2835 women who had been diagnosed with stages 1 to 4 breast cancer between 1992 and 2002. Of these women, 224 deaths (107 of these related to breast cancer) had occurred by the year 2004. Women who were socially isolated before diagnosis had a subsequent 66 per cent increased risk of all-cause mortality and a two-fold increased risk of breast cancer mortality compared with women who were socially integrated. The authors concluded this effect is likely to be caused by their lack of beneficial caregiving from friends, relatives and adult children.

Harding and Higginson (2003) reviewed interventions to support carers in cancer and palliative care. Poor designs and methodology, a lack of outcome evaluation, small sample sizes and a reliance on intervention descriptions and formative evaluations characterized the literature. They suggested that alternatives to 'pure' RCTs would need to be considered in carrying out evaluation research in this domain. As was the case in reviewing interventions for obesity, smoking and drinking (Chapters 7–9) it is apparent that larger-scale studies of higher quality are needed.

The US Institute of Medicine (IOM) (2007a) report, 'Cancer Care for the Whole Patient: Meeting Psychosocial Health Needs', concluded that, despite the evidence for the effectiveness of services, cancer care often fails to meet patients' psychosocial needs. One possible reason for this failure is the tendency of cancer care providers to underestimate patients' distress (Fallowfield, Ratcliffe, Jenkins & Saul, 2001) and to not link patients to appropriate services when their needs are identified (Institute of Medicine, 2007b). The IOM report recommends a model for effective delivery of psychosocial services suggesting a 5-step sequence of processes:

1 identify each patient's psychosocial needs
2 link patients and families to needed psychosocial services
3 support patients and families in managing the illness
4 coordinate psychosocial and biomedical care
5 follow up on care delivery to monitor the effectiveness of services and make modifications if needed

Jacobsen (2009) discusses reasons why evidence-based psychosocial care for cancer patients are not more widely promoted and adopted by clinicians. Firstly, there are inconsistent findings attributable, at least in part, to differences in demographic, disease, and treatment characteristics of the samples, and the type of outcome assessments employed. Considerable variation also exists across studies in the number and content of sessions for interventions that share the same name e.g. relaxation training. This latter issue has been discussed elsewhere (Marks, 2009). The quality of the studies is a second major weakness. Inadequate reporting of study methodology appears to be a major problem. Newell, Sanson-Fisher and Savolainen (2002) found only 3 per cent of trials provided sufficient information to permit evaluation of 10 indicators of study quality. Methodological issues are common, e.g. the majority of studies failing to account for patients lost to follow up in the outcome analyses. This means that it is impossible to calculate with accuracy the odds ratio for a treatment compared to control condition.

Rodin, Katz, Lloyd, Green, Mackay, Wong et al. (2007) carried out a systematic review of pharmacologic and non-pharmacologic treatments for depression in cancer patients. Outcomes of interest included symptomatic response to treatment, discontinuation rate of treatment, adverse effects, and quality of life. Eleven trials (seven with pharmacological, and four of non-pharmacological interventions) were included. On the basis of the review, a Practice Guideline recommended:

1 Treatment of pain and other reversible physical symptoms should be given before or with antidepressant treatment.
2 Antidepressant medication should be considered for moderate-to-severe major depression in cancer patients.
3 Patients with major depression may benefit from a combined approach that includes both psychosocial and pharmacologic interventions.
4 Psychosocial treatments include information and support and therapies aimed at any combination of emotional, cognitive and behavioural factors.

Seitz, Besier and Goldbeck (2009) systematically reviewed psychosocial interventions for adolescent cancer patients. This review summarized four studies of efficacy and effectiveness of psychosocial interventions for adolescent cancer patients. One study reported a significant improvement compared with a waiting list control group. The overall level of distress was reduced with the intervention and knowledge of sexual issues, body image and anxiety about psychosexual issues were also improved. The three remaining studies observed no significant changes in distress and psychosocial functioning. The authors concluded that: 'Taken together, the findings point out that there is a lack of intervention research in psycho-oncology with adolescents. So far, there is only limited evidence for the effectiveness of psychosocial interventions to improve coping with cancer-associated problems in adolescent patients. Future research needs to be done in this population. In order to establish more conclusive results, larger samples and interventions particularly designed for adolescent patients ought to be studied' (Seitz et al., 2009: 683).

CORONARY HEART DISEASE

What Is Coronary Heart Disease?

Coronary heart disease (CHD) or coronary artery disease (CAD) occurs when the walls of the coronary arteries become narrowed by a gradual build-up of fatty material called atheroma (see Figure 20.2). **Myocardial infarction** (MI) occurs when one of the coronary arteries becomes blocked by a blood clot and part of the heart is starved of oxygen. It usually causes severe chest pain. A person having a heart attack may also experience sweating, light-headedness, nausea or shortness of breath. A heart attack may be the first sign of

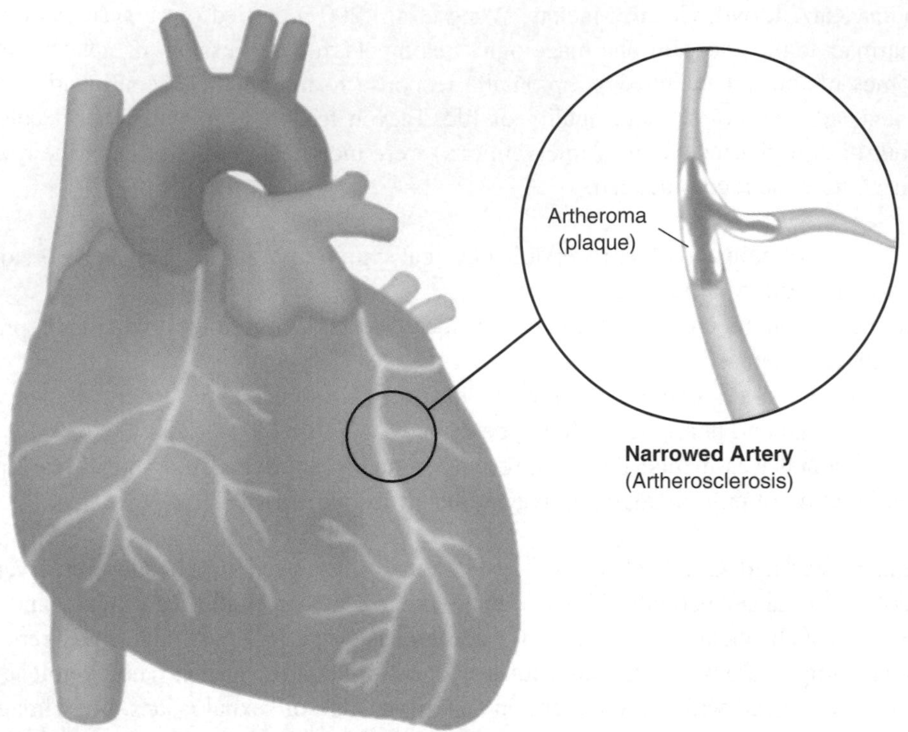

Figure 20.2 CHD (or CAD) occurs when the arteries that supply blood to heart muscle become hardened and narrowed due to the build-up of cholesterol and plaque on the inner surface of their walls. As the build-up develops, less blood can flow through the arteries so that heart muscle is starved of blood and oxygen. This can lead to chest pain (angina) or a heart attack (myocardial infarction)

CHD in many people. Over time, CHD can weaken the heart muscle and cause heart failure and arrhythmias.

Angina is the most common form of CHD. It is characterized by a heavy or tight pain in the centre of the chest that may spread to the arms, necks, jaw, face, back or stomach. Angina symptoms occur when the arteries become so narrow from the atheroma that insufficient oxygen-containing blood can be supplied to the heart muscle when its demands are high, such as during exercise. There are two categories of angina: stable or unstable angina. Stable angina is characterized by chest pain relieved by rest, resulting from the partial obstruction of a coronary artery by atheroma. Unstable angina occurs with lesser degrees of exertion or while at rest. This type increases in frequency and duration and worsens in severity. Unstable angina is an acute coronary syndrome (ACS) that requires immediate medical attention. This is usually caused by the formation of a blood clot at the site of a ruptured plaque in a coronary artery. If left untreated, it can result in heart attack and irreversible damage to the heart.

Risk factors for CHD include:

- increasing age
- male sex
- heredity
- tobacco smoking
- high blood cholesterol
- high blood pressure
- physical inactivity
- obesity and overweight
- diabetes mellitus
- high alcohol consumption
- possibly stress/distressed personality
- possibly depression

The jury is still out with regard to the 'distressed personality' (Denollet, Sys, Stroobant, Rombouts, Gillebert & Brutsaert, 1996) and also depression as risk factors. Nicholson, Kuper and Hemingway (2006) carried out a meta-analysis of depression among 146,538 participants in 54 observational studies of coronary heart disease. Results need to be adjusted for left ventricular function, a risk factor for CHD, but such results were available in only eight studies. It was concluded that depression has yet to be established as an independent risk factor for CHD because of incomplete adjustment for conventional risk factors and severity of coronary disease (see also Chapter 17).

Interventions for CHD

People with suspected CHD usually undergo several different tests for absolute diagnosis and to determine the best treatment to relieve symptoms. These include stress **exercise tolerance test (ETT)**, **electrocardiogram (ECG)** and **coronary angiogram**. Seeking a diagnosis can be a stressful time for people with suspected CHD and their family and friends. Patients commonly feel apprehension about the procedure and find some parts of the procedure unexpected with doctors' technical language being an obstacle to understanding.

Many people with CHD have to make lifestyle changes and take a regime of medication such as **ACE inhibitors**, **statins**, **anticoagulant drugs** and **betablockers**. Clinical guidelines are not always implemented because of a lack of time among physicians who spend an average of about 15 minutes discussing risk factor, lifestyle changes or treatment. This may not be an appropriate time to discuss such issues with a patient who may well feel shocked by the diagnosis of being at risk of CHD and show low levels of compliance with physician advice.

Riesen, Darioli and Noll (2004) acknowledged that, although high rates of compliance with lifestyle changes and lipid lowering agents are reported in clinical trials, rarely are the findings reproduced in regular practice. They recommended the use of educational materials as well as regular telephone contact to improve compliance. However, further research is needed into the causes of poor compliance and methods of improving adherence with lipid-lowering agents.

People living with angina have increased risk of anxiety and depression. Lewin et al. (2002) evaluated the efficacy of a CBT disease management programme, the **Angina Plan** (see Box 20.1), to aid the psychological adjustment of patients with newly diagnosed angina. At six-month follow-up, Angina Plan patients showed a significantly greater reduction in anxiety, depression, frequency of angina, use of *glyceryl trinitrate* and physical limitations. They were also more likely to report a change in diet and increase in their daily walking.

Box 20.1

The Angina Plan – a psychological disease management programme for people with angina (Lewin et al., 2002)

The Angina Plan consists of a patient-held booklet and audio-taped relaxation programme. Before commencing the 30–40 minute Angina Plan session, the patient is sent a questionnaire designed to establish if s/he holds any of the common misconceptions about angina (for example, each episode is a mini heart attack or angina is caused because your heart is worn out). The patient's partner or a friend is invited to the session.

After blood pressure has been taken and body mass index has been recorded, the Angina Plan facilitator discusses any misconceptions that were revealed in the questionnaire with the patient and, if possible, his or her partner in an effort to correct their understanding. Personal risk factors are then identified. Personal goals to reduce the risk factors are then set. They are provided with a relaxation tape and encouraged to use it. The Plan also contains written information such as the role of frightening thoughts and misconceptions in triggering adrenaline release and anxiety and how this can result in poor coping strategies.

The patient is contacted by the facilitator at the end of weeks 1, 4, 8 and 12. During these phone calls, the patient is praised for any success. They are also asked if they want to extend successful goals. Unsuccessful goals can be revisited. Adding procedures that encourage specific implementation intentions to this programme could well improve the success of the Angina Plan.

Other forms of invasive treatment may be necessary when medication alone does not relieve angina. Referral to a cardiologist or a heart surgeon may be required for further treatment to gain effective control of angina symptoms and for some people to prolong life. Invasive **revascularization** treatment may include either a **percutaneous coronary intervention (PCI)** or **coronary artery bypass graft (CABG)** surgery.

Living with CHD

Waiting for invasive treatment to improve or prolong life can be very stressful and have deleterious effects on the quality of daily life. Pre-surgical depression predicts cardiac hospitalization, continued surgical pain, failure to return to previous activity and depression at 6 months (Burg, Benedetto, Rosenberg & Soufer, 2003). Jonsdottir and Baldursdottir (1998) surveyed people on a waiting list for CABG in Iceland. They found that waiting for surgery had negative effects on the work and daily life of the majority of respondents. Prominent symptoms reported included fatigue, shortness of breath, chest pain, anxiety and depression. Eighty-seven per cent reported experiencing stress. The majority reported negative influences of their illness on their spouses and family, with 80 per cent reporting emotional effects. They concluded that pre-operative psychological assessment that focuses on level of stress and anxiety as well as coping skills and social support are needed. Fitzsimons, Parahoo and Stringer (2000) conducted a qualitative analysis into the experience of waiting for a CABG in Northern Ireland. They identified three central themes in this experience – uncertainty, chest pain and anxiety – with six secondary themes: powerless, dissatisfaction with treatment, anger/frustration, physical incapacity, reduced self-esteem and altered family and social relationships, again pointing to a need for psychological intervention during this period.

Arthur, Daniels, McKelvie, Hirsh and Rush (2000) conducted a randomized controlled trial (RCT) of a multidimensional pre-operative intervention on pre-surgery and post-surgery outcomes in low-risk patients awaiting elective CABG. The intervention consisted of individualized, prescribed exercise training twice per week in a supervised environment, education and reinforcement and monthly nurse-initiated telephone calls to answer questions and provide reassurance. Patients who received the intervention spent one day less in the hospital and less time in the intensive care unit. Patients in the intervention group reported a better quality of life during the waiting period than the control group. The improved quality of life continued up to 6 months after surgery. Using outcome measures such as length of hospital stay as well as quality of life measures provides evidence of cost-effectiveness, helpful information for budget holders wondering whether to invest in such interventions.

Rutledge, Reis, Linke, Greenberg and Mills (2006) carried out a meta-analytic review of prevalence, intervention effects, and associations with clinical outcomes of depression in heart failure. Clinically significant depression was present in at least 1 in 5 patients with heart failure but rates can be higher among patients screened with questionnaires. The authors concluded that the relationship between depression and poorer heart failure outcomes is consistent and strong across multiple end points.

Unsurprisingly then, depression is a common response to heart disease. A special committee of the American Heart Association published recommendations for Screening, Referral, and Treatment of depression in heart patients (Lichtman et al., 2008). The committee recommended:

1 Routine screening for depression in patients with CHD in settings, including the hospital, physician's office, clinic, and cardiac rehabilitation centre;
2 Patients with positive screening results should be evaluated by a qualified mental health professional;
3 Patients with cardiac disease who are under treatment for depression should be carefully monitored for adherence to their medical care, drug efficacy, and safety with respect to their cardiovascular as well as mental health.
4 Monitoring mental health may include, but is not limited to, the assessment of patients receiving antidepressants for possible worsening of depression or suicidality, especially during initial treatment when doses may be adjusted, changed or discontinued.
5 Coordination of care between health-care providers is necessary in patients with combined medical and mental health diagnoses.

Of key importance, as always, is social support. Mookadam and Arthur (2004) systematically reviewed social support and its relationship to morbidity and mortality after acute myocardial infarction. The authors were interested in the socio-economic determinants of health, including social change, disorganization and poverty that have been associated with an increased risk of morbidity and mortality. Social support is a possible mediator linking these factors to health and illness. Having low social support networks was a predictor of one-year mortality following acute myocardial infarction. Low social support is equivalent to many 'classic' risk factors, such as elevated cholesterol level, tobacco use and hypertension.

Adaptation to CHD

Cognitive adaptation has been shown to predict psychological adjustment to diseases such as arthritis, cancer, AIDS and heart disease. According to the cognitive adaptation theory, some people who are faced with a chronic illness maintain or develop an optimistic outlook, attempt to regain control or mastery over the event and find ways to restore or enhance their self-esteem (Taylor, 1983). Helgeson and Fritz (1999) tested whether people with high cognitive adaptation scores would be less vulnerable to a new coronary event due to **restenosis** within six months of initial PCI. Three components of cognitive adaptation were measured – self-esteem, optimism and control. Patients with a low cognitive adaptation score were more likely to have a new cardiac event even when demographic and medical variables thought to predict restenosis were statistically controlled.

A large number of MI patients do not return to work or regain normal functioning despite being physically well. There is evidence that cardiac rehabilitation programmes can reduce distress and disability, increase confidence and improve modifiable risk factors. However, many patients do not attend rehabilitation programmes after their MI. Patients' beliefs and perception about their illness are key determinants of recovery after a MI. Petrie, Cameron, Ellis, Buick and Weinman (2002) evaluated a brief hospital intervention designed to alter patients' perceptions about their MI. The content of the intervention was individualized according to the patients' responses on the Illness Perception Questionnaire (Weinman et al., 1996). The intervention caused significant positive changes in patients' views of their MI. The intervention group reported being better prepared for leaving hospital and subsequently returned to work at a significantly faster rate than the control group. At the three-month follow-up, the intervention group reported a significantly lower rate of angina symptoms.

Cooper, Lloyd, Weinman and Jackson (1999) investigated whether the illness beliefs held during their hospital stay by patients who had a MI or who had undergone CABG could predict cardiac rehabilitation attendance. As well as being older, less aware of their cholesterol values and less likely to be employed, non-attenders were less likely to believe their condition was controllable and that their lifestyle may have contributed to their illness. Stewart, Abbey, Shnek, Irvine and Grace (2004) found a difference in the health information needs between men and women recovering from an acute coronary event. Men that had received significantly more information reported a greater satisfaction with health-care professionals meeting their information needs. Women reported wanting more information than men concerning angina and hypertension. Men wanted more information about sexual function. Patients who reported receiving more information reported less depressive symptomatology. Most patients of both sexes preferred a shared decision-making role with their doctor. The majority felt their doctor had made the main decisions. Cardiac rehabilitation that is individualized to patients' needs may be more attractive and effective than current practice of thinking of cardiac rehabilitation as a place to do exercise and be informed about lifestyle changes.

Caring for Someone With CHD

Concordance occurs between men with CHD and their spouses for body mass index, history of smoking, current smoking status, frequency of exercise, miles per exercise session and the amount of fat and fibre in the diet. Behavioural risk factors are correlated among marital partners. Involving partners in lifestyle interventions may be more efficacious than individual patient education strategies.

Moser and Dracup (2004) compared the emotional responses and perception of control of MI and revascularization patients and their spouses and examined the relationship between spouses' emotional distress and patients' emotional distress and psychosocial adjustment to their cardiac event. They found that spouses had higher levels of anxiety and depression than the patients. There were no differences in level of hostility. The patients also had a higher level of perceived control than did the spouses. Spouse anxiety, depression and perceived control were correlated with patient psychosocial adjustment to illness even when patient anxiety and depression were kept constant. The patients' psychosocial adjustment to illness was worse when spouses were more anxious or depressed than patients. Attention should be given to the psychological needs of spouses of patients who have suffered a cardiac event. Moser and Dracup also found that patients' psychosocial adjustment was best when patients were more anxious or depressed than spouses. This finding suggests that interventions that address the psychological distress of spouses may well improve patient outcomes.

Johnston, Foulkes, Johnston, Pollard and Gudmundsdottir (1999) evaluated the effectiveness of a cardiac counselling rehabilitation programme for MI patients and their partners. They found that the programme resulted in more knowledge, less anxiety, less depression and greater satisfaction with care for both patients and their partners and less disability in patients. This study was published five years earlier than the Moser and Dracup (2004) study in the same journal, thus highlighting that it can take a long time for research findings to be disseminated, synthesized and put into practice. Conducting research to influence practice is very time consuming and there are usually many barriers to overcome. In order for research to have an impact, health psychologists must have an awareness of promotional techniques, the politics of the context in which they practise and the power of economical factors.

One problem for evaluation of cardiac patients' experience of QoL is identifying an instrument that is not only reliable and valid but also responsive to change. Instruments that are not very responsive will tend to under-represent the benefits of programme attendance. Research indicates that the most responsive instruments are: Beck Depression Inventory, Global Mood Scale, Health Complaints Checklist, Heart Patients' Psychological Questionnaire and Speilberger State Anxiety Inventory.

Rees, Bennett, West, Davey and Ebrahim (2004) reviewed psychological interventions for coronary heart disease, typically, stress management interventions. They included RCTs, either single modality interventions or a part of cardiac rehabilitation with a minimum follow-up of six months. Stress management (SM) trials were identified and reported in combination with other psychological interventions and separately. The quality of many trials was poor, making the findings unreliable. The authors concluded that psychological interventions showed no evidence of effect on total or cardiac mortality, but small reductions in anxiety and depression in patients with CHD. Similar results were seen for SM interventions when considered separately.

In 2007, the American Heart Association Exercise, Cardiac Rehabilitation, and Prevention Committee and the American Association of Cardiovascular and Pulmonary Rehabilitation reported on the core components of cardiac rehabilitation/secondary prevention programmes (Balady et al., 2007). The associations recommended that all cardiac rehabilitation/secondary prevention programmes should contain baseline patient assessment, nutritional counselling, risk factor management (lipids, blood pressure, weight, diabetes mellitus, and smoking), psychosocial interventions, and physical activity counselling and exercise training. Cardiac rehabilitation services are now routinely offered to patients but many invited patients fail to attend the sessions. Cooper, Jackson, Weinman and Horne (2002) reviewed the literature. The results showed that non-attenders are more likely to be older, to have lower income/greater deprivation, to deny the severity of their illness, are less likely to believe they can influence its outcome or to perceive that their physician recommends cardiac rehabilitation.

HIV/AIDS

What is HIV/AIDS?

HIV/AIDS has become a worldwide pandemic that has infected around 60 million people, and become the fourth largest killer in the world. There are around 3 million new cases each year and about 2 million deaths from **AIDS (acquired immune deficiency syndrome)**. The number of deaths peaked around 2004, and has since declined slightly. **HIV (human immunodeficiency virus)** is a retrovirus that infects and colonizes cells in the immune system and the central nervous system (T-helper and monocyte macrophage cells). Initial flu-like symptoms are followed by a quiescent, asymptomatic period (lasting years) during which the immune system battles the virus. Eventually the virus compromises the immune system and the individual becomes symptomatic. Finally the immune system is overwhelmed and the individual becomes vulnerable to opportunistic diseases, signifying development of the AIDS and eventually likely to result in death.

An HIV particle is around 100–150 billionths of a metre in diameter, one seventieth the size of a human CD4+ white blood cell. HIV particles are coated with fatty material known as the viral envelope or membrane. Seventy-two spikes, formed from the proteins gp120 and gp41, project out of the membrane. Below the viral envelope is a matrix layer, made from protein p17. The core is usually bullet-shaped and made from the protein p24. Inside the core there are three enzymes called reverse transcriptase, integrase and protease together with HIV's genetic material, consisting of two identical strands of RNA.

HIV has nine genes (compared to around 20,000–25,000 in a human). Three HIV genes, gag, pol and env, make proteins for new virus particles. The other six genes, tat, rev, nef, vif, vpr and vpu, govern HIV's ability to infect a cell, produce new copies of virus, or cause disease.

In 1996, the introduction of highly active antiretroviral therapy (HAART) redefined the illness and improved the outlook for infected individuals. However, antiretrovirals do not eliminate the virus, but only suppress it and, currently, only one in ten who need the treatment actually receive it. HIV persistence eventually causes disease in all infected persons (Sleasman and Goodenow, 2003).

Risk factors for HIV are:

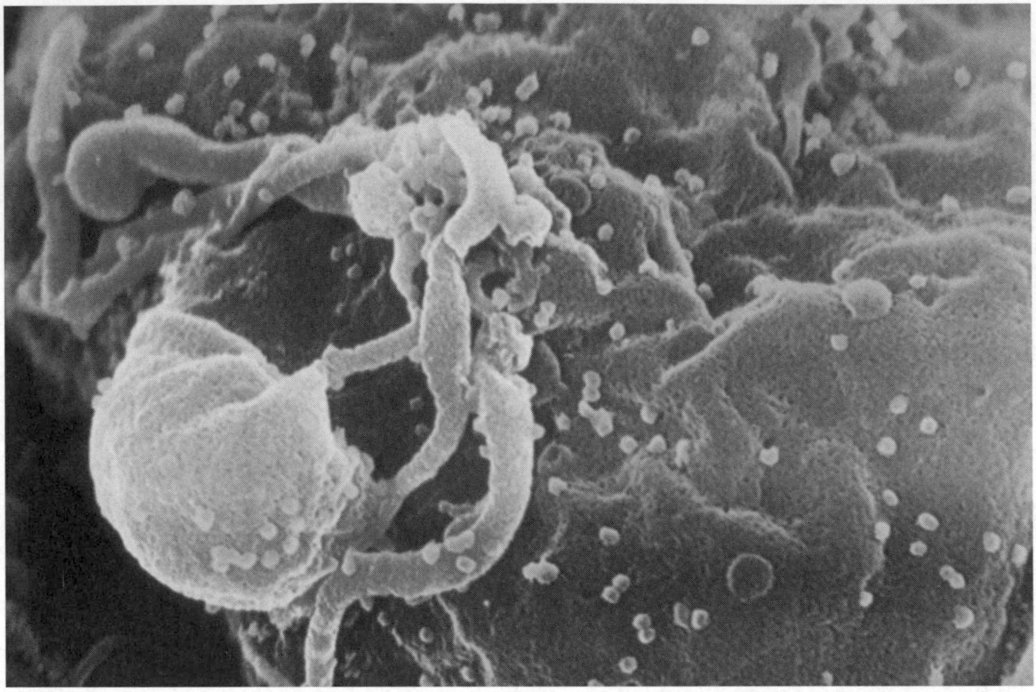

Figure 20.3 The human immunodeficiency virus. Scanning electron micrograph of HIV-1 budding from cultured lymphocyte. Multiple round bumps on cell surface represent sites of assembly and budding of virions

Source: Centers for Disease Control and Prevention, 2010

- Unprotected sex
- Injection drug use
- STIs
- Blood exposure
- Mother–infant transmission
- Breastfeeding transmission
- Mother–to–fetus transmission
- Mother–infant childbirth transmission

Interventions for HIV/AIDS

In the USA, women are one of the fastest growing groups of people with AIDS, among whom women of colour are disproportionately affected (Centers for Disease Control and Prevention, 1999). Mize, Robinson, Bockting and Scheltema (2002) carried out a meta-analysis of the effectiveness of HIV prevention interventions for women. Twenty-four articles from 1989–1997 were included. The authors evaluated five ethnic groupings (All Ethnicities Combined, African–American, White, Hispanic and a Mixed Ethnicity group) over four time periods (post-test, less than two months after the intervention, 2–3 months after the intervention and 6–24 months after the intervention) on three HIV-related sexuality outcome variables (HIV/AIDS knowledge, self-efficacy and sexual risk reduction behaviour). The HIV interventions appeared effective at improving knowledge about HIV/AIDS and increasing sexual risk reduction behaviours for all ethnicities except that the findings for self-efficacy are less consistent. The interventions were less consistently effective for African–American women, for whom significant improvements in feelings of self-efficacy were only seen six months or longer after the intervention.

The HIV virus has a short half-life allowing rapid replication and mutation, which makes vaccine development problematic and increases the likelihood of drug resistance. Absence of a workable vaccine means antiviral medications are the primary treatment for HIV. Combination therapies (HAART) have been shown to decrease an individual's HIV viral load to undetectable levels, reducing associated morbidity and mortality. However, 95–100 per cent adherence is required to produce and maintain successful virologic suppression, with even 80–90 per cent adherence rates showing no viral suppression in some patients. Non-adherence promotes viral drug resistance and cross-resistance, and drug resistant strains can be transmitted to uninfected patients leaving them without effective treatment options. HIV combination drug therapies involve complex, disrupting and challenging medication regimens involving numerous drugs taken several times a day with specific food instructions. In addition, treatment often commences during the asymptomatic phase, drug toxicity commonly results in severe, unpleasant side effects (e.g. vomiting, lipodystrophy) and treatment must continue for the rest of the person's life. Moreover, the long-term treatment stability and maintenance of viral suppression are not certain.

Adherence rates for HAART tend to be sub-optimal. Fogarty, Roter, Larson, Burke, Gillespie and Levy's (2002) review yielded 200 variables associated with adherence to HIV medication regimens falling into four broad categories: regimen characteristics; psychosocial factors; institutional resources; and personal attributes. Of the psychosocial factors reported, positive disease and treatment attitudes, good mental health and adjustment to HIV were positively associated with adherence while perceived negative social climate was negatively associated. Lack of access to institutional resources (financial, institutional, medical) was negatively associated with adherence. Finally, non-adherence was linked to personal attributes of younger age, minority status and history of substance use. Patients' active involvement in their medical care and treatment decision-making also promotes adherence while low health literacy is associated with poor adherence.

Many studies have reported that stress accelerates disease processes in a variety of diseases including HIV. The chronic status of HIV/AIDS and the limited accessibility to HAART for many people living with HIV/AIDS (PLWHA) means that psychosocial support interventions are increasingly important. Programmes of pain management, stress management, coping effectiveness training, sleep disorders and exercise promotion have been found to enhance immune system function, medication adherence and adaptive coping and to decrease anxiety, stress and depression (Chesney, Chambers, Taylor, Johnson & Folkman, 2003). Supportive interventions, especially those that improve function and self-management and maximize independence, represent an essential part of HIV/AIDS treatment.

Interventions to reduce stress among persons living with HIV are an important adjunct to pharmacotherapy. Scott-Sheldon, Kalichman, Carey and Fielder (2008) reviewed stress management interventions for HIV+ adults as evaluated in randomized controlled trials from 1989 to 2006. The authors were interested in measuring the impact of stress-management interventions designed to enhance the psychological, immunological and hormonal outcomes among HIV + adults. The findings indicated that, in comparison to controls, stress-management interventions reduce anxiety, depression, distress, and fatigue and improve quality of life. However, stress-management interventions did not appear to affect immunological or hormonal processes compared with controls.

Living with HIV/AIDS

People living with HIV/AIDS face the general stressors of the chronically ill and may face additional stresses unique to HIV/AIDS, e.g. additional uncertainty and decision-making due to rapidly changing treatment developments/outlook, infectivity persistence, the imperative for major behaviour change (e.g. sexual behaviour), anticipatory grief and the excessive stigma associated with the condition. The quality of life of PLWHA is severely compromised, particularly in the later stages of the disease, due to pain (experienced by 30–90 per cent of PLWHA), discomfort, and mobility difficulties (e.g. Hughes, Jelsma, Maclean, Darder & Tinise, 2004).

The major stressors encountered by PLWHA are summarized in Box 20.2. Different stressors may be experienced at different stages of the illness, with stress peaks at initial diagnosis, onset of symptomology, sudden immune system cell (CD4) count decline, onset of opportunistic infections and diagnosis of AIDS.

Stress has been associated with psychological problems (e.g. anxiety, hopelessness, helplessness, suicidal ideation), psychiatric disorders (e.g. depression, anxiety), negative

Box 20.2

HIV/AIDS related stressors

Disease-related stressors

- Being tested and receiving test results;
- diagnoses – seropositivity, symptomatic phase and AIDS;
- treatment commencement;

- intermittent symptoms and opportunistic disease;
- emergence of new symptoms;
- for children, neurocognitive and emotional developmental problems;
- developing drug resistance and treatment failures;
- co-infections (e.g. hepatitis);
- further exposure to the virus;
- medication side effects;
- pain, discomfort, sexual difficulties, mobility restrictions and progressive physical deterioration;
- complications from ongoing substance use;
- drug trials and drug holidays.

External life-stressors

- Enacted stigma (e.g. ostracism and discrimination);
- disclosure reactions;
- bereavement;
- substance use;
- employment changes;
- reduced income;
- loss/lack of health insurance;
- access to treatment;
- rejection and loss of social support;
- uncertainty.

Emotional/psychological stressors

- Felt stigma (internalization, fear, shame, guilt);
- disclosure decisions;
- reproductive decision-making;
- grief;
- risk behaviour and decision-making;
- anger;
- rejection and isolation;
- changing expectations;
- preparing for death;
- guilt.

health behaviours (e.g. drug use) and disease progression. Sub-clinical distress symptoms, including depression and anxiety, are common in PLWHA though some studies show little difference to comparison HIV-negative populations. Women are increasingly affected by HIV/AIDS and may face 'triple jeopardy', in relation to their individual, reproductive and caregiving roles (Murphy, 2003) and therefore may experience higher levels of psychiatric morbidity (Tostes, Chalub & Botega, 2004).

Few conditions have provoked such unprecedented levels of stigma, fear and uncertainty as HIV/AIDS, even in the well informed. These fears are layered on top of pre-existing stigmas and moral judgements associated with particular groups, including gay men, sex workers, drug users and people with mental illnesses, reinforcing existing social inequalities. PLWHA have been treated as pariahs, discriminated against, abandoned and ostracized. HIV/AIDS has even evoked appeals for mandatory testing and elimination of infected individuals. Stigma can intensify all the stressors and problems of living with the disease and is an obstacle to PLWHA fulfilling their human rights and to HIV/AIDS prevention.

The decision to disclose HIV-positive status is a daunting and multifaceted issue that recurs throughout the course of the disease. Non-disclosure increases the likelihood of infecting others and denies knowledge to previous sexual partners, so represents a major barrier to controlling the epidemic. Non-disclosure also decreases social support and access to services. Disclosure decisions are often conflated with simultaneous disclosure of lifestyle choices (e.g. sexuality, drug use) to family and friends. Disclosure decisions may revert to someone other than the PLWHA, particularly regarding children, when family members make decisions, including whether to tell the child their own serostatus (DeMatteo et al., 2002).

AIDS-related deaths may generate atypical bereavement complicated by a host of factors including survivor guilt, the effects of stigma and inadequate social support. AIDS-related deaths tend to be among relatively younger people. Many people who are affected by HIV/AIDS experience multiple bereavements, increasing distress and psychological problems (e.g. guilt, depression, suicidality, disenfranchised grief, numbing).

Ironson et al. (2002) investigated the relationship between spirituality and religiousness and health outcomes for people living with HIV. Four factors of the Ironson–Woods Spirituality/Religiousness Index were identified: Sense of Peace, Faith in God, Religious Behaviour and Compassionate View of Others. Each of the four sub-scales was related to long survival with AIDS. Also, the Ironson–Woods Index was significantly correlated with lower distress, more hope, social support, health behaviours, helping others, and lower cortisol levels. In a related study, Ironson, Stuetzle and Fletcher (2006) found an increase in religiousness/spirituality in 45 per cent of a sample after HIV diagnosis which predicts slower disease progression over 4 years in people with HIV. Those reporting an increase in spirituality/religiousness after the diagnosis had slower progression.

Adaptation to HIV/AIDS

Post-HAART, HIV/AIDS has been defined as an incurable, chronic and life-threatening illness. Coping with HIV/AIDS is a complex, multidimensional phenomenon that is influenced by personality, contextual and cultural factors. It involves a process of continual adjustment in response to stress, challenging life events, and personal and interpersonal issues. Multiple stressors and negative psychological outcomes are deterrents to successful adjustment. Adaptation is also influenced by health behaviours, which have a bi-directional influence on mood states (e.g. depressed people drink more, which increases depression resulting in increased alcohol consumption, as well as increased risky sex behaviours). An increased number of symptoms and onset of the symptomatic stage are key predictors of adjustment. Factors associated with good psychosocial adjustment to HIV/AIDS include healthy self-care behaviours (medical care, healthy lifestyle, awareness and ability to take action to meet personal needs); a sense of connectedness (one close confidante, openness, disclosure); a sense of meaning and purpose (cognitive appraisal that there is something to live for, optimistic attitude); and maintaining perspective (realistic acceptance e.g. not viewing condition as imminently fatal). Adaptive coping skills have consistently been associated with increased self-esteem, increased self-efficacy and perceived control. They include active behavioural (planning, help and information seeking, relaxation exercises) and cognitive (cognitive reframing, finding meaning, emotion work, problem solving) strategies. Problem-focused coping appears more appropriate for situations that cannot be changed, whereas emotion-focused coping is more suitable where change is not possible (Park, Folkman & Bostrom, 2001).

Adaptive coping strategies along with good social support can mediate the negative effects of stress. Adaptive coping strategies have also been associated with health-related benefits. Finding meaning in the experience of HIV/AIDS has been associated with maintaining immune system cell (CD4) levels, optimism with higher CD4 counts, medication adherence and lower distress, and perceived control, problem-focused coping and social support associated with longer survival. Adaptive and maladaptive coping strategies are not mutually exclusive, co-occuring or changing depending on context. Maladaptive coping strategies have been associated with poor adjustment including lower fighting spirit, higher hopelessness, anxious preoccupation and a fatalistic attitude. Passive and avoidant coping, psychological inhibition and withdrawal have been associated with increased risk behaviours, distress and more rapid disease progression (Stein & Rotheram-Borus, 2004).

Another factor associated with successful adaptation is social support. Zuckerman and Antoni (1995) reported that seven social support criteria were especially related to optimal adjustment to HIV/AIDS: feeling supported, satisfaction with support received, perceived helpfulness of peers, total perceived availability and individual dimensions of support, absence of social conflict, greater involvement of AIDS-related community activities and greater number of close friends. These criteria were related to adaptive coping strategies, increased self-esteem and sense of well-being and decreased depression, hopelessness, anxiety, mood disturbances, dysphoria and risk behaviour. Parental adaptation and support may be the most important influences on the adaptation of children and adolescent PLWHA.

Caring for Someone with HIV/AIDS

The burden of care for people with HIV/AIDS, both formal and informal, is being borne primarily by lay carers within the family or the community, the majority of whom are women and girls (UNAIDS, 2004). There is some evidence, especially in Africa and Asia, that the least acknowledged carers are children (caring for a lone or surviving parent) and that older women, already vulnerable through higher levels of chronic poverty, lack of resources and their own substantial health problems, are disproportionately affected.

Caring involves a broad spectrum of psychological, spiritual, emotional and practical work throughout the course of the illness. It can be a rewarding undertaking from which caregivers derive a sense of purpose and self-esteem. However, the caring literature consistently reports the inherently stressful nature of caring for someone with a chronic illness (e.g. Chesler and Parry, 2001). Many of the stressors and negative psychological outcomes experienced by PLWHA equally affect their carers. Caring is associated with anxiety, depression, overwork, fatigue, fear of death, decreased libido, helplessness, frustration and grief. While other care domains may be similar (e.g. cancer), the greater dependence of PLWHA, and involvement and identification with them, results in increased patient contact and higher intensity of emotional work increasing the negative consequences. Neurological and/or cognitive symptoms associated with HIV/AIDS (from direct effects, opportunistic diseases or other causes) can make the burden of care especially arduous. The effects of multiple bereavements and the carers' own health problems (including own HIV-positive status) also increase mental health problems. The circumscribing effects of stigma create barriers to accessing social support and resources for carers.

The needs of carers are rarely prioritized and 'burnout' is a common problem. Burnout is defined as emotional exhaustion, depersonalization and a damaged sense of personal accomplishment (e.g. Maslach & Jackson, 1981). Emotional support and stress management programmes can help prevent stress, depression and burnout in carers.

END OF LIFE CARE

As noted, increasing age is a risk factor for cancers and CHD, and also dementia. The number of people with chronic illness will increase with the 'greying' of the population (see Figure 2.3). How to best support quality of life in patients and their families is an issue of increasing importance. Yet end-of-life/palliative care tends to be neglected within health psychology.

In this section, we briefly review recent studies of end-of-life care for patients diagnosed with chronic diseases. Specialist palliative care has two main client groups: the majority have a diagnosis of cancer, and a minority are diagnosed with other chronic illnesses. Skilbeck and Payne (2005) provide an analysis of specialist palliative care nursing. They argue that patients dying from chronic, non-malignant disease experience many unmet needs in dealing with symptoms and receipt of psychosocial support. They argued that 'a more coherent approach to research and education is required, in particular strategies that explore how patients and nurses can work together in exploring experiences of illness in order to develop more proactive approaches to care' (p. 325).

In order to provide better patient care, it is helpful firstly to go back to first principles and to work with direct knowledge of people's beliefs about what makes a 'good death'.

Steinhauser, Clipp, McNeilly, Christakis, McIntyre & Tulsky (2000) researched descriptions of what makes a good death from patients, families, and providers using focus group discussions and interviews. The participants identified six components of a good death:

1 pain and symptom management
2 clear decision making
3 preparation for death
4 completion
5 contributing to others
6 affirmation of the whole person

Steinhauser et al. found, unsurprisingly, that physicians held a more biomedical perspective than other people, while patients and families felt that psychosocial and spiritual issues are as important as physiological concerns. Bingley, McDermott, Thomas, Payne, Seymour and Clark (2006) reviewed narratives written since 1950 by people facing death from cancer and other diseases. The search identified 148 narratives since 1950 from which a sub-sample of 63 narratives was reviewed. Bingley et al. found the therapeutic benefits of writing were generally viewed as a way of making sense of dying together with a strong sense of purpose in sharing the story. Common themes were: changes in body image, an awareness of social needs when dying, communication with medical staff, symptom control, realities of suffering, and spiritual aspects of dying. Writing about cancer in comparison to other illnesses showed differences in content and style. The authors suggest that: 'The narrative acts as companion and witness to the encroaching disability and debility, as well as charting the changes in relationships with loved ones, oneself and one's body image' (Bingley et al., 2006: 194).

Lorenz et al. (2008) published a systematic review with clinical guidelines on evidence for improving end of life care. To assess interventions to improve palliative care, Lorenz et al. selected systematic reviews that addressed 'end of life', including terminal illness (e.g., advanced cancer) and chronic, eventually fatal illness with ambiguous prognosis (e.g., advanced dementia), and intervention studies that addressed pain, dyspnea, depression, advance care planning, continuity and caregiving. Lorenz et al. (2008) screened 24,423 titles to find 6381 relevant abstracts and reviewed 1274 articles in detail to finally identify 33 high-quality systematic reviews and 89 relevant intervention studies. This empirical evidence was synthesized into a set of evidence statements:

1 Strong evidence exists for treating cancer pain with opioids, non-steroidals, radionuclides, and radiotherapy; dyspnea (shortness of breath) from chronic lung disease with short-term opioids; and cancer-associated depression with psychotherapy, tricyclics, and selective serotonin reuptake inhibitors.
2 Strong evidence supports multi component interventions to improve continuity in heart failure.

3 Moderate evidence supports advance care planning led by skilled facilitators who engage key decision makers and interventions to alleviate caregiver burden.
4 Weak evidence addresses cancer-related dyspnea management.
5 No evidence addresses non-cancer pain, symptomatic dyspnea management in advanced heart failure, or short-acting antidepressants in terminal illness.
6 No direct evidence addresses improving continuity for patients with dementia.
7 Evidence was weak for improving caregiver burden in cancer and was absent for heart failure.

Habraken et al. (2009) compared health-related quality of life (HRQOL) in patients diagnosed with end-stage chronic obstructive pulmonary disease (COPD) and non-small cell lung cancer (NSCLC) to examine whether COPD patients experience similar or worse disease burden in comparison with lung cancer patients. In fact, NSCLC patients showed higher HRQOL for physical functioning, social functioning, mental health, general health perceptions, dyspnea, activities of daily living, and depression than COPD patients. These findings suggest that COPD patients have a similar need for palliative care to cancer patients.

Spirituality is often a missing factor in studies of end-of-life care. However, the role of spirituality in health is of increasing interest to researchers. Williams (2006) summarized the qualitative literature on spirituality at the end of life. The majority of participants in 11 relevant studies had a diagnosis of cancer but those with HIV/AIDS, cardiovascular disease, and amyotrophic lateral sclerosis were also represented. The studies suggested three main themes within spiritual perspectives at the end of life:

- spiritual despair – alienation, loss of self, dissonance
- spiritual work – forgiveness, self-exploration, search for balance
- spiritual well-being – connection, self-actualization, consonance

Williams' (2006) findings reinforce the importance of spirituality in end-of-life care and highlight the need to consider spiritual health when caring for a terminally ill person.

FUTURE RESEARCH

1 Adherence–research into the optimum time to give information about treatment and how to tailor the content of information for different patients.
2 Research designed to understand the experience of waiting for PCI and other procedures, and how interventions can improve outcomes.

3 We need a better understanding about why some people do not attend cardiac rehabilitation. The focus of the research should be on the content of the programme and how to make it more appealing.
4 More research is needed into the psychological impact of being told a spouse or family member has a serious illness in order to cater for the needs of family members.
5 More longitudinal studies are needed with HAART. The literature spans a short timeframe, and is based on specific populations (e.g. gay men) from developed countries, unrepresentative of the developing world, where the epidemic is at its highest.
6 A variety of psychosocial interventions have been developed for patients with cancer and other life-threatening conditions. Although these studies have shown short-term benefits, in regard to long-term QoL and survival, the evidence to date is disappointing. Large-scale, better-designed evaluation studies are required.
7 Many issues concerning end-of-life care lack high-quality evidence. Future research should address psychosocial support and interventions across different conditions and settings focused on the last part of life.

Summary

1 Chronic illnesses can strike at any age but more often in middle and older age groups and, while they can be fatal, most people diagnosed with a chronic illness live for many years with the condition.
2 Management of fatal or chronic diseases is a principal feature in the lives of 10–15 per cent of the population. This huge amount of informal care occurs almost invisibly to outsiders with little recognition or financial support from society at large.
3 Chronic illness involves restrictions on activities of daily living, and increases in pain and fatigue. 'Juggling' relationships with health professionals, family and friends requires many adaptations and adjustments. Patients may have views about their care and treatment that differ from those of the professionals.
4 Life-threatening diseases are associated with a great variety of metaphors and meanings. Metaphor can be a useful way of coping but may lead to guilt, self-blame and feelings of hopelessness.
5 Stigmatization adheres to people with cancer and chronic diseases. This can be a heavy extra burden for victims to carry.
6 It is important to consider the needs of the family members of people with cancer and chronic diseases.

Cancer

1 Approximately one out of every two men and one out of every three women will have cancer during their lifetime.

(Continued)

(Continued)

2 Cancer occurs when cells keep dividing and forming more cells without internal control or order. This cell growth is known as a tumour or neoplasm and can be benign or malignant.
3 Treatment can aim to cure the cancer, control it, or treat its symptoms. The type of treatment depends on the type of cancer, the stage of the cancer, and individual factors such as age, health status and the personal preferences of the patient and his/her family. The patient ideally is empowered to discuss with the professionals the treatment choices.
4 The four major treatments for cancer are surgery, radiation, chemotherapy and biological therapies such as hormone therapies (e.g. tamoxifen) and transplant options (e.g. with bone marrow or stem cell therapy).
5 Interview and diary studies suggest common themes among long-term survivors: 'authenticity', 'autonomy' and 'acceptance'.

Coronary heart disease

1 CHD is a leading cause of death in western countries.
2 The two main forms of CHD are myocardial infarction and angina.
3 Decreases in the CHD death rates are mainly due to a reduction in major risk factors, principally smoking. Spending on primary prevention does not reflect this finding.
4 Seeking treatment for CHD can be stressful for both people with CHD and their family members. It is important to tailor the information about CHD to the needs of individual patients.
5 Psychological disease management can help angina patients to adjust but psychological services are currently patchy and inadequate.

HIV/AIDS

1 HIV/AIDS has become a worldwide pandemic that has infected around 60 million people, and become the fourth largest killer in the world. There are around 5 million new cases each year.
2 HIV (human immunodeficiency virus) is a retrovirus that infects and colonizes cells in the immune system and the central nervous system (T-helper and monocyte macrophage cells). Initial flu-like symptoms are followed by a quiescent, asymptomatic period (lasting years) during which the immune system battles the virus.
3 The most effective treatment consists of combination therapies (HAART), which have been shown to decrease an individual's HIV viral load to undetectable levels, reducing associated morbidity and mortality.
4 Adaptive coping strategies along with good social support can moderate the negative effects of stress. Finding meaning in the experience of HIV/AIDS has been associated with medication adherence, lower distress and perceived control.
5 Interventions that target adaptive coping skills, emotion work and increasing social support appear to be most effective in helping patients to adapt to living with their illness.

Glossary

ACE (Angiotensin Converting Enzyme) Inhibitor: a drug that is important in the regulation of blood pressure.

Action research: a type of research concerned with the process of change and what else happens when change occurs. Action research is particularly suitable for organizations or systems requiring improvement or change.

Acute: the early stages of a condition; a condition that lasts for less than six months.

Addiction: a term used to describe a person's physical and psychological dependency on an activity, drink or drug, seemingly beyond conscious control. Addiction is said to occur when there is: a strong desire to engage in the particular behaviour (especially when the opportunity to engage in such behaviour is not available); an impaired capacity to control the behaviour; discomfort and/or distress when the behaviour is prevented or ceased; persistence of the behaviour despite clear evidence that it is leading to problems.

Addiction theories: theories based on the construct of addiction used to explain alcoholism and other excessive behaviours (e.g. gambling, shopping, drug use, over-eating).

Adherence (or Compliance): the extent to which a person's behaviour changes as a direct consequence of specific social influence: e.g. a measure of the extent to which patients (or doctors) follow a prescribed treatment plan.

Adipose tissue: tissue in the body in which fat is stored as an energy reserve and which in excess leads to obesity.

Adiposity: the state of being obese.

African health beliefs: beliefs about the causes and correlates of health and illness in African cultures.

Agency: the psychological capacity to act autonomously and instrumentally.

AIDS (acquired immune deficiency syndrome): an advanced HIV infection that generally occurs when the CD4 lymphocyte count is below 200/ml. It is characterized by the appearance of opportunistic infections which take advantage of the weakened immune system due to the reduced number of T-helper cells and includes a variety of serious conditions: pneumocystis carinii pneumonia; toxoplasmosis; tuberculosis; extreme weight loss and wasting; exacerbated by diarrhoea; meningitis and other brain infections; fungal infections;

syphilis; malignancies such as lymphoma, cervical cancer and Kaposi's sarcoma. The virus is transmitted in bodily fluids such as semen and blood, through sexual intercourse, the use of contaminated hypodermic syringes, and placental transfer between mother and fetus. Antiviral drugs can decrease the viral load and subsequent infections in patients with AIDS.

Alcohol dependence syndrome: a psychophysiological disorder characterized by increased tolerance, withdrawal symptoms following reduced consumption, a persistent desire, or unsuccessful efforts to reduce or control drinking.

Angina: the most common form of coronary heart disease. It is characterized by a heavy or tight pain in the centre of the chest that may spread to the arms, neck, jaw, face, back or stomach. Angina symptoms occur when the arteries become so narrow from the *atheroma* that insufficient oxygen-containing blood can be supplied to the heart muscle when its demands are high, such as during exercise.

Angina Plan: a psychological intervention for angina patients. It consists of a patient-held booklet and audio-taped relaxation programme.

Anticipated Regret: the difference between the maximum value one could have achieved in hindsight and the actual value resulting from an action actually taken.

Anticoagulant drugs: drugs that prevent the clotting of blood.

Artefact (Artifact): an uncontrolled and possibly unknown variable or factor causing a misleading, spurious finding in a study.

Assessment: a procedure through which a patient, client, participant or situation can be evaluated against a benchmark or criterion enabling further actions or interventions to be administered, interpreted or understood.

Attitudes: the sum of beliefs about a particular behaviour weighted by evaluations of these beliefs.

Attribution theory: theory of lay causal explanations of events and behaviours.

Attributions: perceived or reported causes of actions, feelings or events.

Audience segmentation: a characteristic of social marketing whereby the target audience is classified into segments so that the intervention can be tailored accordingly.

Authoritarian: a personality type or leadership style favouring obedience rather than freedom of expression.

Autonomy: the capacity to make an informed decision without coercion from others. In health care, respect for the autonomy of patients is an important goal.

Ayurvedic medicine: an integrated system of medicine based on the achievement of balance in body, mind and spirit. This system evolved in India over thousands of years. Therapies used in Ayurvedic medicine are also used on their own as forms of Complementary and Alternative Medicine (CAM), e.g. herbs, massage and specialized diets.

Benign tumour: a growth which is not cancerous.

Betablockers: drugs that block the actions of the hormone adrenaline that makes the heart beat faster and more vigorously.

Between groups design: a research design involving two or more matched groups of participants that receive different conditions, for example, an intervention versus a control condition.

Biomedicine: a health system which identifies the cause of agreed diseases and symptoms as lying in certain physiological processes.

Biopsychosocial model: the view that health and illness are produced by a combination of physical, psychological and cultural factors (Engel, 1977).

Black Report: a report on health inequalities published in the UK in 1980 named after the chairman of the committee who produced the report, Sir Douglas Black.

Body image: the image a person has of her/his own body; a person's perception of their own physical appearance.

Body mass index (BMI): the body weight in kilograms divided by the square of the height in metres; has a normal range of 20 to 25.

Bottom-up: listening to people about what they perceive their needs to be and acting upon that information together in an attempt to meet those needs.

Built Environment: the environment created by humans that provides the setting for human activity, including large-scale civic surroundings, skyscrapers, houses, huts, shanty towns, shops, parks, docks, roads, rubbish dumps, and all other places and spaces created by human intervention.

Bupropion: an antidepressant used both for smoking cessation (Zyban) and for treating depression (Wellbutrin) which blocks the reuptake of dopamine.

Burden of disease: a concept referring to the overall costs associated with a disease measured by the economic, social and psychological resources that are expended during care, treatment and rehabilitation.

Capacity building: an activity or action designed to increase the resources available to tackle a problem.

Carcinogen: any substance that causes cancer.

Case studies: retrospective written reports on individuals, groups or systems.

Case-control study: an epidemiological study in which exposure of patients to factors that may cause their disease (cases) is compared to the exposure to the same factors of participants who do not have the disease (controls).

Catastrophizing: the tendency to become emotional and pessimistic about symptoms, illness or difficulties.

Cause: (1) a reason for an action or condition; (2) something that brings about an effect or a result; (3) a person or event or action that brings something about; (4) personal ideas about aetiology which may include simple single causes or more complex multiple causal models.

Cessation: the process of stopping (ceasing) a specific behaviour, habit or activity; one possible outcome of the *action stage* in the *transtheoretical model of change.*

Chinese medicine: an ancient Chinese system of healing that focuses on achieving internal balance. Practitioners use acupuncture, heat application (moxibustion), herbal preparations, food therapy, massage and exercise (Qi Gong or Tai Chi) to restore the flow of Qi (vital energy) and the balance of Yin and Yang.

Chlamydia: a common sexually transmitted infection (STI) caused by the bacterium, *Chlamydia trachomatis*, which can damage a woman's reproductive organs. Even though symptoms of chlamydia are usually mild or absent, serious complications that cause irreversible damage, including infertility, can occur 'silently' before a woman ever recognizes a problem. Chlamydia also can cause discharge from the penis of an infected man.

Cholesterol: a lipid produced in the body from acetyl-CoA and present in the diet.

Chronic: any condition that continues for at least six months.

Chronic fatigue syndrome (CFS): a syndrome identified in Nevada, USA, 1984, characterized by severe fatigue and other symptoms suggesting a viral infection and persisting over long periods of time. There is much controversy as to whether it is a *psychosomatic disorder* or caused by an as-yet-unidentified virus. CFS is thought to be identical to *myalgic encephalomyelitis (ME).*

Civic literacy: refers to skills that enable people to become aware of public issues and to be involved in the decision-making process.

Classical conditioning: a learning process whereby a previously neutral stimulus (*conditioned stimulus, CS)* comes to evoke a certain response (*conditioned response, CR*) as a result of repeated previous pairings with a stimulus (*unconditioned stimulus, UCS*) which naturally evokes the response (*unconditioned response, UCR*).

Cognitions: thoughts, beliefs and images forming the elements of a person's knowledge concerning the physical and psychosocial environment.

Cognitive-behavioural therapy (CBT): modification of thoughts, images, feelings and behaviour using the principles of *classical* and *operant conditioning* combined with cognitive techniques concerned with the control of mental states.

Common sense: practical, everyday judgement by the common person.

Communitarianism: set of principles that emphasizes the need to balance individual rights and interests with those of the community as a whole, emphasizes the importance of social institutions in the development of individual meaning and identity.

Community: (1) A group of people living in the same locality and under the same government; (2) The district or locality in which such a group lives; (3) A group of people having common interests: *the scientific community; the medical community;* (4) A group viewed as forming a distinct segment of society: *the gay community; the White community; the disabled community.*

Community arts: the application of art and performance directed towards social change.

Community development: the process of helping a community to strengthen itself and develop towards its full potential.

Compensatory conditioned response model: influential model put forward by Siegel (1975) to account for the phenomena of addiction, such as tolerance, dependence and withdrawal, using the principles of *classical conditioning.*

Complementary and alternative medicine (CAM): refers to all non-conventional practices and ideas that aim to prevent or treat illness or promote health and well-being.

Compliance (or adherence): the extent to which a person's behaviour changes as a direct consequence of specific social influence: e.g. a measure of the extent to which patients (or doctors) follow a prescribed treatment plan.

Concordance: model of physician–patient relationship based upon mutual respect and involvement in treatment.

Conditioned stimulus (CS): a stimulus that, because of pairing with another stimulus (*unconditioned stimulus, UCS*) which naturally evokes a reflex response, is eventually able to evoke that response (see *classical conditioning*). The acquisition is believed to occur when there is a positive contingency between two events such that event A is more likely in the presence of event B than in the absence of B.

Conditioning: processes of associating stimuli and responses (see classical conditioning and operant conditioning) producing learning and experience.

Confidence interval: a 95 per cent confidence interval contains the true parameter value on 95 per cent of the occasions that the interval is calculated.

Consequence: the expected effects and outcome of an illness.

Control group: a group of participants assigned to a condition that does not include the specific treatment being evaluated; used for comparative purposes.

Coronary angiogram: an X-ray of the arteries to help to see if any of the arteries are blocked by atheroma.

Coronary artery bypass graft (CABG): an operation that enables a blocked area of the coronary artery to be bypassed so that blood flow can be restored to heart tissue that has been deprived of blood because of coronary heart disease (CHD). During CABG, a healthy artery or vein is taken from the leg, arm, or chest and transferred to the outside of the heart. The new healthy artery or vein then carries the oxygenated blood around the blockage in the coronary artery.

Coronary heart disease (CHD): restriction of the blood flow to the coronary arteries often evidenced by chest pains (angina) and which may result in a heart attack.

Cortisol: also known as hydrocortisone, is a corticosteroid hormone produced by the adrenal cortex, a part of the adrenal gland. It is released in response to stress.

Critical health literacy: the ability to critically evaluate and use information to actively participate in health promotion.

Cross-over or within-participants design: a research design in which participants are placed in two or more conditions; in theory, participants 'act as their own controls'. However, there are sequence effects, practice effects, and other issues that make this design more complicated.

Cross-sectional designs (studies): involve obtaining responses from a sample of respondents on one occasion only. With appropriate randomized sampling methods, the sample can be assumed to be a representative cross-section of the population(s) under study and it will be possible to make comparisons between different sub-groups, e.g. males vs. females, older vs. younger, etc.

Cultural literacy: the ability to recognize and use collective beliefs, customs, worldview and social identity to interpret and act on health information.

Culturally competent health-care systems: health-care systems that have mechanisms in place to adapt to diverse cultural populations.

Culture: a system of meanings and symbols that defines a worldview that frames the way people locate themselves within the world, perceive the world, and find meaning within it.

Cure/Control: beliefs concerning how one recovers from, or controls, an illness.

Death gradient: the variation in mortality that occurs across a population when the population is segmented according to socio-economic status such that the mortality rate is higher among those groups which have lower socio-economic status.

Decisional balance: comparative potential gains and losses. Two decisional balance measures, the *pros* and the *cons*, are constructs in the Transtheoretical Model. The *pros* and *cons* combine to form a decisional 'balance sheet' of comparative potential gains and losses.

Deficit model: an explanation used by health-care professionals to account for low compliance, e.g. women who do not use a screening service may be characterized as lacking in knowledge and concern about their health.

Diary techniques: any data collection method in which the data are linked to the passage of time. They often involve self-report but may also contain information about observations of others.

Direct observation: directly observing behaviour in a relevant setting, e.g. patients waiting for treatment in a doctor's surgery or clinic. The observation may be accompanied by recordings in written, oral, auditory or visual form. Includes casual observation, formal observation and participant observation.

Disability (= disablement): (1) 'A physical or mental impairment that substantially limits one or more major life activities, a record of such impairment, or a perception of such 'impairment' (2) 'Any physical and/or mental impairment that substatially limits one or more of the major life activities (caring for one's self, walking, seeing, hearing, and the like)' (The Americans with Disabilities Act, 1990).

Disability-adjusted life year (DALY): the total amount of healthy life lost, to all causes, whether from premature mortality or from some degree of disability during a period of time. The DALY is the sum of years of life lost from premature mortality plus years of life with disability, adjusted for severity of disability from all causes, both physical and mental (Murray and Lopez, 1997).

Disablement (= Disability): see above.

Discourse: talk or text embedded in social interaction presenting an account of the constitution of subjects and objects; an opinion or position concerning a particular subject.

Discourse analysis: a set of procedures for analysing language as used in speech or texts. It has links with ethnomethodology, conversation analysis and the study of meaning (semiology).

Disease theories: the idea that the control of behaviour such as alcohol consumption or eating is a disease based on personal or inherited characteristics that predispose particular individuals to the condition (e.g. alcoholism or obesity).

Distal: situated farthest away from point of origin, as of an influence or a limb.

Doctor-centred communication style: a communication style which primarily makes use of the doctor's expertise by keeping control of the interview agenda.

Dopamine: a monoamine neurotransmitter found in the brain and essential for the normal functioning of the central nervous system. Bodily functions affected by dopamine include mood, sleep, learning and voluntary movements. Dopamine is available as a medication.

Dorsal Horn: one of the two roots of a spinal nerve that passes dorsally to the spinal cord consisting of sensory fibres.

Ecological approach: a model or theory about health and behaviour that emphasizes environmental influences.

Ecological validity: the extent to which the environment within which behaviour or experience is studied captures the relevant features of the real-world environment.

Effect size: The effect size is a standardized measure of the effect of an intervention (treatment) on outcomes. The effect size represents the change (measured in standard deviations) in an outcome that can be expected if that patient is given the treatment.

Effort-Reward Balance: an imbalance between high efforts and low rewards (e.g. salary, promotion prospects, appreciation, respect, and job security) increases risk of ill-health. A possible risk factor for cardiovascular disease and mental disorders.

E-health: the application of information and communication technology to health or health care.

Electrocardiogram (ECG): a physiological measure used to examine the electrical activity of the heart.

Empowerment: any process by which people, groups or communities can exercise increased control or sense of control over aspects of their everyday lives, including their physical and social environments.

Energy expenditure: use by the body of chemical energy from food and drink or body stores during the processes of metabolism that is dissipated as heat, including heat generated by muscular activity; the day's total energy expenditure is measured in calories of heat lost.

Energy intake: the chemical energy in food and drink that can be metabolized to produce energy in the body; the day's total energy intake is measured in calories supplied by all food and drink consumed.

Epidemiology: the study of their association with patterns of disease in populations and environmental, lifestyle and genetic factors. One basis for scientific or evidence-based medecine.

Ethnicity: pertaining to ethnic group or race.

Ethnocentrism: a bias in perception, thinking or principles stemming from membership of a particular ethnic or cultural group.

Ethnographic methods: seek to build a systematic understanding of a culture from the viewpoint of the insider. Ethnographic methods are multiple attempts to describe the shared beliefs, practices, artefacts, knowledge and behaviours of an intact cultural group. They attempt to represent the totality of a phenomenon in its complete context and naturalistic setting.

Exchange: a characteristic of social marketing which considers the costs and benefits of behaviour change to its target audience.

Exercise tolerance test (ETT): the recording of the heart's electrical activity while it is under the stress of increased physical demand.

Fat: *triglycerides* that are either solid (e.g. butter, lard) or liquid (e.g. vegetable or fish oil) at room temperature.

Fat balance equation: states that the rate of change of fat stores equals the rate of fat intake minus the rate of fat oxidation.

Fetal alcohol syndrome: abnormality found in children whose mothers drink heavily during pregnancy, characterized by facial abnormalities, mental impairment and stunted growth.

Focus groups: discussions in which participants focus collectively upon a topic or issue usually presented to them as a group of questions (or other stimuli) leading to the generation of interactive data.

Functional health literacy: the basic reading and writing skills that can help individuals to function effectively in the health-care context.

Fundamental literacy: reading, writing, speaking and numeracy skills.

Gain-framed appeals: information about a health behaviour that emphasizes the benefits of taking action.

Galenic medicine: health system derived from Greek and Arabic health beliefs.

Gate control theory (GCT): a theory that views pain as a perceptual experience, in which ascending physiological inputs and descending psychological inputs are equally involved. It posits a gating mechanism in the dorsal horn of the spinal cord that permits or inhibits the transmission of pain impulses to the brain.

General adaptation syndrome (GAS): influential three-stage model of the physiological response to stress put forward by Hans Selye but no longer thought to be valid.

Global burden of disease (GBD): the universal totality of economic, social and psychological costs of a disease attributable to both morbidity and mortality over a fixed interval of time.

Gonorrhoea: a sexually transmitted disease (STI) caused by *Neisseria gonorrhoeae*, a bacterium that can grow and multiply easily in the warm, moist areas of the reproductive tract, including the cervix (opening to the womb), uterus (womb), and fallopian tubes (egg canals) in women, and in the urethra (urine canal) in women and men. The bacterium can also grow in the mouth, throat, eyes and anus.

Gradient of reinforcement: principle applied mainly to *operant conditioning* whereby the acquisition of a learned response occurs more quickly, the more rapidly reward follows the occurrence of the response.

Grass roots: a movement founded in groups of local people working cooperatively to achieve greater well-being.

Gross national income (GNI): the total net value of all goods and services produced within a nation over a specified period of time, representing the sum of wages, profits, rents, interest and pension payments to residents of the nation.

Grounded theory analysis: an analysis of transcripts involving coding followed by the generation of categories, using constant comparative analysis within and between interview transcripts. This is followed by memo-writing which requires the researcher to expand upon the meaning of the broader conceptual categories. This in turn can lead to further data generation through theoretical sampling.

Hardiness: personality trait first proposed by Kobasa and consisting of a high level of commitment, sense of control and willingness to confront challenges. Hardiness may protect the individual against the effects of stress.

Hassles scale: life events stress scale designed by Kanner and associates and focusing on everyday events that cause annoyance or frustration. See also *uplifts scale* and *social readjustment rating scale (SRRS)*.

HDL Cholesterol: the cholesterol in high-density lipoproteins; often assumed to be 'good' cholesterol as it reduces fatty deposits (atheroma) in arteries.

Health Belief Model (HBM): psychological model which posits that health behaviour is a function of a combination of factors including the perceived benefits of and barriers to treatment and the perceived susceptibility to and seriousness of the health problem.

Health belief systems: ways of thinking about the causes of health and illness.

Health communication: (1) all interpersonal, organizational or mass communication that concerns health; (2) the field of study concerned with the ways in which communication can contribute to the promotion of health.

Health gradient: the relationship between *socio-economic status (SES)* and mortality or morbidity that normally shows a monotonic increase as SES changes from low to high.

Health literacy: the ability to read and understand information about health and healthcare enabling an individual to take decisions about treatment and prevention.

Health promotion: any event, process or activity which facilitates the protection or improvement of the health of individuals, groups, communities or populations.

High Demand: often linked to stress, a cause of strain on the mind or body.

Historical analysis: the use of data produced from memory, historical sources or artefacts.

HIV (human immunodeficiency virus): the virus that causes acquired immune deficiency syndrome (AIDS); it replicates in and kills the helper T cells. This virus is passed from one person to another through blood-to-blood and sexual contact. In addition, infected pregnant women can pass HIV to their baby during pregnancy or delivery, as well as through breast-feeding. The prevalence of HIV/AIDS in Sub-Saharan Africa was 22.4 million by the end of 2008.

Hypercholesterolemia: the presence of high levels of cholesterol in the blood.

Hysteria (conversion hysteria): physical symptoms which appear to indicate organic disease but where there is no clinical evidence of disease. Believed by some practitioners to be psychologically caused although this is normally denied vehemently by sufferers.

Iatrogenesis: health problems caused by medical or health-care interventions including accidents, inappropriate treatments, incorrect diagnoses, drug side-effects and other problems.

Identity: (1) the collective set of characteristics by which a thing is definitively recognizable or known; (2) the distinctive personality and character of a person; (3) the label of an illness and the symptoms the patient views as being part of the disease.

Illness Perception Questionnaire: a questionnaire used to measure five themes or components which are believed to make up a patient's perception of their illness: identity; cause; time line; consequences; cure-control.

Imagery: quasi-perceptual mental representations of activities, states, persons, objects or conditions in the absence of perception. May be used in therapy to facilitate behaviour change.

Immunization: medical procedure designed to protect susceptible individuals from communicable diseases by the administration of a vaccine. This procedure is aimed at both immediate protection of individuals and also immunity across the whole community where the uptake rate is high.

Incidence: the rate at which new cases of a disease occur in a population during a specified period. In the simplest terms, for example, the incidence of STIs in 2008 was 200 cases per 10,000 people per year in Newtown compared with 150 cases per 10,000 people per year in Oldtown.

Indigenous: belonging to a particular culture, race or tribal group.

Indigenous health: the health of indigenous people.

Individualism: a cultural value that enshrines the personal control and responsibility of the individual.

Interactive health literacy: personal skills that enable individuals to act independently based on knowledge to promote health.

Internal validity: the degree to which the results of a study can be attributed to the manipulations of the researchers and are likely to be free of bias.

Interpretative phenomenological analysis (IPA): a technique for analysing qualitative data which seeks the meaning of experience.

Intervention mix: a characteristic of social marketing where a variety of interventions or methods are used to achieve its goals.

Intervention(s): the intentional and systematic manipulation of variables with the aim of improving health outcomes.

Interviews (structured or semi-structured): a structured interview schedule is a prepared standard set of questions which are asked in person, or perhaps by telephone, of a person or group of persons concerning a particular research issue or question. A semi-structured interview is much more open ended and allows the interviewee scope to address the issues which he/she feels to be relevant to the topics being raised by the investigator.

Ischaemic heart disease: Coronary artery disease is created by a gradual accumulation of fatty deposits (atheroma) in the cells lining the wall of the coronary arteries. These fatty deposits build up in the large branches of the two main coronary arteries which encircle, and are the main source of blood to, the heart. This narrowing or hardening of the blood vessels supplying blood to the heart muscle (the coronary arteries) is called atherosclerosis. The inability to provide adequate oxygen to heart muscle can damage the heart muscle, which is termed 'ischemia'. A total blockage of a blood vessel causes a heart attack (myocardial infarction or 'MI').

Job security: the probability that an individual will keep his or her job.

Ladder of participation: a way of representing the different levels of involvement or engagement of one individual or group in an activity or process of change.

LDL Cholesterol: the cholesterol in low-density lipoproteins; the so-called 'bad' cholesterol; a high level in the blood is thought to be related to various pathogenic conditions.

Leptin: a protein hormone that plays a role in regulating energy intake and energy expenditure, including appetite and metabolism.

Life Events and Difficulties Schedule (LEDS): a psychological measurement of the stressfulness of life events, created by Brown and Harris in 1978. The schedule is based upon an interview which discusses the contextual information around the event.

Liver cirrhosis: frequently fatal form of liver damage usually found among long-term heavy drinkers. Initially fat accumulates on the liver, enlarging it; this restricts blood flow, causing damage to cells, and scar tissue develops, preventing the liver from functioning normally.

Locus of control: personality traits first proposed by social psychologists and then adapted by health psychologists to distinguish between those who attribute their state of health to themselves, powerful others or chance.

Longitudinal designs: involve measuring responses of a single sample on more than one occasion. These measurements may be prospective or retrospective, but prospective longitudinal designs allow greater control over the sample, the variables measured and the times when the measurements take place.

Loss-framed appeals: information about a health behaviour that emphasizes the costs of failing to take action.

Low control: associated with stress, an ability to control demands.

Mammography: a method for imaging breast tissue of women using radiography for detecting early signs of breast cancer.

Medical error: errors in medical diagnosis and treatment.

Medical model: a way of thinking about health and illness that assumes all health and illness phenomena are physiological in nature. According to this model, health, illness and treatments have a purely biological or biochemical basis.

Medicalization: the process by which experiences and practices which do not match those defined as 'natural' and 'healthy' are pathologized and treated as dysfunctional.

Message framing: how information is presented to influence individuals' behavioural decisions.

Meta-analysis: a quantitative literature review that combines the evidence from relevant previous studies, taking account of criteria for quality, allowing high statistical power.

Metastasis: the spread of cancer cells to secondary sites in the body.

Motivational interviewing: brief intervention developed by W.R. Miller for the treatment of alcohol and drug problems, which aims to boost the client's self esteem and motivation to change, in contrast to traditional confrontational approaches.

Multidimensional Health Locus of Control (MHLC) Scale: a popular scale for distinguishing between those who attribute their state of health to themselves, powerful others or chance, originally developed by Wallston et al. (1978).

Myalgic encephalomyelitis (ME): syndrome first observed in an epidemic at the Royal Free Hospital, London, in 1955, now usually thought to be identical to *chronic fatigue syndrome* and controversial for the same reasons.

Myocardial infarction (MI): a form of *coronary heart disease* (CHD) or 'heart attack' that occurs when one of the coronary arteries becomes blocked by a blood clot and part of the heart is starved of oxygen. It usually causes severe chest pain. MI is often the first sign of CHD in many people.

Narrative: structured discourse which connects agents and events over time in the form of a story.

Narrative approaches: set of theories derived from hermeneutic phenomenology that argue that our interpretation of the changing world is organised in narrative form. Narratives can be both personal or shared within a group, organization or society.

Nicotine: an alkaloid found in tobacco with highly addictive properties.

Nicotine Replacement Therapy: a method of smoking cessation that involves the administration of nicotine transdermally (patches) or orally (gum, lozenges or spray).

Obesification: the production of obesity.

Obesity: an excessive accumulation of body fat, usually defined as a body mass index (BMI) greater than 30.

Obesogenic (environment): referring to an environment that exposes the population to, and actively promotes, a large number of foods and drinks that have a high percentage of fats.

Observational studies: a method of data collection using direct observation under field conditions.

Odds ratio: the ratio of the odds of having or being in a condition X in a treatment group relative to the odds of having or being in a condition X in the control group.

Operant conditioning: a learning process whereby a normally voluntary form of behaviour comes to occur with increasing frequency in a particular situation, or in the presence of a particular stimulus, as a result of previously and repeatedly having been rewarded in similar circumstances.

Opportunistic intervention: an attempt to modify health hazardous behaviour, such as smoking or heavy drinking, by a health professional, frequently a doctor, who has been consulted for other reasons.

Participatory action research: is a form of action research that engages its participants in all stages of the research process

Patient informatics: a programme that aims to enable patients to make better use of information and communication technology for health and health care.

Patient satisfaction: a measure of the extent to which patients' expectations of what a medical encounter ought to provide have been met (as judged by the patients).

Patient-centred (communication style): a doctor's communication style which mobilizes the patient's knowledge, experience and involvement through techniques such as silence, listening and reflection.

Perceived barriers: an individual's assessment of the influences that facilitate or discourage adoption of a promoted behaviour.

Perceived benefits: an individual's assessment of the positive consequences of adopting a health protecting behaviour.

Perceived control: the feeling of having control over one's actions in response to others and the environment.

Perceived severity: an individual's assessment of the seriousness of the condition, and its potential consequences.

Perceived susceptibility: an individual's assessment of their risk of getting the condition.

Percutaneous coronary intervention (PCI): a procedure that unblocks narrowed coronary arteries without performing surgery. This may be done with either a balloon catheter to push the atheroma to the side of the artery or a stent inserted to keep the artery open.

Pessimistic explanatory style: tendency of some individuals to blame themselves for everything that goes wrong in their lives, believed to be associated with poor physical health.

Phenomenological: (1) a method of inquiry based on the assumption that reality consists of objects and events as they are perceived or understood in human consciousness and not of anything independent of human consciousness; (2) a movement based on this method, originated by Edmund Husserl.

Photovoice: a method that enables people to define for themselves and others, including policy makers, what is worth remembering and what needs to be changed.

Physical activity: any movement of the body.

Physical dependence: a state resulting from chronic drug or tobacco use that has produced tolerance and will, when usage is reduced or ceased, cause negative physical symptoms of withdrawal.

Placebo: a treatment that consists of nothing other than a simulation of the active treatment, used as a control condition in studies or as a treatment when no better option exists.

Placebo control: a control condition that appears similar to a treatment when in fact it is completely inert.

Positivism: the epistemological position which places scientific method as the sole source of reliable knowledge.

Post-traumatic stress disorder (PTSD): long-term psychological and physiological effects of exposure to traumatic stress, including insomnia, nightmares, flashbacks, problems of memory and concentration, acting or feeling as if the event is recurring and a greatly increased sensitivity to new stressful events.

Poverty: the level of income below which people cannot afford a minimum, nutritionally adequate diet and essential non-food requirements.

Prevalence: the number of people with a disease or behaviour as a proportion of the population or sub-population at any point in time.

Prospect theory: the theory that influenced message framing in health promotion which proposes that people consider their 'prospects' (i.e. potential gains and losses) when making a decision.

Proximal: situated closest to the point of origin, as of an influence or a limb.

Psychological dependency (dependence): a state associated with repeated activity or consumption of a drug or drink which leads to negative affect following reduced consumption or abstinence and a persistent desire or unsuccessful efforts to cut down or control the activity.

Psychoneuroimmunology (PNI): the study of the effects of psychological variables and especially stress on the immune system.

Psycho-oncology: the psychological aspects of cancer care and treatment.

Psychosocial explanations: accounts of events and experiences based on theories and research from psychology and the social sciences.

Psychosomatic (or somatoform) disorders: physical ailments believed to be psychologically caused including *hysteria* and some conditions which have organic features such as ulcers and asthma.

Psychosomatic medicine: a precursor of modern health psychology which flourished from the 1930s to the 1950s, its proponents, including Alexander and Dunbar, believed that psychoanalytic theories about unconscious conflicts could be extended to explain susceptibility to various organic diseases.

Quasi-experimental design: comparison of two or more treatments in as controlled a manner as possible but without the possibility of manipulating an independent variable or randomly allocating participants.

Questionnaires: many constructs in health psychology are measured using questionnaires consisting of a standard set of items with accompanying instructions. Ideally a questionnaire will have been demonstrated to be both a reliable and valid measure of the construct(s) it purports to measure.

Racism: discriminatory beliefs or behaviour against people on the basis of race or skin colour.

Randomized controlled trial(s) (RCTs): these involve the systematic comparison of interventions employing a fully controlled application of one or more interventions or 'treatments' using a random allocation of participants to the different treatment groups.

Reactance theory: a theory concerning the tendency to resist attempts by others to control one's behaviour.

Readability tests: statistical tests used to measure how difficult or easy materials are to read.

Relapse: going back to consumption of tobacco, alcohol or a drug after a period of voluntary abstinence.

Restenosis: coronary artery blockage that occurs following *percutaneous coronary intervention (PCI)*.

Revascularization: a term that describes surgical and catheter procedures that are used to restore blood flow to the heart.

Scientific literacy: competence with fundamental scientific concepts, comprehension of technological complexity, scientific uncertainty, and an understanding that rapid change in the accepted science is possible.

Screening: procedure for the identification of the presence of certain diseases, conditions or behaviours in a community. Those sections of the population who are most at risk of developing a particular disease are examined to see whether they have any early indications. The rationale behind this strategy is that the earlier the disease is identified and treated, the less likely it is to develop into a fatal condition.

Secondhand smoke: smoke produced by cigarette smoking, inhaled by people who are not themselves actively smoking; carcinogenic.

Sedentary: inactive.

Self-concept: a person's beliefs about her/himself.

Self-determination: engaging in activities for their enjoyment or intrinsic motivation.

Self-efficacy: belief that one will be able to carry out one's plans successfully, a personality trait originally proposed by Albert Bandura (1977) and thought to be associated with positive health behaviours.

Self-regulation: process by which individuals monitor and adjust their medication on an ongoing basis.

Self-regulatory model: this model suggests that health-related practices or coping responses are influenced by patients' beliefs or representations of the illness. These illness representations have a certain structure.

Selfways: the way a culture represents human personality.

Sensation seeking: a personality trait or type that is characterized by a strong desire for new sensations.

Sense of coherence: a personality trait originally proposed by Antonovsky (1979) to characterize people who see their world as essentially meaningful and manageable; associated with coping with stress.

Sense of community: a feeling that one belongs to a group located in space and time with a common identity, history and culture.

Sexual behaviour: any activity which arouses sexual arousal for pleasure or procreation.

Sexually transmitted infections (STIs): infections that can be transferred from one person to another through sexual contact through vaginal or anal intercourse, kissing, oral-genital contact, and the use of sexual 'toys', such as vibrators.

Single case experimental designs: investigations of a series of experimental manipulations on a single research participant.

Social capital: the institutions, relationships and norms that shape the quality and quantity of a society's social interactions. Social capital is not just the sum of the institutions which underpin a society – it is the glue that holds them together.

Social cognition: a cognitive model of social knowledge.

Social cognition models (SCMs): theories about the relationship between social cognitions, such as beliefs and attitudes, and behaviour, which aim accurately to predict behaviour or behavioural intentions.

Social constructionism: set of theories that consider how our reality is constructed in everyday social interaction.

Social Darwinism: the concept that competition among all individuals, groups, nations or ideas drives social evolution in human societies.

Social inequality: being treated differently as a consequence of age, race, gender, disability, sexual preference or other attribute.

Social justice: the process of treating a person, group or community fairly and equally.

Social marketing: the application of consumer-oriented marketing techniques in the design, implementation and evaluation of programmes aimed to influence behaviour change for public benefit.

Social readjustment rating scale (SRRS): measurement scale for life events stress developed by Holmes and Rahe and widely used in research on life events stress and illness. See also *hassles scale* and *uplifts scale*.

Social representations (SRs): system of ideas, values and practices specific to a particular community which enables individuals to orient themselves in the world and communicate with each other.

Social representation theory: a theory concerning a system of ideas, values and practices specific to a particular social community.

Social support: informal and formal supportive relationships.

Socio-economic status (SES): position or class based on occupation, education or income.

Specificity Theory: the idea that pain is the result of stimulating a particular kind of neurone.

Spirituality: beyond body and mind, a feeling that nature, the world, the mind, and the body, are an incomplete description of reality.

Statins: drugs used to reduce cholesterol levels.

Stigma: the process of marginalizing a group or class of people by labelling them as different and understanding them in terms of stereotypes and resulting in a loss of social status and discrimination, affecting many areas of life.

Stigmatization: being treated as an object of derision and shame purely as a consequence of others' ignorance and prejudice.

Stress: ambiguous term, sometimes used to refer to environmental pressure and sometimes to a particular type of response to pressure. Currently it is often used to describe an inner state which can occur when either real or perceived demands exceed either the real or the perceived capacity to cope with them.

Stress innoculation training: a self-instructional *cognitive-behavioural* method for stress management developed by Meichenbaum (1985) focusing on changing the way in which participants appraise situations as stressful and cope with stressful events.

Stress management workshops: training programmes in stress management usually delivered to groups, frequently lasting for a whole day or a weekend, and focusing on changing the way in which participants appraise situations as stressful and cope with stressful events.

Subjective norms: the beliefs of other people about the importance of carrying out a behaviour.

Sudden Infant Death Syndrome (SIDS): otherwise known as 'crib' or 'cot death', the sudden and unexpected death of an apparently healthy infant during sleep.

Surveys: systematic methods for determining how a defined sample of participants respond to a set of standard questions attempting to assess their feelings, attitudes, beliefs or knowledge at one or more particular times.

Syphilis: a chronic infectious disease caused by a spirochete *(Treponema pallidum)*, transmitted by direct contact, usually in sexual intercourse, or passed from mother to child in utero, and progressing through three stages characterized respectively by local formation of chancres, ulcerous skin eruptions, and systemic infection leading to general paresis.

Systematic review: review of the empirical literature concerning the efficacy or effectiveness of an intervention that considers all of the relevant studies taking account of quality criteria.

Systems theory approach: a theory concerned with the contextual structures, processes or relationships within communities, groups or families.

Tautological: an empty statement consisting of simpler statements that make it logically true whether the simpler statements are true or false, e.g. the statement: *Either I will wear a condom the next time I have sexual intercourse or I will not.*

Temperance societies: originating in the USA in the nineteenth century, these societies, of which Alcoholics Anonymous is an example, are dedicated to counteracting the harmful effects of drinking, usually advocating teetotalism.

Time line: how long the patient believes an illness will last: acute, chronic or episodic.

Top-down: controlled, directed, or organized from the top using a preconceived theory or model about the processes that are expected to occur.

Toxic environment: a term referring to environmental and social conditions that promote disease, disorder and death.

Triglyceride: the main component of dietary fats and oils and the principal form in which fat is stored in the body; composed of three fatty acids attached to a glycerol molecule which are saturated, monounsaturated and polyunsaturated.

Tumour (benign or malignant): an abnormal new mass of tissue that serves no purpose. A tumour may be malignant or non-malignant depending on whether it is life-threatening or not.

Type A/B personality: the Type A personality, in contrast to the Type B personality, is characterized by intense achievement motivation, time urgency and hostility.

Uplifts scale: life events scale designed by Kanner and associates (1981) to assess desirable events in contrast to their *hassles scale.*

Upstream: the use of policy solutions to change the social, economic, political and community conditions that improve health and well-being.

Varenicline: a prescription medication used to treat smoking addiction.

Viral challenge studies: method of studying the relationship between stress and susceptibility to infectious disease in which volunteers are deliberately exposed to minor viruses, usually colds or flu, to determine whether those who have experienced higher levels of stress prior to exposure are more likely to contract the infection.

Wholistic: a term applied to concepts, systems or methods of health care that assumes that the person should be the target for treatment, not illness.

'Will-Power': a term applied to a person's strength of will to carry out a decision or action.

References

Abraham, C. & Sheeran, P. (2004). Deciding to exercise: the role of anticipated regret. *British Journal of Health Psychology, 9*, 269–278.

Academy of Medical Sciences (2004). *Calling time: the nations drinking as a major health issue.* London: The Academy of Medical Sciences. Washington, DC: Academy Press.

Acheson, D., Barker, D. & Chambers, J. et al. (1998). *Independent inquiry into inequalities in health report.* London: The Stationery Office.

Action on Smoking & Health (2008). *Beyond smoking kills: protecting children, reducing inequalities.* London: Action on Smoking & Health (accessed 4 January 2010 at http://www.ash.org.uk/files/documents/ASH_691/ASH_691.html).

Action on Smoking & Health (2010). *Tobacco explained. The truth about the tobacco industry…in its own words*. Accessed 3 January 2010 at http://old.ash.org.uk/html/conduct/html/tobexpld0.html.

Ad Hoc Committee on Health Literacy (1999). Health literacy: Report of the Council on Scientific Affairs, American Medical Association, *Journal of the American Medical Association, 281*, 552–557.

Adams, S., Pill, R. & Jones, A. (1997). Medication, chronic illness and identity: the perspective of people with asthma. *Social Science & Medicine, 45*, 189–201.

Adams, G. & Salter, P.S. (2007). Health psychology in African settings. A cultural-psychological analysis. *Journal of Health Psychology, 12*, 539–551.

Adler, N.E. & Matthews, K.A. (1994). Health psychology: why do some people get sick and some stay well. *Annual Review of Psychology, 45*, 229–259.

Agostinelli, G. & Grube, J.W. (2002). Alcohol counter-advertising and the media. *Alcohol Research & Health, 26*, 15–21.

AIESEC International (2009). 50% of young people admit they don't know enough about HIV and AIDS. (Accessed on 1 January 2010 at http://www.aiesec.org/cms/aiesec/AI/press.ht.

Airaksinen, O., Brox, J.I., Cedraschi, C., Hildebrandt, J., Klaber-Moffett, J., Kovacs, F., & Zanoli, G. (2006). Chapter 4 – European guidelines for the management of chronic nonspecific low back pain. *European Spine Journal, 15*, S192–S300.

Ajzen, I. (1985). From intention to actions: a theory of planned behavior. In J. Kuhl & J. Beckmann (Eds.), *Action-control: From cognition to behavior*. Heidelberg: Springer. Pp. 11–39.

Ajzen, I. (1991). The theory of planned behavior. *Organizational Behavior & Human Decision Processes, 50*, 179–211.

Ajzen, I. & Fishbein, M. (1980). *Understanding attitudes and predicting social behavior*. Englewood Cliffs, NJ: Prentice-Hall.

Albarracín, D., Gillette, J.C., Earl, A.N., Glasman, L.R., Durantini, M.R. & Ho, M.-H. (2005). A test of major assumptions about behavior change: a comprehensive look at the effects of passive & active HIV-prevention interventions since the beginning of the epidemic. *Psychological Bulletin, 131*, 856–897.

Albarracín, D., Johnson, B.T., Fishbein, M. & Muellerleile, P.A. (2001). Theories of reasoned action and planned behavior as models of condom use: a meta-analysis. *Psychological Bulletin, 127*, 142–161.

Aldwin, C.M. & Park, C.L. (2004). Coping and physical health outcomes: an overview. *Psychology & Health, 19*, 277–281.

Alexander, F. (1950). *Psychosomatic medicine*. New York: Norton.

Allebeck, P., Bolund, C. & Ringback, G. (1989). Increased suicide rate in cancer patients: a cohort study based on the Swedish cancer-environment register. *Journal of Clinical Epidemiology, 42*, 611–616.

American Cancer Society (2003). *Cancer Facts & Figures*. Atlanta: Georgia.

American Cancer Society (2009). *Cancer Facts & Figures*. Atlanta: Georgia.

American College Health Association (2005). *American College Health Association – National College Health Assessment (ACHA-NCHA)*. Web Summary at http://www.acha-ncha.org/data_highlights.html.

American Medical Association (2002). Guidelines for Physician–Patient Electronic Communications. Accessed online 29 July 2009 at http://www.ama-assn.org/ama/pub/about-ama/our-people/member-groups-sections/young-physicians-section/advocacy-resources/guidelines-physician-patient-electronic-communications.shtml.

Anand, S.A. & Chen, L.C. (1996). *Health implications of economic policies: A framework of analysis*. New York: UNDP Working Paper Series.

Andersen, R.E., Franckowiak, S.C., Snyder, J., Bartlett, S.J. & Fontaine, K.R. (1998). Can inexpensive signs encourage the use of stairs? Results from a community intervention. *Annals of Internal Medicine, 129*, 363–369.

Anderson, P. & Baumberg, B. (2006). *Alcohol in Europe: a public health perspective – a report for the European Commission*. London: Institute of Alcohol Studies.

Anderson, I., Crengle, S., Kamaka, M.L., Chen, T., Palafox, N. & Jackson-Pulver, L. (2006). Indigenous health in Australia, New Zealand, and the Pacific. *Lancet, 367*, 1775–1785.

Anderson, G.H., Boyes, D.A., Benedet, J.L., Le Riche, J.C., Matisic, J.P., Suen, K.C., Worth, A.J., Millner, A. & Bennett, O.M. (1988). Organisation and results of the cervical cytology screening programme in British Columbia, 1955–85. *British Medical Journal*, 296, 975–978.

Anderson, L.M., Scrimshaw, S.C., Fullilove, M.T., Fielding, J.E., Normand, J. & the Taskforce on Community Preventive Services (2003). Culturally competent healthcare systems: A systematic review. *American Journal of Preventive Medicine, 24*, 68–79.

Andersson, I., Aspegren, K. & Janzon, L., et al. (1988). Mammographic screening and mortality from breast cancer: the Malmö mammographic screening trial. *BMJ, 297*, 943–948.

Andrus, M.R. & Roth, M.T. (2002). Health literacy: A review. *Pharmacology, 22*, 282–302.

Antilla, T., Helkala, E.-L., Viitanen, M., Kareholt, I., Fratiglioni, L., Winblad, B., & Kivipelto, M. (2004). Alcohol drinking in middle age and subsequent risk of mild cognitive impairment and dementia in old age: a prospective population based study. *British Medical Journal, 329*, 539–545.

Antonovsky, A. (1979). *Health, stress, and coping*. San Francisco: Jossey-Bass.

Apanovitch, A.M., McCarthy, D. & Salovey, P. (2003). Using message framing to motivate HIV testing among low-income, ethnic minority women. *Health Psychology, 22*, 60–67.

Argyris, C. (1975). Dangers in applying results from experimental social psychology. *American Psychologist, 30*, 469–485.

ARIC Investigators (1989). The Atherosclerosis Risk in Communities (ARIC) Study: design and objectives. *American Journal of Epidemiology, 129*, 687–702.

Armitage, C.J. (2009). Is there utility in the transtheoretical model? *British Journal of Health Psychology, 14*, 195–210.

Armstrong, D. (1987). Theoretical tensions in biopsychosocial medicine. *Social Science & Medicine, 25*, 1213–1218.

Armstrong, N. (2007). Discourse and the individual in cervical cancer screening. *Health, 11*, 69–85.

Arnstein, S.R. (1969). A ladder of citizen participation. *Journal of the American Institute of Planners*, 35, 216–224.

Aron, A. & Corne, S. (Eds.) (1994). *Writings for a liberation psychology. Ignatio Martín-Baró*. Harvard: Harvard University Press.

Arrow, K. (1963). *Social choice and individual values* (2nd edn). New York: Wiley.

Arthur, H.M., Daniels, C., McKelvie, R., Hirsh, J. & Rush, B. (2000). Effect of a preoperative intervention on preoperative & postoperative outcomes in low-risk patients awaiting elective coronary artery bypass graft surgery. A randomized, controlled trial. *Annals of Internal Medicine, 133*, 253–262.

Auerbach, S.M. (2001). Do patients want control over their own health care? A review of measures, findings, and research issues. *Journal of Health Psychology, 6*, 191–204.

Auerbach, S.M. & Pegg, P.O. (2002). Appraisal of desire for control over healthcare: Structure, stability, and relation to health locus of control and to the 'Big Five' personality traits. *Journal of Health Psychology, 7*, 393–408.

Austin, R.M. & McLendon, W.W. (1997). The Papanicolaou smear: Medicine's most successful cancer screening procedure is threatened. *JAMA, 277*, 754–755.

Australian Bureau of Statistics. (2006). *Australian social trends, data cube – family and community* (4102.0). Canberra, Australian Capital Territory: Australian Bureau of Statistics.

Avlund, K., Osler, M., Damsgaard, M.T., Christensen, U. & Schroll, M. (2000). The relations between musculoskeletal diseases and mobility among old people: are they influenced by socio-economic, psychosocial and behavioural factors? *International Journal of Behavioural Medicine, 7*, 322–339.

Babor, T.F., Caetano, R., Casswell, S. & Edwards, G. et al. (Alcohol & Public Policy Group) (2003). *Alcohol: no ordinary commodity – research and public policy*. Oxford and London: Oxford University Press.

Babor, T.F. & Winstanley, E.L. (2008). The world of drinking: national alcohol control experiences in 18 countries. *Addiction, 103*, 721–725.

Bachen, E., Cohen, S. & Marsland, A.L. (2007). Psychoimmunology. In S. Ayers, A. Baum, C. McManus, S. Newman, K. Wallston, J. Weinman & R. West (Eds.), *Cambridge handbook of psychology, health and medicine* (2nd ed.). Cambridge University Press. Pp.167–172.

Backett-Milburn, K., Cunningham-Burley, S. & Davis, J. (2003). Contrasting lives, contrasting views? Understandings of health inequalities in differing social circumstances. *Social Science & Medicine, 57*, 613–623.

Baerger, D.R. & McAdams, D.P. (1999). Life story coherence and its relation to psychological well-being. *Narrative Inquiry, 9*, 69–96.

Bagnardi, V., Blangiardo, M., La Vecchia, C. & Corrao, G. (2001). A meta-analysis of alcohol drinking and cancer risk. *British Journal of Cancer, 85*, 1700–1705.

Bailey, J.A., Fleming, C.B., Henson, J.N., Catalano, R.F. & Haggerty, K.P. (2008). Sexual risk behavior 6 months post-high school: associations with college attendance, living with a parent, and prior risk behavior. *Journal of Adolescent Health, 42*, 573–579.

Baker, D.W., Parker, R.M., Williams, M.V., Pitkin, K., Parikh, N.S., Coates, W. & Imara, M. (1996). The health care experience of patients with low literacy. *Archive of Family Medicine, 5*, 329–334.

Baker, D.W., Williams, M.V., Parker, R.M., Gazmararian, J.A. & Nurss, J. (1999). Development of a brief test to measure functional health literacy. *Patient Education and Counseling, 38*, 33–42.

Baker, E.A., Schootman, M., Barnidge, E. & Kelly, C. (2006). The role of race and poverty in access to foods that enable individuals to adhere to dietary guidelines. *Preventing Chronic Disease, 3*, A76.

Baker, S. (2002). Bardot, Britney, bodies and breasts. *Perfect Beat, 6*, 18–32.

Balady, G.J., Williams, M.A., Ades, P.A., Bittner, V., Comoss, P., Foody, J.M., & Southard, D. (2007). Core components of cardiac rehabilitation/secondary prevention programs: 2007 update. *Circulation, 115*, 2675–2682.

Balarajan, R. & Soni Raleigh, V. (1993). *Ethnicity and health: a guide for the NHS*. London: Department of Health.

Balbach, E.D., Smith, E.A. & Malone, R.E. (2006). How the health belief model helps the tobacco industry: individuals, choice, and 'information'. *Tobacco Control, 15*, 37–43.

Balint, M. (1964). *The doctor, his patient and the illness.* New York: International Universities Press.

Balshem, M. (1991). Cancer, control, and causality: talking about cancer in a working class community. *American Ethnologist, 18*, 152–171.

Bancroft, A., Wiltshire, S., Parry, O. & Amos, A. (2003). 'Its like an addiction first thing … afterwards its like a habit': daily smoking behaviour among people living in areas of deprivation. *Social Science & Medicine, 56*, 1261–1267.

Bandura, A. (1977). Self efficacy: towards a unifying theory of behavioural change. *Psychological Review, 84*, 191–215.

Bandura, A. (1986). *Social foundations of thought and action: A social cognitive theory.* Englewood Cliffs, NJ: Prentice-Hall.

Bandura, A. (1994). Self-efficacy. In V. S. Ramachaudran (Ed.), *Encyclopedia of human behavior* (Vol. 4). New York: Academic Press. Pp. 71–81.

Bandura, A. (1995). *Self-efficacy in changing societies*. Cambridge: Cambridge University Press.

Bandura, A. (1997). The anatomy of stages of change. *American Journal of Health Promotion, 12*, 8–10.

Bandura, A. (2001). Social cognitive theory: An agentic perspective. *Annual Review of Psychology, 52*, 1–26.

Barak, A. & Fisher, W.A. (2001). Toward an Internet-driven, theoretically-based, innovative approach to sex education. *Journal of Sex Research, 38*, 324–332.

Bardia, A., Barton, D.L., Prokop, L.J., Bauer, B.A. & Moynihan, T.J. (2006). Efficacy of complementary and alternative medicine therapies in relieving cancer pain: A systematic review. *Journal of Clinical Oncology, 24*, 5457–5464.

Barraclough. J., Pinder, P., Cruddas, M., Osmand, C., Taylor, I. & Perry, M. (1992). Life events and breast cancer prognosis. *British Medical Journal, 304*, 1078–1081.

Bartlett, D. (1998). *Stress: perspectives and processes.* London: Open University Press.

Bass, C. (2007). Psychosomatics. In S. Ayers, A. Baum, C. McManus, S. Newman, K. Wallston, J. Weinman & R. West (Eds.), *Cambridge Handbook of Psychology, Health and Medicine* (2nd Edn.). Cambridge University Press. Pp. 173–177.

Bauld, L., Bell, K., McCullough, L., Richardson, L. & Greaves, L. (2009). The effectiveness of NHS smoking cessation services: a systematic review. *Journal of Public Health, 31*, 1–12.

Baum, F. (2000). Social capital, economic capital & power: further issues for a public health agenda. *Journal of Epidemiology & Community Health, 54*, 409–410.

Beagan, B.L. & Kumas-Tan, Z. (2009). Approaches to diversity in family medicine. *Canadian Family Physician, 55*, e21–28.

Beck, A.T. (1972). *Depression: causes and treatment.* Pennyslyvania: University of Pennsylvania Press.

Beck, N.C., Parker, J.C., Frank, R.G., Geden, E.A., Kay, D.R., Gamache, M., Anderson, S. (1988). Patients with rheumatoid arthritis at high risk for noncompliance with salicylate treatment regimens. *Journal of Rheumatology, 15*, 1081–1084.

Beck, U. (1992). *Risk society: towards a new modernity*. London: Sage.

Becker, M.H. (Ed.) (1974). The health belief model and personal health behavior. *Health Education Monographs, 2*, 324–508.

Becker, M.H. & Mainman, L.A. (1975). Sociobehavioral determinants of compliance with health and medical care recommendations. *Medical Care, 13*, 10–14.

Beisecker, A.E., Murden, R.A., Moore, W.P., Graham, D. & Nelmig, L. (1996). Attitudes of medical students and primary acre physicians regarding input of older and younger patients in medical decisions. *Medical Care, 34*, 126–137.

Bender, B., Milgrom, H., Rand, C. & Anderson, L. (1998). Psychological factors associated with medication nonadherence in asthmatic children. *Journal of Asthma, 35*, 347–353.

Benegal, V. (2005). India: alcohol and public health. *Addiction, 100*, 1051–1056.

Bennett, P. & Murphy, S. (1997). *Psychology and health promotion*. Buckingham: Open University Press.

Benoist, J. & Cathebras, P. (1993). The body: from immateriality to another. *Social Science & Medicine, 36*, 857–865.

Bensing, J. (1991). Doctor–patient communication & the quality of care. *Social Science & Medicine, 11*, 1301–1310.

Benveniste, J., Lecouteur, A. & Hepworth, J. (1999). Lay theories of anorexia nervosa: a discourse analytic study. *Journal of Health Psychology, 4*, 59–69.

Benyamini, Y., Leventhal, E.A. & Leventhal, H. (2009). Self-assessments of health: what do people know that predicts their mortality? *Research on Aging, 21*, 477–500.

Benzeval, M., Judge, K. & Whitehead, M. (Eds.) (1995). *Tackling inequalities in health: an agenda for action*. London: Kings Fund.

Berger, K., Ajani, U.A., Kase, C.S., Gaziano, J.M., Buring, J.E., Glynn, R.J. & Hennekens, C.H. (1999). Light to moderate alcohol consumption and risk of stroke among US male physicians. *New England Journal of Medicine, 341*, 1557–1564.

Berger, P. & Luckmann, T. (1966). *The social construction of reality: a treatise on the sociology of knowledge*. New York: Penguin.

Berghom, I., Svensson, C., Berggren, E. & Kamsula, M. (1999). Patients and relatives opinions and feelings about diaries kept by nurses in an intensive care unit: A pilot study. *Intensive & Critical Care Nursing, 15*, 185–191.

Berkman, L.F., Blumenthal, J., Burg, M., Carney, R.M., Catellier, D., Cowan, M.J., & Schneiderman, N. (2003). Effects of treating depression and low perceived social support on clinical events after myocardial infarction: the Enhancing Recovery in Coronary Heart Disease Patients (ENRICHD) Randomized Trial. *Journal of the American Medical Association, 289*, 3106–3116.

Berman, B.M. (2006). Cochrane Complementary Medicine Field. About The Cochrane Collaboration. Accessed online 24 June 2010 http://www.mrw.interscience.wiley.com/cochrane/clabout/articles/CE000052/frame.html.

Bertakis, K.D., Roter, D. & Putnam, S.M. (1991). The relationship of physician medical interview style to patient satisfaction. *Journal of Family Practice, 32*, 175–181.

Bertholet, N., Daeppen, J.B., Wietlisbach, V., Fleming, M. & Burnard, B. (2005). Reduction of alcohol consumption by brief alcohol intervention in primary care: systematic review and meta-analysis. *Archives of Internal Medicine, 165*, 986–995.

Bigelow, G.E. (2001). An operant behavioural perspective on alcohol abuse and dependence. In N. Heather, T.J. Peters & T. Stockwell (Eds.), *International handbook of alcohol dependence and problems*. London: Wiley.

Bingley, A.F., McDermott, E., Thomas, C., Payne, S., Seymour, J.E. & Clark, D. (2006). Making sense of dying: a review of narratives written since 1950 by people facing death from cancer and other diseases. *Palliative Medicine, 20*, 183–195.

Biondi, M. (2001). Effects of stress on immune functions: An overview. In R. Ader, D.L. Felten & N. Cohen (Eds.), *Psychoneuroimmunology*. London: Academic Press. Pp.189–226.

Bishop, F.L., Yardley, L. & Lewith, G.T. (2007). A systematic review of beliefs involved in the use of complementary and alternative medicine. *Journal of Health Psychology, 12*, 851–67.

Bishop, F.L., Yardley, L. & Lewith, G.T. (2008). Treatment appraisals and beliefs predict adherence to complementary therapies: A prospective study using a dynamic extended self-regulation model. *British Journal of Health Psychology, 13*, 701–718.

Blanchard, J.S., Garcia, H.S. & Carter, R.M. (1989). *Instrumento para diagnosticar lecturas (Espanol-English): Instrument for the diagnosis of reading*. Dubuque, IA: Kendall-Hunt Publishing Co.

Blane, D., Bartley, M. & Davey Smith, G. (1997). Disease aetiology and materialist explanations of socio-economic mortality differentials. *European Journal of Public Health, 7*, 385–391.

Blank, T.O. and Adams-Blodnieks, M. (2007). The who and the what of usage of two cancer online communities. *Computing and Human Behaviour, 23*, 1249–1257.

Blaxter, M. (1983). The causes of disease: women talking. *Social Science & Medicine*, *17*, 59–69.

Blaxter, M. (1990). *Health and lifestyles*. London: Routledge.

Blaxter, M. (1997). Whose fault is it? Peoples' own conceptions of the reasons for health inequalities. *Social Science & Medicine, 44*, 747–756.

Blendon, R.J., DesRoches, C.M., Brodie, M., Benson, J.M. & Rosen, A.B., et al. (2002). Views of practicing physicians and the public on medical errors. *New England Journal of Medicine, 347*, 1933–1940.

Block, G., Patterson, B. & Subar, A. (1992). Fruit, vegetables and cancer prevention: a review of the epidemiological evidence. *Nutrition & Cancer, 18*, 1–29.

Blume, S. (2006). Anti-vaccination movements and their interpretations. *Social Science & Medicine, 62*, 628–642.

Blumhagen, D. (1980). Hyper-tension: a folk illness with a medical name. *Culture, Medicine & Psychiatry, 4*, 197–227.

Bogart, L.M., Collins, R.L., Ellickson, P.L. & Klein, D.J. (2006). Adolescent predictors of college students spontaneous and anonymous sexual experiences. *Journal of Sex Research, 37*, 76–88.

Bogg, T. & Roberts, B.W. (2004). Conscientiousness and health-related behaviors: a meta-analysis of the leading behavioral contributors to mortality. *Psychological Bulletin, 130*, 887–919.

Bon, S.B., Hittner, J.B. & Lawandales, J.P. (2001). Normative perceptions in relation to substance use and HIV-risky sexual behaviors of college students. *Journal of Psychology: Interdisciplinary and Applied, 135*, 165–178.

Bond, C.A. & Monson, R. (1984). Sustained improvement in drug documentation, compliance, and disease control: A four-year analysis of an ambulatory care model. *Archives of Internal Medicine, 144*, 1159–1162.

Borges, G., Cherpitel, C.J., Orozco, R., Bond, J., Ye, Y., Macdonald, S., Giesbrecht, N., Stockwell, T., Cremonte, M., Moskalewicz, J., Swiatkiewicz, G. & Poznyak, V. (2006). Acute alcohol use and the risk of non-fatal injury in sixteen countries. *Addiction, 101*, 993–1002.

Bourdieu, P. (1984). *Distinction: a social critique of the judgement of taste.* London: Routledge & Kegan Paul.

Bourdieu, P. (1986). Forms of capital. In J.G. Richardson (Ed.), *Handbook of theory and research for the sociology of education.* New York: Greenwood Press.

Bowers, K.S. (1968). Pain, anxiety and perceived control. *Journal of Consulting & Clinical Psychology, 32*, 596–602.

Bowling, A. (2001). *Measuring disease: a review of disease-specific quality of life measurement scales.* Buckingham: Open University Press.

Bowling, A. (2004). *Measuring health: a review of quality of life measurement scales.* Buckingham: Open University Press.

Bowman, S.A., Gortmaker, S.L., Ebbeling, C.B., Pereira, M.A. & Ludwig, D.S. (2004). Effects of fast-food consumption on energy intake and diet quality among children in a national household survey. *Pediatrics, 113*, 112–118.

Boyle, M.A. & Morris, D.H. (1999). *Community nutrition in action: an entrepreneurial approach.* Belmont, CA: West/Wadsworth.

Bradley, B.S., Deighton, J. & Selby, J. (2004). The 'Voices' project: Capacity-building in community development for youth at risk. *Journal of Health Psychology, 9*, 197–212.

Brainard, D., Hyslop N.E., Mera, R. & Churchill, J. (1997) Long-term outcome of inpatients with tuberculosis assigned to outpatient therapy at a local clinic in New Orleans. *Journal of Investigative Medicine, 45*, 381–387.

Brawley, L.R., Martin, K.A. & Gyurcsik, N.C. (1998). In J.L. Duda (Ed.), A*dvances in Sport and Exercise Measurement*. Morgantown, WV: Fitness Information Technology. Pp. 37–350.

Bray, S.R., Gyurcsik, N.C., Culos-Reed, S.N., Dawson, K.A. & Martin, K.A. (2001). An exploratory investigation of the relationship between proxy efficacy, self-efficacy and exercise attendance. *Journal of Health Psychology, 6*, 425–434.

Brehm, J.W. (1966). *A theory of psychological reactance*. New York: Academic Press.

Brehm, S. & Brehm, J.W. (1981). *Psychological reactance: A theory of freedom and control*. New York, NY: Academic Press.

Brekke, M., Hjortland, P. & Kvien, T. (2003). Changes in self-efficacy and health status over 5 years: a longitudinal observational study of 306 patients with rheumatoid arthritis. *Arthritis Rheumatology, 49*, 342–348.

Brennan, T.A., Leape, L.L. & Laird, N.M., et al. (1991). Incidence of adverse events and negligence in hospitalized patients: results of the Harvard Medical Practice Study. *New England Journal of Medicine, 324*, 370–376.

Brewer, N.T., Chapman, G.B., Gibbons, F.X., Gerrard, M., McCaul K.D. & Weinstein, N.D. (2007). Meta-analysis of the relationship between risk perception and health behaviour: the example of vaccination. *Health Psychology, 26*, 136–145.

Brewin, C.R., Dalgleish, T. & Joseph, S. (1996). A dual representation theory of posttraumatic stress disorder. *Psychological Review, 103*, 670–686.

Britten, N. (1994). Patients' ideas about medicines: a qualitative study in a general practice population. *British Journal of General Practice, 44*, 465–468.

Britton, A. & Marmot, M. (2004). Different measures of alcohol consumption and risk of coronary heart disease and all-cause mortality 11-year follow-up of the Whitehall II cohort study. *Addiction, 99*, 109–116.

Brocki, J.M. & Wearden, A.J. (2006). A critical evaluation of the use of Interpretative Phenomenological Analysis (IPA) in health psychology. *Psychology & Health, 21*, 87–108.

Bronfenbrenner, U. (1979). *The ecology of human development*. Cambridge, MA: Harvard University Press.

Bronfenbrenner, U. (1986). Ecology of the family as a context for human development. *Developmental Psychology, 22*, 723–742.

Brown, J.A.C. (1964). *Freud and the post-Freudians*. London: Penguin.

Brown, J.B., Stewart, M., Weston, W.W. and Freeman, T.R. (2003). Introduction. In M. Stewart, J.B. Brown, W.W., Weston, I.R. McWhinney, C.L. McWilliam and T.R. Freeman (Eds.), *Patient-centred medicine: Transforming the clinical method*. Oxon: Radcliffe Medical Press. Pp. 1–15.

Brown, M.S. & Goldstein, J.L. (1984). How LDL receptors influence cholesterol and atherosclerosis. *Scientific American, 251*, 52–60.

Brown, S.D. (1996). The textuality of stress: drawing between scientific and everyday accounting. *Journal of Health Psychology, 1*, 173–193.

Brown, R.J. (2004). Psychological mechanisms of medically unexplained symptoms: An integrative conceptual model. *Psychological Bulletin, 130*, 793–812.

Brownell, K. (1991). Personal responsibility and control over our bodies: when expectation exceeds reality. *Health Psychology, 10*, 303–310.

Brownell, K.D. (1994). Get slim with higher taxes. *New York Times*, December 15, A–29.

Brownell, K.D. & Horgen, K.B. (2004). *Food fight: The inside story of the food industry, America's obesity crisis, and what we can do about it.* New York: McGraw-Hill.

Brydon-Miller, M. (2004). Using participatory action research to address community health issues. In M. Murray (Ed.), *Critical health psychology*. New York: Palgrave. Pp. 187–202.

Buller, M.K. & Buller, D.B. (1987). Physicians' communication style and patient satisfaction. *Journal of Health & Social Behavior, 28*, 375–389.

Bullock, H.E. & Lott, B. (2001). Building a research and advocacy agenda on issues of economic justice. *Analyses of Social Issues & Public Policy, 1*, 147–162.

Burg, M.M., Benedetto, M.C., Rosenberg, R. & Soufer, R. (2003). Presurgical depression predicts medical morbidity 6 months after coronary artery bypass graft surgery. *Psychosomatic Medicine, 65*, 111–118.

Burns, M. & Gavey, N. (2004). 'Healthy weight' at what cost? 'Bulimia' and a discourse of weight control. *Journal of Health Psychology, 9*, 549–566.

Bury, M. (1982). Chronic illness as biographical disruption. *Sociology of Health & Illness, 22*, 40–67.

Byrne, A., Ellershaw, J., Holcombe, C. & Salmon, P. (2002). Patients' experience of cancer: Evidence of the role of 'fighting' in collusive clinical communication. *Patient Education and Counseling, 48*, 15–21.

Byrne, D.G. & Espnes, G.A. (2008). Occupational stress and cardiovascular disease. *Stress & Health, 24*, 231–238.

Byrne, P.S. & Long, B.E.L. (1976). *Doctors talking to patients*. London: HMSO.

Cabinet Office, Prime Ministers Strategy Unit (2004). *Alcohol harm reduction strategy for England*, London: Cabinet Office.

Calnan, M. (1987). *Health and illness: the lay perspective*. London: Tavistock.

Calnan, M. & Williams, S. (1991). Style of life and the salience of health: an exploratory study of health related practices in households from differing socio-economic circumstances. *Sociology of Health & Illness, 13*, 506–529.

Cameron, L.D. & Reeve, J. (2006). Risk perceptions, worry, and attitudes about genetic testing for breast cancer susceptibility. *Psychology and Health, 21*, 211–230.

Campbell, A. & Hausenblas, H.A. (2009). Effects of exercise interventions on body image. A meta-analysis. *Journal of Health Psychology, 14*, 780–793.

Campbell, C. (2004a). Editorial: creating environments that support peer education: experiences from HIV/AIDS prevention in South Africa. *Health Education, 104*, 197–200.

Campbell, C. (2004b). Health psychology and community action. In M. Murray (Ed.), *Critical health psychology*. London: Palgrave. Pp. 203–221.

Campbell, C. (2006) *Creating social environments that support the possibility of health.* Commonwealth Health Ministers Reference Report. London: Commonwealth Secretariat.

Campbell, C. & Jovchelovitch, S. (2000). Health, community and development: Towards a social psychology of participation. *Journal of Community & Applied Social Psychology, 10*, 255–270.

Campbell, C. & Murray, M. (2004). Community health psychology: Promoting analysis and action for social change. *Journal of Health Psychology, 9*, 187–915.

Campbell, C., Nair, Y., Maimane, S. & Nicholson, J. (2007a). 'Dying twice': A multi-level model of the roots of AIDS stigma in two South African communities. *Journal of Health Psychology, 12*, 403–416.

Campbell, C., Nair, Y. & Maimane, S. (2007b). Building contexts that support effective community responses to HIV/AIDS. *American Journal of Community Psychology, 39*, 347–363.

Campbell, C., Wood, R. & Kelly, M. (1999). *Social capital and health*. London: Health Education Authority.

Campbell, K., Waters, E., O'Meara, S., Kelly, S. & Summerbell, C. (2002). Interventions for preventing obesity in children (Cochrane Review). In *The Cochrane Library*, Issue 2. CD001871. Chichester: John Wiley.

Campbell, L.C., Clauw, D.J. & Keefe, F.J. (2003). Persistent pain and depression: a biopsychosocial perspective. *Biological Psychiatry, 54*, 399–409.

Cancer Research UK (2010). Cancer Chat. Accessed online 24 June 2010 at http://www.cancerchat.org.uk/

Cannon, W.B. (1932). *The wisdom of the body*. New York: Norton.

Capaldi, E. (1996). Conditioned food preferences. In E.D. Capaldi (Ed.), *Why we eat what we eat: the psychology of eating*. Washington, DC: American Psychological Association. Pp. 53–80.

Car, J. and Sheikh, A. (2004a). Email consultations in health care: 1—scope and effectiveness. *BMJ, 329*, 435–438.

Car, J. and Sheikh, A. (2004b). Email consultations in health care: 2—acceptability and safe application. *BMJ, 329*, 439–442.

Carey, M.P., Braaten, L.S., Maisto, S.A., Gleason, J.R., Forsyth, A.D., Durant, L.E. & Jaworski, B.C. (2000). Using information, motivational enhancement, and skills training to reduce the risk of HIV infection for low-income urban women: A second randomized clinical trial. *Health Psychology, 19*, 3–11.

Carmona, R.H. (2003). Testimony before the Subcommittee on Education Reform Committee on Education and the Workforce U.S. House of Representatives: The obesity crisis in America. Accessed 12 November 2009 at http://www.surgeongeneral.gov/news/testimony/obesity07162003.htm

Carnegie, D. (1913). *How to win friends and influence people*. New York: The World's Work.

Carpenter, M. (2009a). Challenges to local health action. In M. Murray & N. Leighton, N. (Eds.), *Promoting healthy communities*. Keele: North Staffordshire & South Cheshire Public Health Forum.

Carpenter, M. (2009b). The capabilities approach and critical social policy. Lessons from the majority world. *Critical Social Policy, 29*, 351–373.

Cartwright, M., Wardle. J., Steggles, N., Simon, A.E., Croker, H. & Jarvis, M. (2003). Stress and dietary practices in adolescents. *Health Psychology, 22*, 362–369.

Carver, C.S., Scheier, M.F. & Weintraub, J.K. (1989). Assessing coping strategies: a theoretically based approach. *Journal of Personality & Social Psychology, 56*, 267–283.

Caspersen, C.J., Powell, K.E. & Christenson, G.M. (1985). Physical activity, exercise and physical fitness: Definitions and distinctions for health-related research. *Public Health Reports, 100*, 126–131.

Cecil, D.W. & Killeen, I. (1997). Control, compliance and satisfaction in the family practice encounter. *Family Medicine*, 29, 653–657.

Centers For Disease Control and Prevention (1999). HIV/AIDS surveillance report, 11(2), 14, 16, 20, 22, 38.

Centers for Disease Control (2009). *Teen birth rates up slightly in 2007 for second consecutive year.* Press release accessed 26 November 2009 at http://www.cdc.gov/media/pressrel/2009/r090318.htm.

Centers for Disease Control and Prevention (2010). Scanning electron micrograph of HIV-1 budding from cultured lymphocyte. Multiple round bumps on cell surface represent sites of assembly and budding of virions. Accessed on 7 July 2010 at http://commons.wikimedia.org/wiki/File:HIV-budding.jpg

Chacko, M.R., Wiemann, C.M., Kozinetz, C.A., von Sternberg, K., Velasquez, M.M., Smith, P.B. & DiClemente, R. (2010). Efficacy of a motivational behavioral intervention to promote chlamydia and gonorrhea screening in young women: A randomized controlled trial. *Journal of Adolescent Health, 46(2)*, 152–161.

Chalmers, B. (1996). Western and African conceptualizations of health. *Psychology & Health, 12*, 1–10.

Chamberlain, K. (1997). Socio-economic health differentials: from structure to experience. *Journal of Health Psychology, 2*, 399–412.

Chamberlain, K. (2004). Food and health: expanding the agenda for health psychology. *Journal of Health Psychology, 9*, 467–482.

Chamberlain, K. & Zika, S. (1990). The minor events approach to stress: support for the use of daily hassles. *British Journal of Psychology, 81*, 469–481.

Channel 4 (2005). *Jamie's School Dinners*. February–March.

Chapman G.B. & Coups, E.J. (2006). Emotions and preventive health behavior: Worry, regret, and influenza vaccination. *Health Psychology, 25*, 82–90.

Chapman, C.R., Casey, K.L., Dubner, R., Foley, K.M., Gracely, R.H. & Reading, A.E. (1985). Pain measurement: an overview. *Pain, 22*, 1–31.

Charmaz, K. (2008). Grounded theory. In J.A. Smith (Ed.), *Qualitative psychology: a practical guide to research methods*. London: Sage. Pp. 81–110.

Chen, L.M., Miaskowski, C., Dodd, M. & Pantilat, S. (2009a). Concepts within the Chinese culture that influence the cancer pain experience. *Cancer Nursing, 31*, 103–108.

Chen, Y.-H., Tsai, S-Y. & Lin, H.-C. (2009b). Increased risk of acute myocardial infarction for patients with panic disorder: A nationwide population-based study. *Psychosomatic Medicine, 71*, 798-804.

Cheng, Y.H. (1997). Explaining disablement in modern times: hand-injured workers accounts of their injuries in Hong Kong. *Social Science & Medicine, 45*, 739–750.

Chesler, M.A. & Parry, C. (2001). Gender roles and/or styles in crisis: an integrative analysis of the experiences of fathers of children with cancer. *Qualitative Health Research, 11*, 363–384.

Chesney, M.A., Chambers, D.B., Taylor, J.M., Johnson, L.M. & Folkman, S. (2003). Coping effectiveness training for men living with HIV: results from a randomised clinical trial testing a group-based intervention. *Psychosomatic Medicine, 65*, 1038–1046.

Chesterton, L.S., Foster, N.E., Wright, C.C., Baxter, G.D. & Barlas, P. (2003). Effects of TENS frequency. Intensity and stimulation site parameter manipulation on pressure pain thresholds in healthy human subjects. *Pain, 106*, 73–80.

Chida, Y., Hamer, M., Wardle, J. & Steptoe, A. (2008). Do stress-related psychosocial factors contribute to cancer incidence and survival? *Nature Clinical Practice Oncology, 5*, 466–475.

Chida, Y. & Steptoe, A. (2008). Positive psychological well-being and mortality: A quantitative review of prospective observational studies. *Psychosomatic Medicine, 70*, 741–756.

Chopra, M. & Darnton-Hill, I. (2004). Tobacco and obesity epidemics: not so different after all? *British Medical Journal, 328*, 1558–1560.

Chow, E., Tsao, M.N. & Harth, T. (2004). Does psychosocial intervention improve survival in cancer? A meta-analysis. *Palliative Medicine, 18*, 25–31.

Christakis, N.A. & Fowler, J.H. (2007). The spread of obesity in a large social network over 32 years. *New England Journal of Medicine, 357*, 370–379.

Christiannse, M.E., Lavigne, J.V. & Lerner, C.V. (1989). Psychosocial aspects of compliance in children and adolescents with asthma. *Developmental and Behavioral Pediatrics, 10*, 75–80.

Clark, W. (2008). Treatment of substance abuse disorders among Latinos. Invited address presented at the 14th Annual Latino Behavioral Health Institute Conference, Los Angeles, CA, September.

Clark-Carter, D. (1997). *Doing quantitative psychological research: from design to report*. Hove: Psychology Press.

Clark-Carter, D. & Marks, D.F. (2004). Intervention studies: design and analysis. In D.F. Marks & L. Yardley (Eds.), *Research methods for clinical and health psychology*. London: Sage. Pp. 166–184.

Clarke, P. & Eves, F. (1997). Applying the transtheoretical model to the study of exercise on prescription. *Journal of Health Psychology, 2*, 195–207.

Cleland, J., Ali, M.M. & Shah, I. (2006). Trends in protective behaviour among single vs. married young women in Sub-Saharan Africa: the big picture. *Reproductive Health Matters, 14*, 17–22.

Coakley, J. & White, A. (1992). Making decisions: gender and sport participation among British adolescents. *Sociology of Sport Journal, 9*, 20–35.

Coburn, D. (2004). Beyond the income inequality hypothesis: class, neo-liberalism and health inequalities. *Social Science & Medicine, 58*, 41–56.

Cochrane, T., Davey, R.C., Gidlow, C., Smith, G.R., Fairburn, J., Armitage, C.J., Stephansen, H. & Speight, S. (2009). Small area and individual level predictors of physical activity in urban communities: A multi-level study in Stoke-on-Trent, England. *International Journal of Environmental Research and Public Health, 6*, 654–677.

Cockburn, C. (2001). Identities and subculture in relation to sport: an analysis of teenage girls' magazines. In C. Brackenridge, D. Howe & F. Jordan (Eds.), *JUST leisure: Equity, social exclusion and identity.* Leisure Studies Association, Publication No. 72.

Cockburn, C. & Clarke, G. (2002). 'Everybody's looking at you!': Girls negotiating the 'femininity deficit' they incur in physical education. *Womens Studies International Forum, 25*, 651–665.

Coghill, R.C., McHaffie, J.G. & Yen, Y.-F. (2003). Neural correlates of interindividual differences in the subjective experience of pain. *Proceedings of the National Academy of Science, 100*, 8538–8542.

Cohen, J. (1994). The Earth is round (p < .05): The ritual of testing the null hypothesis continues to impede the advance of psychology as a science. *American Psychologist, 49*, 997–1003.

Cohen, S. (2004). Social relationships and health. *American Psychologist, 59*, 676–684.

Cohen, S. & Miller, G.E. (2001). Stress, immunity and susceptibility to upper respiratory infection. In R. Ader, D. Felten & N. Cohen (Eds.), *Psychoneuroimmunology*, 3rd ed. London: Academic Press. Pp. 499–509.

Cohen, S. & Williamson, G.M. (1991). Stress and infectious disease in humans. *Psychological Bulletin, 109*, 5–24.

Collins, R.L. & Bradizza, C.M. (2001). Social and cognitive learning processes. In N. Heather, T.J. Peters & T. Stockwell (Eds.), *International handbook of alcohol dependence and problems.* London: Wiley. Pp. 317–337.

Conner, M. & Armitage, C. (1998). Extending the theory of planned behavior: A review and avenues for further research. *Journal of Applied Social Psychology, 28*, 1429–1464.

Conrad, P. (1985). The meaning of medications: another look at compliance. *Social Science & Medicine, 20*, 29–37.

Cook, C.C.H. & Gurling, H.M.D. (2001). Genetic predisposition to alcohol dependence and problems. In N. Heather, T.J. Peters & T. Stockwell (Eds.), *International handbook of alcohol dependence and problems.* London: Wiley. Pp. 257–280.

Cookson, C. (2002). Benefit and risk of vaccination as seen by the general public and the media. *Vaccine, 20*, S85–S88.

Cooper, A., Lloyd, G., Weinman, J. & Jackson, G. (1999). Why patients do not attend cardiac rehabilitation: role of intentions and illness beliefs. *Heart, 82*, 234–236.

Cooper, A.F., Jackson, G., Weinman, J. & Horne, R. (2002). Factors associated with cardiac rehabilitation attendance: a systematic review of the literature. *Clinical Rehabilitation, 16,* 541–552.

Corin, E. (1995). The cultural frame: context and meaning in the construction of health. In B.C. Amick III, S. Levine, A.R. Tarlov & D. Chapman Walsh (Eds.), *Society and health.* New York: Oxford University Press. Pp. 272–304.

Cornish, F. (2009). Let's get real (with a Small 'r'): For a health psychology that prioritizes the concrete. *Journal of Health Psychology, 14*, 638–642.

Cornwell, J. (1984). *Hard earned lives.* London: Tavistock.

Corrao, G., Bagnardi, V., Zambon, A. & La Vecchia, C. (2004). A meta analysis of alcohol consumption and the risk of 15 diseases, *Preventive Medicine, 38*, 613–619.

Costanza, M.E. (1994). The extent of breast cancer screening in older women. *Cancer, 74*, 2046–2050.

Coulter, A. (1999). Paternalism or partnership. *British Medical Journal, 319*, 719–720.

Coupland, J., Robinson, J.D. & Coupland, N. (1994). Frame negotiation in doctor–elderly patient consultations. *Discourse & Society, 5*, 89–124.

Coyne, C.J., Stefanek, M. & Palmer, S.C. (2007). Psychotherapy and survival in cancer: The conflict between hope and evidence. *Psychological Bulletin, 133*, 367–94.

Cox, T. (1978). *Stress.* London: Macmillan.

Crawford, H.J., Gur, R.C., Skolnick, B., Gur, R.E. & Benson, D.M. (1993). Effects of hypnosis on regional cerebral blood-flow during ischemic pain with and without suggested hypnotic analgesia. *International Journal of Psychophysiology, 15*, 181–195.

Crawford, R. (1980). Healthism and the medicalisation of everyday life. *International Journal of Health Services, 10*, 365–368.

Crombez, G., Bijttebier, P., Eccleston, C., Mascagni, T., Mertens, G., Goubert, L. & Verstraeten, K. (2003). The child version of the pain catastrophizing scale (PCS-C): a preliminary validation. *Pain, 104*, 639–646.

Cropley, M., Ayers, S. & Nokes, L. (2003). People don't exercise because they can't think of reasons to exercise: an examination of causal reasoning with the Transtheoretical Model. *Psychology, Health & Medicine, 8*, 409–414.

Cropper, S., Porter, A., Williams, G., Carlisle, S., Moore, R., O'Neill, M., Roberts, C. & Snooks, H. (Eds.) (2007*). Community health and wellbeing: Action research on health inequalities.* Bristol: Policy Press.

Crossley, M.L. (1999). Making sense of HIV infection: discourse & adaptation to life with HIV positive diagnosis. *Health, 3*, 95–119.

Crossley, M.L. (2003). 'Would you consider yourself a healthy person?' Using focus groups to explore health as a moral phenomenon. *Journal of Health Psychology, 8*, 501–514.

Csikszentmihalyi, M. (1997). *Finding flow: The psychology of engagement with everyday life.* New York: Basic Books.

Cummings, J.H. & Bingham, S.A. (1998). Diet and the prevention of cancer. *British Medical Journal, 317*, 1636–1640.

Cunningham, M. (2009). Health in the United Nations. *State of the World's Indigenous Peoples*. New York: United Nations. Pp. 156–187.

Cunningham, A.J. & Watson, K. (2004). How psychological therapy may prolong survival in cancer patients: new evidence and a simple theory. *Integrative Cancer Therapy, 3*, 214–229.

Curtis, J. & White, P. (1992). Toward a better understanding of the sport practices of Francophone and Anglophone Canadians. *Sociology of Sport Journal,* 9, 403–422.

Curtis, S. & Rees Jones, I. (1998). Is there a place for geography in the analysis of health inequalities? *Sociology of Health & Illness, 20*, 645–672.

Cust, A. E., et al. (2009). Total dietary carbohydrate, sugar, starch & fibre intakes in the European Prospective Investigation into Cancer and Nutrition. *European Journal of Clinical Nutrition, 63 (4)*, S37–S60.

Dahlgren, G. & Whitehead, M. (1991). *Policies and strategies to promote equity and health*. Stockholm: Institute for Future Studies.

Daley, A.J., Copeland, R.J., Wright, N.P. & Wales, J.K.H. (2008). 'I can actually exercise if I want to'. It isn't as hard as I thought: a qualitative study of the experiences and views of obese adolescents participating in an exercise therapy intervention. *Journal of Health Psychology, 13*, 810–819.

Dalton, J.A., Feuerstein, M., Carlson, J. & Roghman, K. (1994). Biobehavioral pain profile: Development and psychometric properties. *Pain, 57*, 95–107.

Dalton, S., Orford, J., Parry, J. & Laburn-Peart, K. (2008). Three ways of talking about health in communities targeted for regeneration: Interviews with community professionals. *Journal of Health Psychology, 13*, 65–78.

Daniels, N., Kennedy, B. & Kawachi, I. (2000). Justice is good for our health: How greater economic equality would promote public health. *Boston Review*, Feb/Mar, 25.

Dar, R., Stronguin, F. & Etter, J.F. (2005). Assigned versus perceived placebo effects in nicotine replacement therapy for smoking reduction in Swiss smokers. *Journal of Consulting & Clinical Psychology, 73*, 350–353.

Dasen, P.R., Berry, J.W. & Sartorius, N. (Eds.) (1988). *Health and cross-cultural psychology: towards applications*. Newbury Park, CA: Sage.

David, T.C., Wolf, M.S., Bass, P.F., Middlebrooks, M., Kennen, E., Baker, D., & Parker, R.M. (2006). Low literacy impairs comprehension of prescription drug warning labels. *Journal of General and Internal Medicine, 21*, 847–851.

Davidson, K.W., Goldstein, M., Kaplan, R.M., Kaufmann, P.G., Knatterund, G.L., Orleans, C.T., & Whitlock, E.P. (2003). Evidence-based behavioral medicine: what is it and how do we achieve it? *Annals of Behavioral Medicine, 26*, 161–171.

Davis, R.B., Duncan, L., Turner, L.W. & Young, M. (2001). Perceptions of human immunodeficiency virus and sexually transmitted disease risk among low-income adults: a pilot study. *Applied Nursing Research, 14*, 105–109.

Davis, T.C., Long, S.W., Jackson, R.H., Mayeaux, E.J., George, R.B., Murphy, P.W. & Crouch, M.A. (1993). Rapid estimate of adult literacy in medicine: a shortened screening instrument. *Family Medicine, 25*, 391–395.

Davison, C., Macintyre, S. & Davey Smith, G. (1994). The potential social impact of predictive genetic testing for susceptibility to common chronic diseases: a review and proposed research agenda. *Sociology of Health & Illness, 16*, 340–371.

De Gruchy, J. and Coppel, D. (2008). 'Listening to reason': A social marketing stop-smoking campaign in Nottingham. *Social Marketing Quarterly, 14*, 5–17.

Deci, E.L. & Ryan, R.M. (1985). *Intrinsic motivation and self-determination in human behavior*. New York: Plenum Press.

Deimling, G.T., Bowman, K.F., Sterns, S., Wagner, L.J. & Kahana, B. (2006). Cancer-related health worries and psychological distress among older adult, long-term cancer survivors. *Psycho-Oncology, 15*, 306–320.

DeMatteo, D., Harrison, C., Arneson, C., Salter Goldie, R., Lefebvre, A., Read, S.E. & King, S.M. (2002). Disclosing HIV/AIDS to children: the paths families take to truthtelling. *Psychology, Health & Medicine, 7*, 339–356.

DeMattia, L. & Denney, S.L. (2008). Childhood obesity prevention: successful community-based efforts. *The ANNALS of the American Academy of Political & Social Science, 615*, 83–99.

Denollet, J., Sys, S.U., Stroobant, N., Rombouts, H., Gillebert, T.C. & Brutsaert, D.L. (1996). Personality as independent predictor of long-term mortality in patients with coronary heart disease. *Lancet, 347*, 417–421.

Denzin, N.K. (2003). *Performance ethnography: critical pedagogy and the politics of culture*. London: Sage.

Department of Health (2000a). *An organization with a memory: report of an expert group on learning from adverse events in the NHS, chaired by the Chief Medical Officer*. London: The Stationery Office.

Department of Health (2000b). *Health Survey for England 1998*. London: The Stationery Office.

Department of Health (2001). *The NHS Plan: a plan for investment, a plan for reform*. London: Stationery Office.

Department of Health (2003). *Tackling health inequalities: A programme for action*. London: HMSO.

Department of Health (2004). *At least five a day: Evidence on the impact of physical activity and its relationship to health*. London: Department of Health.

Department of Health (2008). *Ambitions for Health: A strategic framework for maximising the potential of social marketing and health-related behaviour*. London: NHS.

Desapriya, E., Pike, I. & Subzwari, S. (2006). Injury-related mortality and indigenous people. *Lancet, 368*, 576.

Des Jarlais, D.C., Lyles, C. & Crepaz, N. (2004). Improving the reporting quality of nonrandomized evaluations of behavioral and public health interventions: the TREND statement. *American Journal of Public Health, 94*, 361–366.

Detweiler, J.B., Bedell, B.T., Salovey, P., Pronin, E. and Rothman, A.J. (1999). Message framing and sunscreen use: Gain-framed messages motivate beach goers. *Health Psychology, 2*, 189–196.

Dew, K. (1999). Epidemics, panic and power: representations of measles and measles vaccine. *Health, 3*, 379–398.

DeWalt, D.A. (2007). Low health literacy: Epidemiology and interventions. *North Carolina Medical Journal, 68*, 327–330.

DeWalt, D.A., Berkman, N.D., Sheridan, S., Lohr, K.N. & Pignone, M.P. (2004). Literacy and health outcomes: A systematic review of the literature. *Journal of General Internal Medicine, 19*, 1228–1239.

DeWalt, D.A. & Hink, A. (2009). Health literacy and child health outcomes: A systematic review of the literature. *Pediatrics, 124*, s265–274.

Diamond, J.J. (2007). Development of a reliable and construct valid measure of nutritional literacy in adults. *Nutrition Journal, 6*, 5–8.

Dickerson, S.S. & Kemeny, M.E. (2004). Acute stressors and cortisol responses: A theoretical integration and synthesis of laboratory research. *Psychological Bulletin, 130*, 355–391.

DiClemente, C. & Prochaska, J. (1982). Self change and therapy change of smoking behavior: A comparison of processes of change in cessation and maintenance. *Addictive Behavior, 7*, 133–142.

Diez Roux, A.V., Stein Merkin, S. & Arnett, D. et al. (2001). Neighborhood of residence and incidence of coronary heart disease. *New England Journal of Medicine, 345*, 99–106.

DiMatteo, M.R. (2004). Social support and patient adherence to medical treatment: A meta-analysis. *Health Psychology, 23*, 207–218.

Dishman, R.K. (1986). Exercise compliance: a new view for public health. *Physician and Sports Medicine, 14*, 127–145.

Dixon, H.G., Scully, M.L., Wakefield, M.A., White, V.M. & Crawford, D.A. (2007). The effects of television advertisements for junk food versus nutritious food on children's food attitudes and preferences. *Social Science & Medicine, 65*, 1311–1323.

Doise, W. (1986). *Levels of explanation in social psychology*. Cambridge: Cambridge University Press.

Dolgin, M.J., Katz, E.R., Doctors, S.R. & Siegel, S.R. (1986). Caregivers' perceptions of medical compliance in adolescents with cancer. *Journal of Adolescent Health Care, 7*, 22–27.

Doll, R. & Hill, A.B. (1952). A study of the aetiology of carcinoma of the lung. *British Medical Journal, 2*, 1271–1286.

Donovan, J.L. & Blake, D.R. (1992). Patient non-compliance: deviance or reasoned decision-making? *Social Science & Medicine, 34*, 507–513.

Doran, C.M., Valenti, L., Robinson, M., Britt, H. & Mattick, R.P. (2006). Smoking status of Australian general practice patients and their attempts to quit. *Addictive Behavior, 31*, 758–766.

Dorn, J.M., Hovey, K., Williams, B.A., Freudenheim, J.L., Russell, M., Nochajski, T.H. & Trevisan, M. (2007). Alcohol drinking pattern and non-fatal myocardial infarction in women. *Addiction, 102*, 730–739.

Downing-Matibag, T.M. & Geisinger, B. (2009). Hooking up and sexual risk taking among college students: a health belief model perspective. *Qualitative Health Research, 19*, 1196–1209.

Doyal, L. & Gough, I. (1991). *A theory of need*. London: Macmillan.

Drobes, D.J., Saladin, M.E. & Tiffany, S.T. (2001). Classical conditioning mechanisms. In N. Heather, T.J. Peters & T. Stockwell (Eds.) *International handbook of alcohol dependence and problems*. London: Wiley. Pp. 281–297.

Drummond, D.C., Tiffany, S.T., Glautier, S. & Remington, B. (Eds.) (1995). *Addictive behaviour: Cue exposure theory and practice*. London: Wiley.

DuCharme, K.A. & Brawley, L.R. (1995). Predicting the intentions and behavior of exercise initiates using two forms of self-efficacy. *Journal of Behavioral Medicine, 18*, 479–497.

Duijts, S.F., Zeegers, M.P. & Borne, B.V. (2003). The association between stressful life events and breast cancer risk: A meta-analysis. *International Journal of Cancer, 107*, 1023–1029.

Dumanovsky, T., Nonas, C.A., Huang, C.Y., Silver, L.D. & Bassett, M.T. (2009). What people buy from fast-food restaurants: caloric content and menu item selection, New York City 2007. *Obesity, 17*, 1369–1374.

Duncan, N., Bowman, B., Naidoo, A., Pillay, J. & Roos, V. (2007). *Community psychology: Analysis, context and action*. Cape Town: UCT Press.

Dunton, G.F. & Vaughan, E. (2008). Anticipated affective consequences of physical activity adoption and maintenance. *Health Psychology, 27*, 703–710.

Eaker, E.D., Sullivan, L.M., Kelly-Hayes, M., Agostino, Sr., D. & Benjamin, E.J. (2004). Does job strain increase the risk for coronary heart disease or death in men and women? *American Journal of Epidemiology, 159*, 950–958.

Eardley, A. & Elkind, A. (1990). A pilot study of attendance for breast cancer screening. *Social Science & Medicine, 30*, 693–699.

Eccleston, C. (2001). Role of psychology in pain management. *British Journal of Anaesthesia, 87*, 144–152.

Eccleston, C., Morley, S., Williams, A., Yorke, L. & Mastroyannopoulou, K. (2002). Systematic review of randomised controlled trials of psychological therapy for chronic pain in children and adolescents, with a subset meta-analysis of pain relief. *Pain, 99*, 157–165.

Eccleston, Z. & Eccleston, C. (2004). Interdisciplinary management of adolescent chronic pain: developing the role of physiotherapy. *Physiotherapy, 90*, 77–81.

Edwards, A.G., Hailey, S. & Maxwell, M. (2004). Psychological interventions for women with metastatic breast cancer. *Cochrane Database of Systematic Reviews, 2*, CD004253.

Edwards, D. (1997). *Discourse & cognition*. London: Sage.

EFA (2008). *Education for All Global Monitoring Report 2009: Overcoming Inequality, why governance matters*. Paris: UNESCO.

Egger, G. & Swinburn, B. (1997). An ecological approach to the obesity pandemic. *British Medical Journal, 315*, 477–480.

Eissa, M.A., Poffenbarger, T. & Portman, R.J. (2001). Comparison of the actigraph versus patients diary information in defining circadian time periods for analysing ambulatory blood pressure monitoring data. *Blood Pressure Monitoring, 6*, 21–25.

Elmore, J.G., Barton, M.B., Moceri, V.M., Polk, S., Arena, P.J. & Fletcher, S.W. (1998). Ten year risk of false positive screening mammograms and clinical breast examination. *New England Journal of Medicine, 338*, 1089–1096.

Engels, F. (1845/1958). *The condition of the working class in England in 1844*. London: Lawrence & Wishart.

Engel, G.L. (1959). Psychogenic pain and the pain prone patient. *American Journal of Medicine, 26*, 899–918.

Engel, G.L. (1977). The need for a new medical model: a challenge for biomedicine. *Science, 196*, 129–136.

Engel, G.L. (1980). The clinical application of the biopsychosocial model. *American Journal of Psychiatry, 137*, 535–544.

Estacio, E.V. (2009). Media exploitation, racism and health. *Journal of Health Psychology, 14*, 155–157.

Estacio, E.V. & Marks, D.F. (2007). Health inequity and social injustice for the Aytas in the Philippines: Critical psychology in action. *Journal of Social Action in Counselling and Psychology, 1*, 40–57.

Estacio, E.V.G. & Marks, D.F. (in press). Critical reflections on social injustice and action research: The case of the indigenous Ayta community in the Philippines. WCPCG-2010. *Procedia–Social and Behavioral Sciences.*

Euripides (1954/414BC). *The Bacchae* (P. Vellacott, Trans.) London: Penguin.

European Commission (1999). *A pan-EU survey of consumer attitudes to physical activity, body weight and health*. Luxembourg: EC. DGV/F.3.

Evans, P., Hucklebridge, F. & Clow, A. (2000). *Mind, immunity and health: the science of psychoneuroimmunology.* London: Free Association Books.

Evans, W.D. (2006). How social marketing works in health care. *BMJ, 332*, 1207–1210.

Eysenbach, G. (2003). The impact of the Internet on cancer outcomes. *CA Cancer Journal for Clinicians, 53*, 356–371.

Eysenbach, G., Powell, J., Englesakis, M., Rizo, C. and Stern, A. (2004). Health related virtual communities and electronic support groups: systematic review of the effects of online peer to peer interactions. *BMJ, 328*, 1166–1172.

Eysenck, H.J. (1970). *Fact and fiction in psychology*. London: Penguin.

Eysenck, H.J., Tarrant, M. & Woolf, M. (1960). Smoking and personality. *British Medical Journal, 280*, 1456–1460.

Ezzati, M., Lopez, A.D., Rodgers, A., Hoorn, S.V., Murray, C.J.L. & the Comparative Risk Assessment Collaborating Group (2002). Selected major risk factors and global and regional burden of disease. *Lancet, 360*, 1347–1360.

Ezzy, D. (2000). Illness narratives: Time, hope and HIV. *Social Science & Medicine, 50*, 605–617.

Fallowfield, L., Ratcliffe, D., Jenkins, V. & Saul, J. (2001). Psychiatric morbidity and its recognition by doctors in patients with cancer. *British Journal of Cancer, 84*, 1011–1015.

Falomir-Pichastor, J.M., Toscani, L. & Despointes, L.H. (2008). Determinants of flu vaccination among nurses: The effects of group identification and professional responsibility. *Applied Psychology, 58*, 4–58.

Federal Trade Commission (2007). Bureau of Economics staff report: Childrens exposure to TV advertising in 1977 and 2004. Accessed on 12 November 2009 at http://www.ftc.gov.

Fellowes, D., Barnes, K. & Wilkinson, S. (2004). Aromatherapy and massage for symptom relief in patients with cancer. *Cochrane Database of Systematic Reviews, 2*, CD002287.

Fensham, R. & Gardner, S. (2005). Dance classes, youth cultures and public health. *Youth Studies Australia, 24*, 14–20.

Ferguson, J., Bauld, L., Chesterman, J. & Judge, K. (2005). The English smoking treatment services: one-year outcomes. *Addiction*, Supplement 2, 59–69.

Ferrie, J.E. (2004). *Work, stress and health: the Whitehall II study.* London: Cabinet Office. Accessed on 7 July 2010 at: http://www.ucl.ac.uk/whitehallII/pdf/Whitehallbooklet_1_.pdf

Ferrie, J.E., Shipley, M.J. & Marmot, M.G., et al. (1995). Health effects of anticipation of job change and non-employment: longitudinal data from the Whitehall II study. *British Medical Journal, 311*, 1264–1269.

Ferrie, J.E., Shipley, M.J., Marmot, M.G., Stansfeld, S. & Davey Smith, G. (1998). The health effects of major organisational change and job insecurity. *Social Science & Medicine, 46*, 243–254.

Ferrie, J. E., Shipley, M. J., Stansfeld, S. A., & Marmot, M.G. (2002). Effects of chronic job insecurity and change in job security on self reported health, minor psychiatric morbidity, physiological measures, and health related behaviours in British civil servants: the Whitehall II study. *Journal of Epidemiology & Community Health, 56*, 450–454.

Ferron, C., Narring, F., Cauderay, M. & Michaud, P.-A. (1999). Sport activity in adolescences associations with health perceptions and experimental behaviours. *Health Education Research, 14*, 225–233.

Feste, C. & Anderson, R.M. (1995). Empowerment: from philosophy to practice. *Patient Education & Counseling, 26*, 139–144.

Fieldhouse, P. (1996). *Food and nutrition: customs and culture* (2nd ed.). Cheltenham: Stanley Thornes.

Fillmore, K.M., Stockwell, T., Chikritzhs, T., Bostrom, A. & Kerr, W. (2007). Moderate alcohol use and reduced mortality risk: systematic error in prospective studies and new hypotheses. *Annals of Epidemiology, 17(suppl 5)*, S16–S23.

Fincham, J.E. & Wertheimer, A.I. (1985). Using the Health Belief Model to predict initial drug therapy defaulting. *Social Science & Medicine, 20*, 101–105.

Fine, M. & Asch, A. (1982). The question of disability: no easy answers for the womens movement. *Reproductive Rights National Network Newsletter, 4*, 19–20.

Fine, M. & Barreras, R. (2001). To be of us. *Analysis of Social Issues & Public Policy, 1*, 175–182.

Finkelstein, V. & French, S. (1993). Towards a psychology of disability. In J. Swain, V. Finkelstein, S. French & M. Oliver (Eds.), *Disabling barriers – enabling environments*. London: Sage & Open University Press.

Fishbein, M. & Ajzen, I. (1975). *Belief attitude. Intention and behaviour. An introduction to theory and research.* Menlo Park: Addison-Wesley.

Fisher, J.D. & Fisher, W.A. (1992). Changing AIDS risk behavior. *Psychological Bulletin, 111*, 455–474.

Fisher, J.D. & Fisher, W.A. (2000). Individual level theories of HIV risk behavior change. In J. Peterson & R. DiClemente (Eds.), *Handbook of HIV prevention.* New York: Plenum. Pp. 3–56.

Fisher, J.D., Fisher, W.A., Amico, K.R. & Harman, J.J. (2006). An information-motivation-behavioral skills model of adherence to antiretroviral therapy. *Health Psychology, 25*, 462– 473.

Fitzpatrick, M. (2001). *The tyranny of health*. London: Routledge.

Fitzsimons, D., Parahoo, K. & Stringer, M. (2000). Waiting for coronary artery bypass surgery: a qualitative analysis. *Journal of Advanced Nursing, 32*, 1243–1252.

Flannery, T. (2006). *The weather makers. How man is changing the climate and what it means for life on earth*. New York: Atlantic Monthly Press.

Flannery Pearce, P. (2009). Physical activity: not just for quantitative researchers. *Qualitative Health Research, 19*, 879–880.

Flick, U. (1998). The social construction of individual and public health: contributions of social representations theory to a social science of health. *Social Science Information, 37*, 639–662.

Flick, U. (2002). *An introduction to qualitative research* (2nd ed.). London: Sage.

Flor, H., Fydrich, T. & Turk, D.C. (1992). Efficacy of multidisciplinary pain treatment centers - a meta-analytic review. *Pain, 49*, 221–230.

Flowers, P., Hart, G. & Marriott, C. (1999). Constructing sexual health. *Journal of Health Psychology, 4*, 483–495.

Floyd, D.L., Prentice-Dunn, S. & Rogers, R.W. (2000). A meta-analysis of research on protection motivation theory. *Journal of Applied Social Psychology, 30*, 407–429.

Fogarty, L., Roter, D., Larson, S., Burke, J.G., Gillespie, J. & Levy, B. (2002). Patient adherence to HIV medication regimens: a review of published and abstract reports. *Patient Education & Counseling, 46*, 93–108.

Fogarty, J.S. (1997). Reactance theory and patient non-compliance. *Social Science & Medicine, 45*, 1277–1288.

Folkman, S. & Moskowitz, J.T. (2004). Coping: pitfalls and promise. *Annual Review of Psychology, 55*, 745–774.

Follick, M.J., Smith, T.W. & Ahern, D.K. (1985). The Sickness Impact Profile: a global measure of disability in chronic low back pain. *Pain, 21*, 67–76.

Folta, S.C., Goldberg, J.P., Economos, C., Bell, R. & Meltzer, R. (2006). Food advertising targeted at school-age children: A content analysis. *Journal of Nutrition Education & Behavior, 38*, 244–248.

Food & Agriculture Organization of the United Nations (2006). *The state of food insecurity in the world*. Viale delle Terme di Caracalla, 00153 Rome, Italy.

Food Climate Research Network (2008). *Cooking up a storm. Food, greenhouse gas emissions and our changing climate*. Guildford University of Surrey.

Food Standards Agency (2003). *Does food promotion influence children? A systematic review of the evidence*. London: FSA.

Food Standards Agency (2010). Eat well, be well. Accessed on 8 July, 2010 at http://www.eatwell.gov.uk/healthydiet/fss/salt/

Fortner, B.V., Demarco, G., Irving, G., Ashley, J., Keppler, G., Chavez, J. & Jana Munk, J. (2003). Description and predictors of direct and indirect costs of pain reported by cancer patients. *Journal of Pain and Symptom Management, 25*, 9–18.

Foucault, M. (1976). *The birth of the clinic*. London: Routledge.

Foucault, M. (1979). *The history of sexuality*, Vol. 3: *The care of the self*. London: Allen Lane.

Foucault, M. (1980). *Power/Knowledge: Selected Interviews and Other Writings 1972–1977*, C. Gordon (Ed.). London: Harvester.

Fox, B.H. (1988). Psychogenic factors in cancer, especially its incidence. In S. Maes, D. Spielberger, P.B. Defares & I.G. Sarason (Eds.), *Topics in health psychology.* New York: Wiley. Pp. 37–55.

Foxcroft, D.R., Ireland, D., Lister-Sharp, D.J., Lowe, G. & Breen, R. (2003). Longer term primary prevention for alcohol misuse in young people: A systematic review. *Addiction, 98*, 397–411.

Frank, A.W. (1993). The rhetoric of self-change: illness experience as narrative. *Sociological Quarterly, 34*, 39–52.

Frank, A.W. (1995). *The wounded storyteller: Body, illness and ethics.* Chicago, IL: University of Chicago Press.

Frattaroli, J. (2006). Experimental disclosure and its moderator: A meta-analysis. *Journal of Abnormal Psychology, 96*, 3–13.

Frazier, E.L., Jiles, R.B. & Mayberry, R. (1996). Use of screening mammography and clinical breast examination among Black, Hispanic and White women. *Preventive Medicine, 25*, 118–125.

Freire, P. (1979/1993). *Pedagogy of the oppressed, 20th edn*. New York: Continuum.

French, D.P., Cooke, R., Mclean, N., Williams, M. & Sutton, S. (2007). What do people think about when they answer theory of planned behaviour questionnaires? A 'think aloud' study. *Journal of Health Psychology, 12*, 672–687.

Friedman, H.S., Martin, L.R., Tucker, J.S., Criqui, M.H., Kern, M.L. & Reynolds, C.A. (2008). Stability of physical activity across the lifespan. *Journal of Health Psychology, 13*, 1092–1104.

Friedson, E. (1970). *Profession of medicine*. New York: Harper & Row.

Fulton, J.P., Buechner, J.S., Scott, H.D., DeBuono, B.A., Feldman, J.P., Smith, R.A. & Kovenock, D. (1991) Predictors of breast cancer screening of women ages 40 and older. *Public Health Reports, 106*, 410–420.

Galavotti, C., Pappas-DeLuca, K.A. & Lansky, A. (2001). Modeling and reinforcement to combat HIV: the MARCH approach to behavior change. *American Journal of Public Health, 91*, 1602–1607.

Galindo, R.W. (2004). Fighting hunger in Brazil. *Perspectives in Health – The magazine of the Pan American Health Organization, 9*, Number 2. Accessed on 7 July, 2010, at http://www.paho.org/english/dd/pin/Number20_article05.htm

Gallagher, T.H., Waterman, A.D., Ebers, A.G., Fraser, V.J. & Levinson, W. (2003). Patients and physicians attitudes regarding the disclosure of medical errors. *Journal of the American Medical Association, 2898*, 1001–1007.

Gallant, S.J., Keita, G.P. & Royak-Schaler, R. (Eds.) (1997). *Health care for women: psychological, social & behavioral influences*. Washington, DC: American Psychological Association.

Ganguli, M., Vander Bilt, J., Saxton, J.A., Shen, C. & Dodge, H.H. (2005). Alcohol consumption and cognitive function in late life. *Neurology, 65*, 1210–1217.

Garay-Sevilla, M.E., Nava, L.E., Huerta, J.M., Diaz de Leon, J., Mena, A. & Fajardo, M.E. (1995). Adherence to treatment and social support in patients with non-insulin dependent diabetes mellitus. *Journal of Diabetes & its Complications, 9*, 81–86.

Garbarino, J. (1995). *Raising children in a socially toxic environment*. San Francisco: Jossey-Bass Publishers.

Garcia, J., Ervin, R.R. & Koelling, R.A. (1966). Learning with prolonged delay of reinforcement. *Psychonomic Science, 5*, 121–122.

Gardner, G. & Halweil, B. (2000). *Underfed and overfed: the global epidemic of malnutrition worldwide*. Washington, DC: Worldwide Watch.

Garrison, M.M., Christakis, D.A., Ebel, B.E., Wiehe, S.E. & Rivara, F.P. (2003). Smoking cessation interventions for adolescents. A systematic review. *American Journal of Preventive Medicine, 25*, 363–367.

Gee, G.C., Spencer, M.S., Chen, J. & Takeuchi, D. (2007). A nationwide study of discrimination and chronic health conditions among Asian Americans. *American Journal of Public Health, 97*, 1275–1282.

Geertz, C. (1973). *The interpretation of culture*. New York: Basic Books.

Gil, K.M., Carson, J.W., Sedway, J.A., Porter, L.S., Wilson Schaeffer, J.J. & Orringer, E. (2000). Follow-up of coping skills training in adults with sickle cell disease: analysis of daily pain and coping practice diaries. *Health Psychology, 19*, 85–90.

Gilbert, R.M. (1984). *Caffeine consumption*. New York: Alan R. Liss.

Giles-Corti, B. & Donovan, R.J. (2002). The relative influence of individual, social and physical environment determinants of physical activity. *Social Science & Medicine, 54*, 1793–1812.

Gill, C.J. (2000). Health professionals, disability and assisted suicide: an examination of relevant empirical evidence and reply to Batavia (2000). *Psychology, Public Policy & Law, 6(2)*, 526–545.

Gillies, V. & Willig, C. (1997). 'You get the nicotine and that in your blood': constructions of addiction and control in womens accounts of cigarette smoking. *Journal of Community & Applied Social Psychology, 7*, 285–301.

Ginzel, K.H., Maritz, G.S., Marks, D.F., Neuberger, M., Pauly, J.R., Polito, J.R. & Slotkin, T.A. (2007). Critical review: nicotine for the fetus, the infant and the adolescent? *Journal of Health Psychology, 12*, 215–224.

Glaser, B. & Strauss, A. (1967). *The discovery of grounded theory: strategies for qualitative research*. Chicago: Aldine.

Glaser, B.G. (1992). *Basics of grounded theory analysis: emergence versus forcing*. Mill Valley, CA: Sociology Press.

Glasgow, R.E., Hampson, S.E., Strycker, L.A. & Ruggiero, L. (1997). Personal-model beliefs and social-environmental barriers related to diabetes self-management. *Diabetes Care, 20*, 556–561.

Glass, G.V. (1976). Primary, secondary and meta-analysis of research. *Educational Research, 5*, 3–8.

Gleeson, K. & Frith, H. (2006). (De)constructing body image. *Journal of Health Psychology, 11*, 79–90.

Goffman, E. (1963). *Stigma: Notes on the management of spoiled identity*. London: Penguin.

Goldacre, M.J. & Roberts, S.E. (2004). Hospital admission for acute pancreatitis in an English population, 1963–98: Database study of incidence & mortality. *British Medical Journal, 328*, 1466–1469.

Gooden, R.J. and Winefield, H.R. (2007). Breast and prostate cancer online discussion boards: a thematic analysis of gender differences and similarities. *Journal of Health Psychology, 12*, 103–114.

Gordon, B.O. & Rosenblum, K.E. (2001). Bringing disability into the sociological frame: a comparison of disability with race, sex, and sexual orientation statuses. *Disability & Society, 16(1)*, 5–19.

Gore-Felton, C. & Koopman, C. (2008). Behavioral mediation of the relationship between psychosocial factors and HIV disease progression. *Psychosomatic Medicine, 70*, 569–574.

Gotay, C.C., Shimizu, H., Muraoka, M., Ishihara, Y., Tsuboi, K. & Ogawa, H. (2004). Health attitudes and behaviors: comparison of Japanese and Americans of Japanese and European ancestry. *Health & Place, 10*, 153–161.

Gøtzsche, P.C. & Nielsen, M. (2009). Screening for breast cancer with mammography (Review). *Cochrane Database of Systematic Reviews. Issue 4*, Art. No.: CD001877.

Gracey, M. & King, M. (2009). Indigenous health part 1: Determinants and disease patterns. *The Lancet, 374*, 65–75.

Grafstrom, M. (1994). The experience of burden in the care of elderly persons with dementia. Unpublished doctoral dissertation, Karolinska Institute, Stockholm, Sweden.

Graham, H. (1976). Smoking in pregnancy: the attitudes of expectant mothers. *Social Science & Medicine, 10*, 399–405.

Graham, H. (1987). Women's smoking & family health. *Social Science & Medicine, 25*, 47–56.

Graham, R., Kremer, J. & Wheeler, G. (2008). Physical activity and psychological well-being among people with chronic illness and disability. *Journal of Health Psychology, 13*, 447–458.

Graham, J., Ramirez, A., Love, S., Richards, M. & Burgess, C. (2002). Stressful life experiences and risk of relapse of breast cancer: Observational cohort study. *British Medical Journal, 324*, 1420–1422.

Gram, I.T. & Slenker, S.E. (1992). Cancer anxiety and attitudes toward mammography among screening attenders, nonattenders, and women never invited. *American Journal of Public Health, 82*, 249–251.

Gram, I.T., Lund, E. & Slenker, S.E. (1990). Quality of life following a first positive mammogram. *British Journal of Cancer, 62*, 1018–1022.

Gray, N. & Coughlan, D. (2009). Health literacy is not just reading and writing. *The Pharmaceutical Journal, 283*, 333–336.

Gray, R. & Henderson, J. (2006). *Report to the Department of Health: review of the fetal effects of prenatal alcohol exposure*. University of Oxford: National Perinatal Epidemiology Unit.

Gray, R. & Sinding, C. (2002). *Standing ovation: performing social science research about cancer*. Walnut Creek, CA: Altamira Press.

Gray, R.E., Fergus, K.D. & Fitch, M.I. (2005). Two Black men with prostate cancer: A narrative approach. *British Journal of Health Psychology, 10*, 71–84.

Gray, R.E., Ivonoffski, V. & Sinding, C. (2001). Making a mess and spreading it around: articulation of an approach to research-based theatre. In A. Bochner & C. Ellis (Eds.), *Ethnographically speaking*. Walnut Creek, CA: Altamira Press. Pp. 57–75.

Greene, R. (1995). Survey of prescription anomalies in community pharmacies: (1) prescription monitoring. *Pharmacy Journal, 254*, 476–481.

Greenwald, B.D., Narcessian, E.J. & Pomeranz, B.A. (1999). Assessment of psychiatrists knowledge and perspectives on the use of opiods: review of basic concepts for managing chronic pain. *American Journal of Physical Medicine & Rehabilitation, 78*, 408–415.

Greer, S., Morris, T. & Pettingale, K.W. (1979). Psychological response to breast cancer; effect on outcome. *Lancet, 2*, 785–787.

Gregg, J. & Curry, R.H. (1994). Explanatory models for cancer among African-American women at two Atlanta neighborhood health centers: the implications for a cancer screening program. *Social Science & Medicine, 39*, 519–526.

Gregory, S. & McKie, J. (1991). The smear test: listening to women's views. *Nursing Standard, 5*, 32–36.

Grogan, S. (2006). Body image and health: contemporary perspectives. *Journal of Health Psychology, 11*, 523–530.

Grogan, S. & Richards, H. (2002). Body image: Focus groups with boys and men. *Men and Masculinities, 4*, 219–232.

Grossardt, B.R., Bower, J.H., Geda, Y.E., Colligan, R.C. & Rocca, W.A. (2009). Pessimistic, anxious, and depressive personality traits predict all-cause mortality: The Mayo Clinic cohort study of personality and aging. *Psychosomatic Medicine, 71*, 491–500.

Gual, A. (2006). Alcohol in Spain: is it different? *Addiction, 101,* 1073–1077.

Gueguen, N. & Vion, M. (2009). The effect of a practitioner's touch on a patient's medication compliance. *Psychology, Health & Medicine, 14*, 689–694.

Habraken, J.M., ter Riet, G., Gore, J.M., Greenstone, M.A., Weersink, E.J., Bindels, P.J. & Willems, D.L. (2009). Health-related quality of life in end-stage COPD and lung cancer patients. *Journal of Pain & Symptom Management, 37*, 973–981.

Hackett, A., Boddy, L., Boothby, J., Dummer, T.J.B., Johnson, B. & Stratton, G. (2008). Mapping dietary habits may provide clues about the factors that determine food choice. *Journal of Human Nutrition & Dietetics, 21*, 428–437.

Hagger, M.S., Chatzisarantis, N.L.D. & Biddle, S.J.H. (2002). A meta-analytic review of the theories of reasoned action and planned behaviour in physical activity: predictive validity and the contribution of additional variables. *Journal of Sport & Exercise Psychology, 24*, 3–32.

Hagger, M.S., Chatzisarantis, N.L.D., Culverhouse, T. & Biddle, S.J.H. (2003). The processes by which perceived autonomy support in physical education promotes leisure-time physical activity intentions and behavior: a trans-contextual model. *Journal of Educational Psychology, 95*, 784–795.

Hagger, M.S. & Orbell, S. (2003). A meta-analytic review of the common-sense model of illness representations. *Psychology & Health, 18*, 141–184.

Haines, A.P., Imeson, J.D. & Meade, T.W. (1987). Phobic anxiety and ischaemic heart disease. *British Medical Journal (Clinical Research Edition), 295*, 297–299.

Halkitis, P.N., Kutnick, A.H. & Slater, S. (2005). The social realities of adherence to protease inhibitor regimens: substance use, health care and psychological states. *Journal of Health Psychology, 10*, 545–558.

Hall, J.A., Roter, D.L. & Katz, N.R. (1988). Meta-analysis of correlates of provider behavior in medical encounters. *Medical Care, 26*, 1–19.

Hamajima, N., Hirose, K., Rohan, T. & Calle, E.E., et al. (Collaborative Group on Hormonal Factors in Breast Cancer) (2002). Alcohol, tobacco and breast cancer – collaborative reanalysis of individual data from 53 epidemiological studies. Including 58,515 women with breast cancer and 95,067 women without the disease. *British Journal of Cancer, 87*, 1234–1245.

Hamilton, K. & White, K. (2010). Identifying parents' perceptions about physical activity: A qualitative exploration of salient behavioural, normative, and control beliefs among mothers and fathers of young children. *Journal of Health Psychology, 16*, xx-yy.

Hans, M.B. & Koeppen, A.H. (1989). Huntingtons chorea: its impact on the spouse. *Journal of Nervous & Mental Disease, 168*, 209–214.

Hanson-Divers, E.C. (1997). Developing a medical achievement reading test to evaluate patient literacy skills: a preliminary study. *Journal of Health Care for the Poor and Underserved, 8*, 56–59.

Harding, R. & Higginson, I.J. (2003). What is the best way to help caregivers in cancer and palliative care? A systematic literature review of interventions and their effectiveness. *Palliative Medicine, 17*, 63–74.

Hardy, S. & Grogan, S. (2009). Preventing disability through exercise. Investigating older adults' influences and motivations to engage in physical activity. *Journal of Health Psychology, 14*, 1036–1046.

Hargreaves, D.A. & Tiggemann, M. (2006). 'Body image is for girls' A qualitative study of boys' body image. *Journal of Health Psychology,* 11, 567–576.

Harlan, L.C., Bernstein, A.M. & Kessler, L.G. (1991). Cervical cancer screening: who is not screened and why? *American Journal of Public Health, 81*, 885–890.

Harper, P.S. (1992). Genetic testing, life insurance, and adverse selection. *Philosophical Transactions of the Royal Society, 352*, 1063–1066.

Harré, R. (1979). *Social being*. Oxford: Blackwell.

Harris, J.L., Bargh, J.A. & Brownell, K.D. (2009). Priming effects of television food advertising on eating behavior. *Health Psychology, 28*, 404–413.

Harris, T.O. (2007). Life events and health. In S. Ayers, A. Baum, C. McManus, S. Newman, K. Wallston, J. Weinman and R. West (Eds.), *Cambridge handbook of psychology, health and medicine* (2nd edn.). Cambridge, Cambridge University Press. Pp. 128–132.

Harrison, K. & Marske, A.L. (2005). Nutritional content of foods advertised during the television programs children watch most. *American Journal of Public Health, 95*, 1568–1574.

Hart, C.L., Davey Smith, G., Hole, D.J. & Hawthorne, V.M. (1999). Alcohol consumption and mortality from all causes, coronary heart disease and stroke: results from a prospective cohort study of Scottish Men with 21 years of follow up. *British Medical Journal, 318*, 1725–1729.

Harvey, A.G. & Bryant, R.A. (2002). Acute stress disorder: a synthesis and critique. *Psychological Bulletin, 128*, 886–902.

Hastings, G. & MacFadyen, L. (2000). *Keep smiling, no one's going to die. An analysis of internal documents from the tobacco industrys main UK advertising agencies*. Centre for Tobacco Control Research. (Examples of the documents can be viewed at: www.tobaccopapers.com.)

Haug, M. & Lavin, B. (1983). *Consumerism in medicine: challenging physician authority*. Beverly Hills, CA: Sage.

Hausenblas, H.A., Carron, A.V. & Mack, D.E. (1997). An application of the theories of reasoned action and planned behavior to exercise behavior. *Journal of Sport & Exercise Behavior, 199*, 36–51.

Hausenblas, H.A. & Fallon, E.A. (2006). Exercise and body image: a meta-analysis. *Psychology & Health, 21*, 33–47.

Healey, J. (Ed.) (2006). *Body image and self esteem*. Thirroul, Australia: Spinney Press.

Health Foundation (2004). *The Health Foundation Healthcare Leaders Panel Survey 1: Patient Safety*. London: Health Foundation.

Health Protection Agency (2009). STIs Annual Slide Set 1999–2008, at http://www.hpa.org.uk/HPA/Topics/InfectiousDiseases/InfectionsAZ/1203409656940/.

Heath, A.C. & Madden, P.A.F. (1995). Genetic influences on smoking behavior. In J.R. Turner, L.R. Carden & J.K. Hewitt (Eds.), *Behavior genetic approaches in behavioral medicine*. New York: Plenum Press. Pp. 45–66.

Heath, H. (1998). Keeping a reflective practice diary: a practical guide. *Nurse Education Today, 18*, 592–598.

Heather, N. (2001). Pleasures and pains of our favourite drug. In N. Heather, T.J. Peters & T. Stockwell (Eds.), *International handbook of alcohol dependence and problems*. London: Wiley. Pp. 5–14.

Heather, N. & Robertson, I. (1997). *Problem drinking*. Oxford: Oxford University Press.

Heatherton, T.F., Kleck, R.E., Hebl, M.R. & Hull, J.G. (2000). *The social psychology of stigma*. New York: Guilford.

Heelas, P. & Lock, A. (Eds.) (1981). *Indigenous psychologies: the anthropology of the self*. New York: Academic Press.

Heider, F. (1958). *The psychology of interpersonal relations*. New York: Wiley.

Heidigger, M. (1962). *Being and time*. New York: Harper & Row.

Helgeson, V.S. & Fritz, H.L. (1999). Cognitive adaptation as a predictor of new coronary events after percutaneous transluminal coronary angioplasty. *Psychosomatic Medicine, 61*, 488–495.

Hemingway, H. & Marmot, M. (1999). Psychosocial factors and the aetiology and prognosis of coronary heart disease: systematic review of prospective cohort studies. *British Medical Journal, 318*, 1460–1467.

Henderson, K.A. & Ainsworth, B.E. (2003). A synthesis of perceptions about physical activity among older African American and American Indian women. *American Journal of Public Health, 93*, 313–317.

Henderson, L., Millett, C. & Thorogood, N. (2008). Perceptions of childhood immunization in a minority community: qualitative study. *Journal of the Royal Society of Medicine, 101*, 244–251.

Herbst, J.H., Sherba, R.T., Crepaz, N., DeLuca. J.B., Zohrabyan, L., Stall, R.D. & Lyles, C.M. (2005). A meta-analytic review of HIV behavioral interventions for reducing sexual risk behavior of men who have sex with men. *Journal of Acquired Immune Deficiency Syndromes, 39*, 228–241.

Herr, K., Bjoro, K. & Decker, S. (2006). Tools for assessment of pain in nonverbal older adults with dementia: A state-of-the-science review. *Journal of Pain and Symptom Management, 31*, 170–192.

Herzlich, C. (1973). *Health and illness: A social psychological analysis*. London: Academic Press.

Herzlich, C. & Pierret, J. (1987). *Illness and self in society*. Baltimore, MD: Johns Hopkins University Press.

Herzog, T.A. (2008). Analyzing the transtheoretical model using the framework of Weinstein, Rothman, and Sutton (1998): The example of smoking cessation. *Health Psychology, 27*, 548–556.

Hesketh, T. & Xing, Z.W. (2005). The effect of China's one-child policy after 25 years. *New England Journal of Medicine, 353*, 1171–1176.

Hesse, B.W., Nelson, D.E., Kreps, G.L., Croyle, R.T., Arora, N.K., Rimer, B.K. & Viswanath, K. (2005). Trust and sources of health information. The impact of the Internet and its implications for health care providers: Findings from the first Health Information National Trends Survey. *Archive of Internal Medicine, 165*, 2618–2624.

Heyman-Monnikes, I., Arnold, R., Florin, I., Herda, A., Melfsen, S. & Monnikes, H. (2000). The combination of medical treatment plus multicomponent behavioural therapy is superior to medical treatment alone in the therapy of irritable bowel syndrome. *American Journal of Gastroenterology, 95*, 981–994.

Hirani, S.P., Pugsley, W.B. & Newman, S.P. (2006). Illness representations of coronary artery disease: An empirical examination of the Illness Perceptions Questionnaire (IPQ) in patients undergoing surgery, angioplasty and medication. *British Journal of Health Psychology, 11*, 199–220.

Hittner, J.B. & Kennington, L.E. (2008). Normative perceptions, substance use, age of substance use initiation, and gender as predictors of HIV-risky sexual behavior in a college student sample. *Journal of Applied Biobehavioral Research, 13*, 86–101.

Hittner, J.B. & Kryzanowski, J.J. (2010). Residential status moderates the association between gender and risky sexual behavior. *Journal of Health Psychology, 15*, 634–640.

HMSO (2009). *Chief Medical Officer's Annual Report for 2008*. London: Her Majesty's Stationary Office.

Hodgetts, D. & Chamberlain, K. (2006). Media and health: A continuum concern for health psychology. *Journal of Health Psychology, 11*, 171–174.

Hodgetts, D. and Stolte, O. (2009). Questioning 'Black humour': Racial exploitation, media and health. *Journal of Health Psychology, 14*, 643–646.

Hofrichter, R. (2003). The politics of health inequities: contested terrain. In R. Hofrichter (Ed.), *Health and social justice: politics, ideology, and inequity in the distribution of disease*. San Francisco, CA: Jossey-Bass.

Holbrook, M.L. (1871). *Parturition without pain: A code of directions for escaping the primal curse*. New York: Wood & Holbrook.

Hollis, J.F., Connett, J.E., Stevens, V.J. & Greenlick, M.R. (1990). Stressful life events, Type A behaviour, and the prediction of cardiovascular and total mortality over six years. *Journal of Behavioural Medicine, 13*, 263–281.

Hollway, W. & Jefferson, T. (2000). *Doing qualitative research differently: free association, narrative and the interview method*. London: Sage.

Holmes, T.H. & Rahe, R.H. (1967). The social readjustment rating scale. *Journal of Psychosomatic Research, 11*, 213–218.

Holroyd, K.A. & Coyne, J. (1987). Personality and health in the 1980s: psychosomatic medicine revisited? *Journal of Personality, 55*, 359–376.

Horne, R. (1997). Representations of medication and treatment: Advances in theory and measurement. In K.J. Petrie & J.A. Weinman (Eds.), *Perceptions of health and illness*. Amsterdam: Harwood Academic. Pp. 155–188.

Horne, R., Graupner, L., Frost, S., Weinman, J., Wright, S.M. & Hankins, M. (2004). Medicine in a multicultural society: the effect of cultural background on beliefs about medications. *Social Science & Medicine, 59*, 1307–1313.

Horne, R. & Weinman, J. (1999). Patients' beliefs about prescribed medicines and their role in adherence to treatment in chronic physical illness. *Journal of Psychosomatic Research, 47*, 555–567.

Horne, R. & Weinman, J. (2002). Self-regulation and self-management in asthma: exploring the role of illness perceptions and treatment beliefs in explaining non-adherence to preventive medication. *Psychology & Health, 17*, 17–32.

Horton, R. (2006). Indigenous peoples: time to act now for equity and health. *Lancet, 367*, 1705–1707.

Horton-Salway, M. (2001). Narrative identities and the management of personal accountability in talk about ME: a discursive psychology approach to illness narrative. *Journal of Health Psychology, 6*, 247–259.

House of Commons Health Committee Health Inequalities (2009). *Third report of session 2008–9, vol 1*, HC 286–1. London: The Stationery Office Ltd.

Howarth, C.S. (2001). Towards a social psychology of community: A social representations perspective. *Journal for the Theory of Social Behaviour, 31*, 223–238.

Hu, F.B. (2003). Overweight and obesity in women: health risks and consequences. *Journal of Women's Health, 12*, 163–172.

Hughes, J., Jelsma, J., Maclean, E., Darder, M. & Tinise, X. (2004). The health-related quality of life of people living with HIV/AIDS. *Disability & Rehabilitation, 26*, 371–376.

Hulka, B.S. (1979). Patient–clinician interactions and compliance. In R.B. Haynes, D.W. Taylor & D.L. Sackett (Eds.), *Compliance in health care*. Baltimore, MD: Johns Hopkins University Press. Pp. 63–77.

Hulka, B.S., Cassel, J.C. & Kupper, L.L. (1976). Disparities between medications prescribed and consumed among chronic disease patients. In L. Lasagna (Ed.), *Patient compliance*. Mount Kisco, NY: Futura Publishing. Pp. 123–152.

Human Development Report (2000). *Human rights and human development*. New York: Oxford University Press.

Hunter, K.M. (1991). *Doctors' stories: the narrative structure of medical knowledge*. Princeton, NJ: Princeton University Press.

Hunter, M.S., O'Dea, I. & Britten, N. (1997). Decision-making and hormone replacement therapy: a qualitative analysis. *Social Science & Medicine, 45*, 1541–1548.

Hyman, R.B., Baker, S., Ephraim, R., Moadel, A. & Philip, J. (1994). Health Belief Model variables as predictors of screening mammography utilization. *Journal of Behavioral Medicine, 17*, 391–406.

Idler, E.L. & Banyamini, Y. (1997). Self-rated health and mortality: A review of twenty-seven community studies. *Journal of Health & Social Behavior, 38*, 21–37.

Ikard, F.F., Green, D. & Horn, D. (1969). A scale to differentiate between types of smoking as related to management of affect. *International Journal of the Addictions, 4*, 649–659.

Illich, I. (1976). *Limits to medicine*. London: Calder & Boyars.

Information Centre for Health and Social Care, Lifestyles Statistics (2008). Statistics on NHS Stop Smoking Services: England, April 2007 to March 2008. Accessed on 7 July 2010. http://www.ic.nhs.uk/webfiles/publications/Stop%20smoking%20ANNUAL%20bulletins/SSS0708/SSS%202007-08%20final%20format%20v2.pdf.

Information Centre for Health and Social Care (2009). Statistics on obesity, physical activity and diet: England, February 2009. Accessed on 25 January 2010 at: http://www.ic.nhs.uk/statistics-and-data-collections/health-and-lifestyles/obesity/statistics-on-obesity-physical-activity-and-diet:-england-february-2009.

Ingledew, D.K., Markland, D. & Medley, A.R. (1998). Exercise motives and stages of change. *Journal of Health Psychology, 3*, 477–489.

Insel, K.C., Meek, P.M. & Leventhal, H. (2005). Differences in illness representation among pulmonary patients and their providers. *Journal of Health Psychology, 10*, 147–162.

Institute of Alcohol Studies (2003). *Crime and disorder, binge drinking and the licensing bill.* London: Institute of Alcohol Studies.

Institute of Medicine (IOM) (2000). *To err is human: building a safer health system.* Washington, DC: Institute of Medicine, National Academy of Science.

Institute of Medicine (2004). *Health literacy: Prescription to end confusion.* Accessed on 29 December 2009 at http://books.nap.edu/catalog.php?record_id=10883.

Institute of Medicine (2006). *Progress in preventing childhood obesity: How do we measure up?* USA: Institute of Medicine.

Institute of Medicine (2007a). *Cancer care for the whole patient: meeting psychosocial health needs.* Washington, DC: National Academy Press.

Institute of Medicine (2007b). *Implementing cancer survivorship care planning*. Washington, DC: National Academy Press.

International Association for the Study of Pain (2010). Website accessed on 8 July 2010 at http://www.iasp-pain.org/AM/Template.cfm?Section=PAIN_Jour...isplay.cfm&ContentID=1766.

Ironson, G., Solomon, G.F., Balbin, E.G., O'Cleirigh, C., George, A., Kumar, M., Larson, D. & Woods, T.E. (2002). The Ironson-Woods spirituality/religiousness index is associated with long survival, health behaviors, less distress, and low cortisol in people with HIV/AIDS. *Annals of Behavioral Medicine, 24*, 34–48.

Ironson, G., Stuetzle, R. & Fletcher, M.A. (2006). An increase in religiousness/spirituality occurs after HIV diagnosis and predicts slower disease progression over 4 years in people with HIV. *Journal of General Internal Medicine, 21*, S62–S68.

Iversen, L. & Chapman, V. (2002). Cannabinoids: a real prospect for pain relief? *Current Opinion in Pharmacology, 2*, 50–55.

Jacobsen, P. B. (2009). Promoting evidence-based psychosocial care for cancer patients. *Psycho-Oncology, 18*, 6–13.

Jain, A. & Ogden, J. (1999). General practitioners' experiences of patients' complaints: qualitative study. *BMJ, 318*, 1596–1599.

James, J.E. (1997). *Understanding caffeine: a biobehavioral analysis*. Thousand Oaks, CA: Sage.

Jamner, L.D. & Tursky, B. (1987). Syndrome specific descriptor profiling: A psychophysiological and psychophysical approach. *Health Psychology, 6*, 417–430.

Jarvis, M.J. (2004). Why people smoke. *British Medical Journal, 328*, 277–279.

Jastak, S. & Wilkinson, G.S. (1993). *Wide range achievement test-revised 3.* Wilmington, DE: Jastak Associates.

Jensen, M. & Patterson, D.R. (2006). Hypnotic treatment of chronic pain. *Journal of Behavioral Medicine, 29*, 95–124.

Jensen, M.P., Karoly, P. & Huger, R. (1987). The development and preliminary validation of an instrument to assess patients attitudes toward pain. *Journal of Psychosomatic Research, 31*, 393–400.

Jha, P., Jacob, B., Gajalakshmi, V., Gupta, P.C., Dhingra, N., Kumar, R., & Peto, R. for the RGI–CGHR Investigators (2008). A nationally representative case–control study of smoking and death in India. *New England Journal of Medicine, 358*, 1137–1147.

Joffe, H. (1996). AIDS research and prevention: a social representational approach. *British Journal of Medical Psychology, 69*, 169–91.

Joffe, H. (1999). *Risk and 'the other'*. Cambridge: Cambridge University Press.

Joffe, H. (2002). Social representations and health psychology. *Social Science Information, 41*, 559–580.

Joffe, H. & Bettega, N. (2003). Social representations of AIDS among Zambian adolescents. *Journal of Health Psychology, 8*, 616–631.

Joffe, H. & Haarhoff, G. (2002). Representations of far-flung illnesses: the case of Ebola in Britain. *Social Science & Medicine, 54*, 955–969.

Joffress, M., Reed, D.M. & Nomura, A.M.Y. (1985). Psychosocial processes and cancer incidence among Japanese men in Hawaii. *American Journal of Epidemiology, 121*, 488–500.

Johnson, A.M., Wadsworth, J., Wellings, K. & Field, J. (Eds.) (1994). *Sexual attitudes and lifestyles*. Oxford: Blackwell.

Johnston, M., Foulkes, J., Johnston, D.W., Pollard, B. & Gudmundsdottir, H. (1999). Impact on patients and partners of inpatient and extended cardiac counseling and rehabilitation: a controlled trial. *Psychosomatic Medicine, 61*, 225–233.

Jones, D.R., Goldblatt, P.O. & Leon, D.A. (1984). Bereavement and cancer: Some data on deaths of spouses from the longitudinal study of Office of Population Censuses and Surveys. *British Medical Journal, 289*, 461–464.

Jones, F. & Bright, J. (Eds.) (2001). *Stress: myth, theory and research.* London: Prentice Hall.

Jonsdottir, H. & Baldursdottir, L. (1998). The experience of people awaiting coronary artery bypass graft surgery: the Icelandic experience. *Journal of Advanced Nursing, 27*, 68–74.

Jorenby, D.E., Hays, J.T., Rigotti, N.A., Azoulay, S., Watsky, E.J., Williams, K.E. & Reeves, K.R. (2006). Efficacy of varenicline, an alpha4beta2 nicotinic acetylcholine receptor partial agonist, vs placebo or sustained-release bupropion for smoking cessation: a randomized controlled trial. *Journal of the American Medical Association, 296*, 56–63.

Jovchelovitch, S. & Grevais, M.C. (1999). Social representations of health and illness: The case of the Chinese community in England. *Journal of Community and Applied Social Psychology, 9*, 247–260.

Jylhä, M. (2009). What is self-rated health and why does it predict mortality? Towards a unified conceptual model. *Social Science and Medicine, 69,* 307–316.

Kagee, A., Le Roux, M. & Dick, J. (2007). Treatment adherence among primary care patients in a historically disadvantaged community in South Africa: A qualitative study. *Journal of Health Psychology, 12*, 444–460.

Kamarck, T.W., Muldoon, M.F., Shiffman, S.S. & Sutton-Tyrrell, K. (2007). Experiences of demand and control during daily life are predictors of carotid atherosclerotic progression among healthy men. *Health Psychology, 26*, 324–332.

Kanner, A.D., Coyne, J.C., Schaefer, C. & Lazarus, R.S. (1981). Comparison of two modes of stress measurement: daily hassles and uplifts versus major life events. *Journal of Behavioral Medicine, 4*, 1–39.

Karasek, R. & Theorell, T. (1990). *Healthy work: stress, productivity, and the reconstruction of working life*. New York: Basic Books.

Karlson, S., Nazroo, J.Y., McKenzie, K., Bhui, K. and Weich, S. (2005). Racism, psychosis and common mental disorder among ethnic minority in England. *Psychological medicine, 35*, 1795–1803.

Kart, C.S., Kinney, J.M., Subedi, J., Basnyat, K.B. & Vadakkan, M.F. (2007). Lay explanations and self-management of diabetes in Kathmandu. *Nepal Journal of Aging & Health, 19*, 683–704.

Karus, D., Raveis, V.H., Alexander, C., Hanna, B., Selwyn, P., Marconi. K. & Higginson, I. (2005). Patient reports of symptoms and their treatment at three palliative care projects servicing individuals with HIV/AIDS. *Journal of Pain and Symptom Management, 30*, 408–417.

Kawachi, I., Colditz, G.A., Ascherio, A., Rimm, E.B., Giovannucci, E., Stampfer, M.J. & Willett, W.C. (1994). Prospective study of phobic anxiety and risk of coronary heart disease in men. *Circulation, 89*, 1992–1997.

Kawachi, I., Subramanian, S. & Almeida-Filho, N. (2002). A glossary for health inequalities. *Journal of Epidemiology and Community Health, 56*, 647–652.

Kay, C., Davies, J., Gamsu, D. & Jarman, M. (2009). An exploration of the experiences of young women living with Type 1 diabetes. *Journal of Health Psychology, 14*, 242–250.

Keane, V., Stanton, B., Horton, L., Aronson, R., Galbrath, J. & Hughart, N. (1993). Perceptions of vaccine efficacy, illness, and health among inner-city parents. *Clinical Pediatrics, 32*, 2–7.

Kearney, A.J. (2006). Increasing our understanding of breast self-examination: women talk about cancer, the health care system and being women. *Qualitative Health Research, 16*, 802–820.

Kearney, A.J. & Murray, M. (2009). Breast cancer screening recommendations: Is mammography the only answer*? Journal of Midwifery & Women's Health, 54(5)*, 393–400.

Kearns, R.D., Turk, D.C. & Rudy, T.E. (1985). The West Haven–Yale Multidimensional Pain Inventory. *Pain, 23*, 345–356.

Keefe, R.J., Hauck, E.R., Egert, J., Rimer, B. & Kornguth, P. (1994). Mammography pain and discomfort: a cognitive behavioural perspective. *Pain, 56*, 247–260.

Keegan, A., Liao, L.-M. & Boyle, M. (2003). Hirsutism: A psychological analysis. *Journal of Health Psychology, 8*, 327–346.

Keehn, R.J. (1980). Follow-up studies of World War II and Korean conflict prisoners. III. Mortality to January 1, 1976: *American Journal of Epidemiology, 111*, 194–211.

Kelner, M., Wellman, B., Boon, H. & Welsh, S. (2003). Responses of established healthcare to the professionalization of complementary and alternative medicine in Ontario. *Social Science & Medicine, 59*, 915–930.

Kern, M.L. & Friedman, H.S. (2008). Do conscientious individuals live longer? A quantitative review. *Health Psychology, 27*, 505–512

Kerr, J., Eves, F.F. & Carroll, D. (2001). Getting more people on the stairs: the impact of a new message format. *Journal of Health Psychology, 6*, 495–500.

Key, T.J., Fraser, G.E., Thorogood, M., Appleby, P.N., Beral, V., Reeves, G. & McPherson, K. (1998). Mortality in vegetarians and non-vegetarians: a collaborative analysis of 8,300 deaths among 76,000 men and women in five prospective studies. *Public Health Nutrition, 1*, 33–41.

Keys, A., Anderson, J.T. & Grande, F. (1959). Serum cholesterol in man: diet fat and intrinsic responsiveness. *Circulation, 199*, 201–204.

Khan, L.K. & Bowman, B.A. (1999). Obesity: a major global public health problem. *Annual Review of Nutrition,19*, xiii–xvii.

Kickbusch, I., Wait, S. & Maag, D. (2005). *Navigating health: The role of health literacy*. Accessed 29 December 2009 at http://www.ilonakickbusch.com/health-literacy/NavigatingHealth.pdf.

King, A.C. (1994). Community and public health approaches to the promotion of physical activity. *Medicine & Science in Sports & Exercise, 26*, 1405–1412.

Kirsch, I., Jungleblut, A., Jenkins, L. & Kolstad, A. (1993). *Adult literacy in America: A first look at the results of the National Adult Literacy Survey.* Washington DC: National Center for Education Statistics, US Department of Education.

Kivimäki, M., Leino-Arjas, P., Luukkonen, R., Riihimäki, H., Vahtera, J. & Kirjonen, J. (2002). Work stress and risk of cardiovascular mortality: Prospective cohort study of industrial employees. *British Medical Journal, 325*, 857–860.

Kivits, J. (2006). Informed patients and the internet: A mediated context for consultations with health professionals. *Journal of Health Psychology, 11*, 269–282.

Kleinman, A. (1980). *Patients and healers in the context of culture*. Berkeley, CA: University of California Press.

Klemm, P., Hurst, M., Dearholt, S.L. and Trone, S.R. (1999). Cyber solace: gender differences on Internet cancer support groups. *Computer Nursing, 17*, 65–72.

Klenerman, L., Slade, P.D., Stanley, I.M., Pennie, B., Reilly, J.P., Atchinson, L.E., Troup, J.D.G. & Troup, M.J. (1995). The prediction of chronicity in patients with an acute attack of low back pain in a general practice setting. *Spine, 20*, 478–484.

Köke, A.J.A., Schouten. J.S.A.G., Lamerichs-Geelen, M.J.H., Lipsch, J.S.M., Waltje, E.M.H., van Kleef, M. & Patijn, J. (2004). Pain reducing effect of three types of transcutaneous electrical nerve stimulation in patients with chronic pain: a randomised crossover trial. *Pain, 108*, 36–42.

Koniak-Griffin, D. & Stein, J.A. (2006). Predictors of sexual risk behaviors among adolescent mothers in a human immunodeficiency virus prevention program. *Journal of Adolescent Health, 38*, 297.e1–11.

Konttinen, H., Haukkala, A. & Uutela, A. (2008). Comparing sense of coherence, depressive symptoms and anxiety, and their relationships with health in a population-based study. *Social Science and Medicine, 66*, 2401–2412.

Korp, P. (2006). Health on the internet: Implications for health promotion. *Health Education Research, 21*, 78–86.

Krantz, D.S. & McCeney, M.K. (2002). Effects of psychological and social factors on organic disease: a critical assessment of research on coronary heart disease. *Annual Review of Psychology, 53*, 341–369.

Krause, M. (2003). The transformation of social representations of chronic disease in a self-help group. *Journal of Health Psychology, 8*, 599–615.

Kreps, G.L. (1996). Promoting a consumer orientation to health care and health promotion. *Journal of Health Psychology, 1*, 41–48.

Kreps, G.L. (2001). Consumer/provider communication research: a personal plea to address issues of ecological validity, relational development, message diversity, and situational constraints. *Journal of Health Psychology, 6*, 597–697.

Kreps, G.L. (2003). E-Health: technology-mediated health communication. *Journal of Health Psychology, 8*, 5–6.

Krieger, N. (1987). Shades of difference: theoretical underpinnings of the medical controversy on black/white differences in the United States, 1830–1970. *International Journal of Health Services, 17*, 259–278.

Krieger, N. & Davey Smith, G. (2004). 'Bodies count', and body counts: social epidemiology and embodying inequality. *Epidemiologic Reviews, 26*, 92–103.

Kripalani, S., Henderson, L.E., Chiu, E.Y., Robertson, R., Kolm, P. & Jacobson, T.A. (2006). Predictors of medication self–management skill in low-literacy population. *Journal of General and Internal Medicine, 21*, 852–856.

Kroenke, C.H., Kubzansky, L.D., Schernhammer, E.S., Holmes, M.D. & Kawachi, I. (2006). Social networks, social support, and survival after breast cancer diagnosis. *Journal of Clinical Oncology, 24*, 1105–1111.

Kugelmann, R. (1997). The psychology and management of pain: Gate control as theory and symbol. *Theory & Psychology, 7*, 43–66.

Kugelmann, R. (2000). Pain in the vernacular: psychological and physical. *Journal of Health Psychology, 5*, 305–313.

Kuhlmann, A.K.S., Kraft, J. M., Galavotti, C., Creek, T.L., Mooki, M. & Ntumy, R. (2008). Radio role models for the prevention of mother-to-child transmission of HIV and HIV testing among pregnant women in Botswana. *Health Promotion International, 23*, 260–268.

Kuhn, T.S. (1970). *The structure of scientific revolutions*. Chicago: University of Chicago Press.

Kumanyika, S., Jeffrey, R.W., Morabia, A., Ritenbaugh, C. & Antipatis, V.J. (2002). Obesity prevention: the case for action. *International Journal of Obesity, 26*, 425–436.

Kunesh, M.A., Hasbrook, C.A. & Lewthwaite, R. (1992). Physical activity socialization: peer interactions and affective responses among a sample of sixth grade girls. *Sociology of Sport Journal, 9*, 385–396.

Kuper, H. & Marmot, M. (2003). Job strain, job demands, decision latitude, and risk of coronary heart disease within the Whitehall II study. *Journal of Epidemiology & Community Health, 57*, 147–153.

Kuper, H., Singh-Manoux, A., Siegrist, J. & Marmot, M. (2002). When reciprocity fails: effort–reward imbalance in relation to coronary heart disease and health functioning within the Whitehall II study. *Occupational & Environmental Medicine, 59*, 777–784.

Kvikstad, A. & Vatten, L. (1996). Risk and prognosis of cancer in middle aged women who have experienced the death of a child. *International Journal of Cancer, 67*, 165–169.

Kvikstad, A., Vatten, L. & Tretli, S. (1995). Widowhood & divorce in relation to overall survival among middle-aged Norwegian women with cancer. *British Journal of Cancer, 71*, 1343–1347.

Kwate, N.O.A., Yau, C.-Y., Loh. J.-M. & Williams, D. (2009). Inequality in obesogenic environments: fast food density in New York City. *Health & Place, 15*, 364–373.

Labay, L.E. & Walco, G.A. (2004). Brief report: empathy and psychological adjustment in siblings of children with cancer. *Journal of Pediatric Psychology, 29*, 309–314.

Lai, D.W.L. & Surood, S. (2009). Chinese beliefs of older Chinese in Canada. *Journal of Aging and Health, 21*, 38–62.

Lamb, S. & Sington, D. (1998). *Earth story: the shaping of our world*. London: BBC Books.

Landrine, H. (1997). From the back of the bus. *Journal of Health Psychology, 2*, 428–430.

Lau, R.R. & Hartman, K.A. (1983). Common sense representations of common illnesses. *Health Psychology, 2*, 167–186.

Laubmeier, K.K., Zakowski, S.G. & Bair, J.P. (2004). The role of spirituality in the psychological adjustment to cancer: a test of the transactional model of stress and coping. *International Journal of Behavioral Medicine, 11(1)*, 48–55.

Law, M.R., Frost, C.D. & Wald, N.J. (1991). By how much does dietary salt lower blood pressure? I – Analysis of observational data among populations. *British Medical Journal, 302*, 811–815.

Lawson, K., Wiggins, S., Green, T., Adam, S., Bloch, M. & Hayden, M.R. (1996). Adverse psychological events occurring in the first year after predictive testing for Huntington's disease. *Journal of Medical Genetics, 33*, 856–862.

Lazarus, R.S. & Folkman, S. (1984). *Stress, appraisal and coping*. New York: Springer.

Leichter, H.M. (1997). Lifestyle connectedness and the new secular morality. In A. Brandt & R. Rozin (Eds.), *Morality and health.* New York: Routledge. Pp. 359–378.

Leitch, A.M. (1995). Controversies in breast cancer screening. *Cancer, 76*, 2064–2069.

Lerman, C. (1997). Psychological aspects of genetic testing: introduction to the special issue. *Health Psychology, 16*, 3–7.

Lerman, C. & Rimer, B.K. (1993). Psychosocial impact of cancer screening. In R.T. Croyle (Ed.), *Psychosocial effects of screening for disease prevention and detection.* New York: Oxford University Press.

Lerman, C., Trock, B., Rimer, B.K. & Jepson, C. (1991). Psychological side effects of breast cancer screening. *Health Psychology, 10*, 259–267.

Lerner, W.D. & Fallon, H.J. (1985). The alcohol withdrawal syndrome. *New England Journal of Medicine, 313*, 951–952.

Lesar, T.S., Briceland, L. & Stein, D.S. (1997). Factors related to errors in medication prescribing. *Journal of the American Medical Association, 277*, 312–317.

Leserman, J. (2008). Role of depression, stress, and trauma in HIV disease progression. *Psychosomatic Medicine*, 70, 539–545.

Leshan, L.L. & Worthington, R.E. (1956). Personality as a factor in the pathogenesis of cancer: a review of the literature. *British Journal of Medical Psychology, 29*, 49–56.

Leslie, C. (1976). *Asian medical systems: A comparative study*. Los Angeles: University of California Press.

Lett, H.S., Blumenthal, J.A., Babyak, M.A., Sherwood, A., Strauman, T., Robins, C. & Newman, M.F. (2004). Depression as a risk factor for coronary artery disease: Evidence, mechanisms, and treatment. *Psychosomatic Medicine, 66*, 305–315.

Leventhal, H., Brissette, I. & Leventhal, E.A. (2003). The common-sense model of self-regulation of health and illness. In L.D. Cameron & H. Leventhal (Eds.), *The self-regulation of health and illness behaviour.* London: Routledge. Pp. 42–65.

Leventhal, H. & Cameron, L. (1987). Behavioral theories and the problem of compliance. *Patient Education & Counseling, 10*, 117–138.

Leventhal, H., Diefenbach, M. & Leventhal, E.A. (1992). Illness cognition: Using common sense to understand treatment adherence and affect cognition interactions. *Cognitive Therapy and Research, 16*, 143–163.

Leventhal, H., Leventhal, E.A. & Schaefer, P. (1989). *Vigilant Coping and Health Behaviour: A Lifespan Problem*. New Brunswich, NJ: State University of New Jersey, Rutgers.

Leventhal, H., Meyer, D. & Nerenz, D.R. (1980). The common sense representation of illness danger. In S. Rachman (Ed.), *Contributions to medical psychology—vol 2*. New York: Pergamon Press. Pp. 17–30.

Lewin, K. (1947). Frontiers in group dynamics: II. Channels of group life; social planning and action research. *Human Relations, 1*, 143–153.

Lewin, K. (1948). *Resolving social conflicts: Selected papers in group dynamics*. New York: Harper & Row.

Lewin, R.J., Furze, G., Robinson, J., Griffith, K., Wiseman, S., Pye, M. & Boyle, R. (2002). A randomised controlled trial of a self-management plan for patients with newly diagnosed angina. *British Journal of General Practice, 52*, 199–201.

Lewis, J.E., Miguez-Burbano, M.-J. & Malow, R.M. (2009). HIV risk behavior among college students in the United States. *College Student Journal, 43*, 475–491.

Lexchin, J., Bero, L.A., Djulbegovic, B. & Clark, O. (2003). Pharmaceutical industry sponsorship and research outcome and quality: systematic review. *British Medical Journal, 326*, 1167–1170.

Ley, P. (1979). Memory for medical information. *British Journal of Social & Clinical Psychology, 18*, 245–256.

Li, X., Fang, X., Lin, D., Mao, R., Wang, J., Cottrell, L., Harris, C. & Stanton, B. (2004). HIV/STD risk behaviors and perceptions among rural-to-urban migrants in China. *AIDS Education & Prevention, 16*, 538–556.

Lichtman, J.H., Bigger, J.T., Blumenthal, J.A., Frasure-Smith, N., Kaufmann, P.G., Lespérance, F., & Froelicher, E.S. (2008). Depression and coronary heart disease. *Circulation, 118*, 1768–1775.

Lidbrink, E., Elfving, J., Frisell, J. & Jonsson, E. (1996). Neglected aspects of false positive findings of mammography in breast cancer screening: analysis of false positive cases. *BMJ, 312*, 273–276.

Lidbrink, E., Levi, L., Pettersson, I., Rosendahl, I., Rutqvist, L.E., de la Torre, B., Wasserman, J. & Weige, M. (1995). Singleview screening mammography: psychological, endocrine and immunological effects of recalling for a complete three-view examination. *European Journal of Cancer, 31A*, 932–933.

Lightfoot, N., Steggles, S., Wilkinson, D., Bissett, R., Bakker, D. & Thoms, J., et al. (1994). The short-term psychological impact of organized breast screening. *Current Oncology, 1*, 206–211

Lillard, A. (1998). Ethnopsychologies: cultural variations in theories of mind. *Psychological Bulletin, 123*, 3–32.

Linton, S.J., Buer, N., Vlaeyen, J. & Hellsing, A. (2000). Are fear-avoidance behaviours related to the inception of one episode of back pain? A prospective study. *Psychology & Health, 14*, 1051–1059.

Litt, I.F. (1993). Health issues for women in the 1990s. In S. Matteo (Ed.), *American women in the Nineties: today's critical issues*. Boston: Northeastern University Press.

Lloyd, R. (2008). *Embodying critical pedagogy: a movement towards vitality*, at http://freire.mcgill.ca.

Loewenthal, K.M. & Bradley, C. (1996). Immunization uptake and doctors' perceptions of uptake in a minority group: implications for interventions. *Psychology, Health & Medicine, 1*, 223–230.

Lollis, C.M., Johnson, E.H. & Antoni, M.H. (1997). The efficacy of the Health Belief Model for predicting condom usage and risky sexual practices in university students. *AIDS Education & Prevention, 9*, 551–5263.

Lord, J. & McKillop Farlow, D. (1990). A study of personal empowerment: implications for health promotion. *Health Promotion International, 29*, 2–8.

Lorenz, K.A., Lynn, J., Dy, S.M., Shugarman, L.R., Wilkinson, A., Mularski, R.A. & Shekelle, P.G. (2008). Clinical guidelines. Evidence for improving palliative care at the end of life: a systematic review. *Annals of Internal Medicine, 148*, 147–159.

Low Income Project Team (1996). *Low income, food, nutrition and health: strategies for improvement*. London: Department of Health.

Lowther, M., Mutrie, N. & Scott, E.M. (2007). Identifying key processes of exercise behaviour change associated with movement through the stages of exercise behaviour change. *Journal of Health Psychology, 12*, 261–272.

Lubeck, I. (2005). Beer and women: excessive alcohol consumption and risk of HIV/AIDS among Cambodian beer promotion women ('beer girls'). Presentation at the Universiteit van Leiden, 26 January 2005. Accessed on 10 December 2009 at http://www.fairtradebeer.com/reportfiles/sirchesi/siemreap-newsletter2008.pdf.

Lundahl, B. & Burke, B.L. (2009). The effectiveness and applicability of motivational interviewing: A practice-friendly review of four meta-analyses. *Journal of Clinical Psychology, 65*, 1232–1245.

Lupton, D. (1997). Consumerism, reflexivity and the medical encounter. *Social Science & Medicine, 45*, 373–381.

Lurie, N., Slater, J. & McGovern, P., et al. (1993). Preventive care for women. Does the sex of the physician matter? *NEJM, 329*, 478–482.

Luschen, G., Cockerham, W. & Kunz, G. (1996). The socio-cultural context of sport and health: problems of causal relations and structural interdependence. *Sociology of Sport Journal, 13*, 197–213.

Lykes, M.B. (2000). Possible contributions of a psychology of liberation: whither health and human rights? *Journal of Health Psychology, 5*, 383–398.

Lykes, M.B. (2001). Activist participatory research and the arts with rural Mayan women: interculturality and situated meaning making. In D. Tolman & M. Brydon-Miller (Eds.), *From subjects to subjectivities: a handbook of interpretive and participatory methods*. New York: New York University Press. Pp. 183–197.

Lynch, J.W. & Davey Smith, G. (2002). Commentary: Income inequality and health: the end of the story? *Journal of Epidemiology & Community Health, 31*, 549–551.

Lynch, J., Davey Smith, G., Harper, S., Hillemeier, M., Ross, N., Kaplan, G.A. & Wolfson, M. (2004). Is income inequality a determinant of population health? Part 1. A systematic review. *Milbank Quarterly, 82*, 5–99.

Lynch, J.W., Due, P., Muntaner, C. & Davey Smith, G. (2000). Social capital: is it a good investment for public health? *Journal of Epidemiology & Community Health, 54*, 404–408.

Ma, Q., Ono-Kihara, M., Cong, L., Pan, X., Xu, G., Zamani, S., Ravari, S.M., Kihara, M. (2009). Behavioural & psychosocial predictors of condom use among university students in Eastern China. *AIDS Care, 21*, 249–259.

Macinko, J.A., Shi, L., Starfield, B. & Wulu, J.T. (2003). Income inequality and health: a critical review of the literature. *Medical Care Research & Reviews, 60*, 407–452.

Macintyre, S. & Hunt, K. (1997). Socio-economic position, gender and health. *Journal of Health Psychology, 2*, 315–334.

MacLachlan, M. (2000). Cultivating pluralism in health psychology. *Journal of Health Psychology, 5*, 373–382.

MacLachlan, M. (2004). Culture, empowerment and health. In M. Murray (Ed.), *Critical health psychology*. London: Palgrave. Pp. 101–117.

MacLachlan, M. (2009). Health in the Inter-land. *Journal of Health Psychology, 14*, 647–650.

Macleod, J. & Davey Smith, G. (2003). Psychosocial factors and public health: a suitable case for treatment? *Journal of Epidemiology & Community Health, 57*, 565–570.

Macleod, J., Davey Smith, G., Heslop, P., Metcalfe, C., Carroll, D. & Hart, C. (2002). Psychological stress and cardiovascular disease: Empirical demonstration of bias in a prospective observational study of Scottish men. *British Medical Journal, 324*, 1247–1251.

MacMillan, M. (1997). *Freud evaluated: The completed arc*. Cambridge, MA: MIT Press.

Magni, G., Moreschi, C., Rigatti-Luchini, S. & Merskey, H. (1994). Prospective study on the relationship between depressive symptoms and chronic musculoskeletal pain. *Pain, 56*, 289–297.

Maguen, S., Armistead, L.P. & Kalichman, S. (2000). Predictors of HIV antibody testing among gay, lesbian, and bisexual youth. *Journal of Adolescent Health, 26*, 252–257.

Maguire, P., Fairbairn, S. & Fletcher, C. (1989). Consultation skills of young doctors: benefits of undergraduate feedback training. In M. Stewart & D. Roter (Eds.), *Communicating with medical patients*. London: Sage. Pp. 124–137.

Maier, S.F. & Watkins, L.R. (1998). Cytokines for psychologists: implications of bi-directional immune-to-brain communication for understanding behaviour, mood and cognition. *Psychological Review, 105*, 83–107.

Maniadakis, N. & Gray, A. (2000). The economic burden of back pain in the UK. *Pain, 84*, 95–103.

Mann, T., Sherman, D. and Updegraff, J. (2004). Dispositional motivations and message framing: A test of the congruency hypothesis in college students. *Health Psychology, 23*, 330–334.

Manne, S., Sherman, M., Ross, S., Ostroff, J., Heyman, R.E. & Fox, K. (2004). Couples support-related communication, psychological distress, and relationship satisfaction among women with early stage breast cancer. *Journal of Consulting & Clinical Psychology, 72*, 660–670.

Marcus, B.H., Banspach, S.W., Lefebvre, R.L., Rossi, J.S., Carleton, R.A. & Abrams, D.B. (1992). Using the stages of change model to increase the adoption of physical activity among community participants. *American Journal of Health Promotion, 6*, 424–429.

Marcus, B.H., Eaton, C.A., Rossi, J.S. & Harlow, L.L. (1994). Self-efficacy, decision-making and stages of change: An integrative model of physical exercise. *Journal of Applied Social Psychology, 24*, 489–508.

Marcus, D.A. (2000). Treatment of non-malignant chronic pain. *American Family Physician, 61*, 1331–1338.

Marcus, K.S., Kerns, R.D., Rosenfeld, B. & Breitbart, W. (2000). HIV/AIDS-related pain as a chronic pain condition: implications of a biopsychosocial model for comprehensive assessment and effective management. *Pain Medicine, 1*, 260–273.

Marinker, M. (1997). Writing prescriptions is easy. *British Medical Journal, 314*, 747.

Markova, I. & Wilkie, P. (1987). Representations, concepts and social change: the phenomenon of AIDS. *Journal for the Theory of Social Behaviour, 17*, 389–409.

Marks, D. (1999). *Disability: controversial debates and psychosocial perspectives*. London: Routledge.

Marks, D.F. (1992). Smoking cessation as a testbed for psychological theory: a group cognitive therapy programme with high long-term abstinence rates. *Journal of Smoking-Related Disorders, 3*, 69–78.

Marks, D.F. (1993). *The QUIT FOR LIFE Programme: An easier way to stop smoking and not start again*. Leicester, UK: The British Psychological Society.

Marks, D.F. (1996). Health psychology in context. *Journal of Health Psychology, 1*, 7–21.

Marks, D.F. (1998). Addiction, smoking and health: developing policy-based interventions. *Psychology, Health & Medicine, 3*, 97–111.

Marks, D.F. (2002a) *The health psychology reader*. London: Sage.

Marks, D.F. (2002b). Freedom, responsibility and power: contrasting approaches to health psychology. *Journal of Health Psychology, 7*, 5–199.

Marks, D.F. (2004). Rights to health, freedom from illness: a life and death matter. In M. Murray (Ed.), *Critical health psychology*. London: Palgrave. Pp. 61–82.

Marks, D.F. (2005). *Overcoming your smoking habit*. London: Robinson.

Marks, D.F. (2006). The case for a pluralist health psychology. *Journal of Health Psychology, 11*, 367–372.

Marks, D.F. (2009). Editorial: How should Psychology interventions be reported? *Journal of Health Psychology, 14*, 475–489.

Marks, D.F., Baird, J.M. & McKellar, P. (1989). Replication of trance logic using a modified experimental design: highly hypnotizable subjects in both real and simulator groups. *International Journal of Clinical and Experimental Hypnosis, 37*, 232–248.

Marks, D.F., Murray, M., Evans, B., Sykes, C.M. & Woodall, C. (2005). *Health Psychology. Theory, research and practice* (2nd edn.). London: Sage Publications Ltd.

Marks, D.F. & Sykes, C.M. (2002). A randomized controlled trial of cognitive behaviour therapy for smokers living in a deprived part of London. *Psychology, Health & Medicine, 7*, 17–24.

Marks, D.F. & Yardley, L. (Eds) (2004). *Research methods for clinical and health psychology*. London: Sage.

Markula, P., Grant, B. & Denison, J. (2001). Qualitative research and aging and physical activity: Multiple ways of knowing. *Journal of Aging and Physical Activity, 9*, 245–264.

Markus, H.R., Mullally, P.R. & Kitayama, S. (1997). Selfways: Diversity in modes of cultural participation. In U. Neisser & D. A. Jopling (Eds.), *The conceptual self in context.* New York: Cambridge University Press. Pp. 13–57.

Markwardt, F.C. (1997). *Peabody individual achievement test-revised.* Circle Pines, NM: American Guidance Service.

Marmot, M. (2001). Inequalities in health. *New England Journal of Medicine, 345*, 183–203.

Marmot, M., Shipley, M., Brunner, E. & Hemmingway, H. (2001). Relative contribution of early life and adult socio-economic factors in adult morbidity in the Whitehall II study. *Journal of Epidemiology & Community Health, 53*, 301–307.

Marsh, H. W. (1990). A multidimensional, hierarchical model of self-concept: Theoretical and empirical justification. *Educational Psychology Review, 2*, 77–172.

Marsh, H.W., Papaioannou, A. & Theodorakis, Y. (2006). Causal ordering of physical self-concept and exercise behavior: Reciprocal effects model and the influence of physical education teachers. *Health Psychology, 25*, 316–328.

Marteau, T. (1990). Screening in practice: reducing the psychological costs. *BMJ, 301*, 26–28.

Martín-Baró, I. (1994). *Writings for a liberation psychology*. In A. Aron & S. Corne (Eds.), *Writings for a liberation psychology*. Cambridge, MA: Harvard University Press.

Martinez Cobo, J (1987). *Study of the problem of discrimination against indigenous populations*, Vol 5 UNESCO.

Masek B.J. (1982) Compliance and medicine. In D.M. Doleys, R.L. Meredith & A.R. Ciminero (Eds.) *Behavioral medicine: Assessment and treatment strategies*. New York: Plenum Press.

Maslach, C. & Jackson, S. (1981). The measurement of experienced burnout. *Journal of Occupational Behaviour, 2*, 99–113.

Maslow, A. (1943). A theory of human motivation. *Psychological Review, 50*, 370–396.

Mason, J.W. (1971). A re-evaluation of the concept of 'non-specificity' in stress theory. *Journal of Psychiatric Research, 8*, 323–333.

Mason, J.W. (1975). A historical view of the stress field: Parts 1 & 2. *Journal of Human Stress, 1*, 6–12, 22–36.

Masunaga, R. (1972). *A primer of Soto Zen: a translation of Dogen's Shobogenzo Zuimonki*. London: Routledge.

Masur, H. (1981). Infection after kidney transplantation. *Archives of Internal Medicine, 141*, 1582–1584.

Matarazzo, J.D. (1982). Behavioural health's challenge to academic, scientific and professional psychology. *American Psychologist, 37*, 1–14.

Mathieson, C. & Stam, H. (1995). Renegotiating identity: cancer narratives. *Sociology of Health & Illness, 17*, 283–306.

Matsumoto, D., Pun, K.K., Nakatani, M., Kadowaki, D. & Weissman, M., et al. (1995). Cultural differences in attitudes, values, and beliefs about osteoporosis in first and second generation Japanese-American women. *Women & Health, 23*, 39–56.

McAllister, M., Payne, K., Macleod, R., Nicholls, S., Donnai, D. & Davies, L. (2008). Patient empowerment in clinical genetics services. *Journal of Health Psychology, 13*, 895–905.

McAuley, E. & Jacobson, L. (1991). Self-efficacy and exercise participation in adult sedentary females. *American Journal of Health Promotion, 5*, 185–191.

McCaffery, A.M., Eisenberg, D.M., Legedza, A.T.R., Davis, R.B. & Phillips, R.A. (2004). Prayer for health concerns: results of a national survey on prevalence and patterns of use. *Archives of Internal Medicine, 164*, 858–862.

McCaffery, M. & Thorpe, D. (1988). Differences in perception of pain and development of adversarial relationships among health care providers. *Advances in Pain Research & Therapy, 11*, 113–122.

McCaul, K.D., Dyche Branstetter, A., Schroeder, D.M. & Glasgow, R.M. (1996). What is the relationship between breast cancer risk and mammography screening? A meta-analytic review. *Health Psychology, 15*, 423–429.

McCracken, L.M., Carson, J.W., Eccleston, C. & Keefe, F.J. (2004). Acceptance and change in the context of chronic pain. *Pain, 109*, 4–7.

McCracken, L.M. & Eccleston, C. (2003). Coping or acceptance: what to do about chronic pain? *Pain, 105*, 197–204.

McCrae, R.R. & Costa, P.T. (2003). *Personality in adulthood: A five-factor theory perspective* (2nd edn). New York: Guilford.

McCreanor, T., Caswell, S. & Hill, L. (2000). ICAP and the perils of partnership. *Addiction, 95*, 179–185.

McFadden, E.R. (1995). Improper patient techniques with metered dose inhalers: clinical consequences and solutions to misuse. *Journal of Allergy and Clinical Immunology, 96*, 278–283.

McGee, R. (1999). Does stress cause cancer? *British Medical Journal, 319*, 1015–1016.

McGowan, L., Clark-Carter, D. & Pitts, M.K. (1998). Chronic pelvic pain: a meta-analysis. *Psychology & Health, 13*, 937–951.

McGowan, L., Luker, K., Creed, F. & Chew, C.A. (2007). 'How do you explain a pain that can't be seen': The narratives of women with chronic pelvic pain and their disengagement with the diagnostic cycle. *British Journal of Health Psychology, 12,* 261–274.

McKeown, T. (1979). *The role of medicine*. Princeton, NJ: Princeton University Press.

McKie, L. (1993). Women's views of the cervical smear test: implications for nursing practice–women who have not had a smear test. *Journal of Advanced Nursing, 18*, 972–979.

McKie, L. (1995). The art of surveillance or reasonable prevention? The case of cervical screening. *Sociology of Health & Illness, 17*, 441–457.

McKinlay, A. & McVittie, C. (2008). *Social psychology and discourse.* London: Wiley-Blackwell.

McLeroy, K.R., Norton, B.L., Kegler, M.C., Burdine, J.N. & Sumaya, C.V. (2003). Community-based interventions. *American Journal of Public Health, 93*, 529–533.

McMullan, M. (2006). Patients using the Internet to obtain health information: how this affects the patient-health professional relationship. *Patient Education and Counseling, 63*, 24–28.

McPherron, S.R., Alemseged, Z., Marean, C.W., Wynn, J.G., Reed, D., Geraads, D. & Béarat, H.A. (2010). Evidence for stone-tool-assisted consumption of animal tissues before 3.39 million years ago at Dikka, Ethiopia. *Nature, 466*, 857–860.

McVittie, C. and Goodall, K. (2009). Harry, Paul and the Filipino maid: Racial and sexual abuse in local contexts. *Journal of Health Psychology, 14*, 651–654.

Meade, R. & Shaw, M. (2007) Community development and the arts: reviving the democratic imagination. *Community Development Journal, 42*, 413–421.

Meichenbaum, D. (1985). *Stress innoculation training*. New York: Pergamon.

Meichenbaum, D. & Turk, D.C. (1987). *Facilitating treatment adherence: a practitioner's guidebook.* New York: Plenum Press.

Melzack, R. (1975). The McGill Pain Questionnaire: major properties and scoring methods. *Pain, 1*, 277–299.

Melzack, R. (1999). From the gate to the neuromatrix, *Pain, 82*, S121–126.

Melzack, R. & Wall, P.D. (1988). *The challenge of pain* (2nd ed.). London: Penguin.

Mennella, J.A. & Beauchamp, G.K. (1996). The early development of human flavor preferences. In E.D. Capaldi (Ed.), *Why we eat what we eat: the psychology of eating*. Washington, DC: American Psychological Association. Pp. 83–112.

Merskey, J. (1996). Classification of chronic pain: descriptions of chronic pain syndromes and definitions of pain terms. *Pain, 3(Suppl)*, S1–225.

Meszaros, J.R., Asch, D.A., Baron, J., Hershey, J.C., Kunreuther, H. & Schwartz-Buzaglo, J. (1996). Cognitive processes and the decisions of some parents to forego pertussis vaccination for their children. *Journal of Clinical Epidemiology, 49*, 697–703.

Meyer, T.J. & Mark, M.M. (1995). Effects of psychosocial interventions with adult cancer patients: a meta-analysis of randomized experiments. *Health Psychology, 14*, 101–108.

Meyerowitz, B.E. & Chaiken, S. (1987). The effect of message framing on breast self-examination attitudes, intentions, and behavior. *Journal of Personality and Social Psychology, 52*, 500–510.

Meyerowitz, B.E., Richardson, J., Hudson, S. & Leedham, B. (1998). Ethnicity and cancer outcomes: behavioral and psychosocial considerations. *Psychological Bulletin, 123*, 47–70.

Mezey, G. & Robbins, I. (2001). Usefulness and validity of post-traumatic stress disorder as a psychiatric category. *British Medical Journal, 323*, 561–563.

Michie, S., McDonald, V. & Marteau, T. (1996). Understanding responses to predictive genetic testing: a grounded theory approach. *Psychology & Health, 11*, 455–470.

Mickey, R.M., Durski, J., Worden, J.K. and Danigelis, N.L. (1995). Breast cancer screening and associated factors for low-income African-American women. *Preventive Medicine, 24*, 467–476.

Middleton, D. (1996). A discursive analysis of psychosocial issues: talk in a 'parent group' for families who have children with chronic renal failure. *Psychology & Health, 11*, 243–260.

Midford, R. & McBride, N. (2001). Alcohol education in schools. In N. Heather, T.J. Peters & T. Stockwell (Eds.), *International handbook of alcohol dependence and problems*. London: Wiley. Pp. 785–804.

Mielewczyk, F. & Willig, C. (2007). Old clothes and an older look: The case for a radical makeover in health behaviour research. *Theory & Psychology, 17*, 811–837.

Miles, A. (1981). *The mentally ill in contemporary society*. Oxford: Martin Robertson.

Miller, A.B. (2008). The place for routine mammography screening, commencing at age 40. *Preventive Medicine, 47*, 485–486.

Miller, G.E. & Cohen, S. (2001). Psychological interventions and the immune system: A meta-analytic review and critique. *Health Psychology, 20*, 47–63.

Miller, M.J., Abrams, M.A., McClintock, B., Cantrell, M.A., Dossett, C.D., McCleeary, E.M., & Sager, E.R. (2008). Promoting health communication between the community-dwelling well-elderly and pharmacists: The Ask Me 3 program. *Journal of the American Pharmacists Association, 48*, 784–92.

Miller, G., Chen, E. & Cole, S.W. (2009). Health psychology: Developing biologically plausible models linking the social world and physical health. *Annual Review of Psychology, 60*, 501–524.

Miller, N.H. (1997). Compliance with treatment regimens in chronic asymptomatic disease. *American Journal of Medicine, 102*, 43–49.

Miller, T.Q., Smith, T.W., Turner, C.W., Guijarro, M.L. & Hallet, A.J. (1996). A meta-analytic review of research on hostility and physical health. *Psychological Bulletin, 119*, 322–348.

Miller, W.R. & Rollnick, S. (2002). *Motivational interviewing: preparing people to change addictive behaviours* (2nd edn.). New York: Guilford Press.

Miller, W.R., Walters, G.D. & Bennett, M.E. (2001). How effective is alcoholism treatment in the United States? *Journal of Studies on Alcohol & Drugs, 62*, 211–220.

Miller, W.R. & Wilbourne, P. (2002). Mesa Grande: a methodological analysis of clinical trials of treatments for alcohol use disorders. *Addiction, 97(3)*, 265–277.

Mintz, S. (1997). Sugar and morality. In A.M. Brandt & P. Rozin (Eds.), *Morality and health*. New York: Routledge. Pp. 173–184.

Miovic, M. & Block, S. (2007). Psychiatric disorders in advanced cancer. *Cancer, 110*, 1665–1676.

Mishler, E. (1984). *The discourse of medicine: Dialectics of medical interviews*. Norwood, NJ: Ablex.

Mize, S.J.S., Robinson, B.E., Bockting, W.O. & Scheltema, K.E. (2002). Meta-analysis of the effectiveness of HIV prevention interventions for women. *Aids Care, 14*, 163–180.

Mo, P.K.H., Malik, S.H. and Coulson, N.S. (2009). Gender differences in computer-mediated communication: A systematic review of online health-related support groups. *Patient Education and Counseling, 75*, 16–24.

Modood, T., Berthoud, R., Lakey, J., Nazroo, J., Smith, P., Virdee, S. & Beishon, S. (1997). *Ethnic minorities in Britain: diversity and disadvantage*. London: Policy Studies Institute.

Moher, D., Schultz, K.F., Altman, D.G. & the CONSORT Group (2001). The CONSORT statement: revised recommendations for improving the quality of reports of parallel-group randomized trials. *The Lancet, 357*, 1191–1194.

Montano, D.E. & Taplin, S.H. (1991). A test of an expanded theory of reasoned action to predict mammography participation. *Social Science & Medicine, 32*, 733–741.

Montenegro, R. A. & Stephens, C. (2006). Indigenous health in Latin America and the Caribbean. *Lancet, 367*, 1859–1869.

Mookadam, F. & Arthur, H.M. (2004). Social support and its relationship to morbidity and mortality after acute myocardial infarction: systematic overview. *Archives of Internal Medicine, 164*, 1514–1518.

Mooney, M., White, T. & Hatsukami, D. (2004). The blind spot in the nicotine replacement therapy literature: assessment of the double-blind in clinical trials. *Addictive Behavior, 29*, 673–84.

Moore, S., Barling, N. & Hood, B. (1998). Predicting testicular and breast self-examination: A test of the Theory of Reasoned Action. *Behaviour Change, 15*, 41–49.

Moore, T., Norman, P., Harris, P.R. & Makris, M. (2008). An interpretative phenomenological analysis of adaptation to recurrent venous thrombosis and heritable thrombophilia: The importance of multi-causal models and perceptions of primary and secondary control. *Journal of Health Psychology, 13*, 776–784.

Morinis, C.A. & Brilliant, G.E. (1981). Smallpox in northern India: diversity and order in a regional medical culture. *Medical Anthropology, 5*, 341–364.

Morland, K., Diez Roux, A.V. & Wing, S. (2006). Supermarkets, other food stores, and obesity: The Atherosclerosis Risk in Communities Study. *American Journal of Preventive Medicine, 30*, 333–339.

Morley, S., Eccleston, C. & Williams, A. (1999). Systematic review and meta-analysis of randomized controlled trials of cognitive behaviour therapy and behaviour therapy for chronic pain in adults, excluding headache. *Pain, 80*, 1–13.

Morris, N.S., MacLean, C.D., Chew, L.D. & Littenberg, B. (2006). The Single Item Literacy Screener: Evaluation of a brief instrument to identify limited reading ability. *BMC Family Practice, 7*, 21–26.

Moscovici, S. (1973). Foreword. In C. Herzlich, *Health and illness: a social psychological analysis*. London: Academic Press.

Moscovici, S. (1984). The phenomenon of social representations. In R.M. Farr & S. Moscovici (Eds.), *Social representations*. Cambridge: Cambridge University Press. Pp. 3–70.

Moser, D.K. & Dracup, K. (2004). Role of spousal anxiety and depression in patients psychosocial recovery after a cardiac event. *Psychosomatic Medicine, 66*, 527–532.

Moss-Morris, R., Weinman, J., Petrie, K.J., Horne, R., Cameron, L.D. & Buick, D. (2002). The Revised Illness Perception Questionnaire (IPQ-R). *Psychology & Health, 17*, 1–17.

Mukamal, K.J., Ascherio, A., Mittleman, A.M., Conigrave, K.M., Camargo, C.A., Kawachi, I., Stampfer, M.J., Willett, W.C. & Rimm, E.B. (2005). Alcohol and risk for ischemic stroke in men: the role of drinking patterns and usual beverage. *Annals of Internal Medicine, 142*, 11–199.

Mukamal, K.J., Chiuve, S.E. & Rimm, E.B. (2006). Alcohol consumption and risk for coronary heart disease in men with healthy lifestyles. *Archives of Internal Medicine, 166*, 2145–2150.

Mulatu, M.S. (1995). Lay beliefs about the causes of psychological and physical illness in Ethiopia. *The Canadian Health Psychologist, 3*, 38–43.

Mulatu, M.S. (1999). Perceptions of mental and physical illnesses in north-western Ethiopia: Causes, treatments, and attitudes. *Journal of Health Psychology, 4*, 531–549.

Mulkay, M. (1991). *Sociology of science: a sociological pilgrimage*. Milton Keynes: Open University Press.

Mulrow, C.D. (1987). The medical review article: state of the science. *Annals of Internal Medicine, 106*, 485–488.

Mulveen, R. and Hepworth, J. (2006). An interpretative phenomenological analysis of participation in a pro-anorexia internet site and its relationship with disordered eating. *Journal of Health Psychology, 11*, 283–296.

Munro, S., Lewin, S., Swart, T. & Volmink, J. (2007). A review of health behaviour theories: how useful are these for developing interventions to promote long-term medication adherence for TB and HIV/AIDS? *BMC Public Health, 7*, 104–119.

Muntaner, C., Lynch, J.W., Hillemeister, M., Lee, J.H., David, R., Benach, J. & Borrell, C. (2002). Economic inequality, working class power, social capital, and cause specific mortality in wealthy countries. *International Journal of Health Services, 32*, 629–656.

Murdock, G.P. (1937). Comparative data on the division of labour by sex. *Social Forces*, *15*, 551–553.

Murphy, E.M. (2003). Being born female is dangerous for your health. *American Psychologist, 58*, 205–210.

Murray, C. & Lopez, A. (1997). Global mortality, disability, and the contribution of risk factors: Global Burden of Disease Study. *The Lancet, 349*, 1436–1442.

Murray, D. (2005). The social meanings of prosthesis use. *Journal of Health Psychology, 10,* 425–441.

Murray, M. (1993). Social and cognitive representations of health and illness. In H. Schroder, K. Reschke, M. Johnson & S. Maes (Eds.), *Health psychology – Potential in diversity*. Leipzig, Germany.

Murray, M. (1997). A narrative approach to health psychology: background and potential. *Journal of Health Psychology, 2*, 9–20.

Murray, M. (2000). Levels of narrative analysis in health psychology. *Journal of Health Psychology, 5*, 337–348.

Murray, M. (2002). Connecting narrative and social representation theory in health research. *Social Science Information, 41(4)*, 653–673.

Murray, M. (2008). Narrative psychology. In J.A. Smith (Ed.), *Qualitative psychology: a practical guide to research methods*. London: Sage. Pp. 111–132.

Murray, M. (2009). Telling stories and making sense of cancer. *International Journal of Narrative Practice, 1*, 25–36.

Murray, M. & Campbell, C. (2003). Living in a material world: reflecting on some assumptions of health psychology. *Journal of Health Psychology, 8*, 231–236.

Murray, M. & Crummett, A. (2010). 'I don't think they knew we could do these sorts of things': Social representations of community and participation in community arts by older people. *Journal of Health Psychology, 15*, 777–785.

Murray, M. & Gray, R. (2008). Health psychology and the arts: a conversation. *Journal of Health Psychology, 13*, 147–153.

Murray, M. & McMillan, C. (1988). *Working class women's views of cancer*. Belfast: Ulster Cancer Foundation.

Murray, M. & McMillan, C. (1993a). Gender differences in perceptions of cancer. *Journal of Cancer Education, 8*, 53–62.

Murray, M. & McMillan, C. (1993b). Health beliefs, locus of control, emotional control and womens cancer screening behaviour. *British Journal of Clinical Psychology, 32*, 87–100.

Murray, M. & Poland, B. (2006). Health psychology and social action. *Journal of Health Psychology, 11*, 379–384.

Murray, M. & Tilley, N. (2006). Using community arts to promote awareness of safety in fishing communities: An action research study. *Safety Science, 44*, 797–808.

Murray, M., Jarrett, L., Swan, A.V., & Rumun, R. (1988). *Smoking among young adults*. Aldershot: Gower.

Murray, M., Nelson, G., Poland, B., Maticka-Tyndale, E. & Ferris, L. (2004). Assumptions and values in community health psychology. *Journal of Health Psychology, 9*, 315–326.

Murray, M., Pullman, D. & Heath Rodgers, T. (2003). Social representations of health and illness among 'baby-boomers' in Eastern Canada. *Journal of Health Psychology, 8*, 485–500.

Murray, M., Swan, A.V. & Mattar, N. (1983). The task of nursing and risk of smoking. *Journal of Advanced Nursing, 8*, 131–138.

Murray, R.P., Connett, J.E., Tyas, S.L., Bond, R., Ekuma, O., Silversides, C.K. & Barnes, G.E. (2002). Alcohol volume, drinking pattern and cardiovascular disease morbidity and mortality: Is there a U-shaped function? *American Journal of Epidemiology, 155*, 242–248.

Murray, S., Rudd, R., Kirsch, I., Yamamoto, K. & Grenier, S. (2007). *Health literacy in Canada: Initial results from the International Adult Literacy and Skills Survey*. Ottawa: Canadian Council on Learning.

Mykletun, A., Bjerkeset, O., Dewey, M., Prince, M., Overland, S. & Stewart, R. (2007). Anxiety, depression, and cause-specific mortality: The HUNT study. *Psychosomatic Medicine, 69*, 323–331.

Myrtek, M. (2001). Meta-analyses of prospective studies on coronary heart disease, type A personality and hostility. *International Journal of Cardiology, 79*, 245–251.

Nairn, R., Peaga, F., McCreanor, T., Rankine, J. & Barnes, A. (2006). Media, racism and public health psychology. *Journal of Health Psychology, 11*, 183–196.

Nath, C.R., Sylvester, S.T., Yasek, V. & Gunel, E. (2001). Development and validation of a literacy assessment tool for persons with diabetes. *The Diabetes Educator, 27*, 857–864.

National AIDS Trust (2008). Over 90 percent of the British public do not fully understand how HIV is transmitted. Press release accessed on 26 November 2009 at http://www.nat.org.uk/News-and-Media/Press-Releases/2008/January/over-90-percent-of-the-british-public.aspx.

National Center for Health Statistics (1994). *Healthy people 2000 review, 1993*. Hyattsville, MD: Public Health Service.

National Health Service (2010). Free local NHS stop smoking services. Accessed on 5 January 2010 at http://smokefree.nhs.uk/what-suits-me/local-nhs-services/.

National Institutes of Health (1997). Acupuncture. NIH Consensus Statement, Vol 15 (5). Rockville, MD: US Dept. of HHS Public Health Services.

Neill, R.A., Mainous, A.G. III, Clark, J.R. & Hagen, M.D. (1994). The utility of electronic mail as a medium for patient-physician communication. *Archive of Family Medicine, 3*, 268–271.

Nelson, G., Pancer, S.M., Hayward, K. & Kelly, R. (2004). Partnerships and participation of community residents in health promotion and prevention: Experiences of the Highfield Community Enrichment Project (Better Beginnings, Better Futures). *Journal of Health Psychology, 9*, 213–227.

Ness, A.R. & Powles, J.W. (1997). Fruit and vegetables, and cardiovascular disease: a review. *International Journal of Epidemiology, 26*, 1–13.

Neuberg, S.L., Smith, D.M. & Asher, T. (2000). Why people stigmatize: toward a biocultural framework. In T.F. Heatherton, R.E. Kleck, M.R. Hebl & J.G. Hull (Eds.), *The social psychology of stigma*. New York: Guilford. Pp. 31–61.

New, S.J. & Senior, M. (1991). 'I don't believe in needles': qualitative aspects of study into the update of infant immunisation in two English health authorities. *Social Science & Medicine, 33*, 509–518.

Newell, S.A., Sanson-Fisher, R.W. & Savolainen, N.J. (2002). Systematic review of psychological therapies for cancer patients: overview and recommendations for future research. *Journal of the National Cancer Institute, 94*, 558–584.

Newman, M.F. (2004). Depression as a risk factor for coronary artery disease: Evidence, mechanisms, and treatment. *Psychosomatic Medicine, 66*, 305–315.

Ng, D.M. & Jeffery, R.W. (2003). Relationships between perceived stress and health behaviours in a sample of working adults. *Health Psychology, 22*, 638–642.

Nicholls, S. (2009). Beyond expressive writing: Evolving models of developmental creative writing. *Journal of Health Psychology, 14*, 171–180.

Nicholson, A., Kuper, H. & Hemingway, H. (2006). Depression as an aetiologic and prognostic factor in coronary heart disease: a meta-analysis of 6362 events among 146 538 participants in 54 observational studies. *European Heart Journal, 27*, 2763–2774.

Nielsen, N.R., Zhang, Z.-F., Kristensen, T.S., Netterstrøm, B., Schnohr, P. & Grønbæk, M. (2005). Self reported stress and risk of breast cancer: prospective cohort study. *British Medical Journal, 331*, 548–553.

Nimnuan, C., Rabe-Hesketh, S., Wesseley, S. & Hotopf, M. (2001). How many functional somatic syndromes? *Journal of Psychosomatic Research, 51*, 549–557.

Noar, S.M. (2006). A 10-year retrospective of research in health mass media campaigns: where do we go from here? *Journal of Health Communication, 11*, 21–42.

Noar, S.M., Black, H.G. & Pierce, L.B. (2009). Efficacy of computer technology-based HIV prevention interventions: A meta-analysis. *AIDS, 23*, 107–115.

Norman, C.D. & Skinner, H. (2006). eHEALS: eHealth Literacy Scale. *Journal of Medical Internet Research, 14*, e27.

Norman, P. & Bennett, P. (1996). Health locus of control. In M. Conner & P. Norman (Eds.), *Predicting health behaviour*. Buckingham: Open University Press. Pp. 62–94.

Norman, P., Bennett, P., Smith, C. & Murphy, S. (1998). Health locus of control and health behaviour. *Journal of Health Psychology, 3*, 171–180.

Norman, P. & Brain, K. (2005). An application of an extended health belief model to the prediction of breast self-examination among women with a family history of breast cancer. *British Journal of Health Psychology, 10*, 1–16.

Nutbeam, D. (1998). Health promotion glossary. *Health Promotion International, 13*, 349–364.

Nutbeam, D. (1999). Health promotion effectiveness: the questions to be answered. In International Union for Health Promotion and Education, *The evidence of health promotion effectiveness: shaping public health in a new Europe*. ECSC-EC-EAEC, Brussels–Luxembourg.

Nutbeam, D. (2000). Health literacy as a public health goal: A challenge for contemporary health education and communication strategies into the 21st century. *Health Promotion International, 15*, 259–267.

O'Brien Cousins, S. (2000). 'My heart couldn't take it': Older women's beliefs about exercise benefits and risks. *Journals of Gerontology Series B: Psychological Sciences and Social Sciences, 55*, 283–294.

O'Connor, D.B., Jones, F., Conner, M., McMillan, B. & Ferguson, E. (2008). Effects of daily hassles & eating style on eating behavior. *Health Psychology, 27(1, Suppl)*, S20–S31.

O'Leary, A. (1990). Stress, emotion and human immune function. *Psychological Bulletin, 108*, 363–382.

O'Leary, A. & Helgeson, V.S. (1997). Psychosocial factors and womens health: integrating mind, heart, and body. In S.J. Gallant, G.P. Keita & R. Royak-Schaler (Eds.), *Health care for women: psychological, social, and behavioral influences*. Washington, DC: American Psychological Association. Pp. 25–40.

Oakley, A. (2001). Evaluating health promotion: methodological diversity. In S. Oliver & G. Peersman (Eds.), *Using research for effective health promotion.* Buckingham: Open University Press. Pp. 16–31.

Odom, S.L., Peck, C.A., Hanson, H., Beckham, P.J., Kaiser, K.P., Leiber, J., Brown, W.H., Hom, E.M. & Schwartz, I.S. (1996). Inclusion at the pre-school level: an ecological systems analysis. *Society for Research Child Development, 10(2)*, 18–30.

Oeppen, J. & Vaupel, J.W. (2002). Demography: Broken limits to life expectancy. *Science, 296*, 1029–1031.

Office for National Statistics (2009). Teen pregnancy rates go back up. Accessed on 26 November 2009 at http://news.bbc.co.uk/1/hi/uk/7911684.stm.

Office for National Statistics (2010). *Eating & exercise. 1 in 6 children were obese in 2002*. Accessed on 25 January 10 at http://www.statistics.gov.uk/images/charts/1329a.gif.

Office of Health Economics (2004). *Compendium of Health Statistics, 15th edition*. London: OHE.

Ogden, C.L., Carroll, M.D., Curtin, L.R., McDowell, M.A., Tabak, C.J. & Flegal, K.M. (2006). Prevalence of overweight and obesity in the U. S., 1999–2004. *Journal of the American Medical Association, 295*, 1549–1555.

Ogden, J. (2003). Some problems with social cognition models: a pragmatic and conceptual analysis. *Health Psychology, 22*, 424–428.

Ohenjo, N., Willis, R., Jackson, D., Nettleton, C., Good, K. & Mugarura, B. (2006). Health of Indigenous people in Africa. *Lancet, 367*, 1937–1976.

Ong, L.M.L., de Haes, J.C.J.M., Hoos, A.M. & Lammes, F.B. (1995). Doctor–patient communication: a review of the literature. *Social Science & Medicine, 40*, 903–918.

ONS (2008). *Office for National Statistics: Health Service Quarterly, Winter 2008, No. 40*, 59–60.

Oxman, A.D. & Guyatt, G.H. (1988). Guidelines for reading literature reviews. *Canadian Medical Association Journal, 138*, 697–703.

Oygard, L. & Anderssen, N. (1998). Social influences and leisure-time physical activity in young people; a twelve-year follow-up study. *Journal of Health Psychology, 3*, 59–69.

Ozer, E.J., Best, S.R., Lipsey, T.L. & Weiss (2003). Predictors of posttraumatic stress disorder and symptoms in adults: A meta-analysis. *Psychological Bulletin, 129*, 52–73.

Paasche-Orlow, M.K. & Wolf, M.S. (2007). The causal pathways linking health literacy to health outcomes. *American Journal of Health Behaviour, 31*, S19–26.

Paasche-Orlow, M.K., Schillinger, D., Greene, S.M. & Wagner, E.H. (2006). How health care systems can begin to address the challenge of limited literacy. *Journal of General Internal Medicine, 21*, 884–887.

Paechter, C. (2003). Power, bodies and identity: how different forms of physical education construct varying masculinities and femininities in secondary schools. *Sex Education, 3*, 47–59.

Paljärvi, T., Mäkelä, P. & Poikolainen, K. (2005). Pattern of drinking and fatal injury: a population-based follow-up study of Finnish men. *Addiction, 100*, 1851–1859.

Park, C.L., Folkman, S. & Bostrom, A. (2001). Appraisals of controllability and coping in caregivers and HIV men: testing the goodness-of-fit hypothesis. *Journal of Consulting & Clinical Psychology, 69*, 481–488.

Parker, I. (1997). Discursive psychology. In D. Fox & I. Prilleltensky (Eds.), *Critical psychology: an introduction*. London: Sage.

Parker, I. (Ed.) (1998). *Social constructionism, discourse and realism*. London: Sage.

Parker, R.M., Baker, D.W., Williams, M.V., Gazmararian, J.A. & Nurss, J. (1995). The test of functional health literacy in adults: a new instrument for measuring patients' literacy skills. *Journal of General and Internal Medicine, 10*, 537–541.

Patterson, T.L., Semple, S.J., Fraga, M., Bucardo, J., Davila-Fraga, W. & Strathdee, S.A. (2005). An HIV-prevention intervention for sex workers in Tijuana, Mexico: a pilot study. *Hispanic Journal of Behavioural Sciences, 27*, 82–100.

Paul, E.L., McManus, B. & Hayes, A. (2000). 'Hookups': Characteristics and correlates of college students spontaneous and anonymous sexual experiences. *Journal of Sex Research, 37*, 76–88.

Paulson, S. (2005). The social benefits of belonging to a 'Dance Exercise' group for older people. *Generations Review, 15*, 37–41.

Pavlov, I.P. (1927). *Conditioned reflexes*. Oxford: Oxford University Press.

Paxton, W. & Dixon, M. (2004). *The state of the nation: an audit of injustice in the UK*. London: Institute for Public Policy Research.

Peckham, C., Bedford, H., Senturia, Y. & Ades, A. (1989). *National immunization study: factors influencing immunization uptake in childhood*. Horsham: Action Research for the Crippled Child.

Peele, S. & Grant, M. (Eds.) (1999). *Alcohol and pleasure: a health perspective*. Washington, DC: International Center for Alcohol Policies.

Pennebaker, J.W. (1995). *Emotion, disclosure, and health*. Washington, DC: American Psychological Association.

Pennebaker, J.W. & Beall, S.K. (1986). Confronting a traumatic event: toward an understanding of inhibition and disease. *Journal of Abnormal Psychology, 95*, 274–281.

Penninx, B.W., Guralnik, J.M., Pahor, M., Ferrucci, L., Cerhan, J.R., Wallace, R.B. & Havlik, R.J. (1998). Chronically depressed mood and cancer risk in older persons. *Journal of the National Cancer Institute, 90*, 1888–1893.

Petrie, K. & Revenson, T. (2005). Editorial for special issue on behavioural medicine. *Journal of Health Psychology, 10*, 179–184.

Petrie, K.J., Cameron, L.D., Ellis, C.J., Buick, D. & Weinman, J. (2002). Changing illness perceptions after myocardial infarction: an early intervention randomized controlled trial. *Psychosomatic Medicine, 64*, 580–586.

Petrie, K.J., Weinman, J., Sharpe, N. & Buckley, J. (1996). Role of patients' view of their illness in predicting return to work & functioning after myocardial infarction: longitudinal study. *British Medical Journal, 312*, 1191–1194.

Petticrew, M., Bell, R. & Hunter, D. (2002). Influence of psychological coping on survival and recurrence in people with cancer: Systematic review. *British Medical Journal, 325*, 1066–1069.

Petticrew, M., Fraser, J.M. & Regan, M.F. (1999). Adverse life events and risk of breast cancer: a meta-analysis. *British Journal of Health Psychology, 4*, 1–17.

Pierce, J.P. & Gilpin, E.A. (2002). Impact of over-the-counter sales on effectiveness of pharmaceutical aids for smoking cessation. *Journal of the American Medical Association, 288*, 1260–1264.

Pignone, M.P. & DeWalt, D.A. (2006). Literacy and health outcomes. *Journal of General Internal Medicine, 21*, 896–897.

Pincus, T., Griffith, J., Isenberg, D. & Pearce, S. (1997). The Well-Being Questionnaire: testing the structure in groups with rheumatoid arthritis. *British Journal of Health Psychology, 2*, 167–174.

Pirozzo, S., Summerbell, C., Cameron, C. & Glasziou, P. (2004). Advice on low-fat diets for obesity (Cochrane Review). In *The Cochrane Library*, Issue 2. Chichester: John Wiley.

Plant, M. (2004). Editorial: The alcohol harm reduction strategy for England. *British Medical Journal, 328*, 905–906.

Plant, M. & Plant, M. (2006). *Binge Britain: alcohol and the national response.* Oxford Oxford University Press.

Poag-DuCharme, K.A. & Brawley, L.R. (1993). Self-efficacy theory: use in the prediction of exercise behavior in the community setting. *Journal of Applied Sport Psychology, 5*, 178–194.

Polito, J.R. (2008). Smoking cessation trials. *Canadian Medical Association Journal, 179*, 10.

Pollock, K. (1988). On the nature of social stress: production of a modern mythology. *Social Science & Medicine, 26*, 381–392.

Pomerlau, D.F. (1979). Behavioral factors in the establishment, maintenance, and cessation of smoking. In *Smoking and Health: A Report of the Surgeon General*. Washington, DC: US Department of Health, Education & Welfare. Pp. 161–162.

Popay, J., Bennett, S., Thomas, C., Williams, G., Gatrell, A. & Bostock, L. (2003). Beyond 'beer, fags, egg and chips'? Exploring lay understandings of social inequalities in health. *Sociology of Health and Illness, 25*, 1–23.

Porta, M. (2009). The improbable plunge. What facts refute reasons to expect that the effectiveness of HPV vaccination programs to prevent cervical cancer could be low? *Preventive Medicine, 48*, 407–410.

Porta, M., Gonzalez, B., Marquez, S. & Artazcoz, L. (2008). Doubts on the appropriateness of universal human papillomavirus vaccination: Is evidence on public health benefits already available? *Journal of Epidemiology & Community Health, 62*, 667.

Porter, R. (1997). *The greatest benefit to mankind: a medical history of humanity from antiquity to the present.* New York: Norton.

Posluszny, D., Spencer, S. & Baum, A. (2007). Post-traumatic stress disorder. In S. Ayers, A. Baum, C. McManus, S. Newman, K. Wallston, J. Weinman & R. West (Eds.), *Cambridge handbook of psychology, health and medicine*, 2nd ed. Cambridge: Cambridge University Press. Pp. 814–820.

Potter, J. & Wetherell, M. (1987). *Discourse and social psychology*. London: Sage.

Potvin, L., Camirand, J. & Beland, F. (1995). Patterns of health services utilization and mammography use among women aged 50–59 years in the Quebec medicare system. *Medical Care, 33*, 515–530.

Pound, P., Britten, N., Morgan, M., Yardley, L., Pope, C., Duker-White, G. & Campbell, R. (2005). Resisting medicines: A synthesis of qualitative studies of medicine taking. *Social Science & Medicine, 61*, 133–155.

Powell, L. H., Calvin, J. E. III & Calvin, J. E. Jr. (2007). Effective obesity treatments. *American Psychologist, 62*, 234–224.

Powell, L. M., Szczpka, G., Chaloupka, F. J. & Braunschweig, C. L. (2007). Nutritional content of television food advertisements seen by children and adolescents. *Pediatrics, 120*, 576–583.

Powers, B.J. & Bosworth, H.B. (2006). Revisiting literacy and adherence: Future clinical and research directions. *Journal of General and Internal Medicine, 21*, 1341–1342.

Powers, P. (2003). Empowerment as treatment and the role of health professionals. *Advances in Nursing Science, 26*, 227–237.

Powles, J. (1992). Changes in disease patterns and related social trends. *Social Science & Medicine, 35*, 377–387.

Prescott-Clarke, P. & Primatesta, P. (Eds.) (1998). *Health survey for England 95–97*. London: The Stationery Office.

Prescott-Clarke, P. & Primatesta, P. (1999). *Health survey for England: the health of young people 1995–1997*. London: The Stationery Office.

Priest, P. (2007). The healing balm effect. Using a walking group to feel better. *Journal of Health Psychology, 12*, 36–52.

Prilletensky, I. & Nelson, G. (2004). *Community psychology: In pursuit of liberation and well-being*. London: Palgrave.

Prins, J.T., van der Heijden, F.M., Hoekstra-Weebers, J.E., Bakker, A.B., van de Wiel, H.B., Jacobs, B. & Gazendam-Donofrio, S.M. (2009). Burnout, engagement and resident physicians' self-reported errors. *Psychology, Health & Medicine, 14*, 654–666.

Prochaska, J.O. & DiClemente, C.C. (1982). Trans-theoretical therapy – toward a more integrative model of change. *Psychotherapy: Theory, Research and Practice, 19*, 276–288.

Prochaska, J.O. & DiClemente, C.C. (1983). Stages and processes of self-change in smoking: toward an integrative model of change. *Journal of Consulting & Clinical Psychology, 51*, 520–528.

Project MATCH Research Group (1997). Matching alcoholism treatments to client heterogeneity: Project MATCH post-treatment drinking outcomes. *Journal of Studies on Alcohol, 58*, 7–29.

Putnam, R.D. (2000). *Bowling alone: The collapse and revival of American community*. New York: Simon & Schuster.

Putnam, R.D., Leonarchi, R. & Nanetti, R.Y. (1993). *Making democracy work: civic traditions in modern Italy*. Princeton, NJ: Princeton University Press.

Qi, L., Kraft, P., Hunter, D. J. & Hu, F.B. (2008). The common obesity variant near *MC4R* gene is associated with higher intakes of total energy and dietary fat, weight change and diabetes risk in women. *Human Molecular Genetics, 17*, 3502–3508.

Quintal de Freitas, M. (2000). Voices from the south: the construction of Brazilian community social psychology. *Journal of Community & Applied Social Psychology, 10*, 315–326.

Radley, A. & Billig, M. (1996). Accounts of health and illness: dilemmas and representations. *Sociology of Health & Illness, 18*, 220–240.

Radtke, H.R. & Van Mens-Verhulst, J. (2001). Being a mother and living with asthma: an exploratory analysis of discourse. *Journal of Health Psychology, 6*, 379–391.

Ragland, D.R. & Brand, R.J. (1988). Type A behaviour and mortality from coronary heart disease. *New England Journal of Medicine, 318*, 65–69.

Raistrick, D. (2005). The United Kingdom: alcohol today. *Addiction, 100*, 1212–1214.

Rakowski W., Dube, C.E., Marcus, B.H., Prochaska, J.O., Velicer, W.F. & Abrams, D.B. (1992). Assessing elements of women's decisions about mammography. *Health Psychology, 11*, 111–118.

Raleigh, V.S. (1999). World population and health in transition. *British Medical Journal, 319*, 981–984.

Ramella, M. and de la Cruz, R.B. (2000). Taking part in adolescent sexual health promotion in Peru: community participation from a social psychological perspective. *Journal of Community & Applied Social Psychology, 10*, 271–284.

Ramirez, A., Addington-Hall, J., Richards, M. (1998). ABC of palliative care: the carers. *British Medical Journal, 316*, 208–211.

Randolph, M.E., Pinkerton, S.D., Somlai, A.M., Kelly, J.A., McAuliffe, T.L., Gibson, R.H. & Hackl, K. (2009). Seriously mentally ill womens safer sex behaviors and the theory of reasoned action. *Health Education & Behavior, 36*, 948–958.

Randrianasolo, B., Swezey, T., Van Damme, K., Khan, M.R., Ravelomanana, N., Rabenja, N.L. & Behets, F. (2008). Barriers to the use of modern contraceptives and implications for woman-controlled prevention of sexually transmitted infections in Madagascar. *Journal of Biosocial Science, 40*, 879–893.

Ranney, L., Melvin, C., Lux, L., McClain, E. & Lohr, K.N. (2006). Systematic review: smoking cessation intervention strategies for adults and adults in special populations. *Annals of Internal Medicine, 145*, 845–856.

Rappaport, J. (1987). Terms of empowerment/examples of prevention: towards a theory for community psychology. *American Journal of Community Psychology, 15*, 121–149.

Ravussin, E., Pratley, R.E., Maffei, M., Wang, H., Friedman, J.M., Bennett, P.H. & Bogardus, C. (1997). Relatively low plasma leptin concentrations precede weight gain in Pima Indians. *Nature Medicine, 3*, 238–240.

Rawls, J. (1999). *A Theory of Justice*. Cambridge, MA: Belknap Press.

Reading, R., Colver, A., Openshaw, S. & Jarvis, S. (1994). Do interventions that improve immunisation uptake also reduce social inequalities in uptake? *BMJ, 308*, 1142–1144.

Reason, J. (2000). Human error: models and management. *BMJ, 320*, 768–770.

Reddy, V. (1989). Parents' beliefs about vaccination. *BMJ, 299*, 739.

Reed, D.M., LaCroix, A.Z., Karasek, R.A., Miller, D. & MacLean, C.A. (1989). Occupational strain and the incidence of coronary heart disease. *American Journal of Epidemiology, 129*, 495–502.

Rees, K., Bennett, P., West, R., Davey, S.G. & Ebrahim, S. (2004). Psychological interventions for coronary heart disease. *Cochrane Database of Systematic Reviews, (2)*, CD002902.

Rehse, B. & Pukrop, R. (2003). Effects of psychosocial interventions on quality of life in adult cancer patients: meta analysis of 37 published controlled outcome studies. *Patient Educational Counselling, 50*, 179–186.

Reid, K., Asbury, J., McDonald, R. & Serpell, M. (2003). Dear diary: exploring the utility of diaries as a powerful and multi-functional research tool. *Health Psychology Update, 12(2)*, 7–12.

Reiss, I.L. (1991). Sexual pluralism: ending Americas sexual crisis. *SIECUS Report*, February–March.

Reiter, P.L., Brewer, N.T., Gottlieb, S.L., McRee, A.-L. & Smith, J.S. (2009). Parents' beliefs and HPV vaccination of their adolescent daughters. *Social Science & Medicine, 65*, 1–6.

Remick, A. K., Polivy, J. & Pliner, P. (2009). Internal and external moderators of the effect of variety on food intake. *Psychological Bulletin, 135*, 434–451.

Richards, S.H., Bankhead, C., Peters, T.J., Austoker, J., Hobbs, F.D.R., et al. (2001). Cluster randomised controlled trial comparing the effectiveness and cost effectiveness of two primary care interventions aimed at improving attendance for breast screening. *Journal of Medical Screening, 8*, 91–98.

Riesen, W.F., Darioli, R. & Noll, G. (2004). Lipid-lowering therapy: strategies for improving compliance. *Current Medical Research & Opinion, 20*, 165–173.

Rimal, R.N. (2001). Longitudinal influences of knowledge and self-efficacy on exercise behavior: tests of a mutual reinforcement model. *Journal of Health Psychology, 6*, 31–46.

Rimer, B.K., Keintz, M.K., Kessler, H.B., Engstrom, P.F. & Rosan, J.R. (1989). Why women resist screening mammography: patient related barriers. *Radiology, 172*, 243–246.

Riska, E. (2000). The rise and fall of Type A man. *Social Science & Medicine, 51*, 1665–1674.

Rivers, S.E., Salovey, P., Pizarro, D.A., Pizarro, J. & Schneider, T.R. (2005). Message Framing and Pap Test Utilization among Women Attending a Community Health Clinic. *Journal of Health Psychology, 10*, 65–77.

Robert Wood Johnson Foundation (2006). State action to promote nutrition. Increase physical activity and prevent obesity. *Balance, 2*, 1–135. Accessed on 15 November 2009 at www.rwjf.org/.

Robinson, J.I. & Rogers, M.A. (1994). Adherence to exercise programmes: recommendations. *Sports Medicine, 17*, 39–52.

Robinson, M.K. (2009). Editorial. Surgical treatment of obesity – weighing the facts. *New England Journal of Medicine, 361*, 520.

Roche, A.M. & Freeman, T. (2004). Brief interventions: good in theory but weak in practice. *Drug & Alcohol Review, 23*, 11–18.

Rodin, G., Katz, M., Lloyd, N., Green, E. Mackay, J.A., Wong, R.K.S. and the Supportive Care Guidelines Group of Cancer Care Ontario's Program in Evidence-Based Care (2007). Treatment of depression in cancer patients. *Current Oncology, 14*, 180–188.

Rogers, F. (1975). A protection motivation theory of fear appeals and attitude change. *Journal of Psychology, 91*, 93–114.

Rogers, R.W. (1983). Cognitive and physiological processes in fear appeals and attitude change: A Revised theory of protection motivation. In J. Cacioppo & R. Petty (Eds.), *Social psychophysiology*. New York: Guilford Press. Pp. 153–176.

Room, R., Babor, T. & Rehm, J. (2005). Alcohol and public health. *Lancet, 365*, 519–529.

Rootman, I. & Gordon-El-Bihbety, D. (2008). *A vision for a health literate Canada*. Ottawa: CPHA.

Rose, G. (1992). *The strategy of preventive medicine*. Oxford: Oxford University Press.

Rosengren, A., Tibblin, G. & Wilhelmsen, L. (1991). Self-perceived psychological stress and incidence of coronary artery disease in middle-aged men. *American Journal of Cardiology, 68*, 1171–1175.

Rosenstock, I.M. (1966). Why people use health services. *Milbank Memorial Fund Quarterly, 44*, 94–127.

Rosenstock, I.M., Strecher, V.J. & Becker, M.H. (1988). Social learning theory and the health belief model. *Health Education Quarterly, 15*, 175–183.

Ross, C.E. (2000). Walking, exercising, and smoking: does neighborhood matter? *Social Science & Medicine, 51*, 265–274.

Rossner, S. (2002). Obesity: the disease of the 21st century. *International Journal of Obesity, 26*, S2–S4.

Rothman, A.J., Bartels, R.D., Wlachin, J. & Salovey, P. (2006). The strategic use of gain- and loss – framed messages to promote healthy behaviour: How theory can inform practice. *Journal of Communication, 56*, S202–220.

Rothman, A.J. & Salovey, P. (1997). Shaping perceptions to motivate healthy behaviour: The role of message framing. *Psychological Bulletin, 121*, 3–19.

Rotter, J.B. (1966). Generalised expectancies for internal versus external control of reinforcement. *Psychological Monographs, 80(609)*, 1.

Royal College of Physicians (1962). *Smoking and health*. London: RCP.

Royal College of Surgeons and Anaesthetists (1990). *Commission on the Provision of Surgical Services: Report of the Working Party on Pain After Surgery*. London: RCSA.

Royal College of Surgeons of England (2010). Conference hears of 'unfair and unethical' access to NHS weight loss surgery. Press release, 21 January 2010.

Royal Pharmaceutical Society of Great Britain (1997). *From compliance to concordance: toward shared goals in medicine taking*. London: RPS.

Rozin, P. (1996). Sociocultural influences on human food selection. In E.D. Capaldi (Ed.), *Why we eat what we eat: the psychology of eating*. Washington, DC: American Psychological Association. Pp. 233–263.

Ruitenberg, A., van Swieten, J.C., Witteman, J.C.M., Mehta, K.M., van Duijn, C.M., Hofman, A. & Breteler, M.M.B. (2002). Alcohol consumption and risk of dementia: The Rotterdam study. *Lancet, 359*, 281–286.

Ruiz, P. & Ruiz, P.P. (1983). Treatment compliance among Hispanics. *Journal of Occupational Psychiatry, 14*, 112–114.

Rutledge, T., Reis, V.A., Linke, S.E., Greenberg, B.H. & Mills, P.J. (2006). Depression in heart failure – A meta-analytic review of prevalence, intervention effects, and associations with clinical outcomes. *Journal of the American College of Cardiology, 48*, 1527–1537.

Ryerson, W.N. (2010). The effectiveness of entertainment mass media in changing behavior. Accessed on 1 January 2010 at http://www.populationmedia.org/wp-content/uploads/2008/02/effectiveness-of-entertainment-education-112706.pdf.

Sabido, M. (1981). Towards the social use of commercial television: Mexico's experience with the reinforcement of social values through TV soap operas. Paper presented at the annual conference of the International Institute of Communications (Strasbourg, France). Institute for Communications Research, A.C. (Mexico City, Mexico).

Sackett, D.L. & Snow, J.C. (1979). *Compliance in healthcare.* Baltimore, MD: Johns Hopkins University Press.

Safeer, R.S. & Keenan, J. (2005). Health literacy: The gap between physician and patients. *American Family Physicians, 72*, 463–468.

Saffer, H. & Dave, D. (2002). Alcohol consumption and alcohol advertising bans. *Applied Economics, 34*, 1325–1334.

Salas, J. (2008). Immigrant stories in the Hudson Valley. In R. Solinger, M. Fox & K. Irani (Eds.), *Telling stories to change the world.* New York: Routledge. Pp. 109–118.

Sallis, J.F., Bauman, A. & Pratt, M. (1998). Environmental and policy interventions to promote physical activity. *American Journal of Preventive Medicine, 15*, 379–397.

Sallis, J.F., King, A.C., Sirard, J.R. & Albright, C.L. (2007). Perceived environmental predictors of physical activity over 6 months in adults: Activity counseling trial. *Health Psychology, 26*, 701–709.

Salmon, P. & Hall, G.M. (2003). Patient empowerment and control: a psychological discourse in the service of medicine. *Social Science & Medicine, 57*, 1969–1980.

Sandberg, S., Paton, J., Ahola, S., McCann, D., McGuinness, D., Hillary, C.R. & Oja, H. (2000). The role of acute and chronic stress in asthma attacks in children. *Lancet, 356*, 982–987.

Sanders, K.A., Labott, S.M., Molokie, R., Shelby, S.R. & Desimone, J. (2010). Pain, coping and health care utilization in younger and older adults with sickle cell disease. *Journal of Health Psychology, 15*, 131–137.

Sanders, L.M., Federico, S., Klass, P., Abrams, M.A. & Dreyer, B. (2009). Literacy and child health: A systematic review. *Archive of Pediatric and Adolescent Medicine, 163*, 131–140.

Sarbin, T. (Ed.) (1986). *Narrative Psychology: the storied nature of human conduct.* Santa Barbara, CA: Greenwood Press.

Sayette, M.A. (2007). Alcohol abuse. In S. Ayers, A. Baum, C. McManus, S. Newman, K. Wallston, J. Weinman & R. West (Eds.), *Cambridge handbook of psychology, health and medicine*, 2nd edn. Cambridge: Cambridge University Press. Pp. 534–537.

Schaal, B. & Orgeur, P. (1992). Olfaction in utero: can the rodent model be generalized? *Quarterly Journal of Experimental Psychology, 44*, 245–278.

Schmidt, J.G. (1990). The epidemiology of mass breast cancer screening: a plea for a valid measure of benefit. *Journal of Clinical Epidemiology, 43*, 215–225.

Schober, R. (1997). Complementary and conventional medicines working together. *Canadian Health Psychologist, 5*, 14–18.

Schroeder, D.H. & Costa, P.T. Jr. (1984). Influence of life event stress on physical illness: Substantive effects or methodological flaws? *Journal of Personality & Social Psychology, 46*, 853–863.

Schulz, A., Gravlee, C.C., Williams, D., Israel, B.A., Mentz, G. & Rowe, Z. (2006). Discrimination, symptoms of depression, and self-rated health among African American women in Detroit: Results from a longitudinal analysis. *American Journal of Public Health, 96*, 1265–1270.

Schur, H.V., Gamsu, D.S. & Barley, V.M. (1999). The young persons perspective on living & coping with diabetes. *Journal of Health Psychology, 4*, 223–236.

Schuster, J., et al. (2006). Aids, alcohol and violence against women: strategies for reducing workplace health risks to Cambodian beer-selling women, presented at the XVI International Aids Conference, Toronto, Canada, 13–18 August 2006.

Schwartz, M., Savage, W., George, J. & Emohare, L. (1989). Women's knowledge and experience of cervical screening: a failure of health education and medical organisation. *Community Medicine, 11*, 279–289.

Schwarzer, R. (1992). Self efficacy in the adaptation and maintenance of health behaviours: theoretical approaches and a new model. In R. Schwarzer (Ed.), *Self efficacy: thought control of action*. Washington, DC: Hemisphere. Pp. 217–243.

SCOTH (Scientific Committee on Tobacco and Health) (1998). *Report*. London: The Stationery Office.

Scott-Sheldon, L.A.J., Carey, M.P., Vanable, P.A., Senn, T.E., Coury-Doniger, P. & Urban, M.A. (2010). Predicting condom use among STD clinic patients using the Information-Motivation-Behavioral Skills (IMB) model. *Journal of Health Psychology*.

Scott-Sheldon, L.A.J., Kalichman, S.C., Carey, M.P. & Fielder, R.L. (2008). Stress management interventions for HIV+ adults: A meta-analysis of randomized controlled trials, 1989 to 2006. *Health Psychology,* 27, 129–139.

Searle, A., Norman, P., Thompson, R. & Vedhara, K. (2007). A prospective examination of illness beliefs and coping in patients with type 2 diabetes. *British Journal of Health Psychology, 12*, 621–638.

Seedhouse, D. (1997). *Health promotion: philosophy, prejudice and practice*. England: Wiley.

Segerstrom, S.C. & Miller, G.E. (2004). Psychological stress and the human immune system: A meta-analytic study of 30 years of enquiry. *Psychological Bulletin, 130*, 601–630.

Seitz, D.C.M., Besier, T. & Goldbeck, L. (2009). Psychosocial interventions for adolescent cancer patients: a systematic review of the literature. *Psycho-Oncology, 18*, 683–690.

Selden, C., Zorn, M., Ratzan, S.C. & Parker, R.M. (2000). *Health literacy (online bibliography)*. Accessed on 29 December 2009 at http://www.nlm.nih.gov/archive//20061214/pubs/cbm/hliteracy.pdf.

Selye, H. (1976). *Stress in health and disease.* Reading, MA: Butterworth.

Shahab, L. & McEwen, A. (2009). Online support for smoking cessation: a systematic review of the literature. *Addiction, 104*, 1792–1804.

Shakespeare, T. (1998). Choices and rights: eugenics, genetics and disability equality. *Disability & Society, 13*, 665–681.

Shannon, C.E. & Weaver, W. (1949). *The mathematical theory of communication*. Urbana, IL: University of Illinois.

Shaper, A.G., Wannamethee, G. & Walker, M. (1988). Alcohol and mortality in British men: Explaining the U-shaped curve. *Lancet, 2*, 1267–1283.

Sharpe, K. & Earle, S. (2002). Feminism, abortion and disability: irreconcilable differences? *Disability & Society, 17*, 137–145.

Shaw, S. (1979). A critique of the concept of the alcohol dependence syndrome. *British Journal of Addiction, 74*, 339–348.

Shields, C.A. & Brawley, L.R. (2007). Limiting exercise options: Depending on a proxy may inhibit exercise self-management. *Journal of Health Psychology, 12*, 663–671.

Shorter, E. (1992). *From paralysis to fatigue: a history of psychosomatic illness in the modern era*. New York: Free Press.

Showalter, E. (1997). *Hystories: hysterical epidemics and modern culture*. London: Picador.

Shutty, M.S. Jr, DeGood, D.E. & Tuttle, D.H. (1990). Chronic pain patients' beliefs about their pain and treatment outcomes. *Archives of Physiotherapy & Medical Rehabilitation, 71*, 128–132.

Siegel, S. (1975). Conditioned insulin effects. *Journal of Comparative Physiology & Psychology, 89*, 189–199.

Siegrist, J. & Marmot, M. (2004). Health inequalities and the psychosocial environment – two scientific challenges, *Social Science & Medicine, 58*, 1463–1473.

Siem Reap Citizens for Health, Educational & Social Issues (SiRCHESI) (2008). Newsletter. January 2008. Accessed on 10 December 2009 at http://www.fairtradebeer.com/reportfiles/sirchesi/siemreapnewsletter2008.pdf.

Simpson, N., Lenton, S. & Randall, R. (1995). Parental refusal to have children immunised: extent and reasons. *BMJ, 310*, 225–227.

Singer, P. (1993). *Practical ethics*. Cambridge: Cambridge University Press.

Sinha, S., Curtis, K., Jayakody, A., Viner, R. & Roberts, H. (2007). 'People make assumptions about our communities': sexual health amongst teenagers from Black and Minority Ethnic backgrounds in East London. *Ethnicity & Health, 12*, 423–441.

Skelton, A.M. (1997). Patient education for the millennium: Beyond control and emancipation? *Patient Education and Counseling, 31*, 151–158.

Skilbeck, J.K. & Payne, S. (2005). End of life care: a discursive analysis of specialist palliative care nursing. *Journal of Advanced Nursing, 51*, 325–334.

Skinner, C.S., Champion, V.L., Gonin, R. & Hanna, M. (1997). Do perceived barriers and benefits vary by mammography stage? *Psychology, Health & Medicine, 2*, 65–75.

Slater, A. & Tiggemann, M. (2006). The contribution of physical activity and medic UK during childhood and adolescence to adult women's body image. *Journal of Health Psychology, 11*, 553–565.

Sleasman, J.W. & Goodenow, M.M. (2003). HIV-1 infection. *Journal of Allergy & Clinical Immunology, 111*, S582–592.

Slenker, S.E. & Grant, M.C. (1989). Attitudes, beliefs and knowledge about mammography among women over forty years of age. *Journal of Cancer Education, 4*, 61–65.

Slenker, S.E. & Spreitzer, E.A. (1989). Public perceptions and behaviors regarding cancer control. *Archives of Biochemistry and Biophysics, 275*, 280–288.

Slosson, R.J.L. (1990). *Slosson oral reading test-revised*. East Aurora, NY: Slosson Educational Publishers.

Smedslund, G. (2000). A pragmatic basis for judging models and theories in health psychology: The axiomatic method. *Journal of Health Psychology, 5*, 133–149.

Smee, C., Parsonage, M., Anderson, R. & Duckworth, S. (1992). Effect of tobacco advertising on tobacco consumption: a discussion document reviewing the evidence. London: Economics and Operational Research Division, Department of Health.

Smith, H.E. & Herbert, C.P. (1993). Preventive practice among primary care physicians in British Columbia. *CMAJ, 149*, 1795–1800.

Smith, J. (2004). *Building a safer NHS for patients: Improving medication safety. A report by the Chief Pharmaceutical Officer*. London: The Stationery Office.

Smith, J.A. (1996). Beyond the divide between cognition and discourse: using interpretative phenomenological analysis in health psychology. *Psychology & Health, 11*, 261–271.

Smith, J.A., Flowers, P. & Larkin, M. (2009). *Interpretative phenomenological analysis: theory, method and research*. London: Sage.

Smith, J.A., Jarman, M. & Osborn, M. (1999). Doing interpretative phenomenological analysis. In M. Murray & K. Chamberlain (Eds.), *Qualitative health psychology: theories and methods*. London: Sage. Pp. 218–240.

Smith, J.A. & Osborn, M. (2008). Interpretative phenomenological analysis. In J.A. Smith (Ed.), *Qualitative psychology: a practical guide to research methods*. London: Sage. Pp. 53–80.

Smyth, J.M., Stone, A.A., Hurewitz, A. & Kaell, A. (1999). Effects of writing about stressful experiences on symptom reduction in patients with asthma and rheumatoid arthritis. *Journal of The American Medical Association, 281*, 722–733.

Snyder, L.B. (2007). Health communication campaigns and their impact on behaviour. *Journal of Nutrition Education and Behaviour, 39*, S32–S40.

Solinger, R., Fox, M. & Irani, K. (Eds.) (2008). *Telling stories to change the world*. New York: Routledge.

Somerfield, M.R. (1997). The utility of systems models of stress and coping for applied research: The case of cancer adaptation. *Journal of Health Psychology, 2*, 133–183.

Sontag, S. ([1978, 1988] 2002). *Illness as metaphor and AIDS and its metaphors*. London: Penguin.

Spring, B., Howe, D., Berendsen, M., McFadden, H. G., Hitchcock, K., Rademaker, A. W. & Hitsman, B. (2009). Behavioral intervention to promote smoking cessation and prevent weight gain: a systematic review and meta-analysis. *Addiction, 104*, 1472–1486.

St. Claire, L., Watkins, C.J. & Billinghurst, B. (1996). Differences in meanings of health: an exploratory study of general practitioners and their patients. *Family Practice, 13*, 511–516.

Stainton-Rogers, W. (1991). *Explaining health and illness: An exploration of diversity.* Hemel Hempstead: Wheatsheaf.

Stam, H.J. (2004). A sound body in a sound mind: a critical historical analysis of health psychology. In M. Murray (Ed.), *Critical health psychology*. London: Palgrave.

Stansfeld, S.A., Fuhrer, R., Head, J., Ferrie, J. & Shipley, M. (1997). Work and psychiatric disorder in the Whitehall II Study. *Journal of Psychosomatic Research, 43*, 73–81.

Stanton, A. & Revenson, T.A. (2005). Progress and promise in research on adaptation to chronic illness. In H.S. Friedman & R.C. Silver (Eds.), *The Oxford handbook of health psychology*. New York: Oxford University Press.

Stead, M., Gordon, R., Angus, K. and McDermott, L. (2007). A systematic review of social marketing effectiveness. *Health Education, 2*, 126–191.

Steeg, P.S. (2003). Metastasis suppressors alter the signal transduction of cancer cells. *Nature Reviews Cancer, 3*, 55–63.

Stein, J.A., Fox, S.A., Murata, P.J. & Morisky, D.E. (1992). Mammography usage and the Health Belief Model. *Health Education & Behavior, 19*, 447–462.

Stein, J.A. & Rotheram-Borus, M. (2004). Cross-sectional and longitudinal associations in coping strategies and physical health outcomes among HIV-positive youth. *Psychology & Health, 19*, 321–336.

Steinhauser, K.E., Clipp, E.C., McNeilly, M., Christakis, N.A., McIntyre, L.M. & Tulsky, J.A. (2000). In search of a good death: Observations of patients, families, and providers. *Annals of Internal Medicine, 132*, 825–832.

Steinitz, V. & Mishler, E.G. (2001). Reclaiming SPSSIs radical promise: a critical look at JSIs 'Impact of welfare reform' issue. *Analyses of Social Issues & Public Policy, 1*, 163–173.

Stensland, P. & Malterud, K. (1999). Approaching the locked dialogues of the body: Communicating illness through diaries. *Journal of Primary Health Care, 17*, 75–80.

Stephens, C. (2007a). Participation in different fields of practice: Using social theory to understand participation in community health promotion. *Journal of Health Psychology, 12*, 949–960.

Stephens, C. (2007b). Community as practice: Social representations of community and their implications for health promotion. *Journal of Community & Applied Social Psychology, 17*, 103–114.

Stephens, C. (2009). Racism and Inequalities in Health: Notes towards an Agenda for Critical Health Psychology, *Journal of Health Pscychology, 14*, 655–659.

Stephens, C., Netteleton, C., Porter, J., Willis, R. & Clark, S. (2005). Indigenous peoples' health – why are they behind everyone, everywhere? *Lancet, 366*, 10–13.

Stephens, C., Porter, J., Nettleton, C. & Willis, R. (2006). Disappearing, displaced, and undervalued: a call to action for Indigenous health worldwide. *Lancet, 367*, 2019–2028.

Stewart, D.E., Abbey, S.E., Shnek, Z.M., Irvine, J. & Grace, S.L. (2004). Gender differences in health information needs and decisional preferences in patients recovering from an acute ischemic coronary event. *Psychosomatic Medicine, 66*, 42–48.

Stewart, M.J., Gillis, A., Brosky, G., Johnston, G., Kirkland, S., Leigh, G., Persaud, V., Rootman, I., Jackson, S. & Pawliw-Fry, B.A. (1996). Smoking among disadvantaged women: causes and cessation. *Canadian Journal of Nursing Research, 28*, 41–60.

Stewart, S., Riecken, T., Scott, T., Tanaka, M. & Riecken, J. (2008). Expanding health literacy: Indigenous youth creating videos. *Journal of Health Psychology, 13*, 180–189.

Stewart, W.F., Lipton, R.B., Simon, D., Liberman, J. & Von Korff, M. (1999). Validity of an illness severity measure for headache in a population sample of migraine sufferers. *Pain, 79*, 291–301.

Stokols, D. (1996). Establishing and maintaining healthy environments: toward a social ecology of health promotion. *American Psychologist, 47*, 6–22.

Stokols, D. (1996). Translating social ecological theory into guidelines for community health promotion. *American Journal of Health Promotion, 10*, 282–298.

Stolerman, I.P. & Jarvis, M.J. (1995). The scientific case that nicotine is addictive. *Psychopharmacology, 117*, 2–10.

Stone, G.C., Weiss, S.M., Matarazzo, J.D., Miller, N.E. & Rodin, J. (Eds.) (1987). *Health psychology: a discipline and a profession*. Chicago: University of Chicago Press.

Stone, S.V. & Costa, P.T. (1990). Disease-prone personality or distress-prone personality? The role of neuroticism in coronary heart disease. In H.S. Friedman (Ed.), *Personality and disease*. London: Wiley. Pp. 178–200.

Stone, S.V. & McCrea, R.R. (2007). Personality and health. In S. Ayers, A. Baum, C. McManus, S. Newman, K. Wallston, J. Weinman and R. West (Eds.), *Cambridge Handbook of Psychology, Health and Medicine*, 2nd edn. Cambridge: Cambridge University Press. Pp. 151–155.

Stone, D.H. & Stewart, S. (1996). Screening and the new genetics: a public health perspective on the ethical debate. *Journal of Public Health Medicine, 18*, 3–5.

Strauss, A.L. (1987). *Qualitative analysis for social scientists*. New York: Cambridge University Press.

Stroebe, M.S. & Stroebe, W. (1983). Who suffers more? Sex differences in health risks of the widowed. *Psychological Bulletin, 93*, 279–301.

Sullivan, C.F. (2003). Gendered cybersupport: a thematic analysis of two online cancer support groups. *Journal of Health Psychology, 8*, 83–103.

Sullivan, J., Petronella, S., Brooks, E., Murillo, M., Primeau, L. & Ward, J. (2008). Theatre of the oppressed and environmental justice communities: A transformational therapy for the body. *Journal of Health Psychology, 13*, 166–179.

Sulloway, F.J. (1980). *Freud, biologist of the mind*. London: Fontana.

Suls, J. & Bunde, J. (2005) Anger, anxiety and depression as risk factors for cardiovascular disease: The problems and implications of overlapping affective dispositions. *Psychological Bulletin, 131*, 260–300.

Suls, J. & Rittenhouse, J.D. (1990). Models of linkages between personality & disease. In H.S. Friedman (Ed.), *Personality & Disease*. London: Wiley. Pp. 38–64.

Sulzberger, P. & Marks, D. F. (1977). *Isis smoking cessation programme*. Dunedin, New Zealand: Isis Research Centre.

Summerbell, C.D., Ashton, V., Campbell, K.J., Edmunds, L., Kelly, S. & Waters, E. (2004). Interventions for treating obesity in children (Cochrane Review). In *The Cochrane Library*, Issue 4. Chichester: John Wiley.

Summerfield, D. (2001). The intervention of post-traumatic stress disorder and the social usefulness of a psychiatric category. *British Medical Journal, 322*, 95–98.

Surtees, P., Wainwright, N., Luben, R., Khaw, K-T. & Day, N. (2003). Sense of coherence and mortality in men and women in the EPIC-Norfolk United Kingdom prospective cohort study. *American Journal of Epidemiology, 158*, 1202–1209.

Surtees, P.G., Wainwright, N.W.J., Luben, R.N., Wareham, N.J., Bingham, S.A. & Khaw, K.-T. (2008). Depression and ischemic heart disease mortality: Evidence from the EPIC-Norfolk United Kingdom prospective cohort study. *American Journal of Psychiatry, 165*, 515–523.

Sutton, S. (2000). A critical review of the Transtheoretical Model applied to smoking cessation. In P. Norman, C. Abraham & M. Conner (Eds.), *Understanding and changing health behaviour: From health beliefs to self-regulation*. Amsterdam: Harwood Academic Publishers. Pp. 207–225.

Sutton, S. (2005) Stage theories of health behaviour. In Conner, M. and Norman, P. (Eds.), *Predicting Health behaviour: research and practice with social cognition models*. 2nd edn. Buckingham: Open University Press. Pp. 223–275.

Sutton, S., Bickler, G., Aldridge, J. & Saidi, G. (1994). Prospective study of predictors of attendance for breast screening in inner London. *Journal of Epidemiology & Community Health, 48*, 65–73.

Swartzman, L.C. & Lees, M.C. (1996). Casual dimensions of college students' perceptions of physical symptoms. *Journal of Behavioral Medicine, 19(2)*, 95–110.

Swinburn, B. & Ravussin, E. (1993). Energy balance or fat balance? *American Journal of Clinical Nutrition, 57*, 766S–770S.

Sykes, C.M. & Marks, D.F. (2001). Effectiveness of cognitive behaviour therapy self-help programme for smokers in London, UK. *Health Promotion International, 16*, 255–260.

Syrjala, K.L., Donaldson, G.W., Davis, M.W., Kippes, M.E. & Carr, J.E. (1995). Relaxation and imagery and cognitive-behavioral training reduce pain during cancer treatment: a controlled clinical trial. *Pain, 63*, 189–198.

Taira, D.A., Safran, D.G., Seto, D.B., Rogers, W.H. & Tarlov, A.R. (1997). The relationship between patient income and physician discussion of health risk behaviors. *JAMA, 278*, 1412–1417.

Tataranni, P. A., Harper, I. T., Snitker, S., Del Parigi, A., Vozarova, B., Bunt, J., Bogardus, C. & Ravussin, E. (2003). Body weight gain in free-living Pima Indians: effect of energy intake *vs* expenditure. *International Journal of Obesity, 27*, 1578–1583.

Tatrow, K. & Montgomery, G.H. (2006). Cognitive behavioral therapy techniques for distress and pain in breast cancer patients: a meta-analysis. *Journal of Behavioral Medicine, 29*, 17–27.

Tatzer, E., Schubert, M.T., Timischi, W. & Simbruner, G. (1985). Discrimination of taste and preference for sweet in premature babies. *Early Human Development, 12*, 23–30.

Taylor, C., Carlos Poston, W.S., Jones, L. & Kraft, M.K. (2006). Environmental justice: Obesity, physical activity, and health eating. *Journal of Physical Activity & Health, Suppl. 1*, S30–S54.

Taylor, M.D., Whiteman, M.C., Fowkes, G.R., Lee, A.J., Allerhand, M. & Deary, I.J. (2009). Five factor model personality traits and all-cause mortality in the Edinburgh Artery Study Cohort. *Psychosomatic Medicine, 71*, 631–641.

Taylor, N., Hall, G.M. & Salmon, P. (1996). Is patient controlled analgesia controlled by the patient. *Social Science & Medicine, 43*, 1137–1143.

Taylor, S.E. (1983). Adjustment to threatening events: A theory of cognitive adaption. *American Psychologist, 38*, 1161–1173.

Taylor, S.E., Repetti, R.L. & Seeman, T. (1997). Health psychology: what is an unhealthy environment and how does it get under the skin? *Annual Review of Psychology, 48*, 411–447.

Taylor, T.R., Williams, C.D., Makambi, K.H., Mouton, C., Harrell, J.P., Cozier, Y. & Adams-Campbell, L.L. (2007). Racial discrimination and breast cancer incidence in US black women – The Black Women's Health Study. *American Journal of Epidemiology, 166*, 46–54.

Tessaro, I., Eng, E. & Smith, J. (1994). Breast cancer screening in older African American women: Qualitative research findings. *American Journal of Health Promotion, 8*, 286–292.

Thom, B. (2001). A social and political history of alcohol. In N. Heather, T.J. Peters & T. Stockwell (Eds.), *International handbook of alcohol dependence and problems.* London: Wiley. Pp. 281–297.

Thomas, I. (1979). *The medusa and the snail.* New York: Bantam.

Tibben, A., Frets, P.G., van de Kamp, J.J., Niermeijer, M.F., Vegter-van der Vlis, M., Roos, R.A. & Verhage, F. (1993). Presymptomatic DNA testing for Huntington disease: pre-test attitudes and expectations of applicants and their partners in the Dutch program. *American Journal of Medical Genetics, 48*, 10–16.

Tibben, A., Timman, R., Bannink, E.C. & Duivenvoorden, H.J. (1997). Three year follow up after presymptomatic testing for Huntington's disease in tested individuals and partners. *Health Psychology, 16*, 20–35.

Tickell, O. (2008). *Kyoto2: How to manage the global greenhouse*. London: Zed Books.

Tiggemann, M., Martins, Y. & Churchett, L. (2008). Beyond muscles: unexplored parts of men's body image. *Journal of Health Psychology, 13*, 1163–1172.

Tillotson, K. & Smith, M.S. (1996). Locus of control, social support, and adherence to the diabetes regimen. *The Diabetes Educator, 22*, 133–139.

Todd, K.H., Deaton, C., DAdamo, A.P. & Goe, L. (2000). Ethnicity and analgesic practice. *Annals of Emergency Medicine, 35*, 11–16.

Tolley, K. (1985). *Health promotion: how to measure cost-effectiveness*. London: Health Education Authority.

Tolstrup, J., Jensen, M.K., Tjønneland, A., Overvad, K., Mukamal, K.J. & Grønbæk, M. (2006). Prospective study of alcohol drinking patterns and coronary heart disease in women and men. *British Medical Journal, 332*, 1244–1248.

Tomkins, S.S. (1966). Psychological model for smoking behavior. *American Journal of Public Health, 56*, 17–20.

Tomlinson, A., Ravenscroft, N., Wheaton, B. & Gilchrist, P. (2005). *Lifestyle sports and national sport policy: an agenda for research.* Eastbourne: University of Brighton.

Tong, E.K., England, L. & Glantz, S.A. (2005). Changing conclusions on secondhand smoke in a sudden infant death syndrome review funded by the tobacco industry. *Pediatrics, 115*, 356–366.

Tostes, M.A., Chalub, M. & Botega, N.J. (2004). The quality of life of HIV-infected women is associated with psychiatric morbidity. *AIDS Care, 16*, 177–186.

Townsend, P. & Davidson, N. (1982). *Inequalities in health: the Black report.* London: Penguin.

Trafimow, D. (2009). The theory of reasoned action: a case study of falsification in psychology. *Theory & Psychology, 19*, 501–518.

Trafimow, D., Sheeran, P., Conner, M. & Finlay, K.A. (2002). Evidence that perceived behavioural control is a multidimensional construct: perceived control and perceived difficulty. *British Journal of Social Psychology, 41*, 101–121.

Treharne, G.J., Lyons, A.C. & Kitas, G.D. (2004). Medication adherence in rheumatoid arthritis: effects of psychosocial factors. *Psychology, Health & Medicine, 9*, 337–349.

Trostle, J.A. (1998). Medical compliance as an ideology. *Social Science & Medicine, 27*, 1299–1308.

True, W.R., Heath, A.C., Scherrer, J.F., Waterman, B., Goldberg, J., Lin, N. & Tsuang, M.T. (1997). Genetic and environmental contributions to smoking. *Addiction, 92*, 1277–1287.

Trumbull, R. & Appley, M.H. (1986). A conceptual model for the understanding of stress dynamics. In M.H. Appley & R. Trumbull (Eds.), *Dynamics of stress: physiological, psychological and social perspectives.* New York: Plenum. Pp. 21–45.

Turner, B. (1984). *The body and society: explorations in social theory.* Oxford: Blackwell.

Tversky, A. & Kahneman, D. (1981). The framing of decisions and the rationality of choice. *Science, 221*, 453–458.

Uitterhoeve, R.J., Vernooy, M., Litjens, M., Potting, K., Bensing, J., De Mulder, P. & Van Achterberg, T. (2004). Psychosocial interventions for patients with advanced cancer: a systematic review of the literature. *British Journal of Cancer, 91(6)*, 1050–1062.

UNAIDS (2004). *Report on the global AIDS epidemic*: 4th Global Report. Geneva: Joint United Nations Programme on HIV/AIDS.

UNESCO (2000). *The Dakar Framework for Action, Education for All: Meeting our collective commitments adopted by the World Education Forum (Dakar, Senegal, 26–28 April 2000).* Paris: UNESCO.

United Nations (2009). *State of the World's Indigenous Peoples.* New York: United Nations.

United Nations Development Programme (1995). *Human development report.* New York: Oxford University Press.

Urban, B.J., France, R.D., Steinberger, E.K., Scott, D.L. & Maltbre, A.A. (1986). Long-term use of narcotic/antidepressant medication in the management of phantom limb pain. *Pain, 24*, 1991–1996.

US Census Bureau (2008). World POPClock Projection. Accessed 7 July 2010 at www.census.gov/cgi-bin/ipc/popclockw.

US Census Bureau (2010). Accessed on 7 July 2010 at: http://www.census.gov/population/www/projections/summarytables.html.

US Centers for Disease Control & Prevention (2005). http://www.cdc.gov/nccdphp/ (accessed 7 January 2005).

US Department of Health and Human Services (2000). *Healthy People 2010: Understanding and Improving Health.* Accessed 29 December 2009 at http://www.healthypeople.gov/.

US Department of Health, Education & Welfare (1964). *Smoking and Health. Report of the Advisory Committee to the Surgeon General of the Public Health Service.* Washington, DC. PHS Pub. No. 1103.

US Surgeon General (1989). *Reducing the health consequences of smoking: 25 years of progress: A report of the Surgeon General.* Bethesda, MD: Center for Chronic Disease Prevention & Health Promotion.

US Surgeon General (2004). *The health consequences of smoking: a report of the Surgeon General.* Atlanta, Ga.: Dept. of Health and Human Services, Centers for Disease Control and Prevention, National Center for Chronic Disease Prevention and Health Promotion, Office on Smoking and Health. Washington, DC.

US Surgeon General (2008). *Treating tobacco use and dependence*. 2008 update. Atlanta, Ga.: Dept. of Health and Human Services, Centers for Disease Control and Prevention, National Center for Chronic Disease Prevention and Health Promotion, Office on Smoking and Health; Washington, DC.

Valery, P.C., Coory, M., Stirling, J. & Green, A.C. (2006). Cancer diagnosis, treatment, and survival in Indigenous and non-Indigenous Australians: A matched cohort study. *Lancet, 367*, 1842–1848.

Van Haaften, E.H. & Van de Vijver, F.J.R. (1996). Psychological consequences of environmental degradation. *Journal of Health Psychology, 1*, 411–429.

van Melle, J.P., de Jonge, P., Honig, A., Schene, A.H., Kuyper, A.M., Crijns, H.J. & Ormel, J. (2007). Effects of antidepressant treatment following myocardial infarction. *British Journal of Psychiatry, 190*, 460–466.

Van Uden-Kraan, C.F., Drossaert, C.H.C., Taal, E., Shaw, B.R., Seydel, E.R. & van de Laar, M.A.F.J. (2008). Empowering processes and outcomes of participation in online support groups for patients with breast cancer, arthritis, or fibromyalgia. *Qualitative Health Research, 18*, 405–417.

Vance, Y. & Eiser, C. (2004). Caring for a child with cancer: a systematic review. *Pediatric Blood & Cancer, 42*, 249–253.

Velasquez, M.M., von Sternberg, K., Johnson, D.H., Green, C., Carbonari, J.P. & Parsons, J.T. (2009). Reducing sexual risk behaviors and alcohol use among HIV-positive men who have sex with men: a randomized clinical trial. *Journal of Consulting and Clinical Psychology, 77*, 657–667.

Verhoef, M.J., Love, E.J., & Rose, M.S. (1992). Women's social roles and their exercise participation, *Women's Health, 19*, 15–29.

Vermeire, E., Hearnshaw, H., van Royen, P. & Denekens, J. (2001). Patient adherence to treatment: Three decades of research. A comprehensive review. *Journal of Clinical Pharmacy and Therapeutics, 26*, 331–342.

Viera, A.J., Kshirsagar, A.V. & Hinderliter, A.L. (2007). Lifestyle modification advice for lowering or controlling high blood pressure: who's getting it? *Journal of Clinical Hypertension, 9*, 850–858.

Vincent, C.A., Neale, G. & Woloshynowych, M. (2001). Adverse events in British hospitals: preliminary retrospective record review. *BMJ, 322*, 517–519.

Vlaeyen, J.W.S. & Linton, S.J. (2000). Fear-avoidance and its consequences in chronic musculoskeletal pain: a state of the art. *Pain, 85*, 317–332.

Von Lengerke, T., Vinck, J., Rutten, A., Reitmeir, P., Abel, T., Kannas, L., & Van der Zee, J. (2004). Health policy perception and health behaviours: a multilevel analysis and implications for public health psychology. *Journal of Health Psychology, 9*, 157–175.

Wadden, T.A., Brownell, K.D. & Foster, G.D. (2002). Obesity: responding to the global epidemic. *Journal of Consulting & Clinical Psychology, 70*, 510–525.

Waitzkin, H. (1989). A critical theory of medical discourse: ideology, social control, and the processing of social context in medical encounters. *Journal of Health and Social Behavior, 30*, 220–239.

Wald, N., Kiryluk, S., Darby, S., Doll, R., Pike, M. & Peto, R. (1988). *UK smoking statistics*. Oxford: Oxford University Press.

Wallston, K.A., Wallston, B.S. & DeVellis, R. (1978). Development of multidimensional health locus of control (MHLC) scales. *Health Education Monographs, 6*, 160–170.

Wallwiener, M., Wallwiener, C.W., Kansy, J.K., Seeger, H. and Rajab, T.K. (2009). Impact of electronic messaging on the patient-physician interaction. *Journal of Telemed and Telecare, 15*, 243–250.

Walters, G.D. (2002). The heritability of alcohol abuse and dependence: A meta-analysis of behaviour genetic research. *American Journal of Drug & Alcohol Abuse, 28*, 557–584.

Wang, C. (1999). Photovoice: A participatory action research strategy applied to women's health. *Journal of Women's Health, 8*, 185–192.

Wang, C., Burris, M. & Xiang, Y. (1996a). Empowerment through photo novella: Portraits of participation. *Health Education Quarterly, 21*, 171–186.

Wang, C., Burris, M.A. & Xiang, Y.P. (1996b). Chinese village women as visual anthropologists: A participatory approach to reaching policymakers. *Social Science & Medicine, 42*, 1391–1400.

Wardle, J. & Pope, R. (1992). The psychological costs of screening for cancer. *Journal of Psychosomatic Research, 36*, 609–624.

Wardle, J., McCaffery, K., Nadel, M. & Atkin, W. (2004). Socioeconomic differences in cancer screening participation: comparing cognitive and psychosocial explanations. *Social Science & Medicine, 59*, 249–261.

Wassertheil-Smoller, S., Shumaker, S., Ockene, J., Talavera, G.A., Greeland, P., Cochrane, B. & Dubar-Jacob, J. (2004). Depression and cardiovascular sequelae in postmenopausal women. *Archives of Internal Medicine, 164*, 289–298.

Watson, M., Davidson-Homewood, J., Haviland, J. & Bliss, J. (2003). Study results should not have been dismissed. *British Medical Journal, 326*, 598.

Watson, M., Haviland, J.S., Greer, S., Davidson, J. & Bliss, J.M. (1999). Influence of psychological response on survival in breast cancer: a population-based cohort study. *Lancet, 354*, 1331–1336.

Wear, A. (1985). Puritan perceptions of illness in seventeenth century England. In R. Porter (Ed.), *Patients and practitioners: lay perceptions of medicine in preindustrial society*. Cambridge: Cambridge University Press. Pp. 55–100.

Webb, G.P. (1995). *Nutrition: a health promotion approach*. London: Arnold.

Wechsler, H., Davenport, A., Dowdall, G., Moeykens, B. & Castillo, S. (1994). Health and behavioral consequences of binge drinking in college. A national survey of students at 140 campuses. *Journal of the American Medical Association, 272*, 1672–1677.

Weingart, S.N., Wilson, R., Gibberd, R.W. & Harrison, B. (2000). Epidemiology of medical error. *British Medical Journal, 320*, 774–777.

Weinman, J., Petrie, K.J., Moss-Morris, R. & Horne, R. (1996). The Illness Perception Questionnaire: a new method for assessing the cognitive representation of illness. *Psychology & Health, 11*, 431–446.

Weinman, J., Petrie, K.J., Sharpe, N. & Walker, S. (2000). Causal attributions in patients and spouses following first-time myocardial infarction subsequent lifestyle changes. *British Journal of Health Psychology, 5*, 263–273.

Weinstein, N.D. (1993). Testing four competing theories of health-protective behavior. *Health Psychology, 12*, 324–333.

Weiss, B.D. (2007). *Health literacy and patient safety: Helping patients understand. Manual for clinicians* 2nd ed. Chicago: AMA Foundation.

Weiss, B.D., Mays, M.Z., Martz, W., Merriam-Castro, K., DeWalt, D., Pignone, M., Mockbee, J. & Hale, F.A. (2005). Quick assessment of literacy in primary care: The Newest Vital Sign. *Annals of Family Medicine, 3*, 514–522.

Weitkunat, R., Markuzzi, A., Vogel, S., Schlipköter, U., Koch, H.-J., Meyer, G. & Ferring, D. (1998). Psychological factors associated with the uptake of measles immunization. *Journal of Health Psychology, 3*, 273–284.

Wertheimer, A.I. & Santella, T.M. (2003). Medication compliance research: still so far to go. *Journal of Applied Research in Clinical & Experimental Therapeutics, 3*, 1–11.

West, C. (1984). When the doctor is a "lady": Power, status and gender in physician patient encounters. *Symbolic Interaction, 7*, 87–106.

Westling, E., Garcia, K. & Mann, T. (2007). Discovery of meaning and adherence to medications in HIV-infected women. *Journal of Health Psychology, 12*, 627–635.

Wetherell, M. (1998). Positioning and interpretative repertories: Conversation analysis and post-structuralism in dialogue. *Discourse & Society, 9*, 387–412.

Whiteman, M.C., Fowkes, F.G.R., Deary, I.J. & Lee, A.J. (1997). Hostility, cigarette smoking and alcohol consumption in the general population. *Social Science and Medicine, 44*, 1089–1096.

Whitlock, E.P., Polen, M.R., Green, C.A., Orleans, T. & Klein, J. (2004). Behavioural counseling interventions in primary care to reduce risky/harmful alcohol use by adults: a summary of the evidence for the U.S. Preventive Services Task Force. *Annals of Internal Medicine, 140*, 557–568.

Whittaker, R., Borland, R., Bullen, C., Lin, R.B., McRobbie, H. & Rodgers, A. (2009). Mobile phone-based interventions for smoking cessation. *Cochrane Database of Systematic Reviews*, Issue 4. Art. No, CD006611.

WHO Commission on the Social Determinants of Health (2008).*Closing the gap in a genaration: health equity through action on the social determinants of health. Final report*. Geneva: WHO.

WHO (2007). *World Health Organisation expert committee second report on problems related to alcohol consumption*. Geneva: WHO.

Whooley, M.A. & Browner, W.S. (1998). Association between depressive symptoms and mortality in older women. *Archives of Internal Medicine, 158*, 2129–2135.

Wiggers, L.C., De Wit, J.B., Gras, M.J., Coutinho, R.A. & Van Den Hoek, A. (2003). Risk behavior and social-cognitive determinants of condom use among ethnic minority communities in Amsterdam. *AIDS Education & Prevention, 15*, 430–447.

Wiggins, S., Potter, J. & Wildsmith, A. (2001). Eating your words: discursive psychology and the reconstruction of eating practices. *Journal of Health Psychology, 6*, 5–15.

Wilkinson, R. (1996). *Unhealthy societies*. London: Routledge.

Wilkinson, R. & Pickett, K. (2009). *The spirit level. Why more equal societies almost always do better*. London: Penguin.

Wilkinson, S. (1998). Focus groups in health research: exploring the meaning of health and illness. *Journal of Health Psychology, 3*, 329–348.

Wilkinson, S., Joffe, H. & Yardley, L. (2004). Qualitative data collection: interviews and focus groups. In D.F. Marks & L. Yardley (Eds.), *Research methods for clinical & health psychology*. London: Sage.

Williams, A. (2006). Perspectives on spirituality at the end of life: a meta-summary. *Palliative & Supportive Care, 4*, 407–417.

Williams, D.C., Golding, J., Phillips, K. & Towell, A. (2004). Perceived control, locus of control and preparatory information: effects on the perception of an acute pain stimulus. *Personality & Individual Differences, 36*, 1681–1691.

Williams, D.M., Anderson, E.S. & Winett, R.A. (2005). A review of the outcome expectancy construct in physical activity research. *Annals of Behavioral Medicine, 29*, 70–79.

Williams, D.R. & Collins, C. (1995). US socioeconomic and racial differences in health: patterns and explanations, *Annual Review of Sociology, 21*, 349–386.

Williams, D.R. & Mohammed, S.A. (2009). Discrimination and racial disparities in health: Evidence and needed research. *Journal of Behavioural Medicine, 32*, 20–47.

Williams, D.R., Yu, Y., Jackson. J.S. & Anderson, N.B. (1997). Racial differences in physical and mental health: socio-economic status, stress and discrimination. *Journal of Health Psychology, 2*, 335–351.

Williams, G. (1984). The genesis of chronic illness: narrative reconstruction. *Sociology of Health & Illness, 6*, 175–200.

Williams, G. (2007). Health inequalities in their place. In S. Cropper, A. Porter, G. Williams, S. Carlisle, R. Moore, M. O'Neill, C. Roberts & H. Snooks (Eds.), *Community health and wellbeing: Action research on health inequalities*. Bristol: Policy Press. Pp. 1–22.

Williams, G.H. (2003). The determinants of health: structure, context and agency. *Sociology of Health & Illness, 25*, 131–154.

Williams, S.J. & Calnan, M. (1996). The 'limits' of medicalization?: modern medicine and the lay populace in 'late' modernity. *Social Science & Medicine, 42*, 1609–1620.

Willig, C. (2001). *Introducing qualitative research in psychology*. Buckingham: Open University Press.

Willig, C. (2004). Discourse analysis and health psychology. In M. Murray (Ed.), *Critical health psychology*. London: Palgrave.

Willig, C. (2008). A phenomenological investigation of the experience of taking part in 'extreme sports'. *Journal of Health Psychology, 13*, 690–702.

Willig, C. (2009). 'Unlike a rock, a tree, a horse or an angel ...': Reflections on the struggle for meaning through writing during the process of cancer diagnosis. *Journal of Health Psychology, 14*, 181–189.

Willig, C. & Paulson, S. (2008). Older women and everyday talk about the ageing body. *Journal of Health Psychology, 13*, 106–120.

Willis, P. (1977). *Learning to labour: how working class kids get working class jobs*. Westmead: Saxon House.

Wilson, D.K., Ainsworth, B.E. & Bowles, H. (2007). Body mass index and environmental supports for physical inactivity among active and inactive. *Health Psychology, 26*, 710–717.

Wilson, J. & Jungner, G. (1968). Principles and practice of screening for disease. Geneva, WHO. World Health Organization Public Health Paper 34.

Winefield, H., Murrell, T., Clifford, J. & Farmer, E. (1996). The search for reliable and valid measures of patient-centredness. *Psychology & Health, 11*, 811–824.

Winett, R.A., King, A.C. and Altman, D.G. (1989). *Health psychology and public health*. New York: Pergamon.

Wire, T. (2009). *Fewer emitters, lower emissions, less cost. Reducing future carbon emissions by investing in family planning*. London: London School of Economics.

Woodgate, J. & Brawley, L.R. (2008). Self-efficacy for exercise in cardiac rehabilitation: Review and recommendations. *Journal of Health Psychology, 13*, 366–387.

Woods, L.M., Rachet, B. & Coleman, M.P. (2006). Origins of socio-economic inequalities in cancer survival: a review. *Annals of Oncology, 17*, 5–19.

World Bank (2002). http://www.worldbank.org/poverty/health/data/index.htm.

World Bank (2004). http://www.prb.org/template.cfm?template=InterestDisplay.cfm&Interest CategoryID=206.

World Health Organization (1986). Ottawa Charter for Health Promotion. *Health Promotion, 1*, iii–v.

World Health Organization (1989). *World health statistics annual*. Geneva: WHO.

World Health Organization (1997). The Jakarta Declaration on Leading Health Promotion into the 21st Century. *Health Promotion International, 12*, 261–264.

World Health Organization (2002). *Investing in health: a summary of findings of the Commission on macroeconomics and health*. Geneva: WHO.

World Health Organization (2003). *Global action against cancer*. Geneva: WHO.

World Health Organization (2004). *Palliative care: the solid facts*. Copenhagen: WHO.

Wright, J., MacDonald, D. & Groom, L. (2003). Physical activity and young people: beyond participation. *Sport, Education and Society, 8*, 17–33.

Wu, A.W., Folkman, S., McPhee, S.J. & Lo, B. (1991). Do house officers learn from their mistakes? *JAMA, 265*, 2089–2094.

Wu, P., Wilson, K., Dimoulas, P. & Mills, E. J. (2006). Effectiveness of smoking cessation therapies: a systematic review and meta-analysis. *BMC Public Health, 6*, 300–315.

Wulsin, L.R. & Singal, B.M. (2003). Do depressive symptoms increase the risk for the onset of coronary disease? A systematic quantitative review. *Psychosomatic Medicine*, 65, 201–210.

Yardley, L. (Ed.) (1997). *Material discourses of health and illness*. London: Routledge.

Yardley, L., Sharples, K., Beech, S. & Lewith, G. (2001). Developing a dynamic model of treatment perceptions. *Journal of Health Psychology, 6*, 269–282.

Yaskowich, K.M. & Stam, H.J. (2003). Cancer narratives and the cancer support group. *Journal of Health Psychology, 8*, 720–737.

Yeich, S. (1996). Grassroots organizing with homeless people: a participatory research approach. *Journal of Social Issues, 52*, 111–121.

Young, A. (1995). *The harmony of illusions: inventing post-traumatic stress disorder*. Princeton, NJ: Princeton University Press.

Zarcadoolas, C., Pleasant, A. & Greer, D.S. (2005). Understanding health literacy: An expanded model. *Health Promotion International, 20*, 195–203.

Ziarnowski, K.L., Brewer, N.T. & Weber, B. (2009). Present choices, future outcomes: Anticipated regret and HPV vaccination. *Preventive Medicine, 48*, 411–414.

Zuckerman, M. & Antoni, M.H. (1995). Social support and its relationship to psychological, physical and immune variables in HIV infection. *Clinical Psychology & Psychotherapy, 2*, 210–199.

Zuckerman, M. (1979). *Sensation seeking: beyond the optimal level of arousal*. Hillsdale, NJ: Lawrence Erlbaum.

Name Index

Subject Index

Page numbers in **bold** indicate glossary entries